A THREE-VOLUME SCIENTIFIC EVALUATION OF MODERN NICOTINE PRODUCTS

The Regulation of Vaping

Science, Policy and the Evolution of Global Regulation

EVIDENCE-BASED HARM REDUCTION

VOLUME II

By

Stephen Buss

Cover Design by RageQuitRemedy Ltd Publishing Press

Word Count: 315,015

Ebook ISBN: 978-1-9194567-2-0

Paperback ISBN: 978-1-9194567-6-8

Published in the United Kingdom.
First Edition, 2026

For licensing, media inquiries, academic permissions or professional enquiries, contact:
stephen@vapecompliance.com
www.VapeCompliance.com

SCIENTIFIC DISCLAIMER

This volume is written for scientific, educational, regulatory, professional and public policy discussion. It examines the regulation of vaping and other modern nicotine products through the disciplines of toxicology, analytical science, product stewardship, quality management, manufacturing control, technical documentation, market surveillance and public health policy.

Nothing in this volume should be interpreted as medical advice, legal advice, regulatory approval advice, commercial compliance certification, investment guidance, product endorsement, or an instruction to manufacture, sell, import, distribute or use any nicotine product. Regulatory requirements differ between jurisdictions and may change over time. Any person or organisation making decisions about product compliance, notification, authorisation, importation, retail sale, labelling, advertising, testing or enforcement should obtain current professional advice from appropriately qualified legal, regulatory, scientific and technical specialists.

Nicotine is a pharmacologically active and dependence-forming substance. Products containing nicotine are subject to regulatory control because their use may affect consumers, non-users, young people, public health systems and markets. A discussion of regulatory proportionality or harm reduction should not be read as a claim that nicotine products are without risk, nor as an argument that commercial innovation should proceed without appropriate scientific review, quality control or enforcement.

The regulatory examples discussed in this volume are included for analysis and comparison. References to the Tobacco Products Directive, the MHRA, the FDA, PMTA pathways, the WHO, European Commission working groups, national authorities, public health bodies, technical standards, laboratory methods, quality systems or compliance procedures are provided to explain how regulatory frameworks develop and operate. Their inclusion does not imply institutional endorsement, legal interpretation, official guidance or representation of any regulatory body.

Scientific regulation depends on evidence, but evidence does not apply itself. Data must be generated, validated, interpreted and translated into enforceable systems. Analytical results require method validation. Toxicological assessments require exposure context. Product notifications require accurate ingredient documentation. Quality systems require implementation rather than paperwork alone. Enforcement requires both legal authority and technical competence.

Where uncertainty exists, it is treated as a regulatory problem rather than a rhetorical device. Uncertainty may justify precaution, further research, restrictions, post-market monitoring or adaptive regulation, but it should not be confused with proof. Equally, the absence of a specific prohibition should not be treated as confirmation of safety, quality, compliance or public health suitability.

This volume is therefore not a substitute for legislation, statutory guidance, legal advice, notified body assessment, competent authority engagement, accredited laboratory work, independent toxicological review or properly implemented quality management systems. It is a structured examination of how vaping regulation has developed, how compliance systems are constructed, and how scientific evidence should inform proportionate regulatory decision-making.

AUTHOR'S NOTE

The regulation of vaping has never been a purely administrative subject. From its earliest stages, it has involved a contest between scientific evidence, public health caution, political pressure, commercial urgency, consumer demand and institutional uncertainty. Modern nicotine products entered markets faster than many regulatory systems were prepared to understand them, and the result was a field in which policy frequently had to develop while the science, products and patterns of use were still changing.

This volume approaches regulation as a practical scientific discipline. The central question is not simply whether vaping should be regulated. It must be regulated. The more important question is how regulation can distinguish between real risk and assumed risk, between competent manufacturers and irresponsible operators, between enforceable standards and symbolic restrictions, and between public health protection and policy that unintentionally preserves combustible tobacco use.

Regulation can protect consumers when it is technically literate. It can require ingredient disclosure, emissions testing, toxicological review, manufacturing control, traceability, stability assessment, post-market vigilance and corrective action. It can also fail when it becomes detached from scientific reality, when administrative burden substitutes for risk assessment, or when rules are written without understanding how products are formulated, tested, manufactured, distributed and used.

The vaping sector exposed these tensions sharply. Regulators had to consider nicotine concentration, refill containers, device design, emissions, ingredients, flavours, youth access, labelling, cross-border sales, importation, advertising, toxicology, laboratory data and rapidly evolving market behaviour. At the same time, public health authorities had to decide whether non-combustible nicotine products should be treated primarily as threats, cessation tools, consumer products, tobacco products, medicinal products, or harm reduction technologies.

No single regulatory model has resolved every difficulty. The European approach, the United Kingdom's post-TPD framework, the United States PMTA process, Australian prescription models, New Zealand's harm reduction orientation, Canadian regulation and emerging market controls all reveal different balances between precaution, access, evidence, enforcement and commercial freedom. Each model teaches something about what regulation can achieve, and what it can damage.

This book has been written for readers who want to understand that machinery in detail. It follows the regulatory process from the birth of modern control systems through compliant product development, toxicological assessment, laboratory testing, quality systems, notification dossiers, global models, public health politics, real-world enforcement and the future of adaptive regulation.

Its position is evidence-based but not naïve. Good regulation is necessary. Poor regulation is costly. Over-regulation can drive consumers towards illegal markets or back to smoking. Under-regulation can allow unsafe, non-compliant or counterfeit products to reach the public. The challenge is not to choose between science and regulation, but to build regulation that is competent enough to use science properly.

SERIES PREFACE

Evidence-Based Harm Reduction is a three-volume evaluation of modern nicotine products, structured around science, regulation and future policy. The series begins with the chemistry and toxicology of vaping, moves into the construction of regulatory systems, and concludes with the wider questions of innovation, ethics, consumer choice and evidence-based nicotine policy.

The first volume, The Science of Vaping, examines the technical foundations of the subject: combustion, aerosol formation, formulation science, flavour chemistry, inhalation toxicology, analytical testing, clinical evidence, behavioural science, scientific method, controversies and research gaps. It provides the scientific base on which credible regulation must depend.

The second volume, The Regulation of Vaping, considers how that scientific base is translated into product requirements, technical documentation, laboratory expectations, manufacturing controls, market restrictions, enforcement systems and international policy. It is concerned with the difficult movement from evidence to obligation.

The third volume, The Future of Harm Reduction, looks beyond current rules to the next stage of nicotine policy. It examines risk communication, consumer behaviour, future delivery systems, economics, ethics, artificial intelligence, governance and the framework needed for informed consumer choice.

The sequence is deliberate. Science without regulation may fail to protect the public. Regulation without science may produce burdensome systems that look serious while missing the actual determinants of risk. Harm reduction without ethical clarity may be dismissed as commercial apologetics, while prohibition without proportionality may preserve greater harm by limiting realistic alternatives to smoking.

Modern nicotine products therefore require a multi-disciplinary approach. Chemistry explains what products contain and what they may emit. Toxicology explains why exposure, dose and biological relevance matter. Analytical science determines whether data can be trusted. Quality systems determine whether products can be made consistently. Regulation determines which requirements are enforceable. Public health ethics determine whether adult smokers are allowed access to lower-risk alternatives while young people and non-users are protected.

The purpose of the series is not to remove controversy. Controversy is unavoidable in any field where commercial products, dependence, disease, youth protection, consumer autonomy and public health policy overlap. The purpose is to insist that controversy should be examined through evidence rather than assumption, and through proportionate reasoning rather than ideological certainty.

This trilogy represents the consolidation of almost thirty years of industry, scientific and regulatory experience.

It draws on a career spanning formulation science, chemosensory research, consumer behaviour, toxicology, quality systems, regulatory interpretation, product stewardship and modern nicotine product compliance.

The result is a three-volume scientific evaluation of modern nicotine products: not a promotional account of vaping, and not a simplified argument for or against nicotine use, but a longform examination of chemistry, exposure, toxicology, clinical evidence, behaviour, regulation, ethics and evidence-based harm reduction.

VOLUME PREFACE

The Regulation of Vaping is the second volume in the Evidence-Based Harm Reduction series. It begins from a simple premise: once a nicotine product enters a market, scientific evaluation is no longer enough. The product must be controlled through specifications, documentation, testing, manufacturing standards, submission requirements, labelling rules, distribution controls, enforcement powers and post-market responsibilities.

Regulation is often described as though it exists separately from science. In reality, every serious regulatory requirement contains an implied scientific judgement. A nicotine limit reflects assumptions about exposure and dependence. A testing requirement reflects assumptions about emissions and toxicological relevance. A notification dossier reflects assumptions about what regulators need to know before a product reaches consumers. A restriction on flavour, packaging or sale reflects assumptions about behaviour, youth uptake, risk communication and public health impact.

This volume examines those assumptions. It begins with the origins of modern regulation and the reasons governments intervened in the vaping market. The early regulatory period was shaped by competing pressures: public health concern, industry innovation, tobacco control philosophy, consumer advocacy, uncertainty about long-term effects, and the political need to appear responsive to a fast-growing product category.

The discussion then moves from policy history into product construction. A compliant product is not created at the point of submission. Compliance begins at concept stage, with ingredient selection, supplier qualification, specification development, stability planning, toxicological review, analytical strategy, product stewardship and lifecycle control. When these elements are treated as afterthoughts, regulatory failure becomes likely.

Toxicology and analytical science occupy the centre of the volume because they are the technical foundation of meaningful control. Hazard identification, ingredient assessment, literature review, read-across, weight-of-evidence reasoning, exposure estimation, margin of exposure and animal testing alternatives all influence how a regulator interprets risk. Emissions testing, method validation, laboratory accreditation, carbonyl analysis, heavy metal testing and nicotine verification determine whether the data behind those interpretations are reliable.

Quality systems and manufacturing controls are then considered because no regulatory dossier can compensate for uncontrolled production. ISO 9001 principles, GMP, supplier auditing, CAPA systems, change control, traceability, complaint handling, recalls and continuous improvement are not decorative compliance language. They are the operating structure that determines whether a notified or authorised product remains the same product over time.

The later chapters widen the lens. Product notifications, CAS number control, ingredient databases, toxicological summaries, submission systems and cross-border compliance show how technical evidence becomes regulatory paperwork. Global regulatory models demonstrate that different jurisdictions answer the same questions in different ways. Industry politics, public health organisations, media narratives, consumer advocacy and lobbying reveal that regulation is never formed by evidence alone.

The final chapters consider regulation in practice and the future of regulatory design. Retail compliance, importation, distribution, online sales, border control, counterfeit products, illegal markets and product withdrawals show that the effectiveness of regulation depends on enforceability. Adaptive regulation, artificial intelligence, digital product passports, environmental controls, disposable products, nicotine limits, flavour restrictions and international cooperation point towards the next phase.

This volume does not argue for weak regulation. It argues for competent regulation. A system that cannot distinguish between compliant and non-compliant products, between combustion risk and aerosol risk, between legal markets and illicit supply, or between precaution and disproportionality is unlikely to serve public health well. Evidence-based regulation must be strict where the evidence justifies strictness, flexible where innovation can reduce harm, and honest where uncertainty remains.

Contents

CHAPTER 1

The Birth of Modern Regulation

Electronic cigarettes did not enter a regulatory vacuum because governments had no interest in nicotine, tobacco or consumer safety. They entered a landscape already occupied by some of the most extensive public health controls ever applied to a lawful commercial product. Cigarettes were taxed, labelled, restricted in advertising, excluded from public spaces and governed through an international tobacco-control framework. Medicinal nicotine products were subject to pharmaceutical standards of quality, safety and efficacy. Consumer electrical products, chemicals, packaging and general product safety were each controlled through their own legal systems. What did not yet exist was a settled regulatory category for a consumer product that delivered nicotine without tobacco combustion and did not necessarily claim to treat nicotine dependence.

That ambiguity defined the birth of modern vaping regulation.

The first electronic nicotine products challenged distinctions that had previously appeared comparatively stable. They resembled cigarettes in appearance and patterns of use, but they did not burn tobacco. They contained nicotine, but most were not initially presented as medicines. They were electrical devices, chemical formulations and consumer products simultaneously. They could be used as alternatives to smoking, yet their manufacturers were not always permitted to make explicit claims about smoking cessation or reduced risk. They generated an inhaled aerosol, but the composition of that aerosol depended upon liquid formulation, heating conditions, device design and consumer behaviour. Existing legal systems could regulate parts of the product, but no single system adequately described the whole.

Governments therefore faced a category problem before they faced a detailed scientific one. A product could be classified according to its components, its intended purpose, its presentation, its pharmacological action or its relationship to tobacco. Each approach led towards a different regulatory outcome. Medicines regulation offered rigorous scientific assessment but imposed a demanding authorisation pathway developed for therapeutic products. General consumer-product law provided basic safety obligations but did not address nicotine exposure, emissions, refill liquids or product-specific reporting. Tobacco legislation provided an established public health framework, yet electronic cigarettes did not contain tobacco in the conventional sense and differed fundamentally from combustible products in their mechanism of exposure.

This uncertainty might have remained manageable while the market was small. It became politically unsustainable as vaping expanded. Products diversified, nicotine liquids became widely available, specialist retailers appeared, cross-border internet sales increased and consumer adoption began to alter the visible nicotine market. Governments were no longer dealing with an experimental device used by a limited community. They were confronting a rapidly developing product category operating across national borders, frequently ahead of technical standards and without uniform controls over composition, manufacturing, labelling or sale.

Intervention was therefore inevitable. The important question was not whether regulation would arrive, but what kind of regulation would be constructed and which interpretation of the product would dominate.

From the beginning, regulatory development was shaped by two legitimate but competing concerns. The first was the responsibility to protect consumers and the wider public from poorly characterised products. Early markets contained considerable variation in device quality, nicotine concentration, liquid composition, packaging, instructions and manufacturing control. Regulators could reasonably ask whether consumers knew what they were inhaling, whether products delivered the nicotine concentration stated on the label, whether refill containers were protected against leakage or accidental ingestion, and whether manufacturers had systems for reporting adverse effects or correcting defective products.

The second concern was that excessive restriction could suppress an alternative to combustible smoking before its population-level value had been properly understood. Regulation imposed on the assumption that every nicotine product represented an equivalent form of harm risked ignoring the central toxicological distinction between combustion and non-combustion. A framework that made comparatively lower-risk products inaccessible, unattractive or commercially unviable could protect the established cigarette market by default, even where its stated purpose was public health protection.

This tension between precaution and harm reduction became the central conflict of modern nicotine policy. Public health authorities were required to consider potential long-term risks that could not yet be fully quantified while also recognising the immediate and well-established burden of smoking. Manufacturers argued that innovation was moving faster than legislation and that inappropriate controls would obstruct product improvement. Tobacco-control organisations warned that commercial promotion, youth appeal, dual use and the renormalisation of nicotine behaviour could undermine decades of progress. Consumers increasingly presented their own experience of switching away from smoking as evidence that could not be dismissed. Scientists were asked to interpret an evolving evidence base in which products, methods and patterns of use changed faster than conventional research cycles.

These competing perspectives did not enter the regulatory process with equal institutional weight. Governments and public health bodies inherited regulatory concepts developed through the history of tobacco control. Industry possessed product knowledge and commercial resources but faced questions about conflicts of interest and the legacy of tobacco-company conduct. Independent manufacturers often lacked the influence and infrastructure available to larger corporations. Consumers had direct experience of the products but limited formal access to technical and legislative processes. Researchers contributed scientific evidence, although that evidence was itself shaped by study design, product generation, funding, analytical methodology and the assumptions through which findings were interpreted.

The European Union became one of the principal arenas in which these issues were converted into law. The revision of European tobacco legislation provided a mechanism through which electronic cigarettes could be brought within a harmonised framework rather than left to increasingly divergent national rules. The resulting Tobacco Products Directive, Directive 2014/40/EU, established specific requirements for nicotine-containing electronic cigarettes and refill containers under Article 20. These included product notifications, ingredient and emissions information, nicotine and volume limits, packaging requirements, health warnings, technical protections and obligations relating to adverse effects and corrective action.

The Directive did more than impose a collection of product rules. It gave vaping a durable legal identity within European regulation. Electronic cigarettes were neither treated simply as conventional tobacco products nor left solely within general consumer law. They became "related products" governed through a distinct regulatory architecture situated within tobacco legislation. That placement carried practical advantages because it created harmonised market requirements, but it also embedded vaping within institutions, language and political processes historically designed to reduce tobacco use.

Implementation required national competent authorities to turn broad legislative provisions into operating systems. In the United Kingdom, the Medicines and Healthcare products Regulatory Agency became the competent authority for the notification scheme for nicotine-containing electronic cigarettes and refill containers. Its responsibilities came to include receiving product information, maintaining submission systems, issuing producer guidance and working with other bodies responsible for enforcement and market control. The UK framework also retained a separate medicinal route through which an electronic cigarette or other inhaled nicotine-containing product could seek authorisation as a medicine, subject to pharmaceutical standards of quality, safety and efficacy.

This dual role illustrated the unresolved character of the product. The same general technology could be regulated as a consumer vaping product under tobacco-related legislation or developed as a medicinal nicotine product under medicines law. The distinction depended not merely on chemistry or device function, but on intended purpose, claims, evidence, presentation and the regulatory pathway chosen by the producer. Regulation was therefore not only evaluating products. It was helping to determine what those products were allowed to become.

European policy did not develop in isolation. The World Health Organization and the Conference of the Parties to the WHO Framework Convention on Tobacco Control increasingly considered electronic nicotine delivery systems within the international tobacco-control agenda. At the sixth session of the Conference of the Parties in Moscow in October 2014, Parties considered electronic nicotine delivery systems and adopted guidance that led to further WHO assessment of their health effects, possible role in cessation and impact on tobacco-control efforts.

WHO involvement gave the subject global visibility and provided governments with policy options, terminology and public health objectives. It also reinforced a predominantly precautionary interpretation in many jurisdictions. Countries with limited domestic analytical capacity or product-specific expertise frequently looked towards international guidance when deciding whether to regulate, restrict or prohibit emerging nicotine products. As a result, positions developed within international tobacco-control institutions could influence national policy even where local patterns of smoking, product use, enforcement capacity and healthcare provision differed substantially.

Within Europe, the legal text was only one part of the regulatory machinery. Commission services, Member State representatives, competent authorities, technical groups, scientific advisers and implementation networks had to decide how provisions would operate in practice. Common data formats, notification processes, refill mechanisms, product definitions and reporting expectations required further interpretation. Commission implementing decisions established technical arrangements for the submission of product information and for particular product requirements, demonstrating how apparently simple legal obligations expand into detailed administrative and technical systems.

The creation of those systems exposed the difference between legislation and regulatory science. A law can require manufacturers to provide emissions data, but it does not by itself determine which emissions should be measured, under what operating conditions, using which analytical methods or against what interpretive thresholds. It can require ingredients to be disclosed without resolving how complex flavour mixtures should be identified or toxicologically evaluated. It can demand consistent nicotine delivery while leaving open questions concerning device variability, puffing behaviour and the distinction between laboratory performance and consumer exposure.

Political decisions were therefore often made before the scientific infrastructure needed to support them had fully matured. This was not necessarily evidence of regulatory failure. Legislators cannot always wait for complete evidence where a market is expanding and plausible concerns exist. It does, however, mean that some first-generation controls reflected negotiated political judgements as much as demonstrated toxicological thresholds. Limits on nicotine concentration, container volume and device capacity provided clear and enforceable boundaries, but their numerical precision could create an impression of scientific certainty greater than the evidence underlying them.

Stakeholder consultation became the formal mechanism through which these competing interpretations entered the process. Manufacturers, pharmaceutical companies, tobacco companies, public health organisations, scientists, retailers, consumer groups and individual users sought to influence regulatory design. Lobbying was not confined to commercial actors. Every organised stakeholder attempted to frame the problem in terms favourable to its institutional objectives: consumer protection, tobacco control, market access, smoking cessation, youth prevention, commercial competition or personal autonomy.

The resulting regulation was consequently neither a pure expression of science nor simply a political imposition. It was a negotiated system created under uncertainty. Scientific findings established boundaries around what could reasonably be claimed, but they did not dictate a single policy. Political institutions selected objectives, balanced competing interests and decided how much uncertainty they were prepared to tolerate. Regulators converted those decisions into submission portals, technical guidance, product registers, reporting duties and enforcement procedures. Industry adapted products and business models to the rules. Consumers responded in ways that were not always predicted.

The precautionary principle provided much of the intellectual justification for acting before long-term evidence was complete. Properly applied, precaution allows proportionate measures to be taken where there are credible grounds for concern and where delay could expose the public to avoidable harm. It does not require proof of damage before every intervention. Nor, however, should it permit uncertainty to be treated as proof that the worst outcome will occur. Precaution becomes scientifically weak when it considers only the hypothetical risk of allowing a product while ignoring the foreseeable consequences of restricting it.

For vaping, those consequences included reduced access for adult smokers, slower technological development, market consolidation, increased compliance costs and the possible growth of informal or illegal supply. Conversely, weak regulation could expose consumers to inaccurate labelling, poor manufacturing, unsafe ingredients, defective batteries, uncontrolled nicotine liquids and products for which no responsible economic operator could be identified. The regulatory problem was therefore never reducible to a choice between intervention and freedom. It was a question of where controls should be placed, how strict they should be and whether they addressed the principal determinants of risk.

The first generation of vaping regulation established the foundations still visible today: notification before market entry, ingredient disclosure, emissions reporting, nicotine limits, packaging controls, health warnings, producer responsibilities, market surveillance and restrictions intended to protect children and non-users. In Great Britain, these requirements continue to be administered through the Tobacco and Related Products Regulations and the MHRA notification framework, alongside enforcement by other national and local authorities.

Those foundations were significant achievements. They brought order to a fragmented market, created minimum expectations and made producers accountable for products that had previously entered commerce with limited regulatory scrutiny. They also revealed persistent weaknesses: administrative systems that could receive information without necessarily evaluating every submission in depth; technical requirements unsupported by fully harmonised test methods; restrictions that were easy for compliant businesses to follow but difficult to enforce against unlawful imports; and policy debates in which the risks of vaping were frequently discussed without consistent comparison to the risks of continued smoking.

The birth of modern regulation must therefore be understood as more than the history of a Directive or the creation of a notification scheme. It was the point at which governments attempted to control a technology whose scientific meaning, commercial structure and public health role were still being formed. The rules were written while products evolved, evidence accumulated and institutions competed to define the issue.

The ten discussions that follow examine that process from its principal points of pressure: why intervention became unavoidable; how public health objectives collided with commercial innovation; how the Tobacco Products Directive evolved; how the MHRA assumed its regulatory role; how WHO policy influenced national approaches; how European working groups translated law into practice; how political and scientific drivers interacted; how consultation and lobbying shaped outcomes; how precaution was applied; and what the first generation of regulation ultimately taught.

Those lessons matter because the original regulatory settlement was never an endpoint. It was the first attempt to construct order around a new nicotine technology. Its strengths, compromises and unintended consequences continue to shape every subsequent argument about vaping, harm reduction and the proper limits of public health regulation.

Figure 1.1. The Evolution of Modern Vaping Regulation.

This timeline traces the development of the first generation of vaping regulation from the pre-regulatory period through market growth, legislative intervention, national implementation and later policy adaptation. It shows how the European Tobacco Products Directive, the MHRA, WHO tobacco-control policy, European Commission working groups and the precautionary principle developed in parallel and influenced one another. The figure also identifies the wider drivers behind regulatory intervention, including product innovation, divergent national approaches, uncertainty concerning long-term effects, consumer protection, youth uptake, cross-border sales and the need for harmonised technical requirements.

CHAPTER 1 – THE BIRTH OF MODERN REGULATION

Regulation evolution timeline

From early market emergence to today's taxation, flavour and single-use restrictions.

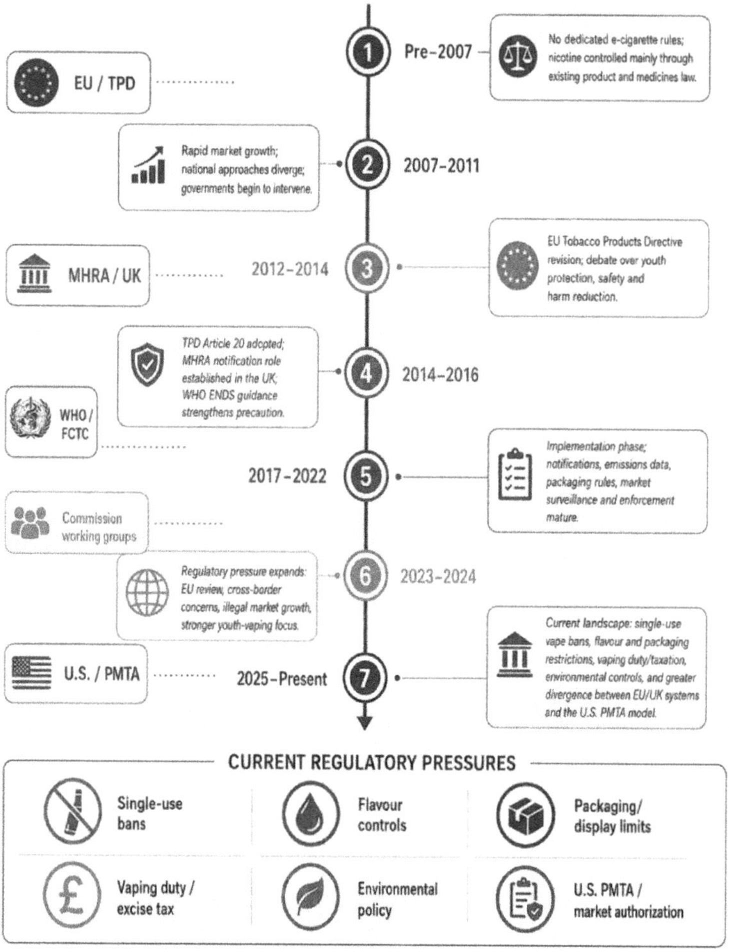

Modern vaping regulation has shifted from early precaution and harmonisation towards a more fragmented era of taxation, youth-protection measures, environmental controls and jurisdiction-specific market access rules.

Why Governments Intervened

Government intervention in the vaping market was not triggered by one decisive scientific discovery, a single public health emergency or a uniform international policy. It arose from the convergence of several pressures that became increasingly difficult for governments to ignore. A rapidly expanding nicotine market was developing outside the regulatory structures traditionally applied to cigarettes, medicines and medical devices. Products varied considerably in their composition, construction, nicotine delivery, packaging and manufacturing quality. They were sold across borders through physical shops and online channels, promoted directly to consumers and used in ways that did not fit comfortably within established legal categories. At the same time, they offered adult smokers a non-combustible alternative to cigarettes, creating a regulatory problem in which intervention could protect consumers but could also obstruct harm reduction.

The earliest products exposed a fundamental weakness in existing law. Governments had extensive systems for regulating tobacco, pharmaceuticals, chemicals, electrical equipment and general consumer goods, but electronic cigarettes combined elements of all of them. The device contained a battery, circuitry, a heating coil and a liquid reservoir. The formulation could contain nicotine, propylene glycol, glycerol, water and multiple flavour compounds. The resulting aerosol was inhaled into the lungs, yet the product was commonly marketed as a consumer good rather than a medicine. It resembled smoking behaviourally, although it did not depend upon the combustion of tobacco.

This unusual combination created uncertainty over which authority should take responsibility. Electrical safety rules could address batteries, chargers and wiring faults, but not necessarily nicotine purity or inhalation toxicology. Chemical legislation could govern the classification and packaging of hazardous substances, but it was not designed to assess the performance of a complete nicotine-delivery system. General product-safety law could require manufacturers to avoid placing unsafe goods on the market, but it offered no detailed framework for ingredient disclosure, emissions testing or nicotine concentration. Medicines legislation could provide rigorous controls, although it was structured around products making therapeutic claims and required standards that many consumer-product manufacturers were not equipped to meet. Tobacco law offered a familiar institutional home, but electronic cigarettes did not operate through tobacco combustion and were not always tobacco products in the literal sense.

The first reason for intervention was therefore legal and administrative rather than purely toxicological. Governments needed to determine what the product was, who was responsible for it and which rules should apply. Without classification, regulators could not establish consistent requirements for market entry, product documentation, advertising, age restrictions, labelling or enforcement. The absence of a settled category also encouraged national divergence. One state might treat a nicotine-containing electronic cigarette as a medicinal product, another as a tobacco-related product and another primarily through consumer law. Manufacturers operating across borders could therefore face incompatible legal interpretations for essentially the same product.

That divergence was particularly problematic within the European Union, where the internal market depends upon the movement of lawful goods under broadly harmonised rules. If Member States imposed substantially different requirements, manufacturers could face fragmented markets, consumers could purchase products across borders and national restrictions could be undermined through online trade. Harmonisation consequently became one of the principal legal justifications for European intervention. Directive 2014/40/EU was expressly designed both to improve the functioning of the internal market for tobacco and related products and to provide a high level of health protection. It entered into force in May 2014 and became applicable across Member States in May 2016.

The second reason for intervention was the variability of early products. The developing market did not consist of one standardised electronic cigarette manufactured to a uniform specification. It included disposable products, refillable devices, cartridge systems, open tanks, different coil materials, varying power outputs and liquids produced under widely differing quality systems. Nicotine concentrations could vary substantially, while flavour formulations ranged from relatively simple mixtures to highly complex blends containing numerous chemical substances. Product labels did not always communicate composition clearly, and the quality of technical documentation differed markedly between suppliers.

Such variability did not prove that every product was unsafe, but it made general assurances difficult to sustain. Regulators needed to know whether the liquid contained the nicotine concentration declared, whether ingredients were adequately identified, whether impurities were controlled and whether the device could operate without overheating or leaking. They also needed to consider whether refill containers could expose children to concentrated nicotine, whether packaging resisted accidental opening and whether users received adequate instructions and warnings.

The distinction between hazard and risk was not always maintained clearly during this period. Nicotine is pharmacologically active and capable of causing adverse effects at sufficient exposure. Certain flavouring chemicals, impurities and thermal degradation products may also present inhalation hazards. However, the existence of a hazardous substance does not by itself establish the magnitude of risk arising from a particular product under normal use. Risk depends upon concentration, delivered dose, frequency, route of exposure and the operating characteristics of the device. Early regulation nevertheless had to be developed before all these variables had been characterised comprehensively.

Governments were therefore responding not only to demonstrated harms but also to incomplete knowledge. The products were new enough that long-term epidemiological evidence did not exist, and analytical methods were still developing. Research findings could differ because investigators used different devices, liquids, puffing regimes, voltages and analytical techniques. Results produced under severe laboratory conditions could be interpreted as representative of normal use, while low measured concentrations could be presented as proof of negligible risk. Regulators had to operate within this uncertainty while the market continued to grow.

The absence of long-term evidence created a familiar public health dilemma. Waiting for definitive epidemiology could require decades, during which millions of products might be sold. Immediate prohibition or severe restriction, however, could remove a potentially valuable substitute for smoking. Governments rarely have the option of postponing all action until science becomes complete. They must instead decide how much evidence is sufficient to justify intervention, which risks require immediate control and which uncertainties can be managed through monitoring, reporting and later revision.

A third driver was the protection of children, young people and non-smokers. Electronic cigarettes were initially discussed principally as alternatives for adults who smoked, but their visibility, flavour variety and consumer-style presentation created concern that they might appeal beyond that population. Governments were especially sensitive to the possibility that nicotine products could establish dependence among people who had never smoked. Even where evidence of progression from vaping to smoking remained disputed, the prospect of youth uptake carried substantial political weight.

Youth protection is one of the strongest and least controversial reasons for nicotine regulation. It supports minimum-age restrictions, responsible retail practices, controls on marketing and enforcement against unlawful sales. The difficulty lies in distinguishing measures that specifically reduce youth access from measures that also reduce the attractiveness or availability of products to adult smokers. A restriction may be justified by reference to children yet affect the entire market. Flavour controls, packaging standardisation, display restrictions and advertising prohibitions illustrate this problem. Each may reduce youth appeal, but each may also alter adult product choice, switching behaviour and the viability of compliant suppliers.

Governments consequently faced a balancing exercise rather than a simple choice between protection and freedom. The question was not whether children should have unrestricted access to nicotine products. They should not. The question was how to protect them without constructing a regulatory system that treated adult smokers, former smokers and never-smokers as though they presented identical policy concerns.

A fourth reason for intervention concerned claims made about smoking cessation and reduced harm. Many consumers reported using electronic cigarettes to reduce or stop smoking, and the products were often discussed publicly as cessation tools. However, commercial claims of therapeutic benefit fall within a legally sensitive area. A product presented as treating nicotine dependence may be regarded as a medicine, requiring evidence of quality, safety and efficacy. A consumer-product manufacturer could not necessarily promote a vape as a clinically proven cessation treatment without entering the medicinal regulatory pathway.

This created a gap between real-world use and permitted commercial presentation. Consumers might use a product to stop smoking even when the manufacturer was not authorised to make that claim. Public health bodies might recognise a harm-reduction role while regulators continued to distinguish consumer vaping products from licensed medicines. Governments therefore needed rules governing claims, presentation and the boundary between consumer and medicinal products.

In the United Kingdom, this distinction eventually produced parallel pathways. Nicotine-containing vaping products sold as consumer goods became subject to notification requirements administered by the MHRA under the Tobacco and Related Products Regulations, while products presented as medicines remained capable of seeking medicinal authorisation. The MHRA is the competent authority for the notification scheme for nicotine-containing vaping products and works with other bodies in implementing relevant provisions.

The existence of these parallel routes demonstrates that government intervention did not resolve the identity of vaping through one universal classification. Instead, regulation created legal pathways based upon intended use and presentation. A vaping product could remain a consumer product subject to tobacco-related controls, or it could be developed as a medicinal product under a more demanding authorisation system. The product's regulatory status was therefore influenced not only by its composition but by what the producer claimed it was for.

A fifth driver was the historical context of tobacco control. Governments did not encounter electronic cigarettes as neutral consumer technology. They encountered them after decades of disease, litigation, marketing controversy and regulatory conflict associated with the tobacco industry. Cigarette manufacturers had previously denied or minimised harms, manipulated product perception and opposed public health controls. This history shaped institutional attitudes towards any new nicotine-delivery system, particularly once major tobacco companies entered the vaping market.

Suspicion was not irrational. Regulatory authorities had reason to scrutinise corporate claims, product research and marketing strategies carefully. However, the transfer of distrust from combustible cigarettes to all non-combustible nicotine technologies also risked obscuring important differences in toxicological exposure. A cigarette is dangerous principally because tobacco is burned and smoke contains a complex mixture of toxic combustion products. An electronic cigarette heats a liquid to produce an aerosol. That aerosol is not harmless, but its composition and risk profile cannot be assumed to be identical to smoke merely because both products contain nicotine.

The central scientific challenge was therefore comparative. Governments were not assessing vaping in isolation. They were regulating it within a market where cigarettes remained widely available and caused a substantial burden of disease. The relevant policy question was not simply whether vaping involved risk, because almost every meaningful consumer exposure involves some degree of risk. It was whether the nature and magnitude of that risk justified particular controls when compared with continued smoking, medicinal nicotine use, abstinence and other available alternatives.

This comparative framework complicated conventional tobacco-control policy. Measures designed to reduce all nicotine consumption might appear coherent from a prevention perspective, but they could conflict with harm reduction where adult smokers were unwilling or unable to achieve complete abstinence. Conversely, presenting vaping too enthusiastically as a safer alternative could encourage use among people who would otherwise avoid nicotine. Governments had to regulate both the absolute risks of vaping and its relative position within the broader nicotine market.

A sixth reason for intervention was the increasing involvement of international public health institutions. The World Health Organization and the Conference of the Parties to the Framework Convention on Tobacco Control considered electronic nicotine delivery systems within the broader tobacco-control agenda. At the sixth session of the Conference of the Parties in 2014, electronic nicotine delivery systems were formally examined, and WHO reporting addressed health effects, cessation, youth use, marketing and possible regulatory options.

This international attention mattered because many countries lacked the domestic scientific or regulatory capacity to develop an independent framework. WHO documents provided terminology, policy options and a public health rationale for intervention. Governments could use those materials when considering bans, age restrictions, advertising controls, product standards or inclusion within smoke-free policies. The international framing also reinforced the idea that electronic cigarettes should not remain ordinary consumer products outside nicotine and tobacco-control policy.

The WHO approach tended to emphasise uncertainty, youth protection and the possibility that electronic nicotine systems could interfere with established tobacco-control objectives. Harm-reduction advocates placed greater emphasis on the difference between smoke and aerosol and on the experience of adult smokers who had switched. These positions were not entirely incompatible, but they placed different weight on potential benefits and potential harms. Governments intervened within this contested space, often adopting precautionary controls while leaving the longer-term role of vaping unresolved.

A seventh driver was the political visibility of the market. Regulation is not produced solely by toxicological evidence. It responds to public concern, media attention, parliamentary pressure, organised advocacy and visible changes in consumer behaviour. Electronic cigarettes became increasingly noticeable in shops, public spaces and advertising. Their resemblance to smoking raised questions about whether they would undermine smoke-free norms. Reports of battery incidents, leaking liquids, inaccurate labels and youth-oriented marketing attracted attention even where the frequency or representativeness of such events was uncertain.

Political institutions tend to act when a new product category becomes sufficiently visible that inaction itself requires explanation. Once electronic cigarettes were widely used, governments could no longer rely upon general consumer law without appearing unprepared. Ministers, regulators and legislators were expected to demonstrate that someone was responsible for product safety, youth access and market oversight. Regulation therefore served an institutional function as well as a public health one: it allocated responsibility and showed that the state was responding.

This does not mean that regulation was merely symbolic. Many early controls addressed genuine weaknesses. Ingredient reporting improved product transparency. Notification created a record of products placed on the market. Packaging and refill requirements reduced certain foreseeable risks. Health warnings communicated nicotine dependence. Producer obligations created mechanisms for corrective action. The problem was that politically attractive measures were not always those most closely linked to the principal determinants of harm.

Numerical limits provide a clear example. A maximum nicotine concentration or container volume is easily understood, written into law and enforced through testing. Such limits create certainty for manufacturers and inspectors. They do not, however, by themselves guarantee low toxicological risk, product quality or successful smoking substitution. A compliant product can still be poorly formulated, manufactured inconsistently or used with an unsuitable device. A numerical rule may therefore be administratively effective without being a complete scientific control.

An eighth reason for intervention was the need for traceability and accountability. In an unstructured market, identifying the responsible producer or importer could be difficult. Products might be manufactured in one country, branded in another, imported through a third and sold online across multiple jurisdictions. Where a defect or safety concern arose, regulators needed to determine who held the formulation data, who controlled manufacturing and who could organise a withdrawal or recall.

The European framework sought to address this through obligations placed upon manufacturers and importers. Article 20 of the Tobacco Products Directive established rules for electronic cigarettes and refill containers sold as consumer products, including notification and information requirements. The associated submission system required structured product information to be provided to national competent authorities. Commission implementing measures subsequently defined common formats and technical arrangements for reporting.

This moved the market away from a position in which products could appear without any formal regulatory record. Notification was not the same as pre-market approval, and inclusion within a database did not necessarily mean that every scientific claim or analytical result had been independently validated. It nevertheless created an auditable relationship between a product and a responsible economic operator. Governments regarded that accountability as essential to effective market surveillance.

A ninth reason for intervention was concern about enforcement asymmetry. Responsible manufacturers might invest in formulation control, laboratory testing, child-resistant packaging and accurate labelling, while less responsible operators could avoid those costs. Without enforceable common standards, poor-quality products could undercut compliant competitors. Regulation was therefore also intended to establish minimum market conditions and prevent safety investment from becoming a commercial disadvantage.

This objective remains difficult to achieve because regulation is only as effective as its enforcement. A detailed technical framework may burden businesses already inclined to comply while leaving illicit traders relatively unaffected. Cross-border internet sales, false declarations, counterfeit products and rapidly changing brands can overwhelm inspection systems. Governments intervened to create legal powers, but those powers did not automatically generate the laboratory capacity, staffing, intelligence or border controls needed to apply them consistently.

The final and most important reason for intervention was that vaping had become too consequential to remain undefined. It could influence smoking prevalence, nicotine initiation, consumer behaviour, pharmaceutical cessation markets, tax revenues and the future structure of the tobacco industry. It raised questions about whether public health should seek the elimination of all non-medical nicotine use or accept continuing nicotine consumption where the method of delivery was substantially less harmful than smoking. Those were not questions that governments could leave entirely to commercial markets.

Intervention was therefore justified by real needs: product characterisation, consumer protection, youth access controls, accountability, harmonisation, quality standards and market surveillance. The more difficult issue was whether the form of intervention was proportionate to the risks and benefits involved. Early regulation often had to convert uncertainty into fixed rules before the evidence base was mature. Some controls addressed credible hazards directly;

others reflected political compromise, institutional caution or the administrative preference for measurable limits.

Governments did not intervene because vaping had been shown to be equivalent to smoking, nor because it had been proved harmless. They intervened because a new nicotine-delivery system had expanded beyond the capacity of existing law to control it coherently. The market combined plausible public health benefit with unresolved product risks, commercial innovation with inconsistent quality, and adult demand with legitimate concern about youth uptake. Once those tensions became visible, non-intervention was no longer a neutral position.

The first regulatory settlement consequently attempted to create order rather than to deliver a final scientific judgement. It defined products, assigned authorities, required information, established technical limits and created mechanisms for enforcement. In doing so, it also shaped the future market. The next question was whether those controls could protect public health without suppressing the commercial innovation that had made non-combustible nicotine products possible in the first place.

Public Health Versus Commercial Innovation

The tension between public health and commercial innovation has shaped vaping regulation from the beginning. Electronic cigarettes emerged because companies identified a demand that existing tobacco and pharmaceutical products were not fully meeting. Adult smokers wanted alternatives that could reproduce some of the behavioural, sensory and social features of smoking without the combustion of tobacco. Commercial developers responded with new devices, liquids, nicotine formats, flavours and delivery systems. Public health institutions, however, were required to consider not only the needs of smokers but also the possible effects on young people, non-smokers, healthcare systems and the wider population.

These objectives were never entirely opposed. Commercial innovation made non-combustible nicotine products possible, while public health regulation created the standards needed to prevent uncontrolled products from reaching consumers. Conflict arose because the two systems operated according to different priorities and timescales. Businesses competed through speed, novelty, product differentiation and consumer appeal. Regulators depended on evidence, consultation, legislative authority and enforceable rules. By the time governments understood one generation of products, the market was often moving towards the next.

Commercial innovation usually begins with an unmet need rather than a completed scientific assessment. Early vaping products were often developed by engineers, entrepreneurs and smokers seeking a practical substitute for cigarettes. Their designs evolved through trial, consumer feedback and competition. Battery capacity increased, atomisers improved, refillable tanks became more reliable and liquid formulations became more varied. These advances were not centrally planned. They emerged from numerous firms testing different approaches in a young market.

This decentralised innovation produced genuine improvements. Devices became easier to use, leakage was reduced, nicotine delivery became more consistent and consumers gained greater control over flavour, concentration and vapour production. Products that provided an unsatisfactory experience were replaced by systems that more closely matched the expectations of smokers. This mattered because a lower-risk product has limited public health value if consumers do not find it acceptable enough to replace cigarettes.

The ability of a vaping product to compete with smoking depends on more than its chemical composition. Cigarettes deliver nicotine rapidly and consistently while also providing familiar sensory cues, rituals and behavioural reinforcement. A viable substitute must address at least some of those functions. Device format, draw resistance, aerosol temperature, flavour, throat sensation, nicotine form and ease of use all influence whether an adult smoker continues using the alternative or returns to cigarettes.

Commercial competition accelerated work in these areas. Manufacturers had a direct incentive to make products more satisfying, reliable and convenient. In public health terms, this could support switching away from combustion. In regulatory terms, however, the same product attributes could also increase uptake among people who had never smoked. Greater palatability, discreetness and ease of use were therefore interpreted as both potential advantages and potential risks.

Flavour illustrates the conflict clearly. For many adult users, flavour provides separation from the taste and smell of cigarettes. It can make switching more acceptable and reduce the appeal of returning to tobacco. A wide flavour range can also allow consumers to find a product they are willing to use consistently. From this perspective, flavour is not merely decorative. It can contribute to product substitution and continued displacement of smoking.

Public health concern arises when flavours, names, packaging or imagery appear designed to attract children. Sweet, fruit and confectionery profiles are not used only by young people, but they are easily framed as youth-oriented.

This has led to calls for restrictions ranging from controls on descriptors and presentation to the prohibition of broad flavour categories. The difficulty is that rules directed at youth appeal may also reduce the products available to adults who have moved away from smoking.

The argument is often presented too simply. One side claims that flavours are essential to harm reduction, while the other treats them primarily as a route into nicotine dependence. Both positions can contain elements of truth. Flavours may assist adult switching and also increase the attractiveness of vaping to adolescents. The regulatory task is not to deny either possibility but to determine which controls reduce youth uptake without unnecessarily weakening the products used by adult smokers.

Packaging creates a similar problem. Commercial brands rely on visual identity to distinguish their products, communicate quality and compete in the market. Public health authorities may view bright colours, stylised graphics and lifestyle branding as mechanisms that normalise nicotine use or appeal to children. Restrictions on packaging, display and advertising can reduce promotional exposure, but they may also make it harder for consumers to distinguish compliant products from illegal or counterfeit ones.

The same conflict appears in device design. Small, simple and convenient products may be particularly useful to smokers who do not want complex refillable systems. They may also be easy for young people to conceal and use. High-capacity rechargeable devices can reduce waste and allow greater control, yet they may require more technical knowledge and maintenance. Disposable or single-use products lowered the practical barriers to trying vaping, but they also created environmental concerns and became associated with rapid youth uptake in several markets.

Innovation therefore changes not only the product but the population using it. A device designed to solve one problem can create another. Regulations written for refillable tank systems may be poorly suited to compact pod products. Rules developed around nicotine concentration may not anticipate changes in nicotine chemistry. Controls based on liquid volume may not reflect improvements in delivery efficiency. Commercial development repeatedly tests the assumptions built into legislation.

Nicotine salts provide one example. Traditional freebase nicotine can become harsh at higher concentrations, limiting the amount that can be delivered comfortably in small devices. Acidified formulations can alter sensory properties and make higher nicotine concentrations more tolerable. This may help some smokers obtain sufficient nicotine from a compact product and move away from cigarettes. It may also increase the ease with which inexperienced users consume nicotine.

The public health interpretation depends heavily on context. For an established smoker, improved nicotine delivery may make a non-combustible product more effective as a substitute. For a nicotine-naive adolescent, the same characteristic may increase the likelihood of repeated use and dependence. Regulation cannot assess the technology solely through the product itself. It must consider who is likely to use it, how it is marketed and what behaviour it may replace or initiate.

Commercial innovation is also shaped by regulation. Once limits, notifications and product standards are introduced, manufacturers redesign products around the legal boundaries. A maximum nicotine concentration encourages firms to compete through device efficiency, aerosol production, formulation and flavour. A container-volume limit affects packaging formats and purchasing behaviour. Restrictions on advertising increase the importance of retail display, brand recognition and social media. Regulation does not stop innovation; it redirects it.

This can produce beneficial outcomes. Safety requirements encourage child-resistant closures, leak resistance, improved battery protection and clearer labelling. Notification obligations promote better ingredient records and product documentation. Restrictions on certain substances can move formulation away from known hazards. Quality-system expectations encourage manufacturers to control suppliers, specifications and production more carefully.

It can also produce unintended effects. When legal limits reduce product performance, manufacturers search for technical workarounds. When compliant market access becomes expensive, smaller firms may withdraw or avoid innovation altogether. When restrictions remove products that consumers value, illegal suppliers may enter the gap. A rule intended to reduce risk may therefore alter competition in ways that favour larger companies or non-compliant operators.

The cost of compliance is central to the relationship between public health and innovation. Scientific testing, toxicological assessment, technical documentation, quality management and regulatory submissions require money and expertise. These costs are justified where they prevent unsafe products from reaching consumers or provide regulators with information necessary for oversight. They become problematic when they are poorly targeted, duplicative or unrelated to meaningful risk.

Large multinational companies can absorb high regulatory costs more easily than small independent manufacturers. They possess legal departments, laboratories, regulatory teams and capital. Smaller firms may have valuable product knowledge and closer relationships with consumers but lack the resources needed to navigate complex submission systems. Regulation can therefore consolidate the market even when it was not designed to do so.

Market consolidation has mixed implications. Larger firms may provide more consistent manufacturing, stronger quality systems and better technical documentation. They may also reduce competition, narrow product diversity and increase the influence of companies with longstanding commercial interests in tobacco. Independent innovation played an important role in the early development of vaping, and a framework that excludes smaller responsible operators may reduce the range of products available to consumers.

The involvement of tobacco companies intensified the debate. Their entry brought investment, manufacturing capability, scientific expertise and distribution networks. It also brought the history of cigarette marketing, political lobbying and public mistrust. Public health organisations were understandably cautious about allowing companies that had profited from smoking to shape the future nicotine market.

Yet excluding tobacco companies from non-combustible innovation creates its own contradiction. If the long-term objective is to reduce or replace cigarette use, companies controlling large parts of the cigarette market may need to participate in the transition. The critical issue is not whether commercial involvement exists but how claims are verified, how products are regulated and whether business incentives align with reducing combustible use rather than sustaining it.

Commercial motives should neither invalidate evidence automatically nor exempt it from scrutiny. Industry-funded research may be technically sound, poorly designed or selectively interpreted, just as non-industry research may be rigorous or flawed. The source of funding is relevant because it may influence study design, publication and communication. It is not a substitute for evaluating methods, data and conclusions.

The same principle applies to public health institutions. Their objectives may be protective, but good intentions do not guarantee effective policy. A measure can be introduced to protect children and still produce unintended harm among adults. A precautionary restriction can appear responsible while strengthening illegal trade. A communication campaign can discourage youth experimentation while also convincing smokers that vaping is no different from smoking.

Risk communication became one of the most contested areas. Manufacturers wanted to explain that their products did not involve tobacco combustion and could expose users to fewer toxicants than cigarettes. Regulators were cautious about allowing reduced-risk claims that might be interpreted as assurances of safety. Public health bodies differed in the extent to which they were willing to communicate relative risk.

The result was often an information gap. Consumers were warned that nicotine products were not risk-free, but they were not always given clear information about differences between product categories. This may have protected against overconfidence, yet it could also leave smokers unable to make informed comparisons. A warning that is technically correct but stripped of context can still mislead.

Commercial communications created the opposite risk. Claims such as "clean", "safe" or "healthy" could imply certainty unsupported by evidence. Even more restrained statements could be used selectively to promote products without acknowledging dependence, uncertainty or the importance of complete switching. Regulators therefore had legitimate reasons to control claims, but those controls needed to preserve the ability to communicate material differences in risk.

Public health and commercial innovation also diverged over speed. Businesses must respond quickly to consumer demand and competitor activity. Product development cycles may be measured in months. Public health evidence develops more slowly, particularly where long-term outcomes are concerned. Legislative change can take several years. This creates a structural mismatch in which the market evolves faster than the system intended to govern it.

A regulator may respond by writing broad, principle-based requirements that can adapt to new technologies. This allows flexibility but may create uncertainty for manufacturers and uneven enforcement. Alternatively, the regulator may specify detailed limits and product rules. These provide clarity but risk becoming obsolete as designs change. The strongest framework combines clear minimum standards with mechanisms for updating technical requirements as evidence and products develop.

Post-market surveillance is essential to this balance. Premarket data cannot answer every question, particularly in a rapidly changing consumer market. Complaints, adverse events, product failures, patterns of youth use, switching behaviour and illegal market activity can reveal effects not predicted during development. Regulation that permits controlled market entry while requiring ongoing monitoring may support innovation more effectively than either unrestricted sale or excessively burdensome pre-authorisation.

The distinction between product innovation and marketing innovation is also important. Improvements in battery safety, emissions control, nicotine consistency and leak prevention can directly reduce risk. New packaging, brand extensions and promotional themes may primarily increase sales. Both are commercial activities, but they should not be treated as equally valuable from a public health perspective.

A proportionate system should reward innovation that improves product quality, consumer understanding or displacement of smoking. It should scrutinise innovation that increases appeal without improving function or safety. This requires regulators to understand the technology in enough detail to distinguish meaningful development from superficial novelty.

Commercial innovation can also support enforcement. Traceability systems, authentication codes, digital product records and better supply-chain controls can help identify legitimate products. Standardised data can improve regulatory review. Manufacturers have practical knowledge of how products are made, distributed and counterfeited. Excluding industry from technical discussion may deprive regulators of information necessary to design workable rules.

Consultation, however, must not become regulatory capture. Companies will naturally argue for rules that protect their products and reduce their costs. Public health organisations may favour restrictions consistent with their institutional mission. Consumer groups may emphasise access and personal experience. Regulators must consider all these perspectives without allowing any single interest to dominate.

The central public health question is whether commercial innovation reduces or increases total harm. That cannot be answered by examining product sales alone. Increased vaping may indicate that smokers are switching, that former smokers are returning to nicotine, that young people are initiating use or that existing users are consuming both cigarettes and vaping products. The same market growth can therefore carry very different meanings.

Population outcomes depend on who uses the product and what they would otherwise have done. An adult smoker who switches completely from cigarettes to a regulated vaping product may reduce exposure to combustion-related toxicants. A person who begins vaping but would never have smoked acquires a risk and may develop nicotine dependence. A dual user who continues smoking may gain less benefit than someone who switches completely, although even that outcome depends on changes in cigarette consumption and exposure.

Policy must therefore consider competing pathways rather than relying on one general narrative. Commercial innovation can support harm reduction, create new dependence or do both within different groups. Public health regulation should seek to maximise substitution among smokers while minimising initiation among non-users. This is more demanding than simply promoting or suppressing the entire category.

The conflict becomes most severe when regulation reduces the features that make products effective substitutes for smoking. Limits on nicotine delivery, flavour, device performance or communication may lower youth appeal but may also reduce adult switching. Conversely, a permissive market may encourage rapid innovation but fail to control quality, marketing and access. Neither extreme provides a satisfactory answer.

The relationship between public health and commercial innovation should therefore be treated as a managed tension rather than a battle in which one side must defeat the other. Public health requires innovation because cigarettes remain difficult to displace through prohibition, taxation and cessation treatment alone. Innovation requires regulation because consumer trust and long-term market legitimacy depend on safety, quality and accountability.

A mature regulatory framework should make responsible innovation easier and irresponsible innovation harder. It should establish clear standards for ingredients, manufacturing, emissions, labelling and youth protection while allowing products to improve. It should demand evidence for claims without preventing truthful communication of relative risk. It should prevent the use of children as a market while preserving viable alternatives for adults who smoke.

The early regulatory debate often treated public health and commerce as opposing forces. In practice, the outcome depends on how their incentives are structured. Commercial competition can improve products when success depends on quality, reliability and effective substitution. It can worsen outcomes when success depends mainly on novelty, aggressive promotion or evasion of controls. Public health regulation can protect consumers when it is technically informed and proportionate. It can preserve smoking-related harm when it restricts lower-risk alternatives without considering what consumers will do instead.

The task is not to choose between regulation and innovation. It is to create conditions in which innovation contributes to the reduction of harm rather than merely the expansion of nicotine consumption.

The Evolution of the Tobacco Products Directive

The Tobacco Products Directive did not begin as legislation for electronic cigarettes. Its origins lay in the European Union's attempt to harmonise national controls over conventional tobacco products while protecting public health and preserving the functioning of the internal market. Electronic cigarettes entered that framework later, when their rapid commercial growth exposed the limits of legislation written principally for cigarettes, roll-your-own tobacco and other established tobacco categories.

European tobacco regulation had developed over several decades through measures addressing product labelling, tar and nicotine yields, oral tobacco, advertising and the movement of goods between Member States. Directive 2001/37/EC consolidated important parts of this earlier framework. It regulated the manufacture, presentation and sale of tobacco products, including maximum yields for cigarette smoke, ingredient reporting and health warnings. Its underlying structure reflected the tobacco market of its time: products were made from tobacco, many were burned, and the dominant public health objective was to reduce smoking and exposure to tobacco smoke.

The early Directive did not contain a purpose-built framework for electronic cigarettes. The modern vaping market had not yet developed sufficiently to require one. As nicotine-delivery devices began appearing across Europe, they were instead assessed through existing national legislation. Depending on the jurisdiction, their presentation and nicotine content, they could be treated as medicines, medical devices, tobacco-related products, chemicals or ordinary consumer goods.

This fragmented position became increasingly difficult to sustain. A nicotine-containing electronic cigarette might be lawfully marketed as a consumer product in one Member State but regarded as an unauthorised medicine in another. National authorities adopted different approaches to nicotine concentration, product classification, advertising and sale. Manufacturers faced uncertainty over which standards applied, while consumers could purchase products across borders or through online retailers operating from other jurisdictions.

The internal-market problem was inseparable from the public health problem. European Union legislation generally requires a legal basis for harmonising national rules, and the free movement of goods is one of the central considerations. Divergent national controls could obstruct trade, but complete freedom of movement without common product standards could leave important health and safety questions unresolved. The eventual revision of the Directive therefore pursued two connected objectives: improving the operation of the internal market and ensuring a high level of health protection.

By the end of the first decade of the twenty-first century, the wider tobacco market had also changed. New products had appeared, packaging and marketing techniques had evolved, and the scientific and political environment surrounding tobacco control had become more demanding. The European Commission concluded that the 2001 framework no longer addressed the market adequately. Its formal proposal for a revised Tobacco Products Directive was adopted in December 2012. The proposal addressed conventional tobacco products, packaging, ingredients, traceability, cross-border distance sales and emerging nicotine-delivery systems.

Electronic cigarettes became one of the most contentious parts of the legislative negotiations. Policymakers agreed that nicotine-containing products required some form of regulation, but there was no agreement initially about the appropriate route. One possibility was to regulate them principally as medicinal products. This would have required manufacturers to demonstrate quality, safety and efficacy under pharmaceutical legislation, particularly where products were presented as smoking-cessation aids.

A medicinal pathway offered clear advantages. It could impose rigorous manufacturing standards, controlled nicotine delivery, formal assessment and post-market pharmacovigilance. Products authorised through this route could potentially make therapeutic claims supported by evidence. The difficulty was that most electronic cigarettes were already developing as consumer products rather than medicines. Their manufacturers, formulations, product cycles and commercial models differed significantly from those of the pharmaceutical industry.

Requiring medicinal authorisation for most or all nicotine-containing electronic cigarettes could therefore have removed a large proportion of the existing market. Smaller manufacturers would have faced substantial costs and lengthy development requirements. Product variation would have been restricted, and the consumer market might have consolidated around a small number of authorised systems. Supporters regarded this as a necessary consequence of applying serious standards to inhaled nicotine. Opponents argued that it would protect cigarettes from effective competition and prevent smokers from accessing products they were already using as alternatives.

The issue became politically prominent during consideration by the European Parliament. The original approach favoured by parts of the European regulatory process would have brought many nicotine-containing electronic cigarettes within medicines legislation, particularly above specified nicotine thresholds. The Parliament rejected a general medicinal classification and supported a separate consumer-product framework, while preserving the medicinal route for products making therapeutic claims or seeking formal medicines authorisation.

The eventual compromise placed consumer electronic cigarettes within the revised Tobacco Products Directive as a distinct category of related product. This was a significant legal development. The products were not treated as conventional cigarettes, but neither were they left under general consumer law. Article 20 of Directive 2014/40/EU created a specific system for electronic cigarettes and refill containers that were not subject to medicinal authorisation.

The revised Directive was adopted on 3 April 2014, entered into force on 19 May 2014 and became applicable in Member States on 20 May 2016. It replaced Directive 2001/37/EC and established a broader regulatory structure for the manufacture, presentation and sale of tobacco and related products.

Article 20 required manufacturers and importers to notify competent authorities before placing electronic cigarettes or refill containers on national markets. Notifications had to include information on ingredients, emissions, toxicological data, nicotine delivery, product components, manufacturing processes and producer responsibility. The Directive did not establish a full pre-market authorisation system. Authorities were not necessarily required to approve every product affirmatively before sale. Instead, manufacturers and importers were required to submit specified information and accept legal responsibility for product quality and safety.

The distinction between notification and authorisation was important. A notified product was not automatically certified as safe, scientifically endorsed or individually approved by the competent authority. Notification created visibility and accountability. It allowed authorities to identify products, examine submitted data, monitor the market and intervene where concerns arose. It also placed manufacturers under a defined set of continuing obligations.

Article 20 established several numerical and technical limits that came to define the European vaping market. Nicotine-containing liquid could not exceed a concentration of 20 milligrams per millilitre. Refill containers were limited to 10 millilitres, while tanks and cartridges were generally limited to 2 millilitres. Products had to be child-resistant and tamper-evident, protected against breakage and leakage, and equipped with a mechanism intended to ensure refilling without leakage. Ingredients other than nicotine were required to meet appropriate purity standards, and products were expected to deliver nicotine consistently under normal conditions of use.

These requirements reflected a mixture of toxicological concern, consumer protection and administrative judgement. The nicotine limit was intended to restrict exposure and dependence potential while allowing products to remain available as alternatives to smoking. Container and tank limits sought to reduce the amount of nicotine liquid available in a single unit and to limit the consequences of accidental exposure. Child-resistant packaging and leak protection addressed practical hazards associated with concentrated nicotine solutions.

The precise limits were not simply direct translations of demonstrated toxicological thresholds. They were negotiated regulatory boundaries created under uncertainty. A 20-milligram-per-millilitre product was not automatically safe, while a marginally stronger formulation was not automatically dangerous. Actual exposure depended on device power, aerosol generation, puffing behaviour, liquid consumption and nicotine absorption. Nevertheless, numerical limits offered legislators a clear and enforceable structure.

The concentration ceiling had wider consequences for product development. Manufacturers working within the European market had to design devices and formulations capable of satisfying smokers without exceeding the legal maximum. Greater attention was directed towards aerosol efficiency, coil design, airflow, nicotine chemistry and sensory properties. The restriction therefore shaped innovation rather than merely limiting it.

The Directive also established packaging and labelling requirements. Nicotine-containing products had to carry health warnings, provide specified consumer information and avoid certain misleading characteristics. Information concerning use, storage, contraindications, possible adverse effects, addictiveness and toxicity had to accompany products. The broader objective was to ensure that nicotine-containing vaping products were not presented as ordinary lifestyle goods without acknowledgement of their pharmacological properties.

Advertising and promotion were restricted through Article 20 and associated national implementation. Cross-border commercial communications in certain media were prohibited or limited, while Member States retained responsibility for aspects of domestic advertising and sponsorship. These rules significantly altered how vaping businesses could communicate with consumers. The framework reduced the risk of unrestricted mass promotion, but it also constrained the ability of manufacturers to explain product differences and relative-risk information.

The revised Directive required more than a legal text. Its operation depended on technical systems capable of receiving and managing product information from manufacturers across Europe. The EU Common Entry Gate, known as EU-CEG, became the electronic submission mechanism through which manufacturers and importers provided information to the authorities of Member States where products were intended to be marketed.

EU-CEG represented an important step in regulatory data collection. It created a common submission architecture for tobacco products, electronic cigarettes and refill containers. In principle, this allowed authorities to compare formulations, identify ingredients, monitor product categories and detect emerging concerns. In practice, the value of the system depended on the quality and consistency of the information submitted.

Ingredient names, chemical identifiers, toxicological descriptions and emissions data could be incomplete or presented inconsistently. Complex flavour formulations were particularly difficult to describe. Manufacturers might depend on confidential information held by flavour suppliers, while authorities had to process large numbers of notifications with differing levels of scientific detail. A centralised entry system solved the problem of data transmission more readily than the problem of data interpretation.

The Commission adopted implementing measures to clarify parts of the Directive. Commission Implementing Decision 2015/2183 established a common format for the notification of electronic cigarettes and refill containers. Commission Implementing Decision 2016/586 addressed technical standards for refill mechanisms. These measures demonstrated how broad legal principles had to be translated into detailed fields, formats and product-engineering expectations before they could operate consistently.

Implementation remained a national responsibility. Each Member State transposed the Directive into domestic law, designated competent authorities and developed its own enforcement arrangements. The harmonised framework created common minimum requirements, but it did not eliminate all national variation. Member States could retain or introduce measures in areas where the

Directive allowed discretion, including aspects of age restriction, domestic advertising, retail licensing, cross-border distance sales and public-place use.

The result was harmonisation without complete uniformity. A manufacturer could use the same basic technical dossier across several markets, but national fees, administrative processes, language requirements and enforcement practices could differ. Some countries imposed additional restrictions or treated the products more cautiously than others. The Directive reduced fragmentation while preserving substantial national influence over the practical conditions of sale.

The Directive also had to survive legal challenge. In the United Kingdom, Totally Wicked challenged the validity of Article 20, arguing that its treatment of electronic cigarettes breached principles including proportionality, equal treatment, legal certainty and subsidiarity. In May 2016, the Court of Justice of the European Union upheld the provisions. The Court accepted that electronic cigarettes possessed different objective characteristics from conventional tobacco products and that the European legislature was entitled to adopt a distinct regulatory regime in response to uncertainty and divergent national rules.

The judgment strengthened the legal foundation of the framework. It confirmed that the Union legislature had broad discretion when regulating a technically complex and evolving field involving public health. It also reinforced the role of precaution. Legislators did not need complete evidence of long-term harm before establishing proportionate controls, particularly where nicotine-containing products were expanding rapidly and national approaches were diverging.

The Directive changed the structure of the European vaping industry. Businesses that had previously operated through general consumer-product obligations were required to maintain formulation records, identify ingredients, commission emissions testing, prepare notifications and manage products through defined regulatory timelines. Packaging had to be redesigned, nicotine strengths adjusted and tank and container capacities brought within the legal limits.

For responsible manufacturers, the framework created clearer expectations and a more stable route to market. It also imposed substantial technical and administrative costs. Smaller companies had to develop regulatory expertise rapidly or depend on specialist consultants and laboratories. Products that could not be documented adequately were removed, reformulated or pushed outside the lawful market.

The six-month notification period influenced commercial planning. New or substantially modified products could not be introduced immediately without prior submission. This reduced the speed at which lawful manufacturers could respond to changing demand. It also created a distinction between regulated innovation and illegal market activity: compliant businesses had to plan ahead, while traders willing to disregard the rules could introduce products more quickly.

As product technology evolved, weaknesses in the Directive became clearer. Article 20 had been designed during the era of cigalikes, early tank systems and comparatively simple refill products. The later market included nicotine salts, compact pod systems, high-puff-count devices, increasingly sophisticated electronics and single-use products that tested the meaning of capacity, refillability and product modification.

The Directive regulated nicotine concentration and container volume more directly than total product performance or likely consumption. A product could comply with the 20-milligram-per-millilitre limit while delivering nicotine efficiently through improved aerosol generation. A small lawful tank could be paired with repeated refilling or replaceable components. Product developers adapted to the rules, illustrating the difficulty of governing a dynamic technology through fixed physical limits.

Enforcement became another source of strain. The legal market was required to comply with detailed composition, notification, packaging and capacity rules, but unauthorised and incorrectly labelled products continued to appear. Products claiming capacities beyond legal limits, unnotified formulations and counterfeit brands could be sold through shops, online marketplaces and informal networks. The Directive created the legal basis for action but did not guarantee sufficient national inspection, testing or border capacity.

In 2021, the European Commission published its first major report on the application of Directive 2014/40/EU. It recognised that the Directive had strengthened tobacco control through larger health warnings, ingredient reporting, traceability and the regulation of electronic cigarettes. It also identified difficulties associated with emerging products, divergent national implementation, enforcement, data quality and rapid market development.

The review confirmed that Article 20 had provided a regulatory foundation but had not resolved every policy question. Member States continued to differ over flavours, taxation, product presentation and the public health role of vaping. New nicotine products did not always fit easily within existing definitions. The distinction between tobacco products, electronic cigarettes, heated products, nicotine pouches and other emerging categories became increasingly important.

The European Commission subsequently began a broader evaluation of the tobacco-control legislative framework, including the Tobacco Products Directive and the Tobacco Advertising Directive. The evaluation was placed within the context of Europe's Beating Cancer Plan and its ambition for a tobacco-free generation. It examined whether the existing framework remained effective, efficient, relevant, coherent and capable of addressing new products and changing market conditions.

This next stage differs from the original development of Article 20. The first regulatory debate concerned whether electronic cigarettes should be regulated and where they belonged within European law. The present debate concerns how strongly they should be controlled whether the existing distinctions between products remain appropriate and how taxation, flavours, environmental policy and youth protection should interact with harm reduction.

The Directive's development also demonstrates the limits of describing it simply as tobacco legislation. Its electronic-cigarette provisions created a technical product-regulation system involving chemistry, toxicology, engineering, information technology, packaging and post-market monitoring. It required manufacturers to translate scientific information into a standardised regulatory format and required authorities to interpret that information within a public health framework.

Its central achievement was to give nicotine-containing consumer vaping products a defined legal route to market across the European Union. Before the revised Directive, their position was fragmented and uncertain. After implementation, manufacturers knew the principal limits, documentation requirements and responsibilities that applied. Consumers gained minimum packaging and product protections, while authorities gained notification data and enforcement powers.

Its central weakness was that the framework could not remain fully aligned with a market that continued to change rapidly. Fixed limits offered clarity but were imperfect proxies for exposure and risk. Notification produced large quantities of information but not necessarily consistent regulatory assessment. Harmonisation reduced national divergence without eliminating it. Legal compliance became more structured, while illegal and cross-border supply remained difficult to control.

The Tobacco Products Directive evolved from legislation governing established tobacco products into the principal European framework for a new class of nicotine technology. That transition was neither seamless nor scientifically complete. It was a negotiated response to market fragmentation, public health uncertainty and political pressure. Article 20 represented a compromise between medicinal authorisation, unrestricted consumer sale and prohibition.

The first version of that compromise established the architecture of modern European vaping regulation. Its concentration limits, notification requirements, packaging rules and producer obligations continue to influence product design and regulatory policy far beyond the European Union. Its continuing evolution reflects a more difficult question: whether a framework created to bring order to an emerging market can adapt without losing the distinction between protecting the public from nicotine-related risk and preserving alternatives to the far greater harm caused by tobacco combustion.

The Role of the MHRA

The Medicines and Healthcare products Regulatory Agency occupies an unusual position in the regulation of vaping in the United Kingdom. Its principal statutory identity is that of a medicines and medical devices regulator, yet it also administers the notification system for nicotine-containing electronic cigarettes and refill containers sold as consumer products. This places the agency at the boundary between pharmaceutical regulation, consumer-product control and tobacco-related legislation.

The MHRA did not become involved because every electronic cigarette was classified as a medicine. Its role developed because nicotine-containing products could enter the market through two distinct routes. A product intended and presented as a consumer vaping product could be regulated under the Tobacco and Related Products Regulations 2016. A product intended to relieve or prevent nicotine withdrawal, support smoking cessation or make medicinal claims could instead seek a marketing authorisation as a medicine. The MHRA became central to both routes, although the standards and legal consequences of each are very different.

This dual structure reflected the unresolved identity of electronic cigarettes during the early regulatory period. Vaping products were being used by many consumers to reduce or stop smoking, but most were not developed as pharmaceutical treatments. They were sold through specialist retailers, convenience stores and online channels rather than supplied primarily through healthcare systems. Requiring every product to obtain a medicines licence would have transformed the market completely. Leaving nicotine-containing inhalation products solely under general consumer law, however, was increasingly considered inadequate.

The Tobacco and Related Products Regulations created a middle route. Consumer vaping products did not have to demonstrate therapeutic efficacy in the manner required of medicines, but producers had to notify products, submit specified information, comply with composition and packaging requirements and accept continuing responsibilities after market entry. The MHRA was selected to manage much of this system because it already possessed experience in nicotine regulation, scientific assessment, product vigilance and the administration of complex regulatory submissions.

The choice was significant. The MHRA brought a pharmaceutical regulatory culture into a consumer market that had developed largely outside traditional healthcare structures. Its institutional approach placed emphasis on documented product identity, responsible producers, structured submissions, adverse-event reporting and traceable regulatory records. These principles were familiar in medicines regulation but relatively new to many early vaping businesses.

The agency's function under the consumer-product route is principally one of notification administration and regulatory oversight rather than conventional medicines approval. Producers must submit information about relevant nicotine-containing products before placing them on the market. The submitted material covers product identity, ingredients, emissions, toxicological information, nicotine delivery, manufacturing processes and declarations concerning producer responsibility. The MHRA receives and processes these submissions and publishes products that have completed the relevant notification process.

This distinction between notification and approval is essential. Publication on the MHRA's notified-products list does not mean that the agency has granted a medicinal licence, certified the product as harmless or independently verified every part of the submitted evidence. It means that a producer has supplied the required information through the applicable system and that the product has passed through the administrative notification process sufficiently to be published.

The language used around notification has sometimes caused confusion. Consumers, retailers and even businesses may interpret an MHRA listing as formal approval. In reality, consumer vaping products are not authorised in the same way as licensed medicines. The notification framework places responsibility for product quality and compliance primarily on the producer. The regulator can examine information, request clarification, identify apparent non-compliance and coordinate action, but the producer remains responsible for ensuring that the product meets the law.

This model differs fundamentally from a pre-market authorisation system. Under full authorisation, the regulator assesses a defined evidence package and decides affirmatively whether the product may be marketed. Under notification, the regulator is informed of the product and receives specified data before market entry, but the depth of assessment may vary according to the information submitted, identified risks and available regulatory resources.

Notification was chosen partly because it offered a proportionate route for a rapidly expanding consumer market. Thousands of product variants could be introduced, often with differences in flavour, nicotine concentration, device configuration or packaging. Requiring a full pharmaceutical-style evaluation for every variation would have demanded very substantial regulatory and commercial resources. The notification system created visibility without converting the entire sector into a medicines market.

The system nevertheless imposed a major change on manufacturers and importers. Before implementation, many businesses had relied mainly on supplier documentation, general product-safety obligations and internally generated technical records. The new framework required them to organise product information in a standardised form and submit it through formal regulatory channels. Ingredient identities, Chemical Abstracts Service numbers, formulation quantities, emissions data and toxicological descriptions had to be assembled into a coherent dossier.

This process exposed weaknesses across the supply chain. Producers did not always possess complete information about flavour formulations. Suppliers sometimes treated ingredient composition as confidential. Chemical identifiers could be inaccurate or inconsistent. Toxicological information designed for food, cosmetics or occupational exposure might be submitted without adequate consideration of inhalation. Emissions testing varied between laboratories and product configurations. The MHRA's notification role therefore encouraged greater discipline, but it also revealed how immature parts of the sector remained.

The agency's publication database became one of the most visible elements of the framework. Consumers and retailers can search for products by identifiers including brand, submitter and product type. The register provides a practical means of checking whether a nicotine-containing product has been notified for lawful supply. It also gives enforcement authorities a reference point when examining products found in the market.

The value of the register depends on how it is understood. It is a record of notification status, not a guarantee that every unit sold under a listed brand is genuine, correctly manufactured or unchanged from the submitted specification. Counterfeit products may copy notified brands. A product may be marketed under a similar name while differing in composition or capacity. Producers may also modify products without managing the change correctly. The database assists traceability, but it cannot replace inspection, analytical testing or supply-chain control.

The MHRA's role also includes issuing detailed guidance to producers, retailers and consumers. Its guidance addresses submission procedures, ingredients, labelling, product presentation, technical requirements, vigilance and the distinction between consumer and medicinal routes. The guidance hub brings these materials together and provides the operational interpretation needed to apply the Tobacco and Related Products Regulations in practice.

This interpretive function is important because legislation rarely answers every technical question. A statutory requirement may state that ingredients must not pose a risk to human health in heated or unheated form, but producers still need to understand what evidence is expected. A rule may require consistent nicotine delivery, yet the law may not define a single test method suitable for every device. Labelling provisions may specify mandatory information while leaving practical questions concerning placement, visibility and product format.

Regulatory guidance fills some of these gaps. It explains how the agency expects information to be submitted and how it interprets particular obligations. Guidance is not identical to legislation, but businesses generally need to follow it unless they can justify an alternative approach that still meets the legal requirement. The result is a regulatory system shaped both by the text of the Regulations and by the agency's operational expectations.

Ingredient control provides a clear example. Producers are required to ensure that nicotine-containing liquids do not contain prohibited additives and that ingredients other than nicotine do not present a human-health risk in heated or unheated form. This obligation places the burden of assessment on the producer rather than the regulator. The MHRA can provide guidance and review submitted information, but it does not formulate the product or select its ingredients.

That burden is scientifically demanding. A flavour ingredient may have an established history of oral use but limited inhalation data. Heating can alter the chemical profile. Mixtures may produce emissions not evident from the unheated formulation. Device operating conditions influence exposure. A producer cannot satisfy the underlying obligation merely by stating that ingredients are food-grade or widely used.

The MHRA's framework therefore pushed the sector towards regulatory toxicology. Producers were expected to describe ingredients, identify relevant hazards and consider exposure. The quality of that work varied, but the requirement itself marked a transition from informal product development to documented scientific responsibility.

The agency also performs a vigilance function. Producers must maintain systems for collecting information about suspected adverse effects on human health and product safety. Where a product may be unsafe, of poor quality or non-compliant, the producer must investigate and take appropriate corrective action. Serious concerns and corrective measures must be reported to the MHRA.

Vigilance is important because pre-market information cannot predict every real-world outcome. Manufacturing defects, leakage, battery failures, unexpected reactions and patterns of misuse may only become visible after distribution. Complaints and adverse-event reports can identify recurring problems that are not apparent from laboratory testing alone.

The Yellow Card system provides a route for reporting suspected adverse reactions and safety concerns associated with nicotine-containing electronic cigarettes and liquids. Reports may come from consumers, healthcare professionals or industry. They do not necessarily prove that a product caused the reported event, but they provide signals that can be reviewed alongside other evidence.

Signal detection requires careful interpretation. A report received after product use establishes a temporal association, not causation. Symptoms may be related to nicotine exposure, another ingredient, an underlying condition, concurrent smoking, an illicit substance or an unrelated event. The value of the system lies in patterns rather than isolated reports. Repeated reports involving similar products, symptoms or defects may justify investigation.

The MHRA can use vigilance data to request information, support product investigation or coordinate corrective action. Producers may need to alter labelling, change manufacturing controls, withdraw affected batches or remove a product from the market. The effectiveness of this process depends on accurate product identification and cooperation across the supply chain.

Market enforcement, however, is not performed by the MHRA alone. The UK system divides responsibilities among several bodies. Trading Standards services play a major role in local enforcement, including product compliance, retail activity and age-of-sale controls. Other bodies may be involved in border control, advertising, environmental requirements, product safety and taxation. The MHRA manages the notification system and relevant technical oversight, but it is not a national retail inspectorate with officers routinely visiting every shop.

This division is both necessary and problematic. Vaping products engage several areas of law simultaneously. A single product may raise questions about notification, nicotine concentration, tank capacity, electrical safety, advertising, age restriction, waste regulation and customs status. No single authority possesses exclusive responsibility for every issue.

Coordination is therefore essential. The MHRA's register and technical guidance can support Trading Standards investigations. Local officers can identify products that appear absent from the notified list, exceed legal capacity limits or carry defective labelling. Border agencies can detect imports. Advertising regulators can examine promotional claims. Information can then be shared across the system.

Fragmentation can nevertheless create enforcement gaps. A retailer may assume that a listed product is entirely compliant. An enforcement officer may lack access to laboratory testing. A product may be notified correctly but sold in a modified or counterfeit form. National and local priorities may differ, producing uneven enforcement between regions.

The rapid growth of illicit and oversized products placed particular pressure on this structure. Products could be labelled as containing lawful capacities while actually holding substantially more liquid. Packaging might display an MHRA-related identifier without corresponding to a valid submission. Brands could introduce frequent variants faster than local authorities could assess them.

The agency's notification function was never designed to police the whole market by itself. It created a regulatory record and a point of accountability. Effective enforcement still required inspection, sampling, product testing, intelligence and sanctions. Where those supporting functions were weak, the existence of a sophisticated submission system could give an appearance of control greater than that achieved in practice.

The relationship between the MHRA and producers also changed after the United Kingdom left the European Union. The Tobacco and Related Products Regulations remained the principal domestic framework, but submission arrangements and market distinctions had to be adjusted. Great Britain developed its own publication and administrative processes, while Northern Ireland retained particular relationships with European rules under post-EU arrangements.

These changes increased the importance of accurate jurisdictional planning. Producers supplying different parts of the United Kingdom could face different procedural requirements. Submission pathways, responsible-person arrangements and market records had to reflect the destination in which products would be supplied. The regulatory burden was no longer simply a matter of completing one European notification and assuming uniform coverage.

The MHRA's continuing role provided some institutional stability. The agency remained the central point for nicotine-vaping notifications and guidance, even as the legal context changed. Businesses familiar with the earlier European system could adapt existing data structures, but they still needed to understand the revised UK processes.

The second major part of the MHRA's role concerns medicinal licensing. An electronic cigarette or other inhaled nicotine-containing product may seek authorisation as a medicine when it is intended to relieve or prevent nicotine withdrawal or to support smoking reduction or cessation. This route requires evidence of quality, safety and efficacy comparable to that expected for medicinal products.

The medicinal route is substantially more demanding than consumer-product notification. The applicant must define the product precisely, control its manufacture, validate analytical methods, demonstrate consistent performance and provide evidence supporting the claimed therapeutic use. Device components may also engage medical-device requirements where relevant. Manufacturing sites, quality systems, stability, pharmacovigilance and benefit-risk assessment become part of the authorisation process.

This higher standard offers important advantages. An authorised medicinal product can make approved therapeutic claims and may potentially be supplied through healthcare pathways. Clinicians and stop-smoking services can rely on a formal assessment rather than a consumer-product notification. Product consistency should be more tightly controlled, and changes must be managed within the medicines regulatory system.

The challenge is commercial feasibility. Consumer vaping markets develop rapidly, with frequent changes in device design, flavour and branding. Medicines development is slower and more expensive. A medicinal product must remain sufficiently stable in specification to support validation, clinical evidence and regulatory assessment. The variety and speed that characterise consumer vaping are difficult to reproduce within a conventional pharmaceutical model.

This helps explain why the availability of authorised medicinal electronic cigarettes has remained limited despite official encouragement. The regulatory route exists, but the scientific and commercial requirements are substantial. Companies must believe that prescription or healthcare supply will justify the investment.

The coexistence of the two pathways produces an unusual policy position. Consumer vaping products may be widely used for smoking cessation without being authorised as cessation medicines. Healthcare professionals may discuss or support vaping while distinguishing consumer products from licensed treatments. The MHRA administers both the consumer notification framework and the potential medicinal route, yet it must preserve the legal boundary between them.

Claims are central to that boundary. A consumer-product manufacturer may describe factual characteristics within the constraints of advertising and consumer law, but explicit claims to treat nicotine dependence or deliver a clinically established cessation benefit may trigger medicines regulation. The same device technology can therefore occupy a different regulatory category depending on its intended purpose and presentation.

The distinction is not merely semantic. Medicinal claims imply that evidence has been assessed and that the benefit-risk balance has been accepted for a defined indication. Consumer products are not held to the same evidential standard. Allowing unlicensed products to make therapeutic claims would undermine the medicines system and could mislead consumers.

At the same time, an excessively rigid approach to communication can create a public health contradiction. If consumers are using vaping products to stop smoking, withholding all discussion of comparative risk or cessation-related use may leave them poorly informed. Regulation must distinguish between unsupported therapeutic promotion and accurate public health communication.

The MHRA is not responsible for determining the entirety of national tobacco-control policy. It does not independently decide taxation, flavour restrictions, retail licensing, advertising law or whether single-use products should be prohibited. Those decisions involve ministers, Parliament, the Department of Health and Social Care, HM Revenue and Customs, environmental departments and other authorities.

Its role is narrower but technically important. It converts legislation into a functioning product-notification system, maintains submission and publication mechanisms, provides technical guidance, receives vigilance reports and supports action where products may present risks or fail to comply. It also preserves the medicinal authorisation route for companies seeking to develop inhaled nicotine products as regulated therapies.

The distinction between policy formation and regulatory administration matters. The MHRA may implement requirements that were politically determined elsewhere. A nicotine concentration limit, warning requirement or submission timetable may originate in legislation rather than an independent agency decision. The agency then has to interpret and operate the rule in a technically coherent manner.

This can create tension between scientific judgement and legal constraint. Regulators may recognise that exposure depends on more than nicotine concentration, yet the law sets a fixed limit. They may understand that product capacity can be manipulated, yet enforcement depends on legal definitions. They may receive large amounts of ingredient and emissions data without possessing a fully harmonised method for comparing every product.

The MHRA's effectiveness must therefore be judged against the powers and resources available to it. It cannot compensate entirely for defective legislation, incomplete producer data or weak market enforcement. Nor can notification alone ensure that every product sold matches the submitted specification.

The strongest aspect of the MHRA model is the regulatory discipline it introduced. Producers were required to identify themselves, document their products, submit structured information and maintain vigilance systems. Products could no longer lawfully enter the nicotine-vaping market with no formal record or responsible economic operator.

Its principal limitation is that administrative visibility does not equal full scientific evaluation. A large notification database can identify products, but the quality of evidence within it may vary. Publication can support enforcement, but it does not prevent counterfeit or altered products from appearing.

Guidance can describe expected practice, but it cannot ensure that every producer follows it.

The MHRA consequently functions as the technical centre of a wider regulatory network rather than as the sole controller of the vaping market. Its work connects producers, laboratories, toxicologists, retailers, enforcement bodies and consumers. It receives product information at the point of notification and safety information after market entry. It maintains the distinction between consumer vaping and medicinal nicotine while operating within a policy environment that increasingly treats vaping as both a harm-reduction tool and a source of youth, environmental and enforcement concern.

The agency's role demonstrates how modern regulation depends on information architecture as much as legal prohibition. Products must be identifiable. Formulations must be documented. Producers must be accountable. Adverse events must be reportable. Corrective action must be possible. Without these elements, regulators cannot distinguish lawful innovation from uncontrolled supply.

The MHRA did not resolve every contradiction surrounding vaping. It created a practical system through which nicotine-containing consumer products could enter the market without being treated automatically as medicines, while retaining a higher evidential route for products seeking therapeutic status. That compromise allowed the consumer market to continue under defined controls, but it also required the agency to administer a product category unlike those at the centre of its traditional remit.

Its continuing importance lies in that bridge between science and administration. The legislation defines what must be controlled; producers generate the technical data; enforcement bodies police the market; and the MHRA provides the regulatory mechanism through which product identity, notification, vigilance and medicinal status are made visible.

WHO Influence on Nicotine Policy

The World Health Organization has exerted substantial influence over the way governments define and regulate modern nicotine products. Its importance does not arise from direct legislative authority within individual countries. WHO cannot itself set national nicotine limits, prohibit flavours, impose taxes or determine which products may be sold in a domestic market. Its influence operates through guidance, technical reports, treaty processes, regional programmes and the policy expectations created around the WHO Framework Convention on Tobacco Control.

The WHO Framework Convention on Tobacco Control, adopted in 2003 and brought into force in 2005, established the first international public health treaty devoted to tobacco control. Its core provisions were developed in response to the health effects of tobacco use, exposure to tobacco smoke, cross-border advertising, illicit trade and the international conduct of the tobacco industry. It created a common structure through which governments could coordinate taxation, advertising restrictions, health warnings, smoke-free measures, ingredient disclosure, cessation support and protection of public health policy from commercial influence.

Electronic cigarettes did not exist as a significant global consumer category when the Convention was negotiated. The treaty was therefore built around tobacco products, smoking and the behaviour of tobacco companies. When electronic nicotine delivery systems expanded later, they entered an international policy system whose language, institutions and assumptions had already been shaped by decades of conflict with the cigarette industry.

This historical context was decisive. WHO did not approach vaping as an isolated engineering innovation or simply as a consumer alternative to smoking. It approached it through tobacco control: a field defined by addiction, commercial manipulation, disease prevention, youth protection and distrust of industry claims. That starting point influenced how uncertainty, relative risk, marketing and harm reduction were interpreted.

The Convention's Conference of the Parties became one of the principal forums in which governments considered electronic nicotine delivery systems. The Conference of the Parties, usually referred to as the COP, is the governing body of the Convention. It brings together Parties to review implementation, adopt decisions and request further work from the Convention Secretariat and WHO. Its decisions are not equivalent to national legislation, but they provide direction and can influence how governments develop domestic policy.

Electronic nicotine delivery systems received significant formal attention at the sixth session of the Conference of the Parties in Moscow in October 2014. WHO presented a report examining health risks, efficacy in smoking cessation, effects on tobacco-control activity and possible regulatory options. The COP subsequently issued guidance concerning electronic nicotine and non-nicotine delivery systems.

The timing was important. The European Union had adopted the revised Tobacco Products Directive earlier that year, while national governments elsewhere were deciding whether to permit, restrict, classify or prohibit vaping products. Many countries had limited laboratory capability, incomplete surveillance data and little regulatory experience with nicotine-containing consumer products. WHO material therefore offered a ready-made policy framework at a moment when governments were under pressure to act.

The early WHO approach identified several objectives: preventing initiation among non-smokers and young people, minimising health risks to users and non-users, preventing unproven health claims and protecting existing tobacco-control activity from commercial interference. It also recognised that products varied greatly and that evidence concerning long-term effects and smoking cessation remained incomplete. The proposed regulatory response was correspondingly broad, covering advertising, youth access, product characteristics, health claims, use in public places and surveillance.

These objectives carried considerable authority because they were presented within an international public health framework rather than as the policy preference of one national regulator. Health ministries could cite WHO positions when introducing restrictions. Civil-society organisations could use them to support advocacy. Regulators in countries without established systems could treat them as an initial template.

WHO influence was especially strong in countries where governments lacked the resources to conduct extensive independent assessment. Evaluating electronic cigarettes requires expertise in aerosol chemistry, toxicology, nicotine pharmacology, behavioural science, epidemiology and market surveillance. Few health ministries possess all these capabilities internally. International guidance can therefore reduce the burden of policy development, but it can also encourage countries with very different smoking patterns and healthcare systems to adopt similar controls.

The terminology used by WHO also shaped policy. Electronic cigarettes were commonly described as electronic nicotine delivery systems, or ENDS, and products without nicotine as electronic non-nicotine delivery systems, or ENNDS. This language placed the mechanism of nicotine delivery at the centre of the discussion. It avoided defining the products as cigarettes in the conventional sense, but it also kept them within a regulatory category associated with dependence and tobacco control.

Terminology matters because regulatory language directs attention. Describing a product as a smoke-free alternative highlights the absence of combustion. Describing it as an electronic nicotine delivery system highlights nicotine administration. Describing it as a tobacco-related product connects it to existing tobacco law. None of these descriptions is entirely false, but each frames the problem differently.

WHO policy generally placed greater emphasis on nicotine initiation, youth appeal, marketing and uncertainty than on consumer-led substitution away from smoking. This reflected its population-level mandate. An international public health organisation must consider effects across users, non-users and future generations rather than focusing only on individual smokers who benefit from switching.

The difficulty is that population-level analysis depends on multiple competing outcomes. Vaping may reduce harm when it replaces smoking. It may create harm when it initiates nicotine use among people who would otherwise remain abstinent. It may produce limited benefit when users continue to smoke heavily alongside vaping. A single policy position must therefore account for substitution, initiation, dual use, relapse, cessation and illegal supply.

WHO has usually treated these uncertainties as reasons for strong control. Its public communications have consistently stressed that e-cigarette aerosol is not harmless, that nicotine is dependence-forming and that products should be kept away from children. Its current public information describes e-cigarettes as products that heat liquids to create inhaled aerosols containing nicotine, additives, flavours and other chemicals that may be harmful.

These statements are scientifically defensible at a general level. Vaping is not risk-free, and nicotine use among children requires control. The more contested question is whether the communication gives sufficient weight to comparative risk. Cigarette smoking exposes users to combustion products that are not present at equivalent levels in vapour aerosols. If all nicotine products are described primarily through harm and addiction, smokers may fail to understand meaningful differences between them.

Relative-risk communication has therefore become one of the sharpest points of disagreement between WHO and harm-reduction advocates. WHO has resisted industry-led claims that electronic cigarettes, heated tobacco products and nicotine pouches should automatically be accepted as public health interventions. It has argued that commercial companies may appropriate the language of harm reduction to expand nicotine markets, protect profits and attract new users.

That concern became more explicit in WHO's 2025 position paper on tobacco control and harm reduction. The paper warned that tobacco and nicotine companies were using the concept of harm reduction to promote products such as electronic cigarettes, nicotine pouches and heated tobacco products. WHO distinguished commercially promoted products from tightly controlled, evidence-based harm-reduction programmes led by health actors and public authorities.

This distinction reflects a fundamental difference in governance philosophy. Under a public-health-led model, harm reduction should be supervised, monitored and directed towards defined health objectives. Under a consumer-market model, smokers select products through retail channels, manufacturers compete to improve them and regulation sets the boundaries within which that market operates.

WHO has generally favoured the first interpretation. It is more willing to recognise harm reduction when it is embedded within a controlled public health programme than when it emerges through ordinary commercial competition. The United Kingdom has taken a more permissive approach, allowing a consumer market to coexist with cessation services and public health messaging. Other countries have adopted prescription-only access, severe restrictions or prohibition.

Neither model is without difficulty. Health-system control can provide greater oversight but may reduce access, choice and product appeal. A broad consumer market can support rapid switching but may increase youth exposure, aggressive promotion and variation in product quality. WHO's influence has encouraged governments to prioritise control, even where that choice may reduce the speed at which smokers move away from cigarettes.

The question of industry involvement sits at the centre of this debate. Article 5.3 of the Framework Convention requires Parties to protect tobacco-control policy from the commercial and other vested interests of the tobacco industry. This provision arose from extensive evidence that tobacco companies had distorted science, opposed effective regulation and interfered with public health policy.

Applying Article 5.3 to modern nicotine products is not straightforward. Large tobacco companies now manufacture electronic cigarettes, heated tobacco products and nicotine pouches. Excluding them from policy influence may be justified by their history and continuing cigarette interests. Yet the same companies possess manufacturing capability, scientific data, distribution systems and technical knowledge relevant to non-combustible products.

Independent vaping manufacturers present a further complication. They may not produce cigarettes or identify themselves as part of the tobacco industry, but they still have commercial interests in nicotine policy. Some regulators and public health bodies distinguish between traditional tobacco companies and independent nicotine businesses; others apply a broad precautionary approach to all commercial actors.

WHO policy has generally treated industry evidence with caution and has encouraged strong protection of policymaking from vested interests. This has helped prevent regulatory capture, but it can also narrow the technical information available to decision-makers. Product developers often hold detailed knowledge about formulations, device performance, manufacturing and consumer use. The challenge is to obtain that knowledge transparently without allowing commercial interests to dictate policy.

The seventh session of the Conference of the Parties in 2016 continued consideration of electronic nicotine and non-nicotine delivery systems. The COP adopted a further decision and maintained the principle that Parties could prohibit or restrict the manufacture, importation, distribution, presentation, sale and use of these products as appropriate to national circumstances and public health objectives.

This approach allowed considerable national variation. WHO did not impose one universal regulatory model. Instead, it provided governments with a range of options, including prohibition, strict regulation and controls modelled on tobacco policy. That flexibility was necessary because Parties differed in legal systems, smoking prevalence, product availability and enforcement capacity.

In practice, however, the available policy options were not neutral. WHO materials often placed prohibition and restrictive control within the range of legitimate public health responses, while giving less institutional support to regulated consumer access as a deliberate smoking-substitution strategy. Countries seeking to ban products could therefore cite WHO guidance more easily than countries seeking to integrate vaping into harm-reduction policy.

The international effect was significant. Some governments prohibited sales entirely. Others restricted imports, advertising, flavours, nicotine concentration or public use. Several classified electronic cigarettes within tobacco law even though the products contained no tobacco. Others treated them as medicines or prescription products.

The resulting global landscape became fragmented. A product lawfully sold as a consumer alternative in one country could be prohibited in another. A flavour permitted in one jurisdiction could be banned in the next. A nicotine concentration considered acceptable under one system could exceed the legal limit elsewhere. WHO's influence contributed to the common principle that electronic cigarettes required control, but it did not produce regulatory harmonisation.

WHO regional offices have also shaped policy. Regional publications adapt global tobacco-control priorities to local circumstances and often focus on youth use, marketing and industry conduct. In 2026, the WHO Regional Office for the Western Pacific issued an updated advocacy brief describing e-cigarette harms, youth uptake and tobacco-industry marketing, while outlining measures available to governments.

Regional emphasis can be appropriate because market conditions differ substantially. Some countries face high smoking prevalence and limited cessation provision. Others have experienced rapid youth uptake of disposable products. Enforcement capacity, illicit trade and cultural attitudes towards nicotine vary widely. A global position that ignores these differences risks becoming too broad to guide proportionate action.

WHO's product-regulation work has expanded alongside the market. Reports prepared for the Framework Convention process now address flavours, nicotine pouches, disposable products and other emerging categories, as well as conventional tobacco and heated tobacco products. A 2024 progress report on Articles 9 and 10 specifically identified flavours, nicotine pouches and disposable electronic nicotine delivery systems as continuing regulatory concerns.

This expansion shows that nicotine policy is no longer centred only on cigarettes or refillable electronic cigarettes. Governments now face a wider ecosystem of nicotine products, each with different exposure profiles, use patterns, environmental consequences and commercial strategies. WHO has responded by favouring controls that can be applied across categories rather than allowing each new product to create a separate regulatory exception.

Cross-category regulation can prevent loopholes. If restrictions apply only to cigarettes, companies may shift promotion towards heated products, pouches or vaping devices. If flavour controls apply to one category but not another, consumers and manufacturers may move accordingly. A consistent framework can reduce regulatory arbitrage.

The risk is that consistency becomes equivalence. Cigarettes, heated tobacco products, nicotine pouches, medicinal nicotine and electronic cigarettes do not create the same exposures. A framework that regulates them identically may be administratively simple but scientifically disproportionate. Product-specific risk must remain visible even where common rules on youth access, marketing and quality are justified.

WHO has also influenced fiscal policy. The Framework Convention recognises taxation and price measures as important tools for reducing tobacco use. As electronic cigarettes and other nicotine products have expanded, governments have increasingly considered whether similar fiscal measures should apply to them.

Taxation can discourage youth uptake and generate revenue for enforcement or public health programmes. It can also reduce the price advantage that non-combustible products hold over cigarettes. If tax policy does not preserve a meaningful differential between more harmful and less harmful products, smokers may have less financial incentive to switch.

WHO's general preference for strong nicotine-product control has encouraged governments to consider taxation as part of a comprehensive response. The public health effect depends on how rates are structured. A risk-proportionate tax system would impose the highest burden on combustible products while maintaining lower rates for non-combustible alternatives. A uniform approach could unintentionally protect cigarette consumption.

Flavour policy has followed a similar path. WHO has repeatedly highlighted flavours as a mechanism through which products may appeal to children and new users. This has strengthened calls for flavour bans or restrictions in numerous jurisdictions.

The youth-protection case is clear where products use child-oriented imagery, confectionery branding or misleading descriptors. The broader scientific question concerns flavour compounds themselves. Adult smokers also use fruit, sweet, mint and beverage flavours, and many report that non-tobacco flavours help separate vaping from the sensory experience of smoking. A prohibition may reduce youth appeal but may also reduce adult product acceptance.

WHO policy tends to place greater weight on prevention of initiation than on preserving product diversity for adult switching. This is understandable within a precautionary framework, but it can produce measures that treat all flavours as marketing devices rather than considering their role in substitution.

Disposable products have brought environmental policy into the same debate. Their small batteries, plastics and mixed materials create waste and recycling difficulties. Their low purchase price, convenience and visual presentation have also been associated with youth uptake. WHO's recent technical work has identified disposable electronic nicotine delivery systems as an emerging regulatory issue.

These concerns have broadened the justification for intervention. Governments no longer rely only on nicotine dependence or inhalation risk. They cite litter, battery waste, product design, illegal capacities and youth visibility. WHO's framework supports this wider interpretation by treating nicotine products as part of a comprehensive public health and regulatory system.

The influence of WHO is strongest when its recommendations align with domestic political priorities. Governments concerned about youth use can cite international guidance when introducing restrictions. Health ministries can use WHO language to justify caution. International reports can strengthen proposals that might otherwise be challenged as lacking evidence.

That influence can be valuable. It gives countries access to technical support, creates common minimum expectations and prevents commercial markets from developing without public health scrutiny. It also gives smaller states a basis for action where national research capacity is limited.

It can become problematic when WHO positions are treated as scientific conclusions rather than policy judgements. Scientific evidence may establish that a product contains nicotine, produces toxic emissions or attracts young users. It does not by itself determine whether the appropriate response is a warning, product standard, flavour restriction, taxation, prescription control or prohibition. Those are policy choices requiring consideration of local smoking rates, enforcement capacity, consumer behaviour and unintended effects.

WHO publications sometimes compress this distinction. Statements about hazard may be followed by broad regulatory recommendations without fully explaining the comparative analysis between vaping, smoking and abstinence. Public communication may emphasise uncertainty around long-term vaping risks while giving less prominence to the established harms of continued smoking.

This can distort public understanding. A smoker deciding whether to switch does not face a choice between vaping and breathing clean air. The realistic alternatives may be vaping, continued smoking, medicinal nicotine, dual use or repeated unsuccessful quit attempts. Relative risk is therefore not a secondary issue; it is central to informed decision-making.

WHO's reluctance to endorse commercially supplied nicotine products as harm-reduction tools reflects legitimate concerns about industry behaviour. It also limits the extent to which the organisation can support countries that view consumer access as part of tobacco control. The disagreement is not simply about whether vaping is harmful. It concerns who should control harm reduction, what evidence is sufficient and whether markets can deliver public health benefits without being treated as public health programmes.

The Framework Convention was built to reduce tobacco use and protect policy from an industry with a documented history of deception. Modern nicotine products challenge that architecture because they may be manufactured by the same companies while exposing users to substantially different chemical hazards. The institutional response has been to preserve caution and extend tobacco-control principles into the new market.

That response has prevented electronic cigarettes from being treated as ordinary consumer gadgets. It has promoted age restrictions, advertising controls, ingredient disclosure, health warnings, surveillance and government oversight. These are important protections.

It has also contributed to policies that may fail to distinguish sufficiently between combustion and non-combustion. Where governments adopt prohibition or severe restriction without controlling cigarette availability, the more harmful product can remain easier to obtain than the alternative. Where public messaging implies equivalence, smokers may see no reason to switch.

WHO influence on nicotine policy is therefore both protective and restrictive. It provides an international counterweight to commercial promotion and reminds governments that innovation does not remove the need for control. At the same time, its institutional emphasis on prevention, industry distrust and precaution can understate the public health value of replacing combustible tobacco.

A stronger international approach would preserve WHO's core protections while applying them according to product risk. Children and non-users should be protected across every nicotine category. Manufacturers should disclose ingredients, control production and substantiate claims. Marketing should not mislead, and policymakers should remain protected from commercial interference. None of these requirements depends on treating all products as equally harmful.

The unresolved issue is whether WHO can accommodate harm reduction as a consumer transition rather than only as a tightly supervised health intervention. That question will shape global nicotine policy for years to come. In countries where smoking remains prevalent, restrictions on lower-risk alternatives can carry consequences as real as the risks those restrictions are intended to prevent.

European Commission Working Groups

The Tobacco Products Directive established the legal framework for electronic cigarettes, but the Directive could not determine every technical, administrative and scientific detail required for implementation. Article 20 set out the principal obligations, including notification, ingredient and emissions reporting, nicotine and volume limits, packaging requirements and producer responsibilities. Turning those provisions into a functioning regulatory system required continuing cooperation between the European Commission, national competent authorities, scientific advisers, information-technology specialists and enforcement bodies.

European Commission working groups became an important part of that process. They provided forums in which Member States could compare interpretation, discuss emerging products, identify enforcement problems and develop common approaches to requirements that were expressed only broadly in the legislation. Their work occurred largely beneath the level of public political debate, but it influenced how manufacturers prepared submissions, how authorities interpreted product data and how the European vaping market operated in practice.

The Commission's role was not to replace national regulators. The Tobacco Products Directive remained a European legal instrument implemented and enforced through Member States. Each country retained responsibility for designating competent authorities, transposing the Directive into national law and applying sanctions. The Commission's task was to support coherent implementation across the Union and to exercise the implementing powers granted to it by the European Parliament and the Council. Those powers allowed it to adopt additional legal acts where detailed rules were needed to make the Directive operational.

This structure created a continuing need for coordination. Without it, Member States could interpret identical provisions differently. One authority might accept a particular notification format, test method or product classification while another rejected it. A device component could be treated as a substantial modification in one market but not in another. A refill mechanism could be considered compliant by one national authority and defective by another. Such divergence would weaken both the internal market and public health protection.

Working groups allowed regulators to identify these differences before they developed into completely separate national systems. Representatives could discuss how legal provisions were being applied, share experience of products found on the market and consider whether further Commission guidance or implementing legislation was necessary. This did not eliminate national variation, but it provided an institutional mechanism for limiting it.

The practical importance of these groups increased sharply before the Directive became applicable in May 2016. Manufacturers and importers had to submit large quantities of information in advance of market entry, yet no common operating system initially existed for receiving it. Regulators needed compatible data structures, agreed identifiers and a process through which submissions could be directed to the relevant Member States.

The EU Common Entry Gate, or EU-CEG, emerged as the central solution. It was designed to provide one electronic gateway through which information on tobacco products, electronic cigarettes and refill containers could be submitted to national authorities. The system covers information including ingredients, emissions and toxicological data and is intended to promote uniform reporting across Member States.

EU-CEG illustrates the practical work required after legislation has been adopted. Article 20 could state that specified information must be notified, but an operational system still needed to determine how products would be identified, which fields would be mandatory, how ingredients would be described, how quantities would be reported and how data would be transmitted securely. These decisions affected thousands of products and became part of daily regulatory practice.

Commission Implementing Decision (EU) 2015/2183 established the common format for notifications concerning electronic cigarettes and refill containers. It converted the requirements of Article 20 into structured reporting fields covering the submitter, product identity, components, ingredients, emissions, toxicological information, nicotine delivery and other technical characteristics.

The common format was intended to improve both comparability and administrative efficiency. A regulator receiving data from many manufacturers needed information arranged consistently enough to permit searching, grouping and comparison. Without standardisation, one producer might describe an ingredient by trade name, another by chemical name and another through a proprietary mixture code. Concentrations might be stated in incompatible units, while emissions results might be generated under different operating conditions.

Standardisation could improve the structure of information, but it could not guarantee scientific comparability. The Implementing Decision acknowledged the absence of agreed Union or international standards for some forms of testing and required producers to describe the methods used and ensure that they were reproducible. It also encouraged the use of agreed standards and compatible components where available.

This limitation was important. Two manufacturers could submit technically complete emissions data while using different puffing regimes, device settings, analytical methods or reporting conventions. Both submissions might pass electronic validation, yet their numerical results might not be directly comparable. The working-group process therefore had to address not only whether data were present but whether the data could support meaningful interpretation.

Electronic validation is primarily administrative. It can confirm that mandatory fields have been completed, that identifiers follow the required format and that files have been transmitted successfully. It cannot determine automatically whether a toxicological argument is scientifically sound, whether a flavour formulation is adequately characterised or whether an emissions test reflects realistic product use. Those questions require expert review.

The volume of information submitted through EU-CEG placed substantial demands on national authorities. The Directive created a mandatory database of product information, but Member States differed in staffing, technical capability and regulatory priorities. Some were able to conduct detailed data analysis, while others used the system mainly to confirm notification status and support targeted enforcement. The Commission's 2021 application report recognised the importance of the system while also identifying problems involving data quality, administrative burden and the practical use of submitted information.

Working groups offered a means of sharing analytical approaches and avoiding duplication. If one authority identified a questionable ingredient, unusual product configuration or pattern of inaccurate reporting, the issue could be raised with other Member States. Regulators could compare whether similar products had been notified elsewhere and whether common action was warranted.

This information-sharing role became increasingly important as the market changed. Early implementation focused heavily on refill liquids, tanks and first-generation electronic cigarettes. Later products included nicotine-salt formulations, compact pod systems, disposable devices, large claimed puff counts and products designed to exploit ambiguities in legal definitions. The regulatory questions became more complex even though the underlying Directive remained largely unchanged.

Disposable electronic cigarettes provided a particularly clear example. By August 2023, approximately 8,200 disposable electronic-cigarette notifications had reportedly been submitted through EU-CEG for Belgium alone. The scale and speed of this expansion created questions concerning liquid capacity, battery design, environmental waste, nicotine delivery, youth appeal and the accuracy of reported product characteristics.

No single Member State could assess the wider European market solely through domestic inspection. Brands and product families circulated across borders, often under slightly different names or configurations. Working-level coordination allowed authorities to compare submissions and identify whether a concern was local or reflected a broader market pattern.

The groups also helped translate legal definitions into practical classifications. The Directive distinguished among tobacco products, electronic cigarettes, refill containers, herbal products for smoking and novel tobacco products. Subsequent market innovation introduced products that did not fit comfortably within those categories. Nicotine pouches, nicotine-free liquids, separate device components and hybrid systems raised questions concerning whether they fell within the Directive and, if so, under which provisions.

Classification determines which data must be submitted, which authority has jurisdiction and whether the product may lawfully be sold. A disagreement over classification is therefore not a minor administrative issue. It can determine whether a product faces notification, prohibition, medicinal regulation or no product-specific European requirement at all.

The Commission could not resolve every borderline case through informal discussion. Where national measures introduced new technical requirements, the Technical Regulation Information System allowed drafts to be notified and examined for potential internal-market effects. This became relevant as Member States considered additional controls on flavours, product categories and nicotine products not fully harmonised under existing European law. Commission responses through this system could raise concerns about proportionality, legal compatibility and the relationship between national restrictions and the Directive.

The relationship between harmonisation and national autonomy remained delicate. The Directive created common requirements, but Article 24 allowed Member States in certain circumstances to prohibit a category of tobacco or related products where justified by public health considerations and the specific national situation. Such measures required notification and scrutiny.

Working groups therefore operated within an unresolved political tension. The Commission was responsible for protecting the internal market and promoting consistent implementation, while Member States retained legitimate public health powers. A country facing rapid youth uptake might seek stronger restrictions than its neighbours. Another might place greater emphasis on adult smoking substitution. Both could claim to be acting within public health objectives.

Technical discussion could not remove these policy differences, but it could clarify their consequences. Representatives could examine whether a proposed national rule would create barriers to trade, whether a product definition was enforceable and whether equivalent controls already existed elsewhere. This helped distinguish genuine technical necessity from measures that were largely political or symbolic.

The development of refill-mechanism standards illustrates how the process could produce concrete legal outcomes. Article 20 required electronic cigarettes and refill containers to include mechanisms ensuring refilling without leakage. The broad requirement did not specify precisely how this should be achieved. Commission Implementing Decision (EU) 2016/586 subsequently established technical standards for refill mechanisms, providing manufacturers and regulators with more detailed expectations. The Commission's implementation materials identify this Decision alongside the common notification format as part of the additional legislation supporting the Directive.

This approach had advantages. A technical requirement could be developed with input from national authorities and specialists rather than being fixed entirely within the original political legislation. It could address a defined safety concern while preserving more than one possible engineering solution.

The weakness was that implementing decisions remained relatively slow compared with product development. By the time a technical issue had been discussed, drafted, reviewed and formally adopted, manufacturers might already have introduced a new generation of devices. European regulatory coordination was therefore often reactive.

Joint initiatives supplemented the Commission's own working structures. The Joint Action on Tobacco Control was launched in 2017 to support Member States in implementing the Tobacco Products Directive. It brought national authorities together around areas including laboratory capacity, product assessment, data analysis and regulatory cooperation.

Joint actions were valuable because formal Commission legislation could not solve every operational problem. Regulators needed practical tools, training, common methodologies and networks of technical specialists. Shared projects could examine data from EU-CEG, develop approaches to priority substances and improve understanding of new products.

The usefulness of EU-CEG data depended heavily on such cooperation. A database containing thousands of formulations has limited regulatory value if authorities cannot search, clean and interpret the information. Ingredient names may be entered inconsistently. Duplicate products may appear under separate identifiers. Proprietary mixtures may obscure individual components. Product variants may differ only slightly yet generate separate records.

Data-analysis projects could identify patterns that were not visible through individual submissions. Regulators could examine the frequency of particular ingredients, compare nicotine concentrations, track growth in product categories and identify products containing substances of concern. This moved EU-CEG beyond its role as a filing system towards its intended function as a market-monitoring tool.

Confidentiality created another area requiring common treatment. Manufacturers were required to disclose commercially sensitive formulation and product information to regulators. At the same time, consumers had a legitimate interest in knowing what products contained. The Implementing Decision required a balance between transparency and the protection of trade secrets.

Working-level agreement was needed over which information could be published, which should remain confidential and how requests for confidentiality should be justified. Excessive secrecy would weaken public accountability. Unrestricted disclosure could expose proprietary formulations and discourage detailed reporting. The resulting system had to protect legitimate commercial information without allowing confidentiality claims to conceal safety-relevant data.

Scientific advisory processes also interacted with Commission coordination. The Commission could request assessments from independent scientific committees where evidence concerning health effects required review. Such assessments informed policy discussion but did not themselves create law. They became one input among epidemiology, market data, Member State experience, stakeholder submissions and political priorities.

The distinction matters because scientific committees answer questions framed by policymakers. The scope of a review, the evidence included and the outcomes measured influence the conclusions reached. A review centred on youth initiation may lead towards different policy implications from one centred on smoking substitution. Working groups and Commission services determine how those scientific findings are translated into regulatory options.

Stakeholder engagement existed alongside the intergovernmental process, but access was unequal. Industry associations, public health organisations, consumer groups, laboratories and technical specialists could contribute through consultations, workshops and written submissions. National authorities and Commission officials, however, retained control over the formal implementation process.

Excluding commercial actors entirely would have deprived regulators of practical product knowledge. Manufacturers understood device architecture, supply chains, formulation constraints and submission problems. Laboratories could explain method limitations. Consumer organisations could describe real-world use and switching behaviour. Public health bodies could identify population concerns and marketing practices.

Participation also created the risk that organised interests would shape technical rules to their own advantage. Large companies could devote more resources to meetings, data submissions and sustained engagement than small manufacturers or consumers. Public health organisations could frame technical questions through a restrictive policy objective. The Commission therefore had to distinguish useful evidence from advocacy while maintaining transparency over who was contributing.

The working-group structure could appear remote to businesses affected by its decisions. Technical interpretations were sometimes communicated indirectly through revised guidance, national authority practice or changes to submission requirements. Manufacturers might discover that an accepted approach had changed without a prominent legislative event.

This created a need for regulatory intelligence. Compliance depended not only on reading the Directive but on monitoring implementing decisions, Commission guidance, EU-CEG updates, national interpretations and enforcement trends. A product that complied with the original text could still face difficulty if working-level interpretation evolved.

The process also revealed the limits of European harmonisation. Common data formats and technical decisions improved consistency, but enforcement remained uneven. One Member State might conduct extensive product testing while another relied mainly on documentary checks. Notification fees differed. Publication practices varied. National restrictions on flavours, online sales and product categories continued to develop.

The Commission's broader evaluation of the tobacco-control legislative framework has brought these issues into the next phase. The evaluation considered the effectiveness, efficiency, relevance, coherence and European added value of both the Tobacco Products Directive and the Tobacco Advertising Directive. It was conducted within the context of Europe's Beating Cancer Plan and the objective of achieving a tobacco-free generation in which fewer than 5 per cent of the population uses tobacco by 2040.

The evaluation drew on Member State authorities, civil-society organisations, economic operators and other stakeholders. It examined whether the framework remained capable of addressing new products and changing market conditions.

Future working groups will have to address a substantially wider policy landscape than the one faced during the original implementation of Article 20. Taxation, flavours, nicotine pouches, disposables, environmental controls, cross-border internet sales and digital traceability now interact with conventional product regulation. The Commission's 2025 proposal to modernise the Tobacco Taxation Directive reflects the movement towards fiscal control of a broader range of products as part of European health and internal-market policy.

The central value of European Commission working groups lies in their ability to connect legislation with technical reality. They allow national authorities to compare experience, develop common systems and respond collectively to market change. Without them, the Directive would be a legal framework lacking the administrative machinery needed for consistent implementation.

Their limitation is that coordination does not automatically produce scientific proportionality or effective enforcement. A common reporting format can standardise data without proving its quality. A shared interpretation can still be technically weak. A detailed database can coexist with widespread illegal sales. Agreement among regulators does not guarantee that a rule addresses the most important determinants of harm.

European Commission working groups occupy the space between political legislation and national enforcement. They do not attract the visibility of parliamentary votes or major public consultations, yet they shape the definitions, submission formats, technical expectations and information flows through which regulation operates. Their decisions determine whether a legal requirement remains an abstract statement or becomes a practical obligation that manufacturers, laboratories and regulators can apply.

The evolution of vaping regulation has shown that this middle layer is indispensable. Modern nicotine products change too quickly and contain too many interacting technical features for legislation alone to govern them effectively. Continuing coordination is necessary, but it must remain transparent, scientifically informed and responsive to real market outcomes. Without those safeguards, technical cooperation can become a mechanism for extending regulatory complexity without demonstrating corresponding public health benefit.

Political Drivers Versus Scientific Drivers

Vaping regulation is frequently presented as though scientific evidence moves directly into law. In practice, science is only one influence among many. Political priorities, public opinion, media attention, institutional history, fiscal interests, electoral pressure and the need for visible government action all shape regulatory decisions. Scientific evidence may define the problem, narrow the available options or expose weaknesses in a proposal, but it rarely determines the final policy by itself.

This distinction does not mean that political influence is illegitimate. Regulation requires value judgements that science cannot make. Evidence can estimate toxicant exposure, nicotine delivery, youth prevalence, cessation outcomes and product failure rates. It cannot decide how much uncertainty society should tolerate, whether adult choice should outweigh a small risk of youth initiation, how public resources should be allocated or whether an environmental concern justifies removing a product from the market. Those decisions belong to elected governments and public institutions.

The difficulty begins when political choices are presented as though they were unavoidable scientific conclusions. A regulator may cite evidence that young people use flavoured products, but the evidence alone does not dictate whether the response should be age-verification enforcement, restrictions on packaging, limitations on descriptors, removal of selected ingredients or a broad flavour prohibition. Each option reflects a different judgement about proportionality, enforceability and acceptable consequences for adults.

Scientific drivers originate in evidence concerning product composition, toxicology, exposure, behaviour and population outcomes. They include measured emissions, nicotine pharmacokinetics, adverse-event data, longitudinal patterns of use, cessation trials, market surveillance and comparative-risk assessment. A scientifically driven intervention should identify a defined problem, establish a plausible causal relationship and select a control capable of reducing the relevant risk.

Political drivers operate differently. They respond to what is publicly visible, easily communicated and institutionally urgent. A sudden rise in brightly packaged disposable products may generate demands for immediate action even before long-term evidence is available. Images of discarded devices, reports of school use or enforcement seizures can move an issue rapidly up the political agenda. Ministers are expected to respond within parliamentary and electoral timescales, while scientific research may require years.

The difference in timescale creates recurring tension. Product markets can transform within months. Epidemiological evidence develops more slowly because meaningful conclusions require adequate follow-up, representative samples and control of confounding factors. By the time a study is published, the products examined may already have been replaced. Governments therefore make decisions using incomplete evidence, provisional data and assumptions about how markets will respond.

Precaution is one way of managing this gap, but it does not remove the political judgement involved. A decision to intervene early reflects a preference for avoiding one type of error: permitting a product that later proves harmful. A decision to preserve access reflects concern about the opposite error: restricting an alternative that could reduce smoking-related harm. Neither position is scientifically neutral.

Youth vaping has become one of the most powerful political drivers. Protecting children commands broad public support and creates a clear basis for intervention. Evidence of underage sales, school use and youth-oriented promotion can justify stronger age controls, retailer sanctions and restrictions on marketing. The problem arises when the political force of youth protection is used to support measures whose effect on youth use has not been demonstrated or whose impact on adult smokers has not been adequately considered.

Policy language often moves rapidly from evidence of youth use to claims that particular flavours, colours or product formats are the cause. Some associations are plausible and supported by survey data, but causal interpretation is difficult. Young people may select sweet flavours because those flavours are widely available, because they are more palatable or because established users prefer them. Product choice after initiation does not necessarily identify the factor that caused initiation.

A scientifically disciplined approach would distinguish between experimentation, regular use and dependence. It would separate never-smokers from young people who already smoke or use other nicotine products. It would examine acquisition routes, family and peer influences, socioeconomic factors and the role of illegal supply. Political debate often compresses these distinctions into one headline prevalence figure.

The resulting policies may be broader than the evidence supports. Restrictions on flavours, packaging and displays can be justified as efforts to reduce youth appeal, but their actual effectiveness depends on implementation and market response. Young users may move to remaining flavours, illegal products, nicotine pouches or cigarettes. Adults may lose products they use to remain smoke-free. A measure can therefore satisfy political demand for action without producing the intended public health outcome.

The United Kingdom's recent legislation illustrates how political and scientific drivers converge. The Tobacco and Vapes Act received Royal Assent in April 2026 and created extensive powers over advertising, sponsorship, packaging, displays, flavours and product standards. The stated objectives include protecting children while retaining access for adults using vaping products to stop smoking. That balance is politically attractive but technically demanding because each future restriction must be designed so that it reduces youth appeal without unnecessarily weakening smoking substitution.

The legislation gives ministers powers to act, but the scientific quality of the eventual regime will depend on how those powers are used. A power to restrict flavours is not itself evidence that a comprehensive flavour ban is necessary. A power to control packaging does not establish which visual features materially influence initiation. Secondary regulations, consultations and impact assessments will determine whether the framework becomes targeted or indiscriminate.

Political action also tends to favour measures that are easily explained. A ban, age limit, numerical cap or tax rate can be communicated clearly. Technical interventions such as improved toxicological review, laboratory surveillance, retailer intelligence or supply-chain traceability are less visible. They may be more effective against specific risks, but they do not provide the same symbolic demonstration of government control.

Single-use vape bans demonstrate this attraction. Disposable products generated concerns involving waste, battery disposal, illegal capacities and youth use. A categorical ban offered a clear response to several problems at once. Yet those problems were not identical. Environmental waste concerns relate to product design and disposal systems. Youth access relates to retail enforcement, price and appeal. Illegal capacity relates to compliance and border control. Combining them into one political intervention simplifies the message but can obscure whether the ban addresses each cause effectively.

Scientific regulation normally seeks specificity. If the problem is lithium battery waste, the control should address battery design, producer responsibility, recyclability and collection. If the problem is youth access, the control should address retailers, online verification and illicit supply. If the problem is misleading capacity claims, it should be addressed through inspection and testing. Political regulation often combines these into a single visible measure because institutional clarity can matter more than causal precision.

Taxation reveals a further divergence. Governments may justify nicotine-product duties through public health, revenue generation or regulatory parity. These objectives can conflict. A high duty may reduce consumption, but it may also narrow the price differential between vaping and cigarettes. A flat-rate duty is administratively convenient, yet it may treat low-strength and high-strength products similarly and may not correspond closely to exposure or risk.

The United Kingdom's Vaping Products Duty, due to commence in October 2026, applies a flat charge to vaping liquid regardless of nicotine concentration. The approach provides a clear fiscal mechanism, but it is not a direct toxicological assessment. The rate is a political and economic choice involving revenue, enforcement, affordability and market behaviour. Whether it improves public health depends partly on how it affects switching, consumption, illicit trade and the relative price of cigarettes.

Political pressure can also arise from institutional targets. The European Commission's evaluation of the tobacco-control framework sits within Europe's Beating Cancer Plan and its objective of a tobacco-free generation with tobacco use below 5 per cent by 2040. Such targets help coordinate policy and maintain momentum. They can also encourage broad control of all nicotine products where the original target concerns tobacco use rather than nicotine use.

A target changes how evidence is interpreted. If success is defined as reducing all nicotine use, vaping uptake may be treated primarily as failure even where smoking declines. If success is defined as reducing disease and premature death, movement from cigarettes to non-combustible products may be viewed more favourably. The same dataset can therefore support different policy conclusions depending on the objective selected.

Institutional mandates reinforce these differences. Tobacco-control bodies are organised to reduce tobacco and nicotine use, medicines regulators to assess quality, safety and efficacy, finance ministries to collect revenue, environmental departments to reduce waste and trading-standards authorities to enforce product law. Each institution sees a different part of the problem.

A public health agency may prioritise youth prevention and population prevalence. A consumer-safety regulator may focus on defective products and accurate labelling. A customs authority may concentrate on undeclared imports. A health service may value products that help smokers quit. Political policy is produced by negotiating among these perspectives, not by applying a single body of evidence.

The institutional history of tobacco control exerts particular influence. Cigarette regulation developed after decades of industry denial and political interference. This created a justified presumption that tobacco-company claims require independent verification. When the same companies entered vaping and heated-product markets, suspicion followed them.

Conflict-of-interest safeguards remain necessary, but they can affect the treatment of evidence. Industry-generated studies may be discounted because of funding source, while evidence from organisations aligned with tobacco-control policy may receive less scrutiny. Scientific quality should not be inferred solely from institutional identity. Study design, analytical method, transparency, reproducibility and relevance remain the appropriate tests.

Political debate rarely applies this standard consistently. Evidence may be accepted when it supports the preferred policy and criticised when it does not. A laboratory study using unrealistic operating conditions may be cited prominently because it demonstrates harm. A cessation trial may be dismissed as unrepresentative because it demonstrates benefit. The reverse can occur within industry advocacy, where favourable findings are amplified and limitations minimised.

The separation between science and advocacy becomes blurred when researchers participate directly in policy campaigns. Scientists have every right to draw policy implications from their work, but those implications contain value judgements. A toxicologist may establish that an aerosol contains a hazardous compound. Recommending prohibition requires additional assumptions about exposure, alternatives, feasibility and acceptable risk.

The media intensify this compression. Complex evidence is translated into claims that vaping is either dangerous or safe, causes or prevents smoking, protects or targets children. Scientific uncertainty is difficult to communicate and performs poorly in political debate. Absolute statements attract attention and are more readily repeated.

A single adverse finding can therefore influence policy disproportionately. An isolated study may receive extensive coverage before replication or methodological review. Government announcements may cite the concern because it supports action already under consideration. Later corrections receive less attention. Regulation can then become anchored to an early narrative even after the evidence changes.

Political framing also determines the comparator. Vaping can be compared with smoking, medicinal nicotine, abstinence or no product use. Each comparison produces a different result. Against smoking, non-combustible vaping is likely to appear substantially less hazardous. Against clean-air exposure and nicotine abstinence, it introduces avoidable risk. Both statements can be true.

For adult smokers, the relevant comparator is often continued smoking. For children and never-smokers, it is non-use. A scientifically coherent policy must hold both comparisons simultaneously. Political arguments frequently choose the comparator that best supports their position.

Harm-reduction advocates focus on smokers who might switch and on differences in toxicant exposure. Prevention advocates focus on non-users who might initiate nicotine use. Governments must consider both groups, but the weighting is political. A small increase in youth initiation may be judged unacceptable even if a larger number of adults stop smoking, or adult substitution may be prioritised because smoking causes immediate and substantial disease.

Population modelling can inform this balance, but models depend on assumptions about initiation, cessation, relapse, dual use and product risk. Small changes in those assumptions can alter conclusions. Models are valuable for exploring scenarios, not for removing judgement from policy.

The United States uses an explicit population standard through the requirement that a new tobacco product be appropriate for the protection of public health. The FDA considers risks and benefits to the population as a whole, including users and non-users. This appears scientifically comprehensive, but the final decision still depends on regulatory assumptions about uptake, switching and marketing.

The PMTA process also shows how evidential requirements can become political through their economic effects. A demanding pre-market standard may prevent weakly documented products from entering the market. It may also favour companies capable of financing extensive applications. The resulting market structure is not merely a scientific outcome; it reflects a policy choice about how much uncertainty and commercial diversity the system will permit.

The FDA's 2026 authorisation of additional electronic nicotine-delivery products demonstrates that the framework can permit products where the agency concludes the evidence meets the statutory standard. Such decisions do not establish that the products are safe or approved in a general sense. They show that the regulator has made a population-level judgement under a defined legal test.

International policy introduces another political layer. WHO guidance influences national regulation through treaty processes, technical positions and public-health advocacy. Its 2025 position on tobacco control and harm reduction proposes minimum controls for electronic cigarettes, heated products and nicotine pouches. These recommendations reflect scientific evidence but also an institutional preference for tightly controlled public-health approaches rather than reliance on commercial consumer markets.

Governments may adopt WHO positions because they regard them as scientifically authoritative, because they align with existing political objectives or because national capacity for independent assessment is limited. International guidance can strengthen good policy, but it can also cause political preferences to acquire the appearance of universal scientific necessity.

The divide between political and scientific drivers is especially visible in the treatment of uncertainty. Science describes uncertainty through confidence intervals, limitations, data gaps and competing hypotheses. Politics often treats uncertainty as a reason either to act immediately or to avoid regulation. Both uses are selective.

Uncertainty concerning long-term inhalation effects is real. So is uncertainty concerning the consequences of restricting products used by smokers. A balanced assessment considers both. Policies that recognise only the uncertainty of permitting vaping apply precaution asymmetrically.

Scientific proportionality requires an explicit chain of reasoning. The regulator should identify the harm, define the exposed population, assess the quality of evidence, select an intervention and evaluate likely unintended effects. The chosen measure should be capable of reducing the identified harm and should not impose greater burdens than necessary.

Political regulation may begin at the opposite end: a preferred measure is announced, and evidence is assembled to justify it. Consultation then becomes a process of refining implementation rather than reconsidering the underlying decision. This is particularly likely where a policy has strong public support or has already been included in a manifesto, ministerial statement or international commitment.

Impact assessment should provide a corrective. It should examine costs, benefits, distributional effects, enforcement requirements and alternative options. In nicotine policy, this must include effects on adult smokers, lawful manufacturers, retailers, illicit markets and enforcement capacity. An assessment that counts only the expected reduction in youth vaping while ignoring changes in smoking or illegal supply is incomplete.

Post-implementation evaluation is equally important. Political attention often moves on once legislation has been enacted. Scientific regulation requires later examination of whether the intervention worked. Youth use may decline, remain unchanged or shift product category. Adult smoking cessation may improve or weaken. Illegal sales may expand. These outcomes should determine whether the measure is retained, modified or reversed.

Regulatory reversibility is rarely politically comfortable. Removing a restriction can be portrayed as weakening public health even where evidence shows that it was ineffective. Governments therefore tend to accumulate controls rather than retire them. Adaptive regulation requires the opposite discipline: rules should change when evidence changes.

Scientific advice can improve this process only if advisory structures are balanced and transparent. Committees need expertise in toxicology, aerosol science, behavioural research, cessation, epidemiology, economics, enforcement and consumer behaviour. A panel dominated by one discipline may produce technically sound but incomplete recommendations.

Consumers also possess relevant evidence. Their experience cannot establish population-level causation, but it can identify why products succeed or fail as substitutes for cigarettes. Ignoring this information can lead to policies that appear logical in theory but do not reflect real use.

Commercial stakeholders hold technical and market data but have direct financial interests. Their participation should be documented and scrutinised rather than either accepted uncritically or excluded automatically. Regulators need access to product knowledge while retaining independent control over policy.

Political influence cannot and should not be removed from regulation. Democratic institutions must decide objectives, distribute burdens and resolve conflicts between individual autonomy and collective protection. The aim is not to replace politics with science but to prevent political preference from masquerading as scientific inevitability.

A credible regulatory decision should make the distinction visible. It should state what the evidence demonstrates, where uncertainty remains and which elements of the decision reflect policy judgement. It should explain why one intervention was chosen over less restrictive alternatives and how success will be measured.

Vaping policy will always involve contested values. Some will prioritise a nicotine-free society; others will prioritise rapid displacement of combustible tobacco. Some will accept a regulated consumer market; others will favour medicinal or state-controlled access. Science can estimate the consequences of these choices, but it cannot select the preferred social objective.

The danger lies in allowing the objective to determine the evidence. Where policy begins with the assumption that all nicotine use must fall, evidence of successful smoking substitution may be undervalued. Where policy begins with commercial expansion, evidence of youth initiation may be minimised. Both approaches replace inquiry with advocacy.

Political drivers provide urgency, legitimacy and direction. Scientific drivers provide accuracy, proportionality and correction. Effective regulation requires both, but their roles must remain distinct. Politics should determine the public objectives openly. Science should test whether the chosen measures are capable of achieving them and expose the costs when they are not.

Stakeholder Consultation and Lobbying

Regulation is rarely written by government in isolation. Before legislation is introduced, amended or implemented, policymakers usually seek evidence from those who will be affected by it. Manufacturers explain how products are designed and supplied. Public health organisations present evidence on disease prevention, youth use and population risk. Consumers describe their experiences of smoking, switching and product access. Retailers identify enforcement problems. Scientists assess the strength and limitations of the evidence. Local authorities explain what can realistically be inspected, tested and prosecuted.

This process is generally described as stakeholder consultation. It can improve policy by bringing practical knowledge into decisions that would otherwise be made at a distance from the market. It can reveal unintended consequences, expose technical errors and identify less burdensome ways of achieving the same public health objective. It can also become an arena in which well-resourced organisations attempt to shape regulation in their own interests.

The boundary between consultation and lobbying is not always clear. A formal response to a government questionnaire is consultation. A private meeting with a minister, regulator or parliamentary adviser may be lobbying. A scientific submission commissioned by an industry association may contain genuine evidence while also advancing a commercial position. A public health campaign may seek stronger controls while presenting itself as an objective interpretation of science. Consumer mobilisation may represent authentic public concern, organised advocacy or a mixture of both.

The relevant distinction is not whether a participant has an interest. Every stakeholder has one. Manufacturers want viable markets. Retailers want workable rules. public health bodies want lower nicotine initiation and disease. Consumers want access, protection or both. Governments want policies that can be defended publicly and implemented within available resources. The important questions are whether those interests are declared, whether the evidence is reliable and whether access to decision-makers is distributed fairly.

Consultation became particularly important during the development of European vaping regulation because legislators were dealing with products they did not fully understand. Electronic cigarettes combined formulations, electrical components, aerosol generation, nicotine delivery and consumer behaviour. Officials could interpret the law, but they often required external knowledge to understand how a proposed rule would affect product design, manufacturing, testing and use.

The revision of the first European Tobacco Products Directive therefore attracted unusually intense participation. The European Commission's 2010 consultation on revision of Directive 2001/37/EC received more than 85,000 responses. This demonstrated the political significance of tobacco regulation and the ability of organised interests to mobilise large numbers of submissions. It also created a problem familiar in modern consultations: response volume did not necessarily correspond to evidential weight. A repeated campaign response and a detailed technical submission were both contributions, but they did not provide the same information.

Large consultation exercises can create an appearance of direct democratic legitimacy. Thousands of responses may be cited as evidence that the public strongly supports or opposes a measure. The meaning of the total depends on how respondents were recruited, whether campaign templates were used, which populations participated and how questions were framed. Consultation results should therefore be analysed rather than treated as a referendum.

The European Commission now evaluates consultation material within its broader tobacco-control review process. Its evaluation of the Tobacco Products Directive and Tobacco Advertising Directive considers effectiveness, efficiency, relevance, coherence and European added value, drawing on public authorities, economic operators, civil society and other stakeholders. The exercise forms part of a wider policy programme linked to Europe's Beating Cancer Plan and the objective of reducing tobacco use below 5 per cent of the population by 2040.

The policy context matters because consultation questions are not neutral. An evaluation framed around achieving a tobacco-free generation may give greatest weight to proposals expected to reduce use, appeal and availability. An evaluation framed around risk-proportionate regulation may give greater attention to differences between combustible and non-combustible products. The evidence submitted may be identical, but the questions asked influence which parts of it become decisive.

Stakeholders also differ in the type of evidence they can provide. Manufacturers possess formulation records, sales data, product testing and knowledge of supply chains. This information can help regulators understand technical feasibility and market response. It may also be incomplete, selectively presented or designed to protect commercial interests.

Public health organisations contribute epidemiology, behavioural research, prevention expertise and experience of tobacco-industry conduct. Their submissions can identify population effects that individual manufacturers are poorly placed to assess. They may also approach new products through an institutional commitment to reducing all tobacco or nicotine use, giving less weight to consumer substitution and relative risk.

Consumers provide evidence of a different kind. They can explain why they began vaping, which products enabled them to stop smoking, why previous cessation attempts failed and how restrictions might affect their behaviour. Such experience is not a substitute for controlled research, but it is relevant to policy. A regulation that appears proportionate in theory may fail because it removes the features that make a product acceptable to smokers.

Consumer testimony is especially important in nicotine policy because substitution is behavioural rather than purely chemical. A product may produce fewer toxicants than cigarettes but have little effect on smoking if consumers reject it. Flavour, nicotine delivery, convenience, ritual and cost influence whether a switch is maintained. These factors are difficult to understand through laboratory evidence alone.

Retailers and enforcement bodies provide another practical perspective. Retailers know how consumers respond to product restrictions, how stock moves through legal and informal channels and which products are being requested. Trading Standards and border authorities understand which rules can be verified, which offences are difficult to prove and how non-compliant suppliers evade controls. Their input can prevent legislation from creating obligations that look precise but cannot be enforced consistently.

Laboratories, toxicologists and regulatory consultants occupy an intermediate position. They may provide independent technical expertise, but many work commercially for manufacturers, trade associations or governments. Their evidence should be judged according to method and transparency rather than treated as automatically neutral or compromised.

The credibility of technical consultation depends heavily on disclosure. A laboratory report should identify who commissioned the work, which products were selected, how testing was performed and whether unfavourable results were omitted. A toxicological assessment should distinguish between evidence and judgement. A consultant presenting policy recommendations should declare relevant clients and commercial relationships.

Consultation can improve regulation only when the authority is genuinely open to more than one outcome. In some cases, governments consult after the main political decision has already been made. The questions then concern implementation rather than principle. Respondents may be invited to comment on how a restriction should operate but not whether it is justified.

This is not necessarily improper. Elected governments may have a mandate to pursue a stated policy. Consultation can still help refine definitions, transition periods and enforcement arrangements. The process becomes misleading when it is presented as an open evidence-gathering exercise despite the outcome being substantially predetermined.

The design of consultation questions can reveal this limitation. A question asking which flavours should be restricted assumes that restriction is required. A question asking how youth appeal can be reduced allows consideration of flavour controls, packaging, age verification, retailer licensing and enforcement. The second structure is more likely to identify alternative interventions.

Consultations may also direct respondents towards politically preferred evidence. Questions concerning the benefits of stronger controls may be detailed, while those concerning adult switching, illegal markets or small-business effects receive less attention. The resulting evidence base then appears to support the chosen policy because contrary considerations were not requested systematically.

The United Kingdom's recent nicotine-policy development has involved several overlapping consultations and calls for evidence. The 2023 consultation on creating a smoke-free generation and tackling youth vaping sought views on generational tobacco restrictions, product measures and enforcement. Later government exercises sought evidence on flavours, ingredients, nicotine strengths and emissions, while further consultation has addressed packaging, flavour descriptions and vape-free places.

These processes show how consultation can extend across several stages. An initial call for evidence identifies the problem. A public consultation tests policy options. Primary legislation creates ministerial powers. Secondary consultation then determines the detailed restrictions. Each stage may involve different respondents and evidence.

The cumulative effect can be difficult to follow. A business may respond to several exercises covering related issues without knowing how the submissions interact. Consumers may participate in one high-profile consultation but not later technical stages where decisive definitions are set. Public health organisations and large companies are more likely to maintain teams capable of responding repeatedly.

This creates an access imbalance. Large organisations can monitor policy developments continuously, employ legal and regulatory specialists and provide detailed responses within short deadlines. Small manufacturers, independent retailers and individual consumers may lack time, expertise or confidence. Consultation remains formally open, but effective participation is unequal.

Resource inequality matters because technical policy is shaped through detail. A proposed ban may attract broad public attention, while the definition of a refillable product, permitted flavour descriptor or duty-stamp requirement receives less. Those technical details determine which products survive and how the market operates.

Lobbying seeks to influence those details outside or alongside formal consultation. It includes meetings with ministers, officials and legislators; parliamentary briefings; commissioned research; public campaigns; coalition-building; media engagement and participation in expert forums. None of these activities is inherently improper. Policymakers need information, and affected parties have a legitimate right to make their case.

Problems arise when influence is hidden, access is unequal or evidence is manipulated. A company may present commercial objectives as consumer protection. A campaign group may cite research selectively. A front organisation may conceal its funding. A scientific expert may fail to disclose a relevant relationship. Repeated access to officials may allow one position to shape the framing of the problem before other stakeholders are consulted.

The European Union's Transparency Register is intended to make some of this activity visible. It records organisations seeking to influence EU lawmaking and policy implementation, together with information about the interests pursued, resources and activities. The register supports public scrutiny but does not capture every informal interaction or indirect route of influence.

Transparency is a minimum requirement rather than proof of balance. A declared meeting may still exert substantial influence. An organisation may be registered but provide selective evidence. Conversely, the fact that a manufacturer has lobbied does not mean that every technical point it raises is wrong. Disclosure allows the argument to be assessed in context; it does not settle its validity.

Tobacco-sector lobbying receives particular scrutiny because of the history of cigarette manufacturers. Evidence accumulated over decades that tobacco companies had challenged established science, delayed regulation and used political influence to protect cigarette sales. This history led to Article 5.3 of the WHO Framework Convention on Tobacco Control, which requires Parties to protect tobacco-control policies from the commercial and other vested interests of the tobacco industry.

The implementation guidelines recommend limiting interactions with the tobacco industry to those strictly necessary for regulation, conducting such interactions transparently and avoiding partnerships or preferential treatment. The principle is intended to prevent the industry from shaping public health policy in ways that conflict with the objectives of the Convention.

Article 5.3 is grounded in a real governance problem, but its application to modern nicotine products is complicated. Major tobacco companies manufacture cigarettes, heated tobacco products, vaping devices and nicotine pouches. Independent vaping companies may have no involvement in combustible tobacco, yet they still possess commercial interests in nicotine regulation. Trade associations may represent a mixture of tobacco-owned and independent businesses.

A policy that excludes all manufacturers from technical discussion may reduce direct commercial influence but also remove detailed product knowledge. A policy that gives manufacturers unrestricted access risks regulatory capture. The more defensible approach is controlled and transparent engagement: obtain information necessary for regulation, record the interaction, test claims independently and prevent commercial actors from determining public-health objectives.

The same scrutiny should apply to indirect lobbying. Commercial interests may fund retailers, consumer groups, scientific meetings or policy institutes. Public health organisations may receive funding from governments or philanthropic foundations with established policy preferences. These relationships do not invalidate the work automatically, but they should be disclosed.

Funding can influence which questions are studied, which results are publicised and which policy outcomes are considered acceptable. A study need not be fraudulent to serve an advocacy purpose. Selecting one comparator, population or outcome can produce findings that are technically valid but incomplete.

Lobbying also occurs through language. Stakeholders compete to define products and policy objectives in terms favourable to their position. "Alternative nicotine products" suggests substitution and reduced exposure. "Novel tobacco and nicotine products" connects them to established tobacco control. "Consumer harm-reduction products" emphasises autonomy and comparative risk. "Addictive products targeting children" emphasises initiation and commercial misconduct.

These descriptions shape the policy problem before evidence is considered. Once a product is framed primarily as a youth epidemic, proposals centred on restriction become more likely. Once it is framed primarily as a smoking alternative, access and proportionality become more prominent. Stakeholder influence therefore begins with terminology, not merely with the eventual legislative text.

Consultation summaries can conceal this contest. Government reports often group thousands of responses into themes such as support, opposition and concerns raised. The process of coding responses involves judgement. A submission arguing for targeted restrictions may be classified as supporting regulation even if it opposes the proposed measure. Technical qualifications may disappear when findings are reduced to headline percentages.

Publication of full responses, where privacy and confidentiality permit, improves accountability. It allows researchers and the public to examine whether the official summary reflects the evidence received. Where only an aggregated report is available, the authority controls both the questions and the interpretation of the answers.

Commercial confidentiality creates a genuine limitation. Manufacturers may need to provide detailed formulations, sales data and supply-chain information that cannot be published openly. Regulators should protect legitimate trade secrets while ensuring that confidentiality does not become a means of shielding safety-relevant evidence or lobbying positions from scrutiny.

Consultation fatigue is another weakness. Repeated exercises can overwhelm smaller participants and reduce response quality. Organisations with permanent policy teams continue to engage, while individuals and small firms withdraw. The apparent consensus may therefore reflect endurance rather than broad agreement.

Digital consultation has lowered barriers to participation but made organised campaigns easier. A template response can mobilise thousands of people quickly. This may demonstrate the intensity of public concern, but the number of identical submissions should not be confused with independent technical analysis.

Campaign responses still have democratic value. A policymaker should know that many people care strongly about an issue. Their role is different from that of expert evidence. Consultation assessment should distinguish between public preference, personal experience, economic impact and scientific evidence rather than collapsing all responses into one count.

Lobbying frequently extends into parliamentary processes. Stakeholders provide briefing notes, suggested amendments and questions for legislators. This can improve scrutiny where parliamentarians lack technical resources. It can also allow complex provisions to be shaped by organisations whose role is not immediately visible to the public.

Draft amendments should therefore be judged on substance and provenance. A technically sound proposal does not become defective because an interested party suggested it. The source matters because it may reveal omitted consequences, but the argument still requires analysis.

The influence of lobbying is often greatest before formal drafting begins. Early meetings can determine which problems enter the policy agenda and which options are considered realistic. Once a proposal has been announced, later consultation may have limited capacity to alter its direction.

Access at this agenda-setting stage is rarely equal. Established organisations know whom to contact and how to present material in a form useful to officials. Consumers and small businesses may become involved only after a proposal is public. By then, the central framing may already be fixed.

Advisory committees can reduce this imbalance where their membership is diverse and their procedures transparent. Scientific, clinical, behavioural, enforcement, industry and consumer knowledge can be brought together under declared conflict-of-interest rules. No member should represent the whole field, and no one perspective should dominate the evidence review.

Conflict management should be proportionate. Financial interests require disclosure, but so do strong institutional and advocacy commitments. A researcher who has publicly campaigned for prohibition or commercial liberalisation may still provide valuable evidence, but that position should be visible. Independence is not established merely by the absence of industry funding.

Stakeholder evidence should be assessed through common criteria. Relevant questions include whether the data are reproducible, whether methods are reported, whether comparisons are appropriate and whether uncertainties are acknowledged. The same standard should apply irrespective of whether the evidence supports stronger or weaker regulation.

This discipline is often lost in polarised debates. Industry evidence may be dismissed without detailed examination, while public health evidence is accepted because its objective appears socially desirable. Industry may respond by treating all restrictive proposals as ideological and elevating consumer testimony above population evidence. Both approaches weaken regulatory reasoning.

Consultation is strongest when disagreement is preserved rather than edited away. Where evidence conflicts, the authority should explain why one interpretation was preferred. Where a measure reflects political judgement rather than scientific consensus, that should be stated. Transparency concerning disagreement increases credibility.

Economic impact requires similar openness. Manufacturers may exaggerate compliance costs or threatened job losses. Governments may understate them. Public health organisations may treat commercial loss as irrelevant even where market consolidation would strengthen large tobacco companies or illegal trade.

The relevant question is not whether regulation has a cost. Effective regulation usually does. The issue is whether the cost is proportionate to the risk addressed and whether smaller responsible operators can comply. An intervention that removes poor-quality suppliers may be beneficial. One that excludes technically competent smaller firms while illicit sellers continue may not be.

Consumer advocacy deserves separate treatment because its role is often contested. Organisations representing people who vape may be accused of acting as industry proxies, especially where they receive commercial support. Some relationships deserve scrutiny, but assuming that all consumer advocacy is manufactured dismisses the experiences of adults who have stopped smoking through vaping.

Consumer groups should disclose funding and governance, as should every organised stakeholder. Their evidence should then be evaluated on its merits. Lived experience cannot establish toxicological safety, but it can reveal behavioural consequences that may not appear in administrative data.

Public health advocacy is also lobbying. Campaigning for advertising bans, flavour restrictions, taxation or prohibition is an attempt to influence policy. The social purpose may differ from commercial lobbying, but the activity should not be treated as though it lies outside stakeholder influence.

Recognising this does not equate public health organisations with tobacco companies. Their interests, conduct and responsibilities are different. It does mean that policy should not assume that one group delivers facts while another delivers advocacy. Most participants provide some combination of evidence, interpretation and preferred outcomes.

The legitimacy of lobbying depends partly on transparency and partly on the quality of government decision-making. Officials who rely on one stakeholder for technical understanding become vulnerable to its framing. Building internal scientific and regulatory capacity reduces this dependence. Authorities that can analyse formulations, market data and behavioural evidence are better able to test claims from every side.

Independent commissioning of research can also help. Where a key question is contested, government can define the protocol, require publication and separate funding from control of the analysis. This is slower and more expensive than relying on stakeholder submissions but may be necessary for major policy decisions.

Consultation should continue after legislation. Stakeholders can identify implementation failures, unintended market shifts and enforcement gaps. Retailers may report that illegal products are replacing restricted ones. Consumers may return to smoking. Regulators may find that a product definition cannot be applied consistently. Manufacturers may identify technical alternatives that achieve the same objective more effectively.

Post-implementation consultation should not become a route for reopening every settled issue indefinitely. It should be connected to measurable outcomes. Where youth use, smoking prevalence, illegal supply, complaints or environmental waste do not respond as predicted, the intervention should be reviewed.

The Vaping Products Duty consultation illustrates the importance of implementation detail. Government engagement addressed duty stamps, supply controls and compliance measures, with the official response explaining how stakeholder views influenced the final arrangements. Fiscal policy may be politically determined, but consultation can still identify practical risks involving stock transitions, registration, imports and enforcement.

The decisive test is whether the authority shows what changed because of consultation. A process that receives submissions but never alters a proposal provides limited evidence of engagement. Government responses should explain which arguments were accepted, which were rejected and why.

Stakeholder consultation and lobbying cannot be removed from nicotine regulation. The products are technically complex, commercially significant and politically contested. Governments need information held outside the state, and affected parties are entitled to participate.

The objective is not to silence interests but to expose and balance them. Meetings should be recorded. Funding and conflicts should be declared. Evidence should be tested through consistent scientific standards. Consumer experience should be heard without being mistaken for epidemiology. Public health advocacy should be recognised as advocacy even where its purpose is protective. Commercial evidence should be scrutinised without being rejected solely because of its source.

Good consultation broadens the evidence available to policymakers. Poor consultation rewards those with the greatest resources, treats response totals as scientific proof and provides legitimacy for decisions already made. Lobbying becomes dangerous when it is concealed or when repeated access allows one stakeholder to define the problem for everyone else.

Nicotine regulation requires a process capable of hearing competing interests without becoming owned by any of them. That requires transparency, internal competence and a willingness to explain where evidence ends and political judgement begins.

The Precautionary Principle in Practice

The precautionary principle allows governments to act where a plausible risk has been identified but scientific knowledge remains incomplete. It is most often invoked when waiting for definitive evidence could expose the public or the environment to serious or irreversible harm. In nicotine policy, the principle has supported intervention before the long-term effects of new products could be measured through decades of epidemiological observation.

Precaution is not intended to replace science. It is a framework for making decisions when science cannot yet provide certainty. The European Commission's formal approach places the principle within risk analysis and states that it should be used where scientific information is insufficient, inconclusive or uncertain and where preliminary evaluation indicates reasonable grounds for concern. Measures taken under it should be proportionate, non-discriminatory, consistent with comparable measures, open to review and accompanied by continuing examination of the evidence. The principle may respond to potential risk, but it should not justify arbitrary action.

This distinction is essential. Precaution does not mean that every theoretical hazard requires prohibition. Nor does uncertainty prove that a product will cause the worst outcome proposed for it. A precautionary decision still requires a credible pathway to harm, an assessment of the available evidence and consideration of the consequences of alternative actions.

Electronic cigarettes presented precisely the kind of uncertainty for which precautionary reasoning was developed. They entered widespread use before long-term health outcomes were available. Formulations varied, devices evolved rapidly and laboratory methods had not yet been harmonised. Regulators could identify nicotine dependence, chemical emissions, battery failures, accidental ingestion and possible youth uptake as legitimate concerns. They could not initially quantify every risk or predict the full population effect.

The absence of long-term evidence did not make government inaction neutral. If serious harms later emerged, delay could leave a large population exposed. Equally, severe restrictions could prevent adult smokers from moving away from combustible tobacco. Precaution therefore had to operate in both directions: against the risk of allowing inadequately controlled products and against the risk of suppressing a less harmful alternative to smoking.

In practice, the first direction received greater regulatory attention. Governments asked what might happen if vaping products were allowed to develop without strong control. They gave less systematic consideration to what might happen if the products were made less accessible, less satisfying or less competitive with cigarettes. This asymmetry became one of the defining weaknesses of early nicotine regulation.

The European Tobacco Products Directive applied a precautionary structure through notification, ingredient disclosure, toxicological information, nicotine limits, container restrictions, health warnings and product-design requirements. These measures did not depend on proof that every unregulated product would cause harm. They reflected the judgement that nicotine-containing inhalation products should not enter a large consumer market without defined controls.

Some of these requirements addressed direct and readily foreseeable risks. Child-resistant packaging reduced the likelihood of accidental access to nicotine liquid. Leak-resistant refill mechanisms addressed dermal exposure, ingestion and product failure. Ingredient reporting allowed regulators to identify substances of concern. Manufacturer and importer responsibilities made corrective action possible.

Other controls were more indirect. The 20 milligram-per-millilitre nicotine limit, 10-millilitre refill-container limit and 2-millilitre tank limit created simple legal boundaries, but they were not complete measures of exposure or risk.

Nicotine delivery depends on concentration, aerosol generation, device efficiency, puff duration, frequency of use and individual behaviour. A lower-concentration liquid used heavily may deliver more nicotine than a stronger liquid used sparingly.

Numerical limits nevertheless appeal to regulators because they are clear and enforceable. A laboratory can measure concentration. An officer can inspect container volume. A court can determine whether a product exceeds a specified limit. The same clarity is harder to achieve with broader requirements such as proportionate exposure, acceptable emissions or consistent delivery under normal use.

Precaution often favours controls that are administratively measurable even where they are scientifically incomplete. This is understandable, but it can create a gap between the stated public health objective and the variable actually regulated. A rule may be easy to enforce without addressing the main determinant of harm.

The European Court of Justice accepted broad legislative discretion in this area when it considered the validity of Article 20 of the Tobacco Products Directive. In the Pillbox 38 case, the Court upheld the electronic-cigarette provisions against challenges based on proportionality, equal treatment, legal certainty and subsidiarity. It recognised that the legislature was dealing with an evolving market, divergent national rules and uncertainty concerning potential health effects.

The judgment confirmed that legislators do not need complete scientific certainty before regulating a new product category. It also demonstrated the legal difficulty of challenging precautionary controls once they have been embedded within a wider public health framework. Courts generally allow political institutions considerable discretion where complex scientific assessment and health protection are involved.

Judicial deference does not establish that every individual rule is scientifically optimal. It means that the legislature acted within the range of choices permitted to it. The distinction matters because legal validity is sometimes treated as proof of scientific proportionality. A court may conclude that a measure is lawful without determining that it is the most effective or least burdensome available intervention.

Precaution has also shaped ingredient policy. Regulators may restrict or discourage substances where inhalation data are limited, even if those substances have a long history of use in food. This reflects the recognised difference between ingestion and inhalation. A compound that can be consumed safely may behave differently when aerosolised, heated and deposited in the respiratory tract.

The absence of inhalation evidence presents a genuine regulatory problem. It does not prove toxicity, but neither does food-use history establish respiratory safety. A precautionary response may require literature review, read-across, exposure estimation, emissions testing or reformulation. Where a credible hazard exists and exposure cannot be justified, exclusion may be reasonable.

The weakness appears when absence of data is treated as evidence of unacceptable risk in itself. This standard can make compliance impossible because complete inhalation datasets do not exist for many flavour compounds. If every data gap leads automatically to prohibition, large parts of the formulation market become untenable without demonstrating that the replacements are safer.

A more disciplined approach distinguishes between different kinds of uncertainty. A substance with structural alerts, known respiratory toxicity or evidence of harmful thermal degradation requires greater caution than one with limited inhalation data but low estimated exposure and no relevant hazard signal. Precaution should be graduated according to the strength of concern.

The same principle applies to emissions. Detecting a chemical in aerosol does not establish that the exposure creates a material risk. Analytical methods can identify substances at extremely low concentrations. Interpretation requires comparison with dose, background exposure, toxicological reference values and the emissions of relevant alternatives.

Precaution becomes distorted when detection alone is treated as proof of danger. It is equally distorted when lower emissions than cigarettes are treated as proof of safety. The appropriate conclusion depends on concentration, exposure and biological relevance.

Youth vaping has become one of the principal justifications for precautionary policy. Governments do not need to wait for a generation of dependent adult users before restricting sales to children, enforcing age limits or controlling marketing directed at them. Early intervention is justified because nicotine dependence may persist and because young people should not be used as a test population for new commercial products.

The difficulty lies in extending that reasoning from targeted controls to market-wide restrictions. A ban on sale to minors directly addresses youth access. A restriction on child-oriented imagery directly addresses promotional appeal. A comprehensive flavour ban or prohibition of an entire device category affects adults as well as young people and requires a broader assessment.

Precaution may support the intervention, but proportionality still requires evidence that the chosen measure is likely to reduce youth use and that less restrictive alternatives would be inadequate. It should also consider whether young users will move towards illegal products, nicotine pouches or cigarettes.

Single-use vape bans illustrate this wider application. Concerns included youth appeal, low price, waste, lithium batteries, illegal capacities and poor recyclability. A categorical ban offered an immediate response to a cluster of problems, but each problem had a different causal pathway. The precautionary case was strongest where product design created unavoidable environmental waste or where lawful controls were repeatedly evaded. It was weaker where enforcement failures were attributed to the entire category rather than to illegal products and retailers.

A ban may still be justified, but its success should be measured against the stated objectives. If youth use shifts to refillable devices, illegal imports continue or battery waste is displaced rather than reduced, the intervention has not fully solved the original problem. Precaution should require review after implementation, not merely action before certainty.

The European Commission's own formulation of the principle includes review in light of new evidence. This feature is often neglected. Precautionary measures tend to become permanent even when the original uncertainty changes. Restrictions are politically easier to introduce than remove because repeal can be portrayed as weakening health protection.

A genuine precautionary system should be adaptive. Measures introduced under uncertainty should contain review dates, defined indicators and mechanisms for amendment. If evidence of harm strengthens, controls can be tightened. If the expected harm does not materialise or the intervention causes greater unintended effects, it should be modified.

The European Commission's 2021 report on the Tobacco Products Directive acknowledged that the framework had created substantial regulatory controls while also identifying problems involving new products, implementation, enforcement and the usefulness of submitted data. The wider evaluation completed in 2026 examined whether the legislation remained effective, efficient, relevant and coherent.

Such reviews are necessary because precautionary rules can become outdated. A restriction designed for early tank systems may not reflect later pod technologies. An ingredient requirement may be overtaken by improved analytical methods. A notification system may collect large amounts of information without enabling meaningful regulatory comparison.

The precautionary principle also influences WHO policy. WHO communications emphasise nicotine dependence, youth protection, harmful aerosol constituents and uncertainty concerning long-term effects. Its policy position supports strong minimum controls across electronic cigarettes, heated products and nicotine pouches.

This approach protects against the assumption that reduced exposure means no risk. It also reflects concern that commercial companies may use uncertainty selectively, demanding proof of harm while promoting products before benefits have been established.

The same standard should apply to restrictive policy. If industry should not claim safety without sufficient evidence, governments should not claim that a ban will improve public health without examining substitution, illicit supply and smoking behaviour. Precaution should not privilege one untested assumption over another merely because it supports intervention.

Risk–risk comparison is therefore essential. Every regulatory option carries consequences. Permitting a product may expose users to uncertain long-term effects. Restricting it may preserve cigarette use, encourage illegal purchasing or reduce successful switching. Taxation may reduce youth demand while narrowing the price advantage over smoking. Flavour restrictions may reduce appeal to non-users while also weakening adult acceptance.

These effects cannot always be quantified precisely, but they should be identified. Precaution is not complete until the risks of the intervention are considered alongside the risks of non-intervention.

Combustible tobacco makes this especially important. Vaping regulation does not operate in a market where the alternative is necessarily abstinence. Cigarettes remain widely available, highly addictive and responsible for established disease. A restriction on vaping may therefore alter the choice between two nicotine products with markedly different toxicological profiles.

For a never-smoker, the appropriate precautionary message is straightforward: avoiding nicotine and inhaled aerosol avoids the associated risks. For an established smoker, the calculation is different. Continued exposure to combustion carries a well-characterised and substantial danger. A precautionary policy that obscures this distinction may discourage movement away from the more harmful product.

Relative risk does not remove the need for product standards. A product can be less harmful than smoking and still be unnecessarily hazardous, poorly manufactured or misleadingly promoted. The correct regulatory objective is to reduce avoidable risk within the non-combustible category without destroying its capacity to displace combustion.

Proportionality should therefore operate at several levels. The severity of the restriction should reflect the credibility and magnitude of the risk. The evidence required should correspond to the type of claim or exposure. Enforcement should focus on products and conduct that create the greatest harm. Policy should distinguish among children, never-users, smokers and former smokers rather than treating them as one population.

A proportionate precautionary measure might require enhanced warnings, ingredient disclosure or post-market monitoring where evidence is incomplete but concern is moderate. Stronger measures may be justified where there is evidence of acute toxicity, widespread mislabelling, deliberate youth targeting or uncontrollable environmental harm. Prohibition should normally require a stronger case because it removes lawful access and is more likely to create substitution and illegal-market effects.

Enforceability is part of this assessment. A precautionary rule that lawful businesses follow but illegal suppliers ignore may increase rather than reduce risk. Compliant products may disappear while untested alternatives remain available. Regulators must therefore assess inspection capacity, border control, online enforcement and retailer behaviour before adopting highly restrictive measures.

The principle should also distinguish temporary controls from permanent settlement. Where evidence is genuinely immature, an interim restriction, enhanced surveillance or controlled market approach may be more defensible than an irreversible ban. Temporary measures preserve the capacity to respond as knowledge develops.

Public communication requires the same discipline. Precautionary warnings should be clear about what is known and unknown. Statements that a product is "not safe" may be technically correct but insufficiently informative where the relevant comparison is smoking. Statements that it is "safer" may also mislead if consumers interpret them as meaning harmless.

The more useful language distinguishes absolute from relative risk. Vaping exposes users to nicotine and aerosol constituents and should not be promoted to non-users. For adults who would otherwise continue smoking, complete substitution is likely to reduce exposure to many combustion-related toxicants. Uncertainty remains concerning long-term use, product variation and population effects.

This form of communication is less dramatic than a simple warning, but it supports informed decision-making. Precaution should not require the public to remain ignorant of established differences between products.

The strongest application of the precautionary principle is structured, evidence-led and reversible. It begins with a plausible risk rather than a speculative fear. It considers exposure and not merely hazard. It compares alternative interventions, including inaction. It selects a measure proportionate to the concern, monitors its consequences and changes course where the evidence requires it.

The weakest application begins with a preferred restriction and uses uncertainty to protect it from challenge. Because no one can prove that long-term harm will never occur, almost any intervention can be defended indefinitely. This converts precaution into a political shield rather than a method of risk management.

Modern nicotine policy needs precaution because products, markets and patterns of use continue to change. It also needs restraint because the more harmful combustible product remains widely available. The principle should protect children, non-users and consumers from poorly controlled innovation while preserving realistic routes away from smoking.

Applied properly, precaution creates a controlled space in which evidence can develop. Applied asymmetrically, it treats every uncertainty associated with innovation as a reason for restriction while ignoring the known harms preserved by that restriction.

Lessons From the First Generation of Regulation

The first generation of vaping regulation established something that had previously been absent: a formal legal identity for nicotine-containing electronic cigarettes, a route through which products could enter the market, a set of minimum technical requirements and a chain of responsibility linking manufacturers, importers, regulators and enforcement authorities. Before that structure existed, the market had expanded through a mixture of general consumer law, chemical controls, electrical standards and inconsistent national interpretation. The revised Tobacco Products Directive and its national implementation brought greater order to that uncertainty. Products became identifiable, producers became accountable, ingredient and emissions information had to be submitted, packaging requirements became enforceable and regulators acquired a clearer basis for intervention. These were substantial achievements. The difficulty is that the framework was designed around an early market and then expected to govern a succession of technologies, commercial models and political pressures that its architects could not fully anticipate.

The most important lesson is that regulation does not merely control a market after it has formed. It changes the direction in which that market develops. The European limits on nicotine concentration, tank capacity and refill-container volume did not simply remove products that fell outside those boundaries. They encouraged manufacturers to redesign devices, alter formulations, improve aerosol efficiency and develop product formats capable of delivering an acceptable experience within the law. Notification requirements changed the timing and cost of product development. Advertising restrictions shifted competition towards packaging, retail presence, branding and product design. The rules became part of the engineering specification. This is unavoidable, but it means that every regulatory requirement should be assessed not only for its immediate protective effect but for the commercial behaviour it is likely to create.

Fixed numerical limits provided clarity during the first phase. A maximum nicotine concentration, tank volume or refill-container size could be understood by manufacturers, checked by laboratories and enforced by authorities. Such limits were administratively attractive because they converted a complex product into a small number of measurable conditions. Their weakness was that they often stood in for variables they did not fully represent. Nicotine exposure is not determined by liquid concentration alone. It depends on aerosol generation, device power, formulation chemistry, puffing behaviour and frequency of use. Liquid capacity does not by itself determine consumption, dependence or toxicological risk. A product can comply with every prescribed volume and concentration limit while still performing poorly, delivering nicotine inconsistently or containing ingredients that deserve closer assessment. The first generation demonstrated that simple limits are useful boundaries, but poor substitutes for a complete understanding of exposure.

The notification model revealed a similar distinction between administrative compliance and scientific evaluation. Requiring producers to submit formulation details, emissions information, toxicological data and manufacturing descriptions brought a level of discipline that had not existed across much of the early market. It encouraged ingredient identification, supplier control, analytical testing and maintenance of technical records. It also created large databases that allowed authorities to identify products and responsible economic operators. Yet notification was never equivalent to product authorisation. The presence of a product on a regulatory list could be mistaken by retailers and consumers for confirmation that it had been individually approved, when in reality the producer retained primary responsibility for the accuracy of the submission and the continuing compliance of the product. The lesson is not that notification failed, but that its meaning must remain precise. A system can record thousands of products without independently validating every formulation, analytical method or toxicological conclusion.

The quality of submitted data became as important as the existence of the data. Structured reporting systems can require every field to be completed, but they cannot ensure that an ingredient has been identified correctly, that a proprietary flavour mixture has been characterised adequately or that an emissions test represents normal product operation. Different laboratories may use different puffing regimes, conditioning procedures, analytical methods and reporting conventions. Two datasets can therefore appear complete while remaining difficult to compare. The first regulatory architecture placed considerable emphasis on information collection, but less emphasis on ensuring that the information could support consistent scientific decisions. A mature system requires common terminology, validated methods, reliable chemical identifiers, exposure-relevant testing and explicit criteria for interpreting results. Data quantity is not regulatory competence.

The early framework also showed that product regulation cannot be separated from manufacturing control. A dossier describes a product at a particular point in time. The consumer receives a manufactured batch produced through a supply chain that may change. Ingredients can be substituted, flavour suppliers altered, coils modified, packaging redesigned and production moved between sites. Each change can affect composition, emissions, performance or compliance. Notification systems are weakened when they focus heavily on initial submission but only lightly on lifecycle management. Change control, supplier qualification, batch release, traceability, complaints, corrective action and recall capability determine whether the product sold six months later remains the product originally described. The first generation brought products into regulatory databases; the next stage must ensure that those records remain connected to the physical goods in the market.

The rapid evolution of the market exposed the limits of legislation tied too closely to one generation of technology. The European framework was developed when cigalike products, refillable tanks and comparatively simple e-liquids dominated discussion. It later had to accommodate nicotine salts, compact pod systems, disposable devices, large claimed puff counts, rechargeable hybrids and products constructed deliberately around narrow readings of refillability or capacity. The problem was not simply that manufacturers innovated quickly. Product developers naturally respond to consumer demand and legal constraints. The problem was that legislation changed far more slowly than the technology it governed. By the time one product configuration had been understood, another had become commercially dominant. The resulting gap encouraged repeated cycles of reinterpretation, enforcement guidance and political intervention.

This experience argues for legislation that defines public health outcomes and core responsibilities clearly while leaving sufficient technical flexibility for standards to evolve. Rules should be specific enough to enforce but not so dependent on a particular construction that minor redesign defeats their purpose. A requirement centred on demonstrable refillability, replaceability, emissions performance or traceability may survive longer than one based entirely on the visible form of a device. Technical requirements should be capable of revision through transparent secondary processes without reopening the whole legislative framework each time the market changes. Adaptability must not mean allowing regulators to rewrite obligations without scrutiny; it means recognising that static product law is poorly suited to rapidly changing technology.

The growth of single-use products exposed this weakness more clearly than any earlier development. These devices combined low purchase cost, convenience and consumer appeal with environmental waste, embedded batteries, rapid brand turnover and widespread concerns about youth use. Their rise demonstrated that a product could comply formally with the core vaping framework while generating problems not fully addressed by that framework. Environmental regulation, waste policy, retail enforcement and youth protection became inseparable from nicotine-product control. The United Kingdom responded by prohibiting the sale and supply of single-use vapes from 1 June 2025, including both nicotine-containing and nicotine-free products. The measure moved beyond the original tobacco-related notification structure and treated product design and disposability as regulatory concerns in their own right.

The single-use ban also illustrates the importance of precise definitions and post-legislative observation. Once a prohibited product category is defined, manufacturers may redesign devices so that they are nominally rechargeable or refillable while preserving much of the commercial model that caused concern. A removable or replaceable component may satisfy the letter of the definition without ensuring meaningful reuse. The rule can therefore redirect product design without necessarily resolving waste, youth appeal or market turnover. This does not prove that the ban was misguided. It shows that regulation must be evaluated through outcomes rather than announcements. Whether waste falls, youth access declines, illicit sales contract and consumers move to genuinely reusable products will determine the measure's success.

Enforcement emerged as the decisive weakness of the first-generation system. Lawful manufacturers were required to manage submissions, testing, packaging, warnings, capacities and product records. Those willing to ignore the rules could sell oversized, unnotified, counterfeit or incorrectly labelled products, often at a lower cost and with faster market entry. The more detailed the compliance obligations became, the greater the potential advantage enjoyed by businesses that avoided them. Regulation intended to improve market quality could therefore create an asymmetry in which responsible companies carried the cost while illegal suppliers competed through non-compliance.

A rule has limited public health value when authorities cannot detect breaches, identify the responsible operator or impose consequences quickly enough to alter behaviour. Notification databases support enforcement, but they do not inspect shops, test products or stop undeclared imports. Local Trading Standards teams, border authorities, laboratories, online platforms and national regulators all hold part of the enforcement chain. Fragmented responsibility can leave gaps between product registration, retail inspection, customs control and prosecution. The first generation demonstrated that legislation without sustained enforcement funding can become a compliance system for the compliant rather than a control system for the market.

This problem becomes more serious as restrictions increase. Flavour controls, advertising prohibitions, packaging rules, duties and retail licensing may each be defensible in isolation, but together they increase the value of illegal supply. Consumers who cannot find a preferred product lawfully may not stop using nicotine; some will switch products, some will return to smoking and some will buy through informal channels. The likely response varies by population, price and availability, but it cannot be ignored. Regulatory design must include the economics of evasion. When the price, convenience or product range available outside the lawful system becomes substantially more attractive, enforcement becomes part of the health intervention rather than an administrative afterthought.

The United States provides a more extreme demonstration of this principle. Its premarket pathway requires new tobacco products to receive a written FDA marketing order before lawful marketing, with applicants expected to show that authorisation would be appropriate for the protection of public health. The system creates a far more demanding evidential threshold than European notification, but the existence of a rigorous authorisation process has not by itself eliminated unauthorised products from the market. The lesson is not that premarket review lacks value. It is that the strength of a legal gateway and the effectiveness of market control are separate variables. An exacting pathway can coexist with widespread unauthorised trade if inspection, border action, retailer compliance and litigation do not keep pace.

Market access requirements also determine who is capable of remaining in the industry. The first generation of European regulation imposed meaningful but generally manageable notification costs. More demanding authorisation systems require extensive chemistry, toxicology, behavioural evidence, manufacturing documentation and legal support. These requirements may improve evidential quality, but they also favour companies with substantial capital and established regulatory departments. Smaller firms can disappear even where their products are competent, not because they fail a scientific test but because they cannot finance the process.

Regulatory burden therefore has a structural public health effect. Market consolidation may improve consistency and accountability where larger firms possess stronger quality systems. It may also reduce competition, narrow product choice and increase the influence of multinational tobacco companies. Independent manufacturers played a major role in the development of early vaping technology, while larger corporations brought manufacturing scale and regulatory resources. A competent framework should not preserve weak operators merely because they are small, but neither should cost become an unstated substitute for scientific assessment. Requirements should be demanding where risk justifies them and proportionate enough that technically capable businesses can comply.

The first generation also showed that product appeal is not peripheral to harm reduction. Early policy often treated flavour, design and sensory performance primarily as commercial characteristics requiring control. For adult smokers, however, these characteristics can determine whether a product replaces cigarettes successfully. Nicotine delivery must be sufficient, the aerosol must be tolerable, the device must be convenient and the experience must be acceptable over time. A lower-risk product that consumers abandon has little population benefit.

This creates an unavoidable tension with youth protection. The same simplicity, palatability and discreetness that make products usable for adults may increase their appeal to adolescents. Regulation cannot solve this conflict by pretending that consumer appeal is either entirely beneficial or entirely harmful. It must distinguish among audiences, marketing practices and product functions. Controls directed at child-oriented imagery, underage sales and irresponsible promotion can be more proportionate than measures that remove broad categories of products used by adults. Broader restrictions may still be justified, but their consequences for smoking substitution should form part of the decision rather than appearing as an afterthought.

The expansion of powers over flavours, packaging, advertising and displays in the United Kingdom shows how far policy has moved beyond the original notification framework. The Tobacco and Vapes Act 2026 created new restrictions and powers intended to protect younger people while maintaining access for adults using vaping products to stop smoking. That stated balance is important, but legislation cannot guarantee it merely by expressing both aims. The detailed rules made under those powers will determine whether the system targets youth exposure precisely or weakens lawful adult access more generally.

The first generation also underestimated the importance of risk communication. Regulations required nicotine warnings and restricted claims, but they did not consistently ensure that consumers understood the relative risks of different products. A warning that a product contains nicotine and is addictive is accurate. It does not explain how the toxicological profile differs from cigarette smoke. Conversely, commercial claims that a product is clean, safe or healthy can minimise genuine uncertainty and dependence.

This gap allowed public understanding to become shaped by polarised messages. Some smokers concluded that vaping was as harmful as smoking, while some users treated it as harmless. Both positions impair informed choice. A mature regulatory system should communicate that non-use remains the lowest-risk option, that vaping is not risk-free and that complete substitution is materially different from continuing to inhale tobacco smoke. Relative risk is not promotional language when it is expressed accurately; it is information necessary to understand the purpose of harm reduction.

The relationship between medicinal and consumer pathways offered another lesson. The United Kingdom preserved the possibility that an electronic cigarette could obtain a medicines authorisation while allowing a broader consumer market under tobacco-related regulation. This recognised that the same general technology could serve different purposes. A medicinal product could make therapeutic claims and enter healthcare pathways, while consumer products could evolve more rapidly and provide greater variety. In practice, the medicinal route remained difficult and commercially unattractive for most manufacturers because pharmaceutical development demands stable specifications, validated performance and substantial evidence.

The limited use of that route shows that regulatory classification affects commercial viability. A theoretically available pathway is not meaningful if its costs, timescales and permitted product formats make it incompatible with the market it is intended to serve. Medicines regulation may be appropriate for products seeking clinical claims and formal healthcare use. It cannot be assumed that it can replace the consumer market without reducing diversity, access and speed of innovation. The first generation's dual structure remains valuable because it recognises more than one legitimate route, but the boundary between them must be clear enough to prevent unsubstantiated therapeutic promotion.

International divergence became another defining feature. The European Union adopted notification and fixed product limits. The United States developed a population-based premarket authorisation system. Australia pursued highly controlled access, while New Zealand adopted a more explicit harm-reduction orientation. Some countries prohibited sales entirely. Others regulated electronic cigarettes as tobacco products, consumer products or medicines. This diversity provided natural experiments, but it also created fragmented supply chains, inconsistent consumer protection and strong incentives for cross-border trade.

No single jurisdiction has yet produced a model that resolves product quality, youth protection, adult access, innovation and enforcement simultaneously. Restrictive systems can limit lawful availability while illegal markets persist. Permissive systems can accelerate switching while struggling with youth uptake and product proliferation. Notification systems can support variety while collecting more data than regulators can evaluate. Authorisation systems can demand strong evidence while concentrating the market. The lesson is not that all models are equally effective, but that every model contains trade-offs that should be assessed honestly.

Taxation has now become part of that wider regulatory settlement. The United Kingdom's Vaping Products Duty is due to take effect on 1 October 2026 and will apply to vaping liquids produced in or imported into the country, alongside a duty-stamp system intended to support control of the taxed market. This marks a significant transition. Vaping is no longer regulated only through product standards, notification and retail restrictions; it is becoming an excisable category with new manufacturing, importation, warehousing and traceability obligations.

Duty can generate revenue, support enforcement and reduce the price advantage that may encourage youth experimentation. It can also alter the relationship between vaping and cigarettes. If taxation narrows the cost difference too far, smokers may have less financial incentive to switch, while illegal products become more profitable. A flat charge on liquid is administratively simpler than a system based on nicotine concentration or toxicological risk, but simplicity does not make it scientifically proportionate. The public health effect will depend on retail prices, cigarette taxation, compliance costs, illicit supply and consumer behaviour after implementation.

Fiscal regulation therefore reinforces the need to evaluate the whole system rather than each measure separately. A product may face notification fees, testing costs, packaging controls, advertising restrictions, flavour limitations, retail licensing and excise duty. The combined burden may differ substantially from the effect predicted for any one rule. Impact assessments that consider measures independently can underestimate cumulative consequences. The next generation of regulation must assess the total route to market and determine whether lawful products remain competitive with both cigarettes and illegal alternatives.

The environmental dimension has also become impossible to separate from nicotine policy. Early vaping regulation concentrated on human exposure, nicotine, ingredients and packaging. The rise of disposable products brought batteries, electronic waste, plastics, resource use and fire risk into the discussion. These concerns are legitimate and may justify product redesign, producer responsibility, collection systems or prohibitions. They should, however, be addressed with the same causal precision expected in health regulation. A device should not be described as environmentally responsible merely because it is technically rechargeable if consumers discard it after brief use. Regulatory definitions need to reflect actual product life and likely behaviour.

The first generation further demonstrated that precaution works best when it is reversible and evidence-sensitive. Early action was justified because governments could not wait decades for complete epidemiology while an inhaled nicotine market expanded. The mistake was not acting under uncertainty. It was allowing provisional assumptions to harden into permanent structures without always reviewing whether the original reasoning remained valid. Rules introduced because data were absent should be reassessed when data become available. Restrictions created for one product generation should be reconsidered when technology changes. A precautionary measure should contain a route for revision, not merely a mechanism for tightening.

The European Commission's evaluation of the tobacco-control framework reflects this need for review. Its 2026 evaluation considered the effectiveness, efficiency and relevance of the Tobacco Products Directive, the Tobacco Advertising Directive and related measures across the Union. The significance of such evaluation lies not only in identifying new risks but in examining whether the existing machinery still performs its intended function. A framework can remain legally intact while becoming technically outdated, administratively burdensome or ineffective against the products actually being sold.

Evidence review must include unintended effects. Youth use, smoking prevalence, complete switching, dual use, illicit trade, retailer compliance, environmental waste and market concentration all belong within the assessment. A policy that reduces one undesirable outcome while worsening several others may still be justified, but the balance must be visible. Regulation becomes weak when it reports only the outcome that supported the original intervention.

The experiences of the first generation also show that consumers are not passive recipients of rules. They adapt. They change products, purchase across borders, mix liquids, retain older devices, seek stronger formulations or return to cigarettes. Retailers adapt by altering stock, branding, component combinations and routes of supply. Manufacturers adapt product design. Illegal traders adapt more quickly because they do not wait for formal approval. Regulation must therefore be built around behavioural response rather than assuming that removing one lawful option removes demand.

This does not mean that governments should avoid strong action for fear of evasion. It means that demand, substitution and enforcement must be part of the intervention from the beginning. Age restrictions require retailer licensing, test purchasing and meaningful penalties. Product bans require border control, marketplace cooperation and clear definitions. Duty requires stamps, registration, audit and action against untaxed goods. Flavour restrictions require an account of how flavours will be classified and how borderline products will be treated. Without that operational layer, legislation can become a declaration of intent rather than a functioning control.

A further lesson concerns institutional coordination. Vaping sits across health, medicines, consumer protection, chemicals, electrical safety, customs, taxation, advertising, environmental law and local enforcement. No single authority can manage every aspect, but fragmented responsibility can create duplication and gaps. The MHRA may hold notification information, Trading Standards may inspect retailers, HMRC may regulate duty, environmental authorities may enforce disposability rules and advertising regulators may examine promotion. Effective control depends on these bodies sharing information and working from compatible definitions.

The next regulatory architecture should treat this network as one system. A product identifier used for notification should connect to customs, duty, retail inspection and recall records. A change in formulation should be visible to the relevant authorities. A failed laboratory sample should be traceable to the importer, batch and retail chain. Digital product passports and authenticated identifiers may support this, but technology cannot compensate for unclear responsibility or weak enforcement.

The first generation also taught that regulation needs internal technical competence. Authorities cannot rely entirely on manufacturers, campaign groups or external laboratories to explain the market. Without sufficient expertise in aerosol science, toxicology, analytical chemistry, formulation, engineering and consumer behaviour, regulators become dependent on stakeholders whose evidence may be selective. Technical capacity allows authorities to challenge poor submissions, interpret laboratory uncertainty and distinguish genuine safety problems from politically convenient claims.

This competence should extend to the drafting of law. Product definitions written without engineering knowledge invite circumvention. Ingredient restrictions written without chemical precision create ambiguity. Emissions requirements written without method standards generate incomparable data. Retail controls written without enforcement input become difficult to prove. The quality of regulation is determined partly by the quality of the people translating policy objectives into technical obligations.

The central lesson is that vaping regulation cannot be judged by the number of restrictions imposed. A strong system is not necessarily the one with the longest legislation, the highest fees or the most extensive submission portal. Its performance lies in whether it reduces avoidable exposure, protects children, enables adults to move away from smoking, maintains product quality, suppresses illegal supply and adapts when evidence changes.

The first generation succeeded in bringing an uncontrolled market within formal public authority. It established minimum expectations and created the language through which modern nicotine products could be regulated. It also revealed the difference between writing rules and controlling outcomes. Administrative compliance could expand while illegal trade remained visible. Data collection could increase without producing consistent scientific assessment. Product limits could be enforced while exposure remained more complex than the limits implied. Restrictions could protect one population while affecting another.

The next generation must retain what worked: identifiable producers, structured product information, ingredient control, manufacturing responsibility, child protection, warnings, vigilance and enforcement powers. It must improve what did not: scientific comparability, lifecycle control, regulatory agility, cross-agency coordination, market surveillance and communication of relative risk. It must also recognise the pressures that now define the market rather than the market that existed when Article 20 was drafted. Those pressures include duties, duty stamps, flavour controls, advertising restrictions, retail licensing, environmental requirements, single-use bans, digital commerce, counterfeit supply and increasingly sophisticated products designed around legal boundaries.

Modern regulation will remain a compromise because the policy objectives are not identical. Preventing youth initiation, preserving adult access, reducing smoking, limiting environmental waste, collecting revenue and controlling illicit trade can point towards different interventions. The quality of the system will depend on whether those conflicts are acknowledged and managed rather than hidden behind general claims of public health protection.

The first generation of regulation was the necessary beginning. It demonstrated that electronic cigarettes could not remain outside formal oversight and that non-combustible nicotine products required rules of their own. Its enduring lesson is that regulation must be judged not by how forcefully it responds to a new product, but by whether it produces a safer and more coherent market than the one it replaced.

CHAPTER 2

Building a Compliant Product

A compliant vaping product is not created at the point of notification, testing or market entry, but through a chain of decisions that begins long before the final formulation is filled, the device is assembled or the packaging is printed. Compliance is the accumulated result of product design, ingredient selection, supplier control, toxicological assessment, engineering judgement, manufacturing discipline, documentation, labelling, testing, submission and post-market responsibility. When these elements are treated as separate administrative tasks, weaknesses appear between them. A formulation may be assessed without sufficient knowledge of the device in which it will be used. A device may be tested under conditions that do not reflect the intended liquid. Packaging may be prepared before the legal product classification has been confirmed. A notification may be completed accurately at the time of submission but become unreliable after an undocumented change in supplier, coil, flavour or manufacturing site. Building a compliant product therefore requires the product itself and the regulatory record describing it to develop together.

The first generation of vaping businesses often approached compliance after product development had already been completed. A device or liquid was created for the market, its commercial potential assessed and its regulatory documentation assembled later. This sequence reflected the speed and informality of the early industry, but it created avoidable problems. Ingredients selected for flavour or sensory performance could prove difficult to justify toxicologically. Components sourced on price or availability could lack adequate specifications. Product variants could multiply faster than technical files could be maintained. Packaging claims might cross the boundary into medicinal presentation or conflict with statutory warning requirements. By the time these issues were identified, reformulation, redesign or withdrawal could be more expensive than addressing them during development.

A more reliable approach begins by defining the intended product clearly. The manufacturer must know what is being placed on the market, who is responsible for it, where it will be sold, how it will be used and which regulatory pathway applies. These questions appear basic, yet they determine almost every later obligation. A nicotine-containing refill liquid, a prefilled pod, a rechargeable device, a nicotine-free liquid and a product presented for therapeutic use do not necessarily follow the same route. Jurisdiction also matters. A product intended for Great Britain may face different administrative requirements from one intended for Northern Ireland, the European Union, the United States or another international market. A compliant product is therefore not an abstract object. It is a defined product placed into a defined legal system by a defined responsible operator.

This definition must extend beyond brand name and flavour description. Regulators require a stable technical identity. The formulation, nicotine concentration, container volume, device architecture, coil resistance, power range, reservoir capacity, materials, packaging configuration and intended method of use all contribute to that identity. Where the product is made from several interacting parts, the relationship between those parts must be understood. A liquid may produce acceptable emissions in one device and undesirable thermal degradation in another. A coil may perform consistently with one formulation but flood, overheat or degrade when used with another viscosity or power setting. Compliance cannot be built around isolated components where consumer exposure arises from the complete system.

The intended consumer also influences product design. A product developed for adult smokers moving away from cigarettes may need to provide sufficient nicotine delivery, ease of use and sensory acceptability to support substitution. Those same features may attract scrutiny where they are associated with youth appeal, concealability or rapid initiation. Compliance therefore includes decisions about presentation, flavour naming, colours, imagery, device form and retail communication as well as chemistry and engineering. A technically lawful product can still create regulatory risk if its presentation appears misleading, irresponsible or directed towards children.

Ingredient selection is one of the earliest points at which compliance can either be strengthened or compromised. Every substance included in a formulation should have a defined function, an established specification and a justification appropriate to inhalation use. The fact that an ingredient is widely used in food, cosmetics or fragrances does not establish that it is suitable for aerosolisation and inhalation. Oral safety and respiratory safety are not interchangeable. Heating may alter chemical structure, create degradation products or change the concentration delivered to the user. The relevant question is therefore not simply whether an ingredient has been used before, but whether its identity, purity, function, concentration, thermal behaviour and likely exposure can be defended within the intended product.

Supplier documentation forms the foundation of this assessment. Certificates of analysis, safety data sheets, compositional declarations, allergen information, impurity limits and manufacturing specifications must be accurate, current and product-specific. Trade names and generic flavour descriptions are insufficient where the regulatory submission requires individual chemical identities and quantities. Proprietary mixtures create particular difficulty because flavour houses may regard their formulations as confidential. Commercial confidentiality can be managed through controlled disclosure, but it cannot remove the producer's responsibility to understand what is present in the product. A manufacturer that cannot identify its ingredients cannot evaluate them adequately, control batch consistency or respond effectively if a substance later becomes restricted.

Nicotine requires equally disciplined control. Its identity, source, assay, purity, impurity profile, storage conditions and stability must be documented. Small errors in nicotine concentration can become significant when repeated across large production batches. The formulation process must therefore account for raw-material strength, density, weighing or volumetric accuracy, mixing efficiency and analytical verification. Where nicotine salts are used, the acid, stoichiometry, resulting pH and sensory consequences become part of the product definition. A label declaration is not a substitute for evidence that the manufactured liquid consistently contains the stated concentration within an appropriate tolerance.

The carrier system also requires control. Propylene glycol, glycerol, water and other formulation components influence viscosity, aerosol formation, flavour release, coil wetting and thermal behaviour. Their ratios may affect leakage, dry-puff potential, aerosol mass and the generation of degradation products. A change made for commercial reasons, such as improving vapour density or flavour intensity, may alter exposure and device performance. Formulation development must therefore be linked to performance testing rather than treated as a matter of blending ingredients to achieve a preferred sensory profile.

Device design introduces another layer of regulatory responsibility. Batteries, circuitry, heating elements, reservoirs, seals, plastics, metals and adhesives must function together under foreseeable conditions of use. Electrical safety, charging behaviour, overheating protection, short-circuit protection and material compatibility are not separate from product compliance. A device that delivers a controlled aerosol under ideal laboratory conditions may behave differently when the coil ages, the liquid level falls, airflow is obstructed or the consumer uses an incompatible charger. Product development must consider normal use, reasonably foreseeable misuse and the consequences of component failure.

Reservoir capacity, refillability, leak resistance and child protection are particularly visible legal requirements, but compliance cannot be reduced to dimensions and closures. A refill mechanism may satisfy the literal wording of a technical standard while remaining difficult to use cleanly. A child-resistant cap may pass a formal test yet fail after repeated opening. A reservoir may remain within the permitted capacity while the wider product architecture allows circumvention. The stronger approach is to design for the purpose of the rule rather than merely its minimum wording.

Materials selection requires similar attention. Metals exposed to liquid or aerosol may contribute trace elements through corrosion, heating or manufacturing residues. Elastomers and plastics may swell, crack or release substances when exposed to particular flavour systems. Wicks and coils can retain processing oils or contaminants if manufacturing controls are poor. These risks are rarely apparent from visual inspection alone. Specifications, supplier qualification, compatibility testing and appropriate analytical review are needed to ensure that the complete device remains stable throughout its intended shelf life and use period.

Testing is often treated as the moment at which compliance is demonstrated, but it is more useful when it guides development. Analytical work should identify weaknesses early enough for the product to be improved. Emissions testing can reveal elevated carbonyls, metals, volatile compounds or inconsistent nicotine delivery. Physical testing can identify leakage, breakage, battery failure or variation between units. Stability studies can show changes in nicotine concentration, colour, flavour, pH or impurity profile over time. Packaging trials can identify interaction between the formulation and the container. Used only at the end of development, testing may confirm that a product has failed after commercial decisions have already been made.

The quality of the test depends on the relevance of the method. Vaping products do not operate under one universal condition. Device power, puff duration, interval, airflow, coil age and liquid composition all affect the result. A test regime must therefore be described clearly and justified in relation to the product. Severe conditions may be useful for identifying failure points, but they should not be presented as representative of ordinary exposure without explanation. Mild conditions may underestimate reasonably foreseeable use. A compliant technical file should distinguish between routine operating conditions, stress testing and misuse assessment rather than combining them into one undifferentiated dataset.

Analytical results also require interpretation. Detecting a substance does not by itself establish that the product presents an unacceptable risk, just as failing to detect a short list of compounds does not prove that the product is safe. Concentration, exposure, toxicological significance, method sensitivity and comparison with relevant benchmarks all matter. The purpose of testing is not to produce reassuring numbers or to satisfy a checklist, but to determine whether the product contains avoidable hazards, whether performance is consistent and whether identified exposures can be justified.

Manufacturing converts the designed product into the product that reaches the consumer. This stage is where theoretical compliance can be lost through variation. Raw materials may arrive outside specification. Operators may use incorrect quantities. Mixing times may be shortened. Components may be substituted. Filling equipment may drift. Labels may be applied to the wrong strength. Batches may be released without adequate review. A compliant formulation produced through an uncontrolled process is not a compliant product in any reliable sense.

Quality management therefore provides the structure through which compliance is maintained. Approved specifications, controlled procedures, trained personnel, calibrated equipment, batch records, line clearance, in-process checks, finished-product testing and documented release decisions are not bureaucratic additions to manufacturing. They are the evidence that the product sold corresponds to the product assessed and notified. Where production is outsourced, the legal responsibility does not disappear. The producer or importer must still understand the process, qualify the manufacturer, define acceptance criteria and retain access to the records needed to investigate problems.

Change control is one of the most important parts of this system. Products evolve continuously. A supplier changes an ingredient source, a flavour is reformulated, a coil is replaced, a battery specification changes or a filling site is moved. Each change must be assessed for its effect on composition, emissions, performance, stability, labelling and regulatory status. Some changes may be minor and remain within the existing product definition. Others may create a substantially modified product requiring a new or amended notification. The decision should be documented rather than left to commercial convenience.

Packaging and labelling complete the physical product but also communicate its legal identity. Mandatory warnings, ingredient information, nicotine content, batch details, storage instructions, contact information and instructions for use must be accurate and legible. Claims must remain within the permitted regulatory category. A consumer vaping product should not be presented in a manner that implies medicinal authorisation, guaranteed cessation or absence of risk unless the relevant evidential and legal requirements have been met. At the same time, warnings should not be so disconnected from relative risk that they prevent smokers from understanding why non-combustible products differ from cigarettes.

Presentation also affects enforcement and traceability. Clear product identifiers, batch numbers, manufacturer or importer details and tamper evidence help distinguish lawful goods from counterfeit or altered products. Weak identification makes recalls difficult and allows non-compliant products to borrow the appearance of legitimate brands. Packaging should therefore serve not only marketing and statutory warning functions but also supply-chain control.

The regulatory submission brings together the information generated throughout development. It should describe the product that actually exists, not an idealised specification assembled for administrative purposes. Ingredient quantities, component details, emissions data, toxicological reasoning, manufacturing descriptions and declarations must be internally consistent. The device listed in one section should be the device used for testing. The formulation notified should match the formulation manufactured. The nicotine concentration on the label should correspond to the analytical specification. Inconsistency between these elements is often a stronger indication of weak compliance than any single missing field.

Submission does not transfer responsibility to the regulator. A notified product remains the responsibility of the manufacturer or importer. Publication in a database does not convert the product into an approved medicine or remove the need for continuing quality control. The technical file must remain current, and the producer must be able to provide supporting evidence when requested. Regulators may review the information, identify concerns and take enforcement action, but they do not manufacture the product or maintain its specification.

Market entry begins a new stage rather than ending the compliance process. Complaints, adverse effects, leakage reports, battery incidents, labelling errors and unexpected patterns of use must be collected and assessed. Individual reports may not establish causation, but repeated signals can reveal problems not detected during development. Producers need systems for identifying affected batches, investigating root causes, implementing corrective action and communicating with regulators where necessary.

Corrective action may involve changes to instructions, packaging, manufacturing control or formulation. More serious problems may require withdrawal or recall. A company that cannot trace products through the supply chain cannot act effectively when a defect is found. Distribution records, batch identification and customer communication procedures are therefore part of the original compliance architecture, not emergency measures invented after a problem appears.

Compliance also depends on the behaviour of importers, distributors and retailers. A manufacturer may produce a lawful product, but the supply chain can introduce risk through incorrect storage, relabelling, counterfeit substitution or sale into an unintended jurisdiction. Retailers may assume that the presence of a regulatory identifier proves complete conformity. Distributors may alter packaging or combine components in ways not covered by the original submission. Contracts, training, supply-chain audits and clear responsibilities are needed to preserve the product's regulatory identity after it leaves the factory.

Online marketplaces and cross-border trade make this more difficult. Products can be offered in markets for which they were never notified, accompanied by translated packaging that omits mandatory information or sold through traders with no effective domestic presence. A compliant producer must understand where its products are distributed and take reasonable steps to prevent diversion. Regulatory responsibility cannot be managed solely at the point of manufacture where the commercial route to the consumer is uncontrolled.

The economic pressure to accelerate launch, reduce testing or multiply product variants will remain present throughout development. Compliance is strongest where the business model recognises regulatory work as part of product creation rather than an external cost imposed after commercial decisions. A technically disciplined company can still innovate quickly, but it does so within controlled specifications, justified ingredients and documented change. A weak company treats compliance as a file assembled to support sales.

Building a compliant product therefore requires integration. Legal classification determines the route to market. Formulation science determines composition and stability. Toxicology determines whether ingredients and emissions can be justified. Engineering determines how the product behaves in use.

Manufacturing determines whether the specification is reproduced. Quality systems preserve that specification over time. Labelling communicates the product accurately. Notification makes the product visible to regulators. Vigilance connects real-world experience back to design and control.

When these functions operate separately, the technical file becomes disconnected from the product and compliance becomes fragile. When they are integrated, the regulatory record becomes a faithful account of the product's composition, manufacture, performance and responsibility. That is the foundation on which lawful market access, consumer confidence and effective enforcement depend.

Figure 2.1 Building a Compliant Product: Concept-to-Compliance Lifecycle

Compliance starts at concept, not submission.

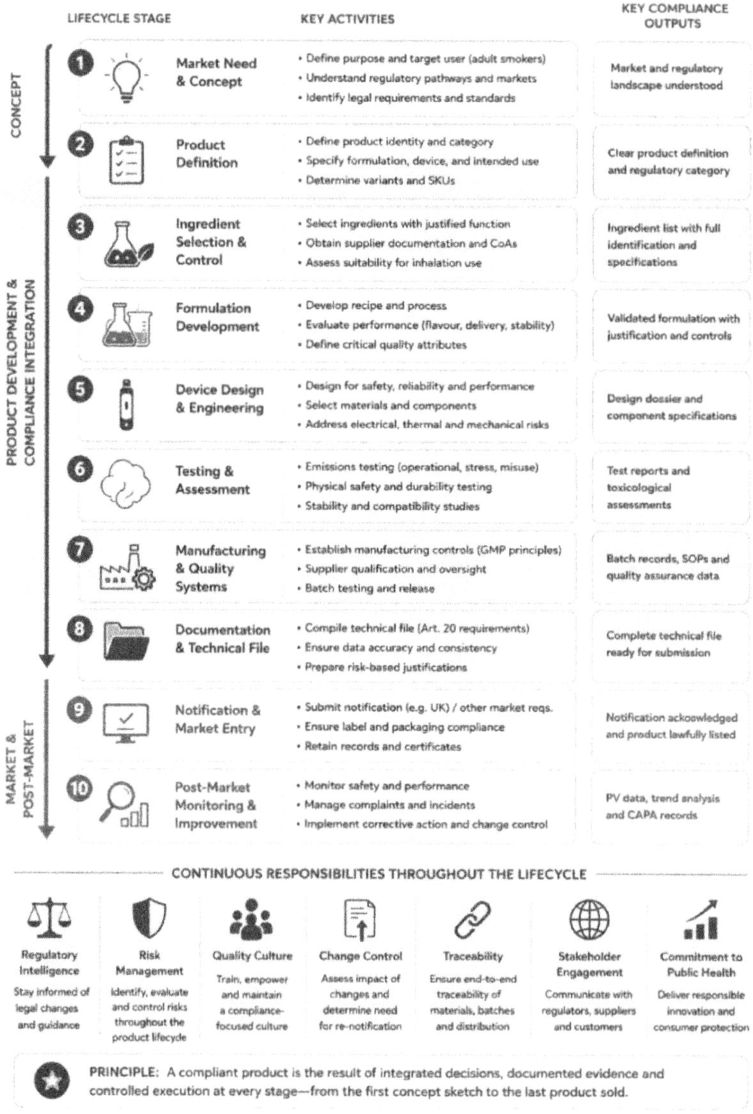

Figure 2.1. Building a Compliant Product: Concept-to-Compliance Lifecycle.

The concept-to-compliance lifecycle shows how regulatory responsibility begins at the earliest stage of product planning and continues through development, manufacture, notification and post-market control. Each stage produces a defined compliance output, including a clear product category, controlled ingredient list, validated formulation, design dossier, test evidence, manufacturing records, technical documentation and market-entry record. Regulatory intelligence, risk management, quality culture, change control, traceability, stakeholder engagement and public health responsibility continue across the whole lifecycle. The figure emphasises that a compliant product is the result of integrated decisions and controlled execution from the first product concept to the final unit supplied.

The discussions that follow examine the principal stages of that process: defining the product and its regulatory category; selecting and controlling ingredients; assessing formulations and emissions; designing compliant hardware; establishing manufacturing and quality systems; preparing technical documentation; managing notifications and substantial modifications; constructing lawful packaging and claims; maintaining vigilance and corrective action; and ensuring that compliance survives beyond launch. Together, these elements show that a compliant product is not created by one test, one submission or one certificate, but by a controlled system capable of demonstrating that the product placed on the market remains the product that was designed, assessed and declared.

Regulatory Strategy from Concept

Regulatory strategy should begin at the moment a product idea is first defined, because the earliest commercial and technical decisions determine which legal pathway will apply, what evidence will be required and whether the product can be placed on the intended market without costly redesign. A vaping product is not regulated only through its final formulation or finished device. Its classification can depend on nicotine content, intended use, presentation, claims, packaging, route of supply, jurisdiction and the relationship between the liquid and the hardware. A concept that appears commercially attractive may become difficult to defend if those factors are considered only after development has progressed. The stronger approach is to treat regulatory strategy as part of product architecture, ensuring that the concept is designed within an identified legal route rather than forced into one at the end.

The first task is to define the product in terms that are precise enough to support both development and regulatory assessment. Broad descriptions such as refill liquid, pod system, disposable alternative or cessation product are not sufficient. The business must determine whether the product contains nicotine, whether it is open or closed, whether it is refillable or prefilled, whether it includes electrical components, whether it is intended for repeated use, whether it will be supplied with accessories and whether it is presented as a consumer product or as a product intended to treat nicotine dependence. Each answer changes the legal analysis. A nicotine-containing refill container may fall within one regulatory category, while a nicotine-free liquid, a rechargeable device, a medicinally presented inhalation product or a separately sold component may engage different obligations.

Intended purpose is particularly important because regulators classify products partly through what they are presented as doing. A consumer vaping product may be used by adults to stop smoking without being authorised as a medicine. Once the manufacturer makes explicit claims to treat addiction, relieve withdrawal or deliver a clinically proven cessation effect, the product may move towards medicines regulation. The technology may be similar, but the evidential standard changes substantially. A consumer-product route may require notification, technical documentation, ingredient disclosure and compliance with product limits, while a medicinal route requires formal demonstration of quality, safety and efficacy. Regulatory strategy must therefore control claims from the beginning. Marketing language, packaging, website content, training materials and sales presentations all contribute to intended purpose and cannot be separated from product classification.

Jurisdiction must be defined at the same stage. A product is not compliant in the abstract; it is compliant for a specified market under a specified legal framework. The requirements in Great Britain differ from those in the European Union, the United States and other international jurisdictions. Even where legislation shares common origins, submission systems, responsible-person requirements, fees, timelines, labelling, language and enforcement expectations may differ. A product developed for several markets may require one core design with controlled regional variants, or it may require materially different formulations, capacities, warnings or documentation. Failing to resolve this early can produce a product that fits one jurisdiction but requires substantial modification for another.

Market selection therefore becomes a regulatory decision as much as a commercial one. A company may wish to launch simultaneously across several countries, but the evidence package, administrative burden and lead time may make a staged strategy more realistic. The first market may be chosen because its legal pathway is clearer, its requirements are proportionate or its notification process provides a workable route to launch. Later markets can then be added using the existing technical file as a foundation, provided the product is reviewed against local requirements rather than assumed to be transferable automatically.

The responsible economic operator must also be identified from the outset. Regulators need to know which legal entity places the product on the market and accepts responsibility for its conformity. The manufacturer, importer, brand owner and distributor may be different organisations, but responsibility cannot remain ambiguous. Contracts should define who controls formulation, who owns the technical documentation, who submits notifications, who holds manufacturing records, who manages complaints and who can initiate corrective action. A commercial arrangement that leaves these functions divided without clear authority creates regulatory risk even where the physical product is technically sound.

This issue is especially important where manufacturing is outsourced. A brand owner may rely on a third-party factory for formulation, device assembly, filling or packaging. Outsourcing production does not outsource legal responsibility. The company placing the product on the market must still have access to specifications, batch records, test data, supplier information and change notifications. It must be able to investigate complaints and determine whether the product supplied matches the product described in the technical file. A regulatory strategy that depends entirely on a distant manufacturer's assurances is fragile because the brand owner may be unable to verify changes, challenge inconsistencies or respond effectively when authorities request evidence.

The intended user should be defined alongside the product and market. A vaping product aimed at adult smokers requires a different development rationale from one positioned as a general lifestyle product. The intended user influences nicotine delivery, ease of use, instructions, warnings, flavour presentation and the assessment of foreseeable misuse. It also influences the way the product should be presented commercially. A product intended to support substitution away from smoking may need sufficient sensory and functional performance to be credible, but it must not be packaged or promoted in a way that appears directed towards children or nicotine-naive consumers.

This distinction should be documented in the initial product brief. The brief should identify the target user, the behaviour the product is intended to replace or support, the expected method of use and the boundaries of the intended population. These definitions provide a basis for later decisions concerning formulation, device performance, packaging and risk communication. They also allow the manufacturer to test whether commercial proposals remain aligned with the original regulatory position. A change in branding, format or promotional strategy can alter the way the product is perceived even if the formulation remains unchanged.

Early regulatory strategy should also establish the legal and technical requirements that will shape design. These may include nicotine concentration limits, container capacities, refillability criteria, child-resistance, tamper evidence, leakage control, warning statements, ingredient restrictions, emissions reporting and notification periods. These are not matters to be checked only when the product is complete. They should become design inputs. A device that exceeds a permitted reservoir capacity, a refill bottle that cannot support the required closure or a packaging concept that cannot accommodate mandatory information is already defective from a regulatory perspective before testing begins.

The same applies to the formulation. Ingredient selection should be guided by the intended regulatory route and the evidence likely to be required. A flavour system containing poorly identified proprietary mixtures may be commercially attractive but difficult to assess or notify. A nicotine source with incomplete impurity data may create later analytical problems. A formulation that depends on a substance restricted in one target jurisdiction may undermine a multi-market strategy. Regulatory review at concept stage can prevent these decisions from becoming embedded in the product.

The initial regulatory assessment should therefore produce a set of design constraints rather than a general statement that the product must comply with applicable law. Those constraints should be specific enough to guide developers, suppliers and commercial teams. They may include maximum nicotine concentration, approved ingredient categories, prohibited substances, required container format, target shelf life, minimum documentation standards, intended device range and required evidence for market entry. Once defined, these constraints become part of the product specification and change-control system.

Evidence planning is another essential part of concept-stage strategy. Each regulatory requirement should be linked to the type of evidence needed to demonstrate compliance. Ingredient identity may require supplier specifications, certificates of analysis and compositional disclosure. Nicotine concentration may require validated analytical testing. Stability may require real-time or accelerated studies. Emissions may require product-specific analytical work under justified operating conditions. Child resistance, leak resistance and electrical safety may require physical or standards-based testing. Claims may require scientific support proportionate to their wording.

This evidence should be mapped before development begins because data generation affects time, cost and product design. A six-month or twelve-month stability programme cannot be created retrospectively shortly before launch. Emissions testing cannot be interpreted properly if the device, formulation or operating conditions are still changing. Supplier qualification cannot be completed if commercial sourcing remains unstable. The regulatory plan must therefore identify which decisions need to be fixed early and which can remain flexible until later stages.

The concept stage is also the correct point to identify critical quality attributes. These are the characteristics that must remain controlled for the product to perform as intended and remain compliant. They may include nicotine concentration, formulation ratio, pH, viscosity, liquid volume, coil resistance, reservoir capacity, battery output, aerosol mass, leakage performance and labelling accuracy. Critical attributes provide a link between development, manufacturing and release. Without them, product quality remains described in general terms and batch acceptance becomes difficult to justify.

The regulatory strategy should distinguish between the core product and its variants. Commercial teams often seek multiple flavours, strengths, colours and device formats. Each variation can affect the regulatory burden. A new flavour may require separate ingredient assessment, toxicological review and notification. A different coil or power setting may alter emissions. A new bottle size may change packaging and capacity compliance. A minor branding change may be administratively simple, while a change in formulation or device architecture may create a substantially modified product.

Variant planning should therefore be deliberate. The company should determine which elements can vary within a controlled family and which changes create a new regulatory identity. This reduces unnecessary proliferation and prevents technical files from becoming disconnected from the product range. A disciplined launch portfolio may be commercially narrower at first but easier to support with robust evidence and consistent manufacturing.

Timelines must also be built around regulatory lead times rather than only commercial launch dates. Notification systems may require submission several months before market entry. Authorities may request clarification. Packaging cannot be finalised until the product identity, formulation and warning requirements are stable. Manufacturing scale-up may reveal changes requiring further assessment. If the launch date is fixed before these dependencies are understood, regulatory work is forced into the final stages and shortcuts become more likely.

A realistic plan works backwards from the intended market date and identifies the final date by which formulation, device, packaging and testing must be locked. It includes time for data review, corrective action, resubmission and manufacturing preparation. It also recognises that delays are sometimes necessary where evidence is incomplete. A postponed launch is less damaging than placing a product on the market with a weak technical foundation and then managing enforcement, withdrawal or reputational consequences.

Commercial confidentiality should be addressed within the strategy. Product development often involves flavour houses, device manufacturers, testing laboratories and regulatory consultants, each holding part of the information needed for compliance. Confidentiality agreements can protect intellectual property, but they must not prevent the responsible operator from obtaining the data needed to assess and document the product. The company must know enough about proprietary mixtures, manufacturing processes and component materials to fulfil its legal obligations.

A supplier's statement that information is confidential is not a complete regulatory answer. Mechanisms may be needed for direct confidential disclosure to regulators, controlled access by toxicologists or contractual obligations to notify composition changes. The product cannot be managed responsibly where critical information remains permanently inaccessible to the entity placing it on the market.

Risk assessment should begin at concept stage and continue throughout development. Early assessment does not require complete data, but it should identify foreseeable hazards and uncertainty. These may include nicotine exposure, accidental ingestion, battery failure, thermal degradation, leakage, material incompatibility, incorrect use and youth appeal. The purpose is not to produce a final safety conclusion before the product exists, but to direct development towards the most important controls.

The risk register should evolve as evidence becomes available. A theoretical concern may be closed after testing, while an unexpected issue may require redesign. The regulatory strategy should define who reviews risks, who has authority to stop development and how decisions are documented. Without this structure, risk assessment can become a paper exercise completed after commercial commitment has already been made.

Claims strategy requires equal discipline. Product descriptions, comparative statements and public-health language should be reviewed before marketing concepts are finalised. Claims such as cleaner, safer, healthier or clinically proven may carry legal and evidential consequences. Even technically accurate statements can mislead if they omit context. A product may emit fewer selected toxicants than cigarettes under defined conditions, but that does not justify an unqualified claim of safety.

The regulatory strategy should therefore distinguish permitted factual statements from prohibited or higher-risk claims. It should define the evidence required for each statement and ensure consistency across packaging, websites, social media, retailer materials and training. Claims control is not the responsibility of marketing alone. It requires coordination between regulatory, scientific, legal and commercial functions.

The intended route to post-market control should also be planned before launch. The company needs systems for complaint intake, adverse-event review, incident escalation, batch tracing and corrective action. These systems depend on product identifiers, distribution records and contractual access to manufacturing information. They cannot be created effectively after the first serious complaint occurs.

Post-market planning should include thresholds for investigation, recall and regulatory notification. It should define who reviews reports, how causality is considered and how trends are identified. The regulatory strategy should also anticipate product review after launch, using complaints, returns, test results and market intelligence to determine whether changes are needed. This makes compliance an active lifecycle process rather than a static pre-market exercise.

Governance determines whether the strategy remains effective. Product development involves commercial, scientific, engineering, quality, regulatory and marketing teams, each with different priorities. Commercial teams may prioritise speed and differentiation. Engineers may prioritise performance. Formulators may prioritise sensory quality. Regulatory and quality teams must ensure that these decisions remain within the defined route to market. No single function can build a compliant product alone.

A formal product-development process should therefore include regulatory decision points. Concept approval should confirm classification, market and intended user. Development approval should confirm ingredient and design suitability. Design freeze should confirm that testing reflects the final product. Launch approval should confirm that documentation, notification, packaging and manufacturing controls are complete. These gates prevent the product from moving forward on commercial momentum alone.

The regulatory strategy should be documented in a living plan. It should record the product definition, jurisdictions, classification, legal basis, evidence requirements, responsible parties, submission route, key risks, critical milestones and post-market obligations. It should be revised when the product, market or law changes. A brief plan maintained actively is more valuable than a lengthy document written once and ignored.

Change control must protect the original strategy after development begins. A change in supplier, ingredient, device component, nicotine source, packaging or claim can alter the regulatory position. The change should be assessed before implementation to determine whether new testing, documentation or notification is required. Commercial urgency should not bypass this assessment.

The strongest regulatory strategies also consider future development. A product may begin with one strength or format, but the company may anticipate line extensions, new flavours or entry into additional markets. Designing the technical file, specifications and data systems with future expansion in mind can reduce later duplication. This does not mean overbuilding the initial product, but it does mean avoiding decisions that make every extension a complete redevelopment.

Regulatory intelligence supports this planning. Laws, guidance, enforcement priorities and technical expectations change. A product strategy based on current rules must include a process for monitoring developments that could affect future compliance. Proposed flavour restrictions, packaging controls, duties, environmental rules or changes to notification systems may alter the commercial viability of a concept before launch.

Intelligence should not be limited to formal legislation. Enforcement notices, regulator guidance, market seizures, standards development and policy consultations can indicate the direction of travel. Early awareness allows the company to adapt before a requirement becomes mandatory or a product becomes politically exposed. This is particularly important in nicotine regulation, where product categories and policy priorities evolve rapidly.

A concept may therefore be rejected for regulatory reasons even where it is technically feasible and commercially attractive. That is not a failure of innovation. It is evidence that regulatory strategy is functioning. Resources should be directed towards products that can be supported, manufactured consistently and maintained lawfully. Persisting with a concept that depends on uncertain classification, inaccessible supplier data or unsupported claims creates avoidable risk.

Regulatory strategy from concept is ultimately a method of controlling uncertainty. It does not eliminate legal change, scientific gaps or market risk. It ensures that these are identified early, assigned to responsible functions and addressed before the product becomes commercially fixed. It connects the intended user, product design, evidence plan, manufacturing system and market pathway into one controlled structure.

A compliant product begins with a concept that has been defined honestly and developed within known boundaries. Every later stage depends on that foundation. Ingredient assessment, stability, testing, technical documentation, notification and stewardship are more reliable when the regulatory route is already clear. Where strategy begins only at submission, compliance becomes a process of repairing earlier decisions. Where it begins at concept, compliance becomes part of the product itself.

Ingredient Selection

Ingredient selection is one of the earliest and most consequential stages in the development of a compliant vaping product because the final safety, stability, emissions profile and regulatory defensibility of the formulation all depend on the substances chosen at the outset. A product cannot be made compliant simply by testing it after development if its ingredients were selected without sufficient knowledge of identity, purity, function and inhalation relevance. The strongest approach is to require every ingredient to have a clear technological or sensory purpose, a defined specification and a documented justification for use at the intended concentration. Ingredients should not be included merely because they are commercially available, widely used in food or capable of improving flavour. Their suitability must be considered within the complete aerosol-generating system in which they will be heated, transferred and inhaled.

The distinction between oral and inhalation exposure is central to this assessment. Many flavouring substances have established histories of use in food, beverages, cosmetics or fragrances, but that history does not establish respiratory suitability. The lungs and gastrointestinal tract differ in structure, metabolism, protective mechanisms and tolerance. A compound consumed safely at a particular oral dose may behave differently when aerosolised and deposited repeatedly within the respiratory tract. Heating may also alter the original substance or produce secondary compounds that were not present in the unheated liquid. Ingredient selection must therefore move beyond statements such as food-grade, naturally derived or generally recognised as safe. These descriptions may provide useful background information, but they are not substitutes for inhalation-focused assessment.

Full chemical identification is the starting point. Each ingredient should be linked to an unambiguous name, Chemical Abstracts Service number where available, concentration range, functional role and supplier specification. Proprietary flavour mixtures require particular attention because their commercial names reveal little about composition. A manufacturer cannot assess toxicological suitability, detect restricted substances or maintain batch consistency without knowing what is present. Where flavour houses wish to protect intellectual property, confidential disclosure arrangements may be used, but the responsible economic operator must still be able to obtain sufficient information for regulatory submission, toxicological review, change control and investigation of complaints.

Purity is equally important. Nicotine, propylene glycol, glycerol, acids, water and flavouring materials may contain impurities arising from raw-material production, storage, degradation or contamination. Supplier certificates of analysis should therefore be reviewed against defined acceptance criteria rather than filed without scrutiny. The specification should identify relevant assay values, water content, residual solvents, heavy metals, degradation products and microbiological limits where appropriate. The absence of a contaminant from a supplier certificate does not prove that it is absent unless the material has been tested for that contaminant using a suitable method.

Ingredient function should be documented clearly because every component changes the product in some way. Nicotine determines pharmacological activity and influences sensory harshness. Propylene glycol and glycerol control viscosity, aerosol formation and flavour delivery. Water affects fluidity and coil wetting. Acids can alter nicotine form, pH and inhalation experience. Flavour compounds shape taste and odour but may also influence thermal stability and emissions. Sweeteners can improve palatability while increasing residue formation or thermal degradation. Colourants, vitamins, oils and other additives may create additional concerns without delivering a necessary function. A disciplined formulation includes only what can be justified technically and toxicologically.

Concentration matters as much as identity. A substance that is acceptable at a low level may become difficult to justify at a higher one. Ingredient assessment should therefore consider the actual amount used, the likely transfer into aerosol and the expected pattern of consumer use. Hazard information alone is insufficient because risk depends on exposure. The formulation should avoid using excessive concentrations to compensate for poor flavour design or weak device performance. Where the same sensory effect can be achieved with a lower quantity or a better-characterised alternative, the more conservative formulation is generally easier to defend.

Known respiratory sensitisers, irritants and substances with evidence of inhalation toxicity require particular caution. Compounds associated with bronchiolar injury, significant respiratory irritation, genotoxicity, carcinogenicity or harmful thermal decomposition should not be included merely because they are lawful in another product category. Structural alerts and read-across from related chemicals may also justify exclusion where direct inhalation data are absent. The objective is not to demand complete toxicological datasets for every flavour molecule, which may be unrealistic, but to apply a consistent hierarchy of evidence and precaution.

Thermal behaviour should be considered during ingredient selection rather than deferred entirely to emissions testing. Aldehydes, ketones, esters, sugars, acids and other flavour-related compounds may react or degrade when heated. Some can alter coil deposits, aerosol composition or the formation of carbonyl compounds. Compatibility with the intended device and operating range is therefore essential. An ingredient may appear stable in the bottle yet behave differently under repeated heating, high power or poor liquid supply. Screening at formulation stage can prevent the inclusion of substances likely to create avoidable emissions problems later.

Supplier control is inseparable from ingredient selection. An acceptable ingredient from one qualified source is not necessarily interchangeable with a material sold under the same name by another supplier. Differences in purity, carrier system, concentration, processing method and impurity profile may alter the final product. Approved supplier lists, written specifications and change-notification agreements should therefore be established before commercial manufacture. Substitution should not occur solely because another material is cheaper or more readily available. Any proposed change must be reviewed for its effect on composition, stability, emissions and regulatory documentation.

Natural extracts and complex botanical materials create additional challenges because their composition may vary with source, season, extraction method and storage. They may contain numerous unidentified or variable constituents and can be difficult to standardise. The term natural provides no assurance of safety, purity or consistency. Where such materials are used, the manufacturer must define the extract sufficiently, control key constituents and assess whether the variability can be managed within a stable product specification.

Ingredient selection should also support the intended shelf life. Some substances oxidise, hydrolyse, darken or interact over time. Nicotine can degrade, flavours can fade or transform and acids can alter the behaviour of other components. The chosen ingredients and packaging system must therefore remain compatible throughout storage. A formulation that meets specification at manufacture but changes materially before the end of its labelled shelf life is not adequately controlled.

The final ingredient list should represent a deliberate and documented balance between function, sensory performance, inhalation suitability, stability and regulatory acceptability. It should be capable of being traced from supplier records through the master formulation, batch documentation, technical file and notification. Each component should be known, justified and controlled. Where uncertainty remains, it should be identified honestly and managed through additional testing, reduced use levels, tighter specification or substitution.

A compliant product begins with restraint as much as innovation. Ingredient selection is strongest when unnecessary complexity is removed, poorly characterised materials are excluded and every remaining substance contributes a clear and defensible function. Once those principles are established, later toxicological assessment, stability testing and regulatory documentation become more reliable because the formulation has been designed to withstand scrutiny rather than merely to satisfy taste.

Supplier Qualification

Supplier qualification is the process through which a manufacturer determines whether a supplier is capable of providing materials, components or services that consistently meet the product specification and support continuing regulatory compliance. It extends beyond checking price, availability or a single certificate of analysis. A supplier becomes part of the product-control system because the quality of nicotine, solvents, flavour materials, acids, packaging, coils, batteries and testing services directly affects the composition, performance and legal status of the finished product. Where supplier control is weak, the manufacturer may believe that a product remains unchanged while critical inputs have already shifted.

The first stage is to define what the supplier is expected to provide. Each raw material or component should have an approved specification covering identity, grade, purity, concentration, relevant impurities, physical characteristics, packaging, storage conditions and required documentation. For complex materials such as flavour blends, the specification should also address compositional disclosure, carrier systems, restricted substances and change notification. For device components, it may include dimensions, materials, electrical characteristics, resistance tolerances, battery performance and compatibility with the intended formulation. Qualification cannot be meaningful where the purchasing description is vague.

Initial supplier assessment should examine technical capability, quality systems, regulatory awareness, manufacturing controls and traceability. The depth of review should reflect the importance of the supplied item. A nicotine supplier, flavour house, coil manufacturer or battery producer may require a more detailed assessment than a supplier of low-risk secondary packaging. Relevant evidence can include quality certificates, audit reports, manufacturing descriptions, complaint history, test methods, regulatory declarations and examples of batch documentation. Certification may support confidence, but it does not remove the need to assess whether the supplier's actual controls are suitable for the specific product.

Documentation should be reviewed for substance as well as presence. A certificate of analysis is useful only if it relates to the correct batch, uses appropriate test methods and reports results against agreed acceptance criteria. A safety data sheet may describe broad hazards but provide little information about trace impurities or inhalation relevance. A declaration that a flavour is food-grade does not establish its suitability for vaping. Supplier records should therefore be assessed against the manufacturer's own regulatory and technical requirements rather than accepted as complete merely because they appear formal.

Supplier qualification should include confirmation of identity and consistency. Initial verification testing may be necessary for critical materials, particularly nicotine, propylene glycol, glycerol, acids and complex flavour systems. The purpose is to confirm that the material received corresponds to the supplier's description and that key parameters remain within specification. The frequency and scope of testing can later be adjusted according to supplier performance, but early reliance on documentation alone may leave important differences undetected.

Change control is one of the most important elements of the supplier relationship. Suppliers may alter raw-material sources, manufacturing sites, extraction methods, carrier systems, specifications or sub-suppliers without recognising that the change could affect the finished product. Written agreements should therefore require advance notification of changes that may influence composition, purity, performance, stability or regulatory documentation. The manufacturer must then assess whether the change is acceptable, whether new testing is required and whether the product notification or technical file must be updated.

Supplier substitution should never be treated as an administrative purchasing decision where the input is critical to product performance or safety. Two materials sold under the same name may differ in impurity profile, concentration, moisture content or processing history. Two coils of the same nominal resistance may use different metals, wick materials or manufacturing residues. Two flavour blends with the same commercial description may not have the same composition. Any proposed substitute should therefore be evaluated against the approved specification and, where necessary, tested in the complete product.

Ongoing monitoring is required after approval. Supplier performance should be reviewed through incoming inspection results, batch failures, deviations, complaints, late deliveries, documentation quality and responsiveness to investigations. A supplier that repeatedly provides incomplete certificates, changes specifications without notice or fails to support root-cause analysis should not remain approved simply because supply is commercially convenient. Qualification is not a one-time decision but a continuing judgement based on evidence.

Auditing may form part of this oversight. The need for an on-site or remote audit depends on risk, supplier importance and available evidence. Audits can examine raw-material control, production processes, laboratory capability, calibration, traceability, deviation handling, cleaning, contamination prevention and change control. The objective is not to impose an identical quality system on every supplier, but to determine whether the supplier can reliably meet the agreed requirements and disclose problems promptly.

Contracts and quality agreements should define responsibilities clearly. These may cover specifications, testing, documentation, complaint support, retention samples, record retention, confidentiality, audit rights, change notification and corrective action. Where proprietary information is involved, the agreement should permit controlled disclosure to the manufacturer, toxicologist or regulator where necessary. Commercial confidentiality cannot be allowed to prevent lawful assessment of the product.

Supplier qualification also applies to service providers. Testing laboratories, consultants, contract manufacturers, filling sites and packaging companies can all influence the integrity of the technical file. Laboratories should be assessed for method suitability, competence, sample handling and reporting quality. Contract manufacturers should be able to reproduce the approved formulation and maintain batch records. Consultants should work from complete and accurate data. A weak service provider can create regulatory risk even where the underlying product is well designed.

The final qualification decision should be documented with a clear rationale. The supplier may be approved, approved with conditions or rejected. Conditional approval may require enhanced incoming testing, restricted use, corrective action or a follow-up audit. The decision should identify which materials or services are covered, because approval for one product does not automatically extend to all products supplied by the same company.

A compliant supply chain depends on transparency, consistency and control. The manufacturer must know what is being supplied, where it comes from, how it is tested and when it changes. Supplier qualification provides the evidence that these expectations are being met. Without it, the product specification is only theoretical, because the materials and components entering production may no longer correspond to those originally assessed.

Product Specifications

A product specification is the controlled technical definition of what the product is, what it must contain, how it must perform and which limits determine whether it can be released to market. It connects formulation, device design, packaging, manufacturing, testing and regulatory documentation within one approved standard. Without a robust specification, compliance remains dependent on assumptions because there is no stable reference against which incoming materials, production batches, finished products or later changes can be judged. The specification therefore acts as the central point of control between the product originally conceived, the product submitted to regulators and the product ultimately supplied to consumers.

The specification should describe the complete product rather than one isolated element. For a refill liquid, this includes the formulation, nicotine concentration, carrier ratio, flavour system, container, closure, fill volume, labelling and storage conditions. For a prefilled pod or complete device, it must also include reservoir capacity, coil type, resistance, power characteristics, materials, battery, airflow, charging arrangement and the interaction between liquid and hardware. A specification that defines only the liquid while leaving the intended device uncontrolled is incomplete because emissions, nicotine delivery and user exposure arise from the product system as a whole.

Product identity must be unambiguous. The specification should include the product name, internal code, variant, nicotine strength, flavour, intended market, regulatory category and version status. Where several products belong to one family, each shared and variable feature should be identified clearly. This prevents confusion between products that may appear commercially similar but differ materially in composition, strength or device configuration. Accurate coding also supports traceability, notification, batch documentation and recall.

The formulation section should list every ingredient by approved name, function and target concentration, together with acceptable manufacturing tolerances. Raw-material grades and approved suppliers should be referenced where relevant. For proprietary flavour systems, the controlled formulation should be linked to a detailed confidential compositional record rather than relying on a trade name alone. Nicotine form, assay, salt composition, acid ratio, pH target and carrier balance should be specified where they affect performance or regulatory identity. The finished formulation must be defined precisely enough that another qualified manufacturer could reproduce it consistently from the approved record.

Tolerances require careful judgement. A formulation cannot be manufactured to an infinitely exact value, but excessively broad tolerances can undermine product consistency and label accuracy. The permitted range should reflect process capability, analytical uncertainty, toxicological significance and the declared product characteristics. Nicotine concentration, for example, should remain within a justified range around the label claim. The same principle applies to fill volume, resistance, liquid ratio and other measurable attributes. Tolerances should not be selected merely to make batch release easier; they should describe the variation that can be accepted without altering product performance, exposure or legal status.

Physical and chemical characteristics should also be included where they are relevant to identity, stability or manufacture. These may include appearance, colour, odour, density, viscosity, pH, refractive index and water content. Not every parameter requires routine testing, but each selected attribute should have a clear purpose. Density may support formulation verification and fill control. Viscosity may influence coil wetting and leakage. pH may affect nicotine form, harshness and stability. Appearance and odour may reveal contamination or degradation. A good specification includes the characteristics most capable of confirming that the product remains within its approved design.

The device specification should define the hardware sufficiently to control both safety and aerosol performance. Important features may include dimensions, reservoir volume, coil material, wick material, nominal resistance, resistance tolerance, battery capacity, voltage or power range, airflow, firmware, charging input and protection features. Materials in contact with the liquid or aerosol should be identified. Where a component may be replaced, compatible versions should be listed. The intention is not to record every cosmetic detail, but to control those features that can influence function, exposure or compliance.

Nominal values should be distinguished from actual acceptance limits. A coil sold as 1.0 ohm may have an approved manufacturing range around that value. A reservoir declared as 2 millilitres must remain within the applicable legal capacity. A battery may have a stated capacity but require additional limits for charge behaviour, current and temperature. The specification should define which values are descriptive and which are release criteria. This reduces ambiguity during testing and supplier qualification.

Packaging forms part of the product specification because it protects the formulation, communicates legal information and preserves traceability. The bottle, pod, carton, closure and label should be linked to approved drawings or component codes. Child resistance, tamper evidence, leak protection and material compatibility should be specified where required. Label content should be controlled by version, including warning statements, nicotine declaration, batch code, responsible operator details, instructions and storage conditions. Packaging changes must be assessed because a different bottle, seal or label can affect shelf life, leakage, legal presentation or market identity.

Storage and shelf-life conditions should appear within the specification and should be supported by stability evidence. The product should have a defined manufacturing date, expiry or best-before period where applicable, storage temperature range and protection requirements such as avoidance of light or heat. Shelf life cannot be selected solely for commercial convenience. It should reflect the period during which nicotine concentration, flavour, appearance, packaging integrity and other critical attributes remain within specification.

The specification should identify critical quality attributes and critical process outputs. These are the characteristics most directly connected to product safety, performance and regulatory conformity. Examples include nicotine concentration, absence of restricted substances, correct fill volume, reservoir capacity, coil resistance, leak resistance, label accuracy and batch traceability. Identifying them allows quality control to focus effort where failure would be most consequential.

Acceptance criteria must be linked to suitable test methods. A requirement such as correct nicotine strength is not complete unless the method of determination is defined or referenced. The same applies to pH, density, leak testing, resistance, fill volume and physical inspection. Test methods should be sufficiently clear to produce reproducible decisions. Where a compendial, standardised or validated method exists, it should be used or justified against an alternative. Method uncertainty should be considered when setting release limits.

Sampling should also be defined. Testing every unit may be impossible, but testing too few may fail to detect meaningful variation. The specification or associated quality plan should state how batches are sampled, which tests are applied routinely and which are periodic or verification-based. The sampling approach should reflect batch size, process capability, supplier history and risk. A stable automated filling process may require a different control strategy from a manual small-batch operation.

The specification must remain aligned with the regulatory submission. Ingredient quantities, nicotine strength, device parameters, reservoir capacity, packaging and product identifiers should correspond to the notified or authorised product. A technical file that describes one configuration while the factory produces another creates a direct compliance failure. Document control should ensure that only the current approved specification is used and that obsolete versions are withdrawn from production.

Version control is therefore essential. Every specification should have a unique number, revision status, effective date, approval history and summary of changes. Revisions should not overwrite the historical record. The manufacturer should be able to demonstrate which version applied to each batch and when any change took effect. This is particularly important where a change requires new testing, updated notification or revised packaging.

Change control protects the specification after approval. Proposed changes to ingredients, suppliers, device components, manufacturing methods, packaging, claims or tolerances should be assessed before implementation. The assessment should consider quality, toxicology, stability, emissions, labelling and regulatory impact. A change may be acceptable within the existing specification, may require a formal revision or may create a new product requiring separate notification. The decision should be documented and approved by the appropriate functions.

The specification should also distinguish between mandatory requirements and internal targets. A legal maximum, such as a nicotine concentration or reservoir capacity, is non-negotiable. An internal target may be set more tightly to provide operating margin and reduce the risk of borderline failure. This is often good practice because manufacturing and analytical variation can make a product designed exactly at the legal limit vulnerable to non-compliance. Internal controls should therefore be capable of ensuring that released product remains comfortably within statutory boundaries.

Finished-product release depends on comparison with the specification. Batch records, analytical results, physical checks and packaging verification should be reviewed before approval. Deviations must be investigated rather than ignored because the batch appears commercially usable. A batch outside specification should not be released without a documented assessment and lawful justification. Repeated deviations may indicate that the specification is unrealistic or that the process is not capable of meeting it consistently.

The specification also supports post-market investigation. When a complaint arises, the manufacturer can compare the returned product and batch records with the approved requirements. Leakage, unusual flavour, weak nicotine delivery or device failure can be assessed against defined criteria. Without a clear specification, investigations become subjective and corrective action becomes difficult to justify.

A well-constructed product specification is therefore more than a formulation sheet or manufacturing instruction. It is the controlled technical identity of the product across its entire lifecycle. It links approved ingredients, qualified suppliers, device characteristics, packaging, test methods, acceptance limits, regulatory records and change control. When maintained correctly, it ensures that the product placed on the market remains the product that was designed, assessed and declared.

Stability Studies

Stability studies determine whether a vaping product remains within its approved specification throughout storage and use, rather than only at the point of manufacture. A product may be correctly formulated, accurately filled and fully compliant when released, yet change progressively as nicotine oxidises, flavours degrade, water is lost or gained, packaging interacts with the liquid or device components deteriorate. Stability assessment therefore links formulation science, packaging, storage conditions, shelf life and regulatory control. Its purpose is to establish how long the product can be expected to remain chemically, physically and functionally acceptable under defined conditions and to provide evidence for the storage instructions and expiry period applied to the finished product.

The first requirement is to define which product is being studied. Stability data are meaningful only when they relate to the final formulation, final packaging and intended device configuration. Testing a bulk liquid in a laboratory bottle does not necessarily support the shelf life of the same liquid stored in a commercial refill container, pod or integrated device. Oxygen exposure, headspace, light transmission, closure integrity, polymer composition and contact with metals or elastomers can all influence degradation. The stability programme should therefore use production-representative batches filled into the packaging system intended for market supply.

The study design should reflect the nature of the product and the intended commercial shelf life. Real-time studies provide the most direct evidence because products are stored under the labelled conditions for the full proposed period. Accelerated studies expose products to elevated temperature, humidity or other stress conditions to increase the rate of change and identify likely degradation pathways more quickly. Accelerated data can support development decisions and provide early indications of stability, but it should not be treated automatically as equivalent to real-time evidence. Chemical reactions do not always accelerate uniformly, and elevated temperatures may create changes that would not occur under ordinary storage.

A combined approach is usually more informative. Accelerated studies can begin during development, allowing unstable formulations, unsuitable closures or vulnerable packaging materials to be identified before launch. Real-time studies should continue in parallel to confirm that the product remains within specification under its recommended storage conditions. Intermediate conditions may also be useful where products are likely to experience warmer retail, transport or domestic environments.

The stability protocol should define the batches, storage conditions, time points, test parameters, methods and acceptance criteria before the study begins. This prevents the programme from being altered later to accommodate unfavourable results. The number of batches should be sufficient to distinguish a reproducible product trend from an isolated manufacturing variation. Early development may use pilot batches, but commercial shelf-life claims should be supported by batches representative of the final manufacturing process.

Nicotine concentration is one of the principal stability attributes. Nicotine can oxidise over time, leading to reduced assay, colour change and the formation of degradation products. The rate of change may be influenced by oxygen, light, temperature, pH, water content, packaging permeability and the presence of other ingredients. A stability study should therefore monitor not only the declared nicotine concentration but also visible changes and, where relevant, known impurities or degradation markers. A product that remains close to label claim while developing an unacceptable impurity profile may still be unsuitable for release or continued sale.

Colour change is often one of the first visible signs of nicotine oxidation or flavour degradation. Darkening does not by itself prove that the product has become unsafe, but it may indicate chemical change and can affect consumer acceptance. Colour should therefore be assessed against defined criteria rather than described subjectively. Photographic standards, instrumental colour measurement or controlled visual comparison may be used depending on the product and available methods.

Flavour stability requires equal attention because volatile compounds, esters, aldehydes and other flavour constituents may degrade, react or evaporate over time. The sensory profile can flatten, shift or become harsh even when the formulation remains chemically within broad limits. Where flavour performance is central to product identity, sensory assessment may form part of the stability programme, provided the method is controlled and reproducible. Analytical tracking of selected marker compounds may also support evaluation of flavour consistency.

The carrier system may change through water exchange, evaporation or interaction with packaging. Variations in propylene glycol, glycerol and water content can alter density, viscosity, aerosol formation, leakage and coil wetting. Viscosity should therefore be monitored where it is critical to device performance. A liquid that thickens may no longer wick correctly, while one that becomes less viscous may leak more readily. Physical stability is therefore directly connected to both user experience and emissions behaviour.

pH can change as nicotine and flavour components degrade or interact. This may alter throat sensation, nicotine form, chemical stability and the behaviour of the formulation within the device. Where pH is relevant to product performance or toxicological assessment, it should be measured at appropriate intervals using a defined method. The same applies to density, refractive index or other physical parameters used as identity or quality indicators.

Packaging compatibility is a major part of stability assessment. The liquid may extract substances from plastic, attack seals, soften elastomers, corrode metals or weaken adhesives. Packaging may also permit oxygen or moisture transfer. Visual inspection should therefore include the bottle, closure, pod, reservoir, seals and labelling as well as the liquid itself. Signs of swelling, cracking, leakage, discolouration, delamination or closure failure should be documented and investigated.

Container-closure integrity should remain effective throughout the claimed shelf life. A child-resistant closure is not sufficient if the seal loses integrity during storage. A pod may be leak-free initially but fail after repeated temperature cycling. Stability studies can include upright and inverted storage, transport simulation, vibration or temperature cycling where these conditions are relevant to distribution and use. The purpose is to establish whether the complete packaging system remains protective under foreseeable conditions.

Device-integrated products require additional assessment because the liquid remains in prolonged contact with coils, wicks, metals, plastics and adhesives. The formulation may corrode components, absorb manufacturing residues or change in response to the internal environment. Device functionality should therefore be checked at intervals, including activation, charging where relevant, leakage, aerosol generation and consistency of delivery. A chemically stable liquid is not sufficient if the integrated device fails before the end of shelf life.

Stability after opening may differ from unopened shelf life. Refill containers are repeatedly opened and exposed to air, light and contamination. Open systems may also experience water loss or oxidation more quickly. Where the product is likely to be used over an extended period after first opening, an in-use stability study may be appropriate. This can assess whether the product remains acceptable under a realistic pattern of opening, closing, handling and storage.

Microbiological stability is generally less problematic in high-propylene-glycol or high-glycerol formulations with low water activity, but it should not be assumed without consideration. Products containing higher water levels, botanical extracts or other supportive materials may require microbiological assessment. Manufacturing hygiene and packaging integrity remain important because contamination can occur even where the formulation does not readily support microbial growth.

Acceptance criteria should be based on the approved product specification and the characteristics necessary for safe and consistent use. These may include nicotine assay, appearance, colour, pH, viscosity, packaging integrity, leakage, device function and selected impurity limits. The criteria should be defined before testing and should reflect analytical uncertainty. A product should not be considered stable merely because every result remains close to the initial value if one critical attribute moves outside its justified range.

Trend analysis is more informative than isolated pass-or-fail results. A parameter may remain within specification at the current time point while showing a consistent movement towards failure. Monitoring the rate and direction of change can reveal whether the proposed shelf life is realistic. Trend data can also identify differences between batches, packaging formats or storage conditions.

Out-of-trend results should be investigated even where they remain within formal limits. An unexpected change in one batch may indicate supplier variation, filling error, packaging defect or analytical inconsistency. Stability programmes should therefore link to deviation control and corrective action rather than operating as separate laboratory exercises.

Shelf life should be assigned conservatively from the evidence available. Commercial pressure may favour a longer period, but the claim must remain supportable. Where full real-time data are not yet available, a provisional shelf life may be used if justified by accelerated data, formulation knowledge and continued monitoring. The product should then be reviewed as further real-time results become available.

The labelled storage conditions must reflect the study. If a product is tested under controlled room-temperature conditions, the label should not imply that it can tolerate prolonged exposure to heat, direct sunlight or freezing without evidence. Storage instructions should be practical and clear, particularly where the product is sensitive to temperature or light.

Stability data must remain connected to change control. A new flavour supplier, nicotine source, bottle material, closure, coil or manufacturing site may alter the stability profile. Not every change requires a complete new programme, but each should be assessed for its likely impact. Bridging studies may be appropriate where the change is limited and well understood. Major formulation or packaging changes may require a new study.

The stability report should document the protocol, batches, methods, storage conditions, results, trends, deviations and conclusion. It should explain how the proposed shelf life was derived and identify any limitations. The report should also state whether the product remained within its complete specification, not merely whether nicotine concentration was acceptable.

A robust stability programme demonstrates that compliance continues beyond the day of manufacture. It confirms that the formulation, packaging and device remain capable of meeting their intended function throughout distribution, storage and use. Without that evidence, the expiry period is little more than a commercial estimate. With it, shelf life becomes a controlled and defensible part of the product specification.

Technical Documentation

Technical documentation is the structured body of evidence that describes the product, explains how it was developed and demonstrates why it is considered suitable for lawful market placement. It is not a collection of disconnected certificates assembled shortly before notification. It is the controlled record linking the product specification, ingredients, suppliers, formulation, device, manufacturing process, testing, labelling and post-market responsibilities. Where that record is incomplete or inconsistent, the manufacturer may be unable to show that the product sold is the same product that was assessed, tested and declared.

The technical file should begin with an unambiguous product identity. This includes the product name, internal code, variant, flavour, nicotine strength, device type, intended market, regulatory category and version status. The responsible manufacturer, importer or other economic operator should be identified clearly, together with the legal entity responsible for the submission and continuing compliance. Where several businesses participate in manufacture, filling, packaging or distribution, their roles should be recorded so that responsibility does not become fragmented.

The product description should explain the complete system rather than only its most visible component. For a refill liquid, this includes the formulation, container, closure, fill volume, label and intended use. For a pod or complete device, it should also cover reservoir capacity, coil, wick, battery, power characteristics, airflow, materials, charging system and compatibility between liquid and hardware. Drawings, photographs, component lists and approved specifications can be used to make the product identity clear. The purpose is to ensure that the technical record corresponds to the product placed on the market and can be understood by someone who was not involved in its development.

Formulation documentation should identify every ingredient by approved name, concentration, function and supplier. Chemical identifiers, raw-material grades, nicotine form, acids, carrier ratios and flavour-system details should be included where relevant. Proprietary mixtures should be supported by controlled compositional records rather than trade names alone. The formulation record should correspond to the master manufacturing formula and the data used for toxicological assessment, stability work and notification. Any discrepancy between these records creates uncertainty over which product was actually assessed.

Supplier evidence should support the formulation and component list. Certificates of analysis, specifications, quality agreements, declarations, safety data and change-notification commitments should be linked to the correct material or component. The file should distinguish between current approved documents and superseded versions. Retaining historical records is important because a product complaint or regulatory query may relate to a batch manufactured under an earlier supplier specification.

The toxicological section should explain how ingredient and emissions risks were considered. It should not consist only of copied hazard statements. The assessment should identify relevant hazards, expected exposure, available inhalation data, thermal behaviour, impurity concerns and any important uncertainty. Where read-across, exposure thresholds or other scientific approaches are used, the rationale should be stated. The conclusion should explain why each ingredient and the complete formulation are considered acceptable for the intended product and use, rather than merely asserting compliance.

Emissions documentation should describe the product tested, sample condition, device settings, puffing regime, analytical methods, target compounds, limits of detection and results. The test configuration must match the notified or marketed product. Where several device settings or variants exist, the file should justify which conditions were selected and whether they represent normal use, worst-case operation or stress testing. Laboratory reports should be interpreted rather than filed without comment, particularly where results vary between replicates or approach internal action limits.

Stability records should show how the proposed shelf life and storage conditions were derived. Protocols, batch details, packaging configuration, storage conditions, time points, results, trends, deviations and final conclusions should be retained. If a provisional shelf life was used before the completion of full real-time studies, the basis for that decision and the plan for continuing review should be documented. Later stability results should be added to the same controlled record so that the conclusion remains current.

Device and packaging evidence should include the specifications and tests relevant to safety and performance. Depending on the product, this may cover reservoir capacity, leak resistance, child resistance, tamper evidence, electrical safety, charging behaviour, coil resistance, battery protection, materials compatibility and refill mechanism performance. Approved drawings and component codes should identify the exact versions used. Packaging artwork should be controlled in the same way as a formulation or device component because warning statements, nicotine declarations, responsible-operator details and batch information form part of legal conformity.

Manufacturing documentation should explain how the approved product is reproduced consistently. Process descriptions, master batch records, mixing instructions, filling parameters, in-process checks, line-clearance procedures, cleaning, equipment calibration, release testing and final approval should be included or referenced. Where manufacture is outsourced, the file should contain the relevant quality agreement and evidence that the contract manufacturer has been qualified. The technical file should demonstrate not only what the product contains but how the manufacturer controls the process that creates it.

Batch traceability is an essential part of this record. Every released batch should be linked to the applicable formulation, raw-material lots, component lots, packaging version, production date, test results and release decision. This connection allows a complaint or defect to be investigated accurately. Without it, the technical file may describe the nominal product while providing no evidence about the particular units supplied to consumers.

Risk management should be documented throughout the file rather than added as a final generic statement. The manufacturer should identify foreseeable hazards involving nicotine exposure, leakage, accidental ingestion, battery failure, overheating, material incompatibility, thermal degradation, incorrect use and youth appeal where relevant. The record should show which controls were introduced, what evidence supports them and whether any residual risks remain. Risk assessment should be updated when new information emerges or when the product changes.

The regulatory submission should be generated from the technical documentation rather than maintained as a separate version of the truth. Product identifiers, ingredient quantities, device details, emissions information, manufacturing descriptions and declarations should match the controlled file.

Where submission portals require abbreviated or standardised fields, the underlying technical evidence should remain available to support those entries. Any later correction or update should be reflected both in the submission and in the source documentation.

Document control determines whether the file remains reliable. Every controlled document should have a unique identifier, title, revision number, approval status, effective date and change history. Obsolete versions should be withdrawn from active use but retained for traceability. Access should be controlled so that authorised personnel can use the current version while preventing uncontrolled alteration. Electronic systems may be used, but they should preserve version history, approvals and retrieval.

Cross-referencing is important because the file may contain hundreds of records. The product specification should link to the formulation, test methods and packaging drawings. The toxicological assessment should identify the ingredient list and exposure data used. Stability reports should state the batch and packaging configuration. Laboratory reports should identify the device and operating conditions. A technical file becomes difficult to defend where documents are individually present but cannot be shown to relate to the same product version.

The file should also record deviations, investigations and decisions. A failed test, out-of-trend result or manufacturing deviation should not disappear from the record after corrective action. The investigation, root cause, impact assessment and disposition should be retained. This demonstrates that the quality system identified the issue and responded appropriately. A file containing only successful results can appear less credible where the product has undergone substantial development or manufacture.

Change control must remain connected to the documentation. Proposed changes to ingredients, suppliers, nicotine source, device components, manufacturing site, packaging, claims or test methods should be assessed before implementation. The assessment should determine which documents require revision, whether new testing is necessary and whether the regulatory notification must be updated. The file should preserve the evidence supporting the decision, including the reason why a change was considered minor or substantial.

Post-market information should become part of the technical record after launch. Complaints, adverse events, returns, product failures, regulatory correspondence, market surveillance and corrective actions may reveal weaknesses not apparent during development. Periodic review can determine whether the original risk assessment remains valid and whether the specification or instructions require amendment. The technical file should therefore remain active for as long as the product is supplied and for the retention period required afterward.

The depth of documentation should be proportionate to the complexity and risk of the product, but proportionality does not mean informality. A simple refill liquid may require fewer engineering records than a rechargeable device, yet it still needs a controlled formulation, supplier evidence, toxicological assessment, stability support, packaging records and batch traceability. A complex integrated product requires a wider file because more components and interactions can affect exposure and performance.

Technical documentation also protects the manufacturer commercially. It provides evidence during regulatory inspection, customer due diligence, distributor review, complaint investigation and product transfer. It reduces dependence on individual employees because the rationale and history of the product remain available when personnel change. It also supports future development by showing which ingredients, materials, methods and suppliers have already been assessed.

A strong technical file is coherent rather than merely large. Every important claim should be supported by evidence, every record should relate to the correct product version and every change should be traceable. The documentation should allow the manufacturer to answer four fundamental questions: what is the product, how is it made, why is it considered compliant and how is that status maintained after market entry. Where those answers are clear and supported, the technical file becomes a working demonstration of product control rather than an administrative archive.

Notification Planning

Notification planning determines how and when a completed product is translated into the formal information required by the competent authority before market placement. It should begin well before the final submission date because the notification depends on stable product identity, complete technical records, confirmed formulation data, finished packaging and evidence that the product has been tested in its final configuration. A submission prepared too early may describe a product that is still changing, while one prepared too late can delay launch or create pressure to file incomplete information. Effective planning connects product development, documentation, manufacturing and commercial timing so that the notification reflects the product that will actually be supplied.

The first requirement is to confirm the applicable regulatory route and jurisdiction. A nicotine-containing consumer vaping product may require notification under tobacco-related legislation, while a product making medicinal claims may require a medicines authorisation. Nicotine-free products, hardware components and accessories may fall under different legal regimes. The route must therefore be established before the submission timetable is set. A company planning to sell in several jurisdictions should identify whether one technical data package can support multiple filings or whether separate systems, formats, fees, responsible operators and language requirements will apply.

The notification plan should identify the responsible submitter and the legal entity placing the product on the market. This is especially important where the brand owner, manufacturer, importer and distributor are different organisations. The submitter must have authority to provide the product information and access to the underlying evidence. It must also be able to maintain the record, respond to regulator queries and update the submission when the product changes. A filing made by an entity that lacks control over formulation, manufacturing or documentation creates continuing risk.

Product scope should then be defined carefully. Each flavour, nicotine strength, device configuration or packaging format may require separate treatment depending on the jurisdiction and notification system. Commercial teams often view closely related variants as one product family, but regulatory systems may require distinct identifiers and records. Planning should therefore establish which features are common across the range and which create a separate notification. This avoids both unnecessary duplication and the greater risk of combining materially different products under one record.

The submission timetable must be built around the legal lead time for market entry. Where notification is required several months before sale, that period should be treated as a fixed development constraint. Product formulation, device configuration and core technical information must be sufficiently stable before filing. Packaging, manufacturing and distribution planning should also account for the possibility that the authority may request clarification or that data problems may need correction. Launch dates should not be set solely by commercial preference if the regulatory pathway cannot support them.

A notification readiness review should be completed before submission. This review should confirm that product identifiers, formulation records, ingredient quantities, device specifications, emissions data, toxicological information, manufacturing descriptions and packaging details all correspond to the same approved version. It should also confirm that the product has not changed since testing. A common weakness is that the final commercial product differs from the version assessed because a flavour, coil, supplier or packaging component was altered late in development.

Ingredient data usually require particular attention. The notification may require chemical names, CAS numbers, quantities, functions, supplier information and toxicological descriptions. Proprietary mixtures should be resolved before submission rather than entered through vague trade names or incomplete placeholders. Where confidential disclosure is necessary, the process should be agreed with the supplier early enough to avoid delaying the filing. The responsible operator should also ensure that ingredient quantities in the submission match the master formulation and finished-product specification.

Device and component information should be equally precise. Reservoir capacity, resistance, battery characteristics, materials, airflow, power range and refill mechanism may all affect product identity and compliance. The submitted device should be the device used for emissions and performance testing. If several devices are intended to be compatible with one liquid or pod, the submission strategy should explain how those combinations are controlled and whether additional evidence is needed.

Emissions and toxicological records should be reviewed for relevance and consistency before they are converted into portal fields. Laboratory reports may use terminology or units that differ from the notification format. Data may need to be summarised without losing important context. The company should confirm that operating conditions, test methods and product identifiers are recorded accurately. A numerical result entered into a system without the supporting method and product context may be technically complete but scientifically weak.

The manufacturing section should describe the process sufficiently to demonstrate control without becoming disconnected from the actual production arrangement. The manufacturing site, principal process stages, quality controls and responsible entities should be identified. Where production is outsourced, the notification should remain consistent with the quality agreement and technical file. The submitter should not describe an idealised process that differs from the one used by the contract manufacturer.

Packaging and labelling should be reviewed as part of notification planning because product names, nicotine strengths, warnings, volumes and responsible-operator details must align with the submitted record. A late branding change can create inconsistency between the database, carton and product label. Artwork should therefore be controlled by version and linked to the relevant notification. Regional packaging differences should be managed carefully where the same product is sold in more than one market.

Data entry should be subject to quality review. Notification systems often require large numbers of structured fields, and administrative errors can create significant consequences. Incorrect units, decimal placement, duplicate identifiers, incomplete ingredient records or mismatched product names can make the submission unreliable. A second-person review should compare the entered data with the approved source documents before filing.

Submission records should be retained in a controlled form. The company should preserve copies of the final data package, confirmation of submission, product identifiers, correspondence, fees and any regulator queries. Portal access should be managed so that responsibility does not depend on one employee or consultant. Login credentials, account ownership and authorised users should be controlled securely because loss of access can prevent updates or delay responses.

Notification planning should also anticipate questions from the authority. The technical file should be capable of supporting every substantive entry. Where the submission contains a scientific conclusion, the underlying assessment should be available. Where a field is not applicable, the reason should be clear. A company that can only reproduce what was entered into the portal but cannot explain the basis of the entry is not adequately prepared.

The filing should be treated as a controlled regulatory event. Final approval should confirm that the product is ready for notification, that the data are complete and that all relevant functions have signed off. Regulatory, quality, technical and commercial teams should agree on the product version and intended launch market. This prevents one function from continuing to change the product after another has submitted it.

Post-submission control is as important as the original filing. The notified product must remain aligned with the market product. Changes to flavour composition, nicotine source, supplier, device component, capacity, packaging or manufacturing site should be assessed before implementation. The company should determine whether the change is administrative, whether the existing notification must be updated or whether a new submission is required. This decision should be documented through formal change control.

Notification databases should also be reviewed after publication. Product names, identifiers and public information should be checked for accuracy. Any error should be corrected promptly because retailers, distributors and enforcement authorities may rely on the public record. Publication should not be assumed to confirm that every aspect of the product has been approved; it is evidence that the notification process has been completed, not a substitute for continuing manufacturer responsibility.

Commercial launch should not occur until the required notification period has passed and all applicable conditions have been met. Inventory planning must account for this. Producing large quantities before submission is secure can create financial pressure to release product prematurely. A staged manufacturing approach may be more prudent, particularly for new markets or complex products.

A well-planned notification process reduces regulatory delay because it is built from controlled product information rather than assembled through last-minute reconstruction. It ensures that the regulator receives a coherent account of the product and that the manufacturer retains the evidence needed to support it. The strongest notification is not the one completed fastest, but the one that remains accurate after launch because the product, technical file and regulatory record continue to describe the same controlled system.

Risk Assessment

Risk assessment provides the structured reasoning through which a manufacturer identifies the hazards associated with a vaping product, estimates the likelihood and severity of harm and determines which controls are necessary before market entry and throughout the product lifecycle. It should not be reduced to a generic statement that the product is intended for adult smokers or that it complies with applicable legislation. A credible assessment must relate to the actual formulation, device, packaging, manufacturing process, intended user and foreseeable patterns of use. Its purpose is to show that relevant risks have been identified, understood and reduced as far as reasonably practicable without undermining the product's intended function.

The first stage is to define the scope of the assessment. The product should be evaluated as a complete system rather than as a collection of isolated parts. The formulation, nicotine concentration, device architecture, power characteristics, reservoir, coil, battery, packaging and instructions all contribute to the final exposure and use profile. A refill liquid may present a different risk when used in a low-power pod than in a high-power open system. A device may be safe with one formulation but prone to leakage, overheating or poor wicking with another. Risk assessment must therefore consider the intended combinations and identify where uncontrolled compatibility could create additional hazards.

Hazard identification should be systematic. Relevant categories may include nicotine toxicity, accidental ingestion, dermal or ocular exposure, inhalation of harmful emissions, respiratory irritation, sensitisation, thermal degradation, battery failure, overheating, fire, leakage, breakage, material migration, contamination, mislabelling, incorrect nicotine strength, foreseeable misuse and youth appeal. The objective is not to list every theoretical possibility but to identify those that are credible for the product and capable of causing meaningful harm.

Nicotine-related risks require particular attention because nicotine is pharmacologically active and can cause adverse effects at sufficient exposure. The assessment should consider the concentration present, total quantity available in the product, potential for accidental access, likelihood of leakage and the clarity of warnings. Child-resistant closures, restricted fill volumes, secure pod construction and clear storage instructions may reduce risk, but their effectiveness should be supported by design evidence rather than assumed. For higher-strength products, the consequences of leakage or ingestion may require tighter controls.

Inhalation risk must be assessed through both ingredient and emissions evidence. The presence of a substance in the liquid does not establish the amount inhaled, while the absence of concern in the unheated formulation does not exclude harmful degradation during aerosol generation. The assessment should therefore consider ingredient identity, concentration, inhalation hazard, thermal behaviour, transfer into aerosol and the operating conditions of the device. Where emissions testing identifies carbonyls, metals, volatile compounds or other substances of concern, the results should be interpreted in relation to exposure, method conditions and relevant toxicological benchmarks.

Device-related risks should be considered with equal depth. Batteries can fail through short circuit, overcharging, physical damage or use of incompatible chargers. Heating systems can overheat when liquid supply is insufficient. Coils may vary outside resistance tolerance. Reservoirs can leak, seals can fail and plastics may crack or deform. The risk assessment should identify the control features built into the product, including protection circuitry, charging limits, temperature management, material selection, leak resistance and user instructions. Where the product depends on firmware or electronic controls, failures in those systems should also be considered.

Foreseeable misuse should be distinguished from extreme or deliberate abuse. Consumers may overfill a tank, use the wrong charger, operate a device at an unsuitable power level, allow liquid to run low or store the product in a hot vehicle. These behaviours may not be intended, but they are plausible and should be addressed through design and instructions. A risk assessment that considers only ideal laboratory use is incomplete because products are used in uncontrolled domestic and retail environments.

The intended user population must be defined clearly. A product designed for adult smokers or existing nicotine users presents a different benefit–risk context from one used by nicotine-naive individuals. The assessment should consider whether the product's nicotine delivery, presentation, flavour naming, colours, imagery or format could increase appeal to children or non-users. Youth appeal is not solely a marketing issue; it is a product-stewardship risk because initiation among people who would otherwise avoid nicotine changes the population impact of the product.

Risk estimation should assess both severity and likelihood. A rare battery fire may have severe consequences, while minor throat irritation may occur more frequently but carry lower severity. The method used can be qualitative or semi-quantitative, but it should be consistent. Risk matrices may assist prioritisation, provided they do not create false precision. The score is less important than the reasoning used to determine which hazards require stronger control.

Existing controls should then be evaluated. These may include ingredient exclusion, concentration limits, child-resistant packaging, tamper evidence, leak-resistant design, battery protection, supplier qualification, incoming testing, manufacturing controls, warning statements and post-market monitoring. The assessment should explain how each control reduces likelihood, severity or exposure. A control should not be credited merely because it exists on paper; there should be evidence that it functions as intended.

Residual risk is the risk remaining after controls have been applied. It should be accepted only where the product's intended benefits and function justify it and where further reduction would be impracticable or would materially impair performance. Residual risk should not be hidden by describing the product as compliant. Legal compliance establishes minimum requirements, but it does not prove that every avoidable risk has been controlled.

Comparative risk may be relevant where the product is intended for adults who would otherwise continue smoking. In that context, the assessment should recognise the difference between aerosol exposure and tobacco combustion while avoiding unsupported claims of safety. A product may present lower exposure to many combustion-related toxicants and still require control of nicotine, emissions, materials and device failure. Comparative reasoning should inform proportionality, not replace product-specific assessment.

The risk assessment should be linked directly to the product specification and technical documentation. Each identified critical risk should have a corresponding control, test, acceptance criterion or monitoring activity. If leakage is identified as significant, the file should contain leak testing and closure specifications. If carbonyl formation is a concern, the emissions programme should address relevant operating conditions. If nicotine accuracy is critical, the manufacturing and release methods should reflect that priority.

Risk assessment should also influence supplier control. Critical materials and components should be subject to greater qualification, testing and change-notification requirements. A supplier of nicotine, flavour systems, coils or batteries may carry more risk than a supplier of secondary packaging. The assessment can therefore support a risk-based approach to auditing, incoming testing and documentation review.

Manufacturing risks must be included because an acceptable design can become unsafe through process failure. Incorrect weighing, cross-contamination, wrong labels, underfilled or overfilled containers, unapproved component substitution and inadequate mixing can all change the product materially. Process controls, line clearance, batch records, calibration, release testing and independent verification reduce these risks. The assessment should identify where human error is possible and where additional control is needed.

Labelling and instructions form part of the risk-control system. Warnings should address nicotine, age restriction, storage, accidental exposure and safe device use where relevant. Instructions should be clear enough to reduce misuse without becoming so dense that consumers ignore them. Where a safety feature depends on the user taking a particular action, that dependency should be recognised as a weaker control than one built into the product.

The assessment should be completed before launch but should not end there. Complaints, adverse events, returns, enforcement findings and market surveillance may reveal risks that were not predicted during development. Post-market data should therefore feed back into the risk record. A pattern of leakage, battery incidents or consumer confusion may require redesign, stronger instructions, supplier action or withdrawal.

Change control must trigger risk review. A new ingredient, supplier, coil, battery, packaging material or manufacturing site can alter the risk profile. Even a change presented as equivalent may affect impurities, stability, emissions or performance. The assessment should therefore be revised when changes are proposed and before they are implemented.

The document should show who performed the assessment, which evidence was reviewed, what assumptions were made and how conclusions were reached. It should identify uncertainties honestly rather than presenting a level of certainty the evidence cannot support. Where data are limited, the appropriate response may be additional testing, tighter controls, restricted use or removal of the questionable feature.

A strong risk assessment is practical, specific and connected to decision-making. It identifies where harm could arise, determines which controls are necessary and confirms whether those controls remain effective. It should enable the manufacturer to explain not only that the product is compliant, but why its remaining risks are considered acceptable for the intended use and how those risks will continue to be monitored after market entry.

Product Stewardship

Product stewardship is the continuing responsibility to ensure that a vaping product remains controlled, supportable and appropriately managed after development and market entry. It extends beyond compliance with the initial notification because products continue to move through manufacturing, distribution, retail, consumer use and disposal long after the regulatory submission has been completed. Stewardship connects technical documentation, quality management, market surveillance, complaint handling, corrective action, responsible marketing and environmental responsibility within one lifecycle approach. Its purpose is to ensure that the manufacturer or responsible operator continues to understand the product, monitor its effects and intervene where evidence shows that the original controls are no longer sufficient.

The foundation of product stewardship is ownership. A named legal entity must remain responsible for the product throughout the period in which it is supplied. This responsibility should not become diluted between the brand owner, contract manufacturer, importer, distributor and retailer. Commercial partners may perform different functions, but someone must retain authority over the product specification, technical file, notifications, complaints, investigations, recalls and regulatory communication. Where ownership is ambiguous, emerging problems can remain unresolved because each party assumes that another organisation is responsible.

Stewardship begins before launch by defining the systems that will operate afterward. The company should establish how complaints will be received, recorded, categorised, investigated and closed. It should determine how adverse events, battery incidents, leakage, incorrect nicotine strength, packaging failures and consumer misuse will be escalated. It should also ensure that distribution records and batch identifiers are sufficient to trace affected products. These arrangements should exist before the first unit is sold rather than being improvised after a serious incident.

Complaint handling is one of the most important sources of post-market information. A single complaint may reflect isolated misuse, transport damage or an individual preference, but repeated reports can reveal a wider product defect. Complaints should therefore be coded consistently so that trends can be identified. Categories may include leakage, weak or excessive nicotine effect, burnt taste, device failure, charging problems, damaged packaging, label errors, unusual odour, adverse respiratory effects and accidental exposure. The system should preserve both the consumer's description and the technical interpretation applied during review.

Investigation should be proportionate to the seriousness and frequency of the issue. Minor complaints may be resolved through replacement and routine monitoring, while significant incidents may require retention-sample testing, review of batch records, examination of returned products, supplier investigation or laboratory analysis. The investigation should identify whether the problem arose from design, manufacture, transport, storage, consumer use or deliberate alteration. Conclusions should be supported by evidence and should not default automatically to user error where the underlying cause remains uncertain.

Adverse-event review requires particular care because reports may involve incomplete information and uncertain causality. The manufacturer should record the product involved, timing, pattern of use, other nicotine exposure, relevant medical history where voluntarily provided, symptoms and outcome. A report does not prove that the product caused the event, but it may still contribute to a signal when considered alongside similar cases. Serious or unexpected events should be escalated promptly and reported to the relevant authority where required.

Trend analysis allows isolated records to become useful regulatory intelligence. Complaint rates should be considered in relation to sales volume, product age, market, batch and device configuration. An increase in leakage complaints from one production period may indicate a closure or seal defect. Burnt taste reports linked to a particular coil lot may suggest resistance variation or poor wicking. Charging incidents associated with one component supplier may justify immediate containment. Stewardship depends on recognising these patterns before they develop into widespread harm.

Batch traceability supports this work. Every market unit should be linked to the applicable formulation, raw-material lots, component lots, packaging version, manufacturing date and release record. Distribution records should identify where batches were supplied. Traceability does not need to follow every unit to an individual consumer, but it should allow affected stock to be located efficiently. Without this connection, targeted corrective action becomes difficult and a limited defect may require a much broader withdrawal.

Market surveillance extends beyond complaints submitted directly to the company. Retailer feedback, distributor reports, online reviews, regulator notices, laboratory findings, product returns and competitor incidents can all provide useful information. Social media should not be treated as scientifically reliable evidence on its own, but repeated descriptions of the same failure may justify investigation. Stewardship requires the company to remain attentive to the way the product behaves outside controlled development conditions.

Regulatory intelligence should also continue after launch. Ingredient restrictions, labelling rules, environmental obligations, tax requirements, standards and enforcement priorities may change. A product that was compliant when notified may require reformulation, revised packaging or withdrawal under a later rule. The responsible operator should monitor relevant legislative and technical developments and assess their effect on the existing portfolio. This process should be documented so that action is based on structured review rather than late reaction.

Product review should occur periodically even where no serious complaint has emerged. The review may include complaint trends, adverse events, batch failures, stability data, supplier performance, manufacturing deviations, regulatory changes and sales information. The purpose is to determine whether the original risk assessment remains valid, whether the specification is still appropriate and whether any preventive action is justified. A product that has remained on the market for several years should not continue solely because it has not yet triggered enforcement.

Continued stability monitoring is part of stewardship. Real-time studies may still be in progress after launch, and their results should be reviewed as they become available. Market-retained samples can also be examined to determine whether commercial storage and distribution produce changes not observed under controlled conditions. If later data show faster nicotine degradation, packaging interaction or device deterioration than expected, the shelf life or storage instructions may need revision.

Supplier performance should remain under review because changes in raw materials or components can alter the product after launch. Certificates of analysis, incoming results, deviations, complaint support and change notifications should be assessed regularly. A supplier that was suitable at initial qualification may become less reliable through ownership change, process transfer, raw-material substitution or declining quality control. Product stewardship therefore includes requalification, auditing and replacement where necessary.

Change control protects the marketed product from uncontrolled modification. Commercial pressure may encourage cost reductions, new suppliers, revised flavours, altered coils or different packaging. Each proposed change should be assessed for its effect on formulation, emissions, stability, safety, labelling and notification status. Stewardship requires that the decision be made from the perspective of the whole lifecycle rather than only immediate cost or availability.

Corrective and preventive action should follow where evidence identifies a weakness. Corrective action addresses the specific problem, while preventive action reduces the chance of recurrence or similar failure elsewhere. Actions may include supplier correction, revised manufacturing controls, tighter specifications, additional testing, packaging redesign, updated instructions, retraining, notification amendment or market withdrawal. The effectiveness of each action should be checked rather than assumed.

Recall and withdrawal procedures should be established in advance. A recall may be necessary where a product presents a significant safety or compliance concern, while a withdrawal may remove non-conforming stock before it reaches consumers. The procedure should define authority, decision criteria, communication, stock control, regulator contact, effectiveness checks and final reconciliation. Delayed action can increase harm and regulatory exposure, particularly where internal approval chains are unclear.

Stewardship also includes responsible communication. Product claims, retailer materials, online content and consumer guidance should remain consistent with the product's evidence and regulatory category. Marketing should not overstate reduced-risk findings, imply medicinal authorisation or minimise nicotine-related risks. Where new information changes the understanding of the product, communications should be revised. A company cannot claim to exercise stewardship while promoting the product in a manner disconnected from its technical evidence.

Youth access and unintended uptake form part of this responsibility. Age-verification systems, retailer controls, product presentation, flavour naming, imagery and sponsorship should be assessed for their potential to attract minors or nicotine-naive consumers. Stewardship does not require the product to become commercially invisible, but it does require active consideration of who is likely to be reached by the marketing and how the product is framed. A product designed for adult smokers should be presented consistently with that intended population.

Consumer education can reduce misuse and improve product performance. Clear instructions on filling, charging, coil replacement, storage, handling leaks and disposal may prevent avoidable incidents. Information should be practical and proportionate rather than buried within technical language. Where users commonly make the same error, the company should consider whether the design or instructions are inadequate rather than simply repeating warnings.

Environmental responsibility is increasingly connected to product stewardship. Batteries, electronics, plastics, nicotine residues and packaging may create waste-management concerns. The producer should consider recyclability, take-back schemes, component separation, labelling and compliance with relevant waste obligations. Single-use products create particular scrutiny because their commercial convenience can conflict with environmental policy. Stewardship therefore includes decisions about product format as well as end-of-life instructions.

Counterfeit and diverted products can also affect the reputation and safety profile of the legitimate brand. Packaging security, traceable identifiers, authorised distribution and retailer education can help distinguish genuine products from imitations. Reports of suspected counterfeit goods should be investigated because consumers may attribute failures to the legitimate manufacturer. Cooperation with enforcement bodies may be necessary where illicit products use the same branding.

Stewardship should be risk-based across the product portfolio. Products with higher nicotine content, more complex electronics, larger sales volume or a history of complaints may require more intensive monitoring. New products may need enhanced surveillance during the first months of sale. Mature, stable products may justify lower review frequency, provided that no new signal or regulatory change has emerged. Resources should be directed towards the products and issues capable of causing the greatest harm.

Governance is essential because stewardship crosses regulatory, quality, technical, commercial and customer-service functions. Responsibilities should be assigned clearly, with defined escalation routes and authority to stop supply where necessary. Senior management should receive meaningful information about significant incidents, trends and unresolved risks. A stewardship system cannot function where quality concerns are routinely overridden by sales pressure.

Records should demonstrate the operation of the system. Complaint logs, investigation reports, trend analyses, regulatory reviews, CAPA records, recall exercises, supplier reviews and periodic product assessments should be retained in the technical file or linked quality system. These documents show whether the company has maintained control after launch. They also provide evidence during inspection that post-market responsibility is active rather than nominal.

The original risk assessment should be treated as a living document. New evidence may alter the likelihood or severity assigned to a hazard. A rare failure may become more important after market expansion increases exposure. A previously unknown material interaction may emerge through ageing. Conversely, sustained experience may show that some anticipated risks are effectively controlled. The assessment should evolve with the evidence rather than remaining fixed at the pre-market stage.

Product stewardship is ultimately the practical expression of continuing responsibility. It recognises that no development programme can predict every condition of real-world use and that compliance must be maintained through observation, review and intervention. A product is not responsibly managed simply because it passed its initial tests or appeared in a notification database. It is responsibly managed when the company remains capable of tracing it, understanding its performance, correcting its weaknesses and withdrawing it when continued supply can no longer be justified.

Maintaining Compliance Through the Product Lifecycle

Maintaining compliance through the product lifecycle requires the manufacturer or responsible operator to preserve alignment between the product originally designed, the product documented in the technical file, the product notified to the regulator and the product actually supplied to consumers. Compliance can be lost after launch even where the initial submission was accurate. Ingredients may change, suppliers may alter specifications, device components may be substituted, packaging may be revised, manufacturing processes may drift and new regulatory requirements may emerge. Lifecycle compliance therefore depends on continuing control rather than a one-time demonstration of conformity.

The central principle is that the marketed product must remain the same controlled product that was assessed and declared. This does not mean that no change is permitted. Products may need to evolve in response to supply constraints, performance improvements, regulatory developments or market feedback. The requirement is that each change is identified, assessed, approved and documented before implementation. The company must understand whether the proposed modification affects product identity, safety, emissions, stability, labelling, notification status or manufacturing control. Informal changes made through purchasing, production or marketing can create regulatory divergence without being recognised as such.

Change control is therefore the main mechanism through which lifecycle compliance is preserved. Every proposed change should enter a formal process that records what is changing, why it is necessary, which product versions and markets are affected and what evidence is required. The review should involve the relevant technical, quality, regulatory and commercial functions. A supplier change may require new certificates, incoming testing and stability bridging. A coil change may require emissions or performance testing. A new bottle may require compatibility, child-resistance and leakage assessment. A revised claim may require legal and scientific review. The decision should be completed before the change reaches production.

Changes should be classified according to significance. Some may be administrative, such as correction of a typographical error that does not alter legal meaning. Others may be minor but still require documentation, such as a controlled artwork adjustment or equivalent packaging source. More substantial changes may affect formulation, nicotine concentration, device performance, reservoir capacity, emissions or intended use. These may require updated notification, a new submission or a separate product identity. The classification should be justified rather than selected to avoid additional regulatory work.

The product specification must remain current throughout this process. Approved ingredient lists, component drawings, manufacturing instructions, test methods, packaging artwork and acceptance criteria should be revised together where necessary. Partial updates create inconsistency. A formulation may be changed in the production record while the toxicological assessment and notification still describe the previous version. A label may be revised while the technical file retains obsolete warnings. Document control should ensure that all dependent records are identified and updated as part of the same change.

Version control allows the company to demonstrate which product configuration was supplied at any point in time. Every specification, formulation, label and technical record should carry a revision number, effective date and approval history. Historical versions should remain retrievable. Batch records should show which approved version was used. This is essential during complaint investigation, inspection and recall because the current specification may not describe a product manufactured months or years earlier.

Supplier management remains active after launch. Approved suppliers should be monitored through incoming inspection, certificates of analysis, audit findings, deviations, complaints and responsiveness to technical questions. Requalification may be necessary where performance declines or where a supplier undergoes significant change. Written agreements should continue to require advance notification of changes to raw-material source, processing method, manufacturing location, carrier system, specification or sub-supplier.

The manufacturer should not assume that a material remains unchanged because the trade name and catalogue number are the same. Flavour compositions, nicotine sources, plastics, adhesives, coils and batteries may be altered without obvious commercial distinction. Supplier declarations should therefore be reviewed critically, and critical materials may require periodic verification testing. Where a change is discovered after implementation, the company should assess affected batches, determine whether the technical file remains valid and decide whether market action is required.

Manufacturing control also requires periodic review. A process that performed consistently at launch may drift over time through equipment wear, operator variation, maintenance gaps or increased production volume. In-process results, batch failures, yield changes and release data should be trended. Repeated small deviations can indicate loss of control before a formal out-of-specification result occurs. Preventive maintenance, calibration, training and process verification should therefore continue throughout the product's commercial life.

Scaling production may introduce new risks. A formulation developed in small batches may mix differently at commercial volume. Filling accuracy may change with faster equipment. New manufacturing sites may use different environmental controls or process sequences. Each scale or site transfer should be assessed and validated to confirm that the approved product can still be reproduced consistently. The existence of an established formula does not guarantee equivalent manufacture under different conditions.

Finished-product testing should remain proportionate to risk and process performance. Routine release testing may include nicotine concentration, fill volume, appearance, leakage, resistance, packaging checks and label verification. Periodic testing may cover parameters that are less likely to vary batch by batch but remain important, such as emissions, material verification or selected impurities. Testing frequency can be adjusted where justified by historical control, but it should not be reduced solely for cost reasons.

Ongoing stability studies provide evidence that the marketed product continues to meet its shelf-life claim. Real-time data should be reviewed as they become available, particularly where the original launch relied partly on accelerated results. Annual or periodic stability commitments may be appropriate for selected production batches. Trends in nicotine degradation, colour, pH, leakage, packaging integrity and device function should be assessed against the approved limits. A stability failure may require reduced shelf life, revised storage instructions or withdrawal of affected stock.

Figure 2.2. Building a Compliant Product: Product Specification Map.

The product specification is the controlled description of the formulation, device, packaging and intended use. It links ingredient selection and toxicological justification with approved suppliers, raw-material specifications, certificates of analysis and change notification. Stability and compatibility evidence support shelf life, storage conditions and the continued suitability of the formulation, container and closure system. Documentation connects the master specification to test reports, technical files, labels and batch records, while product stewardship maintains traceability, vigilance, corrective action and periodic review after market entry. The specification is therefore more than a recipe: it is the central record connecting product composition, evidence, manufacturing control and continuing regulatory responsibility.

Figure 2.2 Building a Compliant Product: Product Specification Map

Links ingredient selection, suppliers, stability, documentation and stewardship.

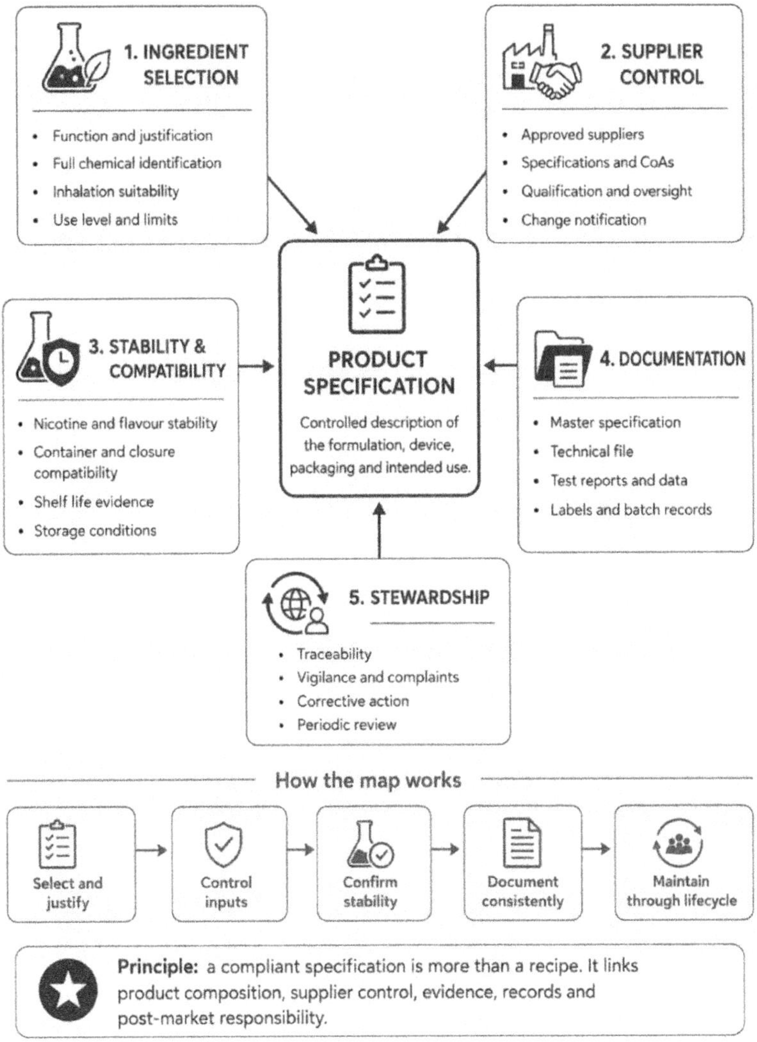

Post-market data should be integrated into lifecycle control. Complaints, adverse events, returns, distributor feedback, retailer reports and regulator findings may reveal issues not detected during development. These records should be trended by product, batch, market and failure type. A single report may not justify action, but repeated patterns can indicate a design, supplier, manufacturing or labelling problem. The company should define thresholds for escalation and ensure that serious incidents are reviewed promptly.

Periodic product review can bring these data together. A structured review may examine production performance, deviations, complaints, adverse events, supplier changes, stability data, regulatory developments and corrective actions. The review should determine whether the product specification remains appropriate, whether the original risk assessment is still valid and whether additional control is required. The frequency may depend on sales volume, complexity and risk, but every active product should be subject to continuing oversight.

Risk assessment should be updated whenever new information changes the understanding of the product. A hazard considered unlikely at launch may become more significant after wider use. A packaging failure may increase accidental exposure risk. A new toxicological finding may alter the assessment of an ingredient. A regulatory authority may identify an emerging concern involving a component or product category. Lifecycle risk management requires the company to respond to this evidence rather than relying permanently on the original assessment.

Regulatory intelligence is equally important. Laws, guidance, technical standards, tax rules, environmental obligations and enforcement priorities change. A product can become non-compliant even if its composition remains unchanged. The responsible operator should monitor relevant developments in every market where the product is sold. Proposed restrictions may require early reformulation or packaging redesign, while new reporting requirements may require changes to data systems or submission records.

Regulatory monitoring should include more than enacted legislation. Consultations, draft standards, authority notices, court decisions, enforcement actions and industry alerts can provide advance warning of change. Early review allows the company to assess commercial impact, plan development and avoid abrupt withdrawal. The process should be assigned to named personnel and recorded so that relevant developments are not dependent on informal awareness.

Notification maintenance is part of lifecycle compliance. The product record should be updated where required to reflect approved changes, corrected information or new responsible-operator details. Public databases should be checked for accuracy. Submission accounts and product identifiers should remain accessible even when staff or consultants change. Regulatory correspondence, confirmation receipts and update histories should be retained within the technical file.

The company should also monitor whether the product is being sold in the markets and configurations originally intended. Cross-border distribution, online marketplaces and unauthorised resellers may place products into jurisdictions for which they were not notified or labelled. Diversion can expose the manufacturer to regulatory and reputational risk. Distribution agreements, market checks and product coding can help identify where stock is moving and whether regional variants are being supplied correctly.

Packaging and claims require continuing control because marketing materials often evolve more quickly than technical products. Websites, social media, retailer content and promotional campaigns should remain consistent with the approved product position. New claims should be reviewed for evidential support and legal classification. A consumer vaping product can acquire medicinal or unsupported risk claims through marketing even where the physical product remains unchanged. Compliance review should therefore extend beyond the carton and label.

Instructions should also be revised where post-market experience shows that consumers are misunderstanding the product. Repeated charging errors, leakage caused by overfilling or confusion over coil replacement may indicate that the instructions or design are inadequate. The response should not be limited to blaming user behaviour. The company should assess whether clearer communication, redesign or additional control is necessary.

Corrective and preventive action connects identified problems to improvement. Corrective action addresses the immediate non-conformity, while preventive action reduces the risk of recurrence or similar failure elsewhere. Actions may involve supplier correction, process change, additional testing, retraining, specification tightening, design modification, packaging revision or notification update. Each action should have an owner, target date and effectiveness check.

A corrective action is not complete merely because a new procedure has been issued. The company should confirm that the action worked. Complaint rates may need to be monitored, new batches tested or supplier performance reviewed. Where the action fails, the investigation should be reopened. This discipline prevents recurring defects from being closed administratively without genuine resolution.

Recall and withdrawal readiness must be maintained throughout the product lifecycle. Contact lists, decision authority, batch records, distribution data and communication templates should remain current. Mock recalls can test whether affected stock can be identified and recovered within an acceptable period. A company that cannot locate its product in the supply chain cannot manage serious non-compliance effectively.

The decision to recall should be based on risk, legal obligation and evidence rather than commercial reluctance. Where a defect presents a meaningful safety concern, incorrect nicotine concentration, prohibited ingredient, battery hazard or material labelling failure, prompt action may be required. The scope should be proportionate to the affected batches and markets, but uncertainty should not be used to justify delay where the potential consequences are serious.

Environmental and end-of-life obligations can also change during the commercial life of the product. Requirements concerning batteries, electronic waste, packaging, producer responsibility and single-use formats may be introduced or strengthened. Product stewardship should therefore consider whether the design remains viable from an environmental and regulatory perspective. A product that becomes difficult to recycle, recover or lawfully dispose of may require redesign even if its immediate performance remains acceptable.

Counterfeit products and unauthorised modifications create additional lifecycle challenges. Consumers may refill closed pods, combine incompatible components or purchase imitation products bearing the same branding. These behaviours may produce incidents attributed to the legitimate manufacturer. Security features, clear compatibility instructions, authorised distribution and cooperation with enforcement bodies can help reduce the risk, although they cannot eliminate it entirely.

Training should remain current across the organisation. Regulatory, quality, manufacturing, customer-service, sales and marketing teams need to understand the controls relevant to their roles. New employees should not rely on informal knowledge. Training records should show that changes in specifications, procedures and legal requirements have been communicated. A well-designed system can still fail where personnel do not understand how or why it operates.

Senior management oversight is necessary because lifecycle compliance often competes with commercial pressure. Supply shortages, launch commitments and cost reductions may encourage uncontrolled substitution or delayed action. Management should receive information on significant deviations, complaint trends, regulatory changes and unresolved risks. It should also ensure that quality and regulatory functions have authority to stop production or supply where necessary.

Product discontinuation should be managed as carefully as launch. Remaining stock, stability, complaints, regulatory records, spare components and customer support may continue after production ends. The company should determine how long documentation will be retained, how market stock will be monitored and how late complaints or incidents will be investigated. Notifications may need to be withdrawn or marked inactive, while legal record-retention periods may extend for several years.

The technical file should therefore remain available after the final unit has been sold. Historical specifications, batch records, test results, supplier records and post-market data may still be required by regulators or during litigation and complaint investigation. Closure of a supplier, manufacturer or brand does not eliminate the need for traceable records where the responsible entity continues to exist.

Maintaining compliance through the product lifecycle is ultimately a process of preserving control while the product, market and regulatory environment continue to change. The manufacturer must be able to recognise when the product has changed, when the evidence has changed and when the law has changed. It must then determine whether existing controls remain adequate and act before divergence becomes non-compliance.

A product remains compliant not because it once passed testing or completed notification, but because every subsequent batch, change, claim and market decision remains connected to the approved specification and supporting evidence. Lifecycle compliance is therefore the continuing demonstration that the product supplied today is still understood, controlled and justified on the same disciplined basis as the product originally placed on the market.

CHAPTER 3

Toxicology Within Regulation

Toxicology enters regulation at the point where scientific uncertainty must be converted into a decision that can be defended. The regulator, manufacturer and toxicologist rarely have the luxury of complete evidence, particularly for products built from complex mixtures, rapidly changing formulations and devices capable of altering exposure through heat, power, airflow and consumer behaviour. A vaping product may contain dozens of identified ingredients, hundreds of flavour constituents and a hardware system that introduces further variables through metals, polymers, wicks, coils and electrical controls. Some substances have extensive toxicological histories, others have been studied only through oral exposure, and many have little or no useful inhalation evidence. The aerosol may also contain compounds that were absent from the original liquid because they formed during heating, oxidation or interaction with the device. Regulation must nevertheless reach a conclusion: whether the product can enter the market, whether its composition is sufficiently characterised, whether its remaining risks are acceptable and whether further evidence or control is required. Toxicology within regulation is therefore not the search for a single declaration of safety. It is the disciplined construction of an evidence-based position from hazards, exposures, uncertainties, analogies and limitations that are rarely distributed evenly across the product.

The starting point is hazard identification, but hazard is only the beginning of the regulatory question. A substance may be corrosive, sensitising, genotoxic, carcinogenic, systemically toxic or capable of causing respiratory irritation, yet the significance of that property depends on the route, concentration, duration and pattern of exposure. Regulatory toxicology must distinguish the inherent capacity to cause harm from the conditions under which harm becomes plausible. That distinction is essential in vaping because ingredient lists can appear alarming when read as inventories of isolated chemical hazards, while apparently reassuring formulations can conceal relevant risks if exposure, heating and device performance are ignored. The presence of a hazardous substance does not automatically establish unacceptable product risk, but neither does a low nominal concentration remove the need to understand aerosol transfer or repeated use. Hazard identification should therefore be broad enough to recognise structural alerts, known respiratory effects, impurities, degradation products and foreseeable interactions, while remaining connected to the actual product rather than becoming a catalogue of every theoretical effect ever reported for its constituent chemicals.

Ingredient risk assessment develops that initial screen into a product-specific evaluation. Each ingredient must be considered by identity, purity, function, concentration, likely aerosol transfer, thermal behaviour and relevance to inhalation. Food use, fragrance use or cosmetic acceptance may provide information about identity and systemic toxicity, but it does not establish respiratory suitability. The gastrointestinal tract, skin and respiratory system present different barriers, metabolic capacities and patterns of exposure, and substances that are tolerated after ingestion may irritate or damage respiratory tissue when deposited directly in the airway. The same caution applies to labels such as natural, botanical or food-grade, which describe source or commercial quality rather than inhalation safety. A credible assessment asks why the ingredient is present, whether a better-characterised alternative exists, what evidence supports its use and whether the chosen concentration is the lowest reasonably necessary to achieve the intended function. Ingredient review should also recognise that flavour systems are not passive additions. They can alter pH, viscosity, sensory response, aerosol generation, coil deposits and the production of secondary emissions, making formulation toxicology inseparable from device performance.

The literature review is the principal mechanism through which existing knowledge is assembled, but its reliability depends on how the evidence is searched, selected and interpreted. A regulatory review should not begin with a desired conclusion and collect only those publications that support it. It should define the substances, endpoints, routes and exposure conditions of interest, search across relevant databases and distinguish primary studies from reviews, alerts, opinions and secondary reporting. Study quality matters as much as study outcome. Experimental concentration, test system, species, duration, analytical confirmation, controls and relevance to human inhalation must all be considered. A dramatic cellular response at a concentration far beyond plausible exposure may identify a biological hazard without predicting real-world risk. Conversely, a negative study using an insensitive assay or poorly characterised material may provide little reassurance. Vaping research presents additional difficulties because products and methods vary greatly. Results obtained from an obsolete high-voltage device, unrealistic dry-coil conditions or an uncharacterised liquid cannot be transferred automatically to all products. Literature review must therefore separate what a study demonstrates directly from what it merely suggests, while preserving evidence that may still be valuable for identifying mechanisms, susceptible endpoints or priorities for further testing.

Where direct data are missing, read-across methodologies offer a way to use information from structurally or biologically related substances, but similarity must be demonstrated rather than asserted. Two chemicals may share a functional group yet differ substantially in volatility, reactivity, metabolism or respiratory potency. A defensible read-across identifies the source and target substances, explains the basis of similarity, compares physicochemical properties, considers common metabolites or mechanisms and addresses differences that could make the target more hazardous. It should also explain why the selected analogue is more appropriate than other available candidates. Read-across becomes particularly important for flavour ingredients because many have limited inhalation datasets, while related compounds may have useful information from occupational toxicology, repeated-dose studies, irritation testing or metabolic research. Its purpose is not to manufacture certainty where none exists, but to make structured use of relevant evidence while recording uncertainty openly. Modern regulatory practice increasingly accepts grouping, read-across and other non-animal approaches when they are scientifically justified, although weak analogies remain vulnerable to rejection because structural resemblance alone does not establish equivalent toxicological behaviour.

A weight-of-evidence approach becomes necessary when no single study can answer the regulatory question. Evidence may come from chemical structure, physicochemical properties, in vitro assays, human observations, occupational exposure, animal studies, computational models, analytical emissions data and information from related substances. These sources differ in reliability and relevance, and they should not be counted as though each contributes equally. A well-reasoned assessment gives greater weight to evidence that is methodologically sound, directly relevant to the route and product and consistent with other findings. Conflicting results should be examined for differences in material identity, exposure conditions, dose, model sensitivity and study quality rather than averaged into an artificial compromise. Consistency strengthens a conclusion, but inconsistency can also be informative where it reveals a threshold, susceptible condition or methodological limitation. Weight of evidence is not a phrase used to conceal judgement. It is a transparent explanation of how multiple incomplete sources were combined, why some were given greater influence and how uncertainty affected the final decision.

Exposure assessment is the point at which the product itself becomes inseparable from toxicology. Ingredient concentration in the liquid is not the same as concentration in the aerosol, and aerosol concentration is not the same as the dose deposited in the user. Transfer depends on volatility, formulation, device power, coil temperature, puff duration, airflow, liquid supply and chemical reaction during heating. Consumer use introduces further variability through puff frequency, intensity, device maintenance, product switching and compensatory behaviour. An exposure estimate must therefore define the product, operating conditions, analytical method and assumptions used. It may calculate exposure per puff, per session, per day or over a longer period, but the chosen metric should match the toxicological endpoint being evaluated. Conservative assumptions can protect against underestimation, although excessive conservatism can produce exposure scenarios so remote from real use that they cease to support proportionate decision-making. The strongest assessment uses measured product-specific emissions where available, realistic upper-bound use patterns and clearly separated normal-use and stress conditions.

Margin-of-exposure analysis provides one method of relating estimated human exposure to a dose associated with a defined toxicological effect. The margin is commonly derived by comparing a point of departure, such as a benchmark dose or no-observed-adverse-effect level, with the estimated exposure from the product. A larger margin generally indicates greater separation between the experimental effect level and anticipated human exposure, but the numerical result cannot be interpreted without understanding the evidence behind both sides of the calculation. The point of departure may come from oral rather than inhalation data, from a short-duration study, from a different species or from an endpoint of uncertain relevance. The exposure estimate may depend on transfer assumptions, body weight, frequency of use and analytical sensitivity. Uncertainty factors may be required to account for interspecies differences, human variability, duration and database limitations. Margin of exposure is therefore a decision-support tool rather than a universal pass-or-fail threshold. It can help prioritise substances, compare formulation options and identify where exposure reduction is needed, but it should not be used to create false precision from weak inputs.

Missing inhalation data remain one of the defining limitations of vaping toxicology. The number of possible flavour compounds and combinations is far greater than the number supported by robust repeated-inhalation studies, and conventional testing cannot realistically fill every gap one substance at a time. This creates a tension between the need to protect consumers and the ethical, scientific and practical limits of generating new animal data. The appropriate response is not to treat absence of evidence as proof of safety or proof of harm, but to apply a tiered strategy. Existing information can be screened for respiratory hazards, structural alerts and occupational limits; computational methods can identify likely reactivity or metabolism; in vitro respiratory models can assess irritation, cytotoxicity, oxidative stress and other relevant responses; analytical studies can determine whether the substance transfers to aerosol or generates harmful products; and exposure-based considerations can establish whether predicted doses are sufficiently low to reduce concern. Higher-tier testing should be reserved for questions that remain important after these stages. ECHA continues to identify read-across and new approach methodologies as important means of generating hazard and exposure information while reducing unnecessary animal testing, reflecting a broader regulatory movement towards evidence integration rather than automatic reliance on traditional whole-animal studies.

Animal testing alternatives are therefore not a concession made after conventional toxicology has failed, but an increasingly central part of modern evidence generation. Human-relevant cell systems, reconstructed airway tissues, organotypic cultures, organ-on-chip platforms, computational toxicology, quantitative structure–activity relationships and adverse outcome pathways can examine mechanisms that conventional studies may detect only indirectly. These approaches can compare formulations rapidly, identify high-risk ingredients and support decisions before products reach advanced development. Their limitations must still be understood. In vitro systems may not reproduce whole-body metabolism, chronic adaptation, immune interactions or long-term disease development, while computational predictions depend on the quality and applicability of their training data. A non-animal method is not automatically superior because it is modern, just as an animal study is not automatically decisive because it is traditional. Regulatory value depends on validation, biological relevance, exposure realism and integration with the wider evidence base.

The final difficulty lies in the distance between regulatory interpretation and scientific reality. Regulation requires categories, deadlines, documentary standards and decisions that can be enforced consistently, while science often produces probabilities, ranges and conclusions that remain conditional. A regulator may need to decide whether a product dossier is sufficient even when long-term epidemiology is unavailable. A manufacturer may need to reformulate because an ingredient cannot be justified, despite the absence of direct evidence that it has harmed consumers. A study may identify cellular effects without demonstrating clinical disease, while policy debate may present the result as proof of either danger or safety. The toxicologist working within regulation must resist both simplification and paralysis. Scientific uncertainty should not be hidden, but neither should it be used to prevent every decision. The task is to distinguish known hazard from plausible risk, plausible risk from speculative concern and genuine data gaps from demands for evidence that no realistic product could ever satisfy.

This chapter examines how that judgement is constructed in practice, beginning with hazard identification and progressing through ingredient assessment, literature review, read-across, weight of evidence, exposure estimation and margins of exposure before confronting the persistent absence of inhalation data and the expanding role of non-animal methods. These elements do not operate as separate exercises. Hazard information guides literature searching; literature determines whether read-across is necessary; read-across contributes to weight of evidence; exposure determines the relevance of identified hazards; margins of exposure help translate evidence into risk-management priorities; and data gaps determine whether further testing, reformulation or precaution is justified. Regulatory interpretation then brings those strands together and decides what the evidence is sufficient to support. Toxicology within regulation is therefore neither pure laboratory science nor administrative compliance. It is the controlled point at which chemical evidence, product exposure, public-health purpose and legal responsibility are required to meet.

Figure 3.1. Toxicology Within Regulation: Regulatory Toxicology Pathway.

The regulatory toxicology pathway begins with hazard identification and product-specific ingredient assessment before progressing through literature review, read-across, weight-of-evidence evaluation and exposure assessment. Margin-of-exposure analysis then helps place identified hazards into the context of likely consumer exposure. Missing inhalation data do not interrupt the process but increase reliance on structured read-across, exposure-based reasoning and integrated evidence, while validated non-animal methods can contribute mechanistic and screening information across several stages. The final regulatory interpretation brings these strands together to determine whether the available evidence supports market entry, additional controls, reformulation, further testing or rejection of the product.

Toxicology Within Regulation

Regulatory toxicology pathway

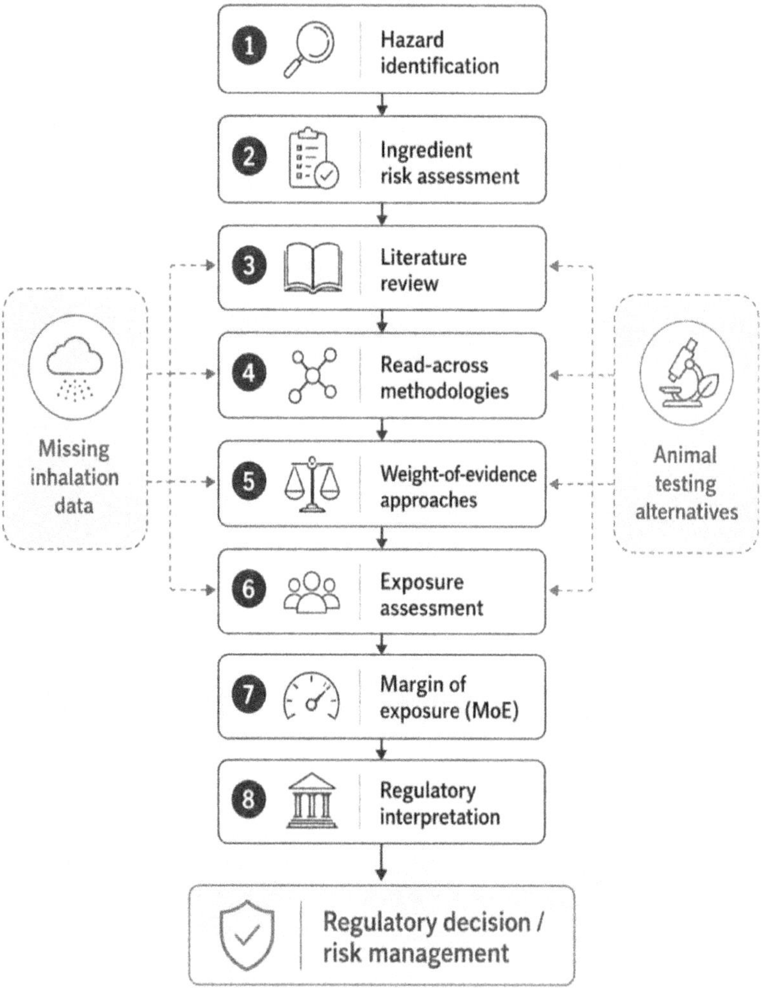

Hazard Identification

Hazard identification is the first formal stage of regulatory toxicology because no meaningful assessment can begin until the potentially harmful properties of the product, its ingredients, its emissions and its constituent materials have been recognised and described. The task is broader than listing substances that appear on a formulation sheet and narrower than attempting to predict every possible adverse outcome under every conceivable condition. It requires the toxicologist to identify which chemical, physical and biological hazards are relevant to the actual product, the route of exposure and the intended pattern of use, while distinguishing credible concerns from remote theoretical possibilities. In vaping products this process is particularly demanding because the product presented to the consumer is not simply the liquid placed in a bottle or pod. It is a dynamic aerosol-generating system in which formulation, device power, coil material, wick behaviour, airflow, temperature, puffing pattern and user maintenance interact to determine what is ultimately inhaled. Hazard identification must therefore begin with the complete product as used, not with the unheated liquid considered in isolation.

The first distinction that must be preserved is the difference between hazard and risk. Hazard describes the inherent capacity of an agent or condition to cause harm, while risk describes the likelihood and severity of that harm occurring under defined exposure circumstances. Nicotine is intrinsically pharmacologically active and toxic at sufficient dose, but the risk associated with a specific product depends on concentration, total available quantity, packaging, route of exposure and actual use. A flavouring substance may be a respiratory irritant, yet the relevance of that hazard depends on how much transfers into the aerosol and how often the product is used. A metal may be present in a device component without appearing at a meaningful level in emissions, while another metal may migrate into aerosol through heating, corrosion or manufacturing residue. Hazard identification should therefore be deliberately sensitive, because failing to recognise a relevant hazard at the outset weakens every later stage, but it should not collapse immediately into a conclusion that the product is unacceptable. The purpose is to identify what requires evaluation, control or further evidence.

The starting point is a complete and accurate description of the product. Hazard identification cannot be reliable where the formulation is incomplete, proprietary mixtures are only described by trade name, component materials are unknown or the intended device configuration has not been fixed. Each ingredient should be identified by a recognised chemical name, Chemical Abstracts Service number where available, concentration, function, purity and supplier specification. The device should be described in terms of coil composition, wick material, reservoir, battery, electrical controls, plastics, seals, adhesives and any other materials in contact with the liquid or aerosol pathway. Packaging should also be considered because interaction with containers, closures and elastomers can introduce migration, leakage or contamination hazards that are not apparent from the formulation alone. The quality of hazard identification is therefore dependent on the quality of product definition; a vague product identity produces an equally vague toxicological conclusion.

Ingredient hazards form the most obvious part of the assessment. Nicotine, propylene glycol, glycerol, water, acids, flavour compounds, sweeteners and processing aids each require consideration, but their toxicological significance differs considerably. Nicotine presents pharmacological and acute toxicity concerns, particularly through accidental ingestion, dermal contact or exposure of children. Propylene glycol and glycerol are widely used substances with substantial histories of exposure, but heating can generate aldehydes and other degradation products under certain conditions. Acids used to form nicotine salts may alter pH, sensory response and aerosol chemistry. Flavour compounds can include aldehydes, ketones, esters, alcohols, lactones, terpenes and other substances with widely varying toxicological profiles. Some have known irritation or sensitisation potential, some possess structural alerts, some are poorly studied by inhalation and some may be relatively unremarkable at the exposure levels expected. Hazard identification requires the assessor to examine each substance without assuming that a common commercial category implies common safety.

The route of exposure is fundamental. A substance may have a long history of safe use in food and still require careful consideration when inhaled because the lungs are not simply another route of administration. Oral exposure involves digestion, intestinal absorption, first-pass metabolism and elimination pathways that differ from those operating in the respiratory tract. The airway epithelium is directly exposed to aerosol droplets and vapour, and substances may interact with mucus, cilia, immune cells and delicate gas-exchange surfaces. A compound that is rapidly metabolised in the liver after ingestion may persist locally in respiratory tissue, while another that is harmless on the skin may irritate the airways when aerosolised. Hazard identification should therefore distinguish route-specific evidence from general toxicological information. Food-use status, fragrance approval or cosmetic history can contribute to understanding identity and systemic effects, but none can be treated as direct evidence of inhalation suitability.

Known classifications provide one important source of hazard information. Substances classified as carcinogenic, mutagenic, toxic to reproduction, acutely toxic, corrosive, sensitising or specifically toxic to target organs require particular scrutiny. Regulatory classifications, harmonised hazard statements, occupational exposure limits and authoritative evaluations can identify substances that should be excluded or tightly controlled. However, classification systems were often developed for industrial handling, oral exposure or high-dose scenarios rather than consumer inhalation through vaping products. Their relevance must therefore be interpreted carefully. A hazard classification should trigger investigation, not automatic extrapolation without regard to concentration, route or exposure. Equally, the absence of formal classification does not establish that a substance is safe, especially where the database is sparse or the substance has not been assessed comprehensively.

Respiratory irritation is one of the most relevant hazard categories because vaping products deliver aerosol directly to the airways. Irritants can cause coughing, throat discomfort, bronchial reactivity or inflammatory responses, and repeated low-level exposure may have different consequences from a single acute exposure. Ingredient assessment should examine evidence from inhalation studies, occupational reports, human sensory data, in vitro respiratory models and structurally related compounds. The concentration at which irritation occurs matters, as does the difference between local discomfort and tissue injury. Some ingredients may be included specifically because they produce a sensory effect, yet excessive harshness can indicate irritation rather than desirable product performance. Hazard identification should therefore consider whether the formulation relies on irritation to produce satisfaction and whether that effect can be reduced without undermining the intended function.

Sensitisation requires separate attention because the consequences of repeated exposure may increase over time rather than remain proportional to dose. A respiratory sensitiser can trigger immune-mediated responses after an individual becomes sensitised, and subsequent exposure may provoke symptoms at comparatively low concentrations. Direct inhalation data are often limited, so evidence may come from occupational settings, skin sensitisation data, structural alerts or related chemicals. Skin sensitisation does not automatically establish respiratory sensitisation, but it may indicate electrophilic reactivity or immune potential requiring further review. Where an ingredient has known sensitising properties and no compelling technical necessity, exclusion is usually easier to defend than reliance on uncertain exposure thresholds.

Genotoxicity and carcinogenicity represent high-concern endpoints because the possibility of irreversible harm changes the evidential standard. Genotoxic substances may damage DNA directly or indirectly, while carcinogenic substances may act through genotoxic or non-genotoxic mechanisms. Hazard identification should examine authoritative classifications, in vitro and in vivo genotoxicity data, metabolic activation, structural alerts and impurities. The significance of positive in vitro findings depends on assay quality, concentration, cytotoxicity and biological relevance, but they cannot be dismissed simply because consumer exposure is expected to be low. Where a substance presents a credible genotoxic concern, the preferred regulatory approach is generally avoidance or reduction to the lowest reasonably achievable level, particularly where the ingredient is not essential.

Reproductive and developmental toxicity may also be relevant because nicotine products can be used by individuals of reproductive age, including during unrecognised pregnancy. Nicotine itself has recognised developmental concerns, and packaging and warnings should reflect that hazard. Other ingredients may have reproductive or developmental data from animal studies or occupational exposure, although these datasets are often oral or systemic rather than inhalational. Hazard identification should record such evidence and consider whether estimated exposures are materially below effect levels. The assessment should not imply that adult-only marketing removes the need to consider pregnancy or reproductive risk, because actual consumer populations are rarely as controlled as intended-use statements suggest.

Systemic toxicity must be considered where substances can cross the respiratory epithelium and enter circulation. Potential target organs include the nervous system, liver, kidneys, cardiovascular system and blood. Nicotine is the clearest example because it has systemic pharmacological effects, but flavour constituents and contaminants may also contribute. Hazard identification should examine repeated-dose studies, toxicokinetics and evidence of bioavailability. The absence of visible local irritation does not exclude systemic toxicity, just as the presence of low systemic exposure does not exclude local airway effects. Local and systemic hazards should therefore be evaluated separately.

Thermal decomposition introduces a second layer of hazard beyond the original ingredient list. The chemistry of the liquid can change during aerosol generation, particularly under high power, poor wicking, low liquid level, restricted airflow or aged-coil conditions. Propylene glycol and glycerol can generate carbonyl compounds such as formaldehyde, acetaldehyde and acrolein. Flavour ingredients may degrade into aldehydes, acids or reactive intermediates. Sugars and sweeteners can contribute to deposits and alter coil temperature. Acids may influence decomposition pathways and nicotine volatility. Hazard identification should therefore include known and plausible thermal products, not merely parent compounds. This requires information from emissions testing, thermal screening, published literature and chemical reasoning.

The device can create hazards that do not arise from the formulation. Heating coils may release metals through corrosion, erosion or manufacturing residues, while solder, connectors and other metallic components can contribute additional elements. Plastics and elastomers may migrate compounds into the liquid or aerosol pathway, particularly under prolonged contact or elevated temperature. Wicks can retain processing residues, and adhesives may degrade or volatilise. Hazard identification should consider materials of construction and whether they are appropriate for repeated thermal cycling and contact with the formulation. A chemically acceptable liquid can become problematic in an inadequately controlled device, which is why device and formulation toxicology cannot be separated completely.

Battery and electrical hazards sit partly outside conventional chemical toxicology but remain relevant to the overall regulatory risk assessment. Overheating, short circuit, thermal runaway, fire and explosion can cause acute injury. The toxicologist may not be responsible for electrical engineering analysis, but hazard identification should ensure these risks are recognised and assigned to appropriate technical functions. The same applies to mechanical hazards such as sharp components, breakage, leakage or accidental activation. Regulatory toxicology should not become so focused on molecules that it overlooks the physical routes through which harm can occur.

Contamination and impurities also require systematic review. Raw materials may contain residual solvents, heavy metals, tobacco-specific nitrosamines, pesticides, microbial contaminants or process-related impurities. Nicotine quality can vary according to source and purification. Flavour systems may contain undeclared carriers or impurities. Manufacturing equipment may introduce cleaning residues, lubricants or cross-contamination from other products. Hazard identification should therefore examine supplier specifications, certificates of analysis, analytical verification and process controls. An ingredient may be acceptable in principle but unsuitable in practice because the supplied material does not meet the purity assumed in the toxicological assessment.

Degradation during storage adds another source of hazard. Nicotine oxidation, flavour breakdown, pH shift, interaction with oxygen and migration from packaging can alter the product over time. Some degradation products may affect sensory quality only, while others may have toxicological significance. Hazard identification should therefore be linked to stability studies and should consider the product at the end of its proposed shelf life, not merely when freshly manufactured. A product that becomes more irritating or chemically unstable during storage cannot be judged solely on initial release data.

Microbiological hazards are generally less prominent in conventional propylene-glycol and glycerol formulations because low water activity may inhibit growth, but they should not be dismissed automatically. Products containing higher water levels, botanical extracts or poorly controlled materials may be more vulnerable. Contamination can also arise from manufacturing environments, reusable containers or consumer handling. The relevance depends on formulation, process and packaging, but hazard identification should include microbiological risk where the product characteristics justify it.

Foreseeable misuse expands the hazard landscape because products are not always used exactly as intended. Consumers may operate devices at excessive power, use incompatible liquids, overfill reservoirs, continue using burnt coils, charge with unsuitable equipment or modify components. Closed systems may be refilled despite instructions. Products may be stored in hot vehicles, exposed to sunlight or left accessible to children. Hazard identification should distinguish plausible misuse from extreme abuse, but it should not assume perfect compliance with instructions. A risk that can arise predictably from normal consumer behaviour should be addressed through design, labelling or compatibility control rather than dismissed as misuse.

Accidental exposure routes require separate consideration because the risks differ from inhalation. Liquid nicotine may be swallowed, splashed into the eyes or absorbed through the skin. Leakage from pods or bottles can increase these hazards. The total nicotine content, concentration, closure design, fill volume and packaging integrity all influence severity and likelihood. Hazard identification should recognise that a product designed for inhalation can create its most serious acute hazard before aerosolisation occurs. This is particularly relevant where concentrated nicotine-containing liquids are supplied in forms that can be opened, spilled or transferred.

Population-specific hazards should also be recorded. Children, pregnant women, individuals with cardiovascular disease, people with asthma or respiratory sensitivity and nicotine-naive users may respond differently from the intended adult smoker population. A regulatory assessment may reasonably focus on intended users, but it should not ignore foreseeable exposure among others. Vulnerable groups may influence warning statements, packaging design, age restrictions and marketing controls. Hazard identification should not be distorted into a claim that every product must be safe for every individual, but it should recognise where certain populations face materially greater risk.

Youth appeal and initiation are not toxicological hazards in the narrow chemical sense, yet they influence regulatory interpretation because exposure among nicotine-naive adolescents changes the public-health context. Flavour naming, device appearance, concealability, packaging and promotional style can increase the likelihood of use by people for whom the product was not intended. Hazard identification in a broader product-stewardship framework should therefore include behavioural and population-level hazards alongside chemical and physical ones. This is not a substitute for exposure toxicology, but it recognises that the same product can produce different overall consequences depending on who uses it and why.

The literature review supporting hazard identification should be systematic enough to avoid selective interpretation. Sources may include regulatory databases, safety assessments, peer-reviewed studies, occupational reports, in vitro data, animal studies, case reports and information from structurally related substances. Each source should be evaluated for reliability and relevance. A study using an unidentified e-liquid, extreme device conditions or concentrations far above plausible exposure may still identify a hazard, but its value for product-specific risk assessment may be limited. Negative findings should also be scrutinised for assay sensitivity, exposure duration and analytical confirmation. Hazard identification is strengthened when it distinguishes between evidence of absence and absence of evidence.

Structural alerts and computational tools can help identify hazards where direct data are sparse. Chemical structures may indicate electrophilic reactivity, mutagenic potential, sensitisation or likely metabolism. Quantitative structure–activity relationships can support screening, but predictions depend on the applicability domain of the model and the quality of the underlying data. A positive prediction should trigger review rather than automatic rejection, while a negative prediction should not override strong empirical evidence. Computational methods are most useful when integrated with other evidence rather than treated as standalone conclusions.

Read-across can also contribute at the hazard-identification stage, particularly where related compounds share metabolic pathways or reactive functional groups. The choice of analogue should be justified carefully because superficial structural similarity can be misleading. Differences in volatility, lipophilicity, reactivity or metabolism may produce different respiratory outcomes. Hazard identification should use read-across to identify plausible concerns and data needs, while later stages determine whether the analogy is strong enough for quantitative assessment.

The output of hazard identification should be a structured hazard profile rather than a simple pass-or-fail statement. The profile should identify each relevant hazard, the evidence supporting it, the route of concern, the affected endpoint, the uncertainty and the next regulatory action. Some hazards may be controlled through concentration limits, supplier specifications, packaging or device design. Others may require emissions testing, additional literature review, read-across or exposure assessment. High-concern hazards may justify exclusion of the ingredient or component entirely. The process should therefore lead directly into risk assessment and product design decisions.

Prioritisation is essential because not every hazard warrants the same level of effort. Substances with severe endpoints, credible respiratory relevance, high concentration, high aerosol transfer or major data gaps should receive greater scrutiny. Low-level ingredients with extensive reassuring evidence may require less. Device-related hazards should be prioritised according to likelihood and consequence. A risk-based approach prevents the assessment from becoming an indiscriminate accumulation of data while ensuring that the most important issues are addressed thoroughly.

Hazard identification should also be iterative. New emissions data, stability results, supplier changes, complaints or scientific publications may reveal hazards not recognised initially. A formulation change can remove one concern and introduce another. A new coil can alter metal emissions or thermal behaviour. Post-market incidents may expose failure modes not observed during development. The hazard profile should therefore remain a living part of the technical file rather than a static document completed before launch and never revisited.

Documentation should make the reasoning transparent. The assessor should record which substances and components were reviewed, which evidence sources were used, how conflicting information was handled and why certain hazards were considered relevant or not relevant. Uncertainty should be described directly. Where no inhalation data exist, the document should say so and explain what alternative evidence supports the assessment. Where a hazard is controlled by low exposure, the exposure analysis should be referenced rather than implied. A strong hazard-identification record allows another competent reviewer to understand how the conclusions were reached and where the remaining weaknesses lie.

The most serious failure in hazard identification is not necessarily the presence of uncertainty, because uncertainty is unavoidable in complex product assessment. The greater failure is unrecognised uncertainty, particularly where incomplete composition, inadequate supplier disclosure or unsupported assumptions create false confidence. A robust process accepts that some evidence will remain imperfect but ensures that important gaps are visible and connected to conservative design, additional testing or restricted use. Scientific honesty is therefore a regulatory control in its own right.

Hazard identification ultimately determines the shape of the entire toxicological assessment. It defines which ingredients require closer review, which emissions need measurement, which analogues may be used, which endpoints should drive exposure analysis and which product features require engineering or packaging controls. Performed superficially, it reduces toxicology to a checklist of familiar hazards and leaves important interactions unexplored. Performed properly, it creates a coherent map of the ways in which the product could cause harm and the evidence needed to determine whether those possibilities are materially relevant.

The regulatory objective is not to demonstrate that the product contains no hazardous substances, because almost every functional consumer product involves substances or conditions capable of harm under some circumstances. The objective is to identify the hazards accurately enough that avoidable ones can be removed, necessary ones can be controlled and residual ones can be evaluated against realistic exposure. In this sense hazard identification is both scientific and practical. It converts the composition and operation of the product into a set of testable regulatory questions and establishes the foundation on which ingredient risk assessment, exposure assessment, margin-of-exposure analysis and final regulatory interpretation depend.

Ingredient Risk Assessment

Ingredient risk assessment converts the broad hazard profile of a vaping product into a substance-specific evaluation of whether each component can be justified at the concentration, purity and mode of use proposed. Hazard identification establishes what a chemical is capable of doing under some set of conditions, but ingredient risk assessment asks whether those hazardous properties are materially relevant within the finished product and whether the evidence is sufficient to support continued inclusion. The assessment must therefore move beyond simple ingredient lists, supplier declarations or generic statements of food use. It must connect chemical identity, toxicological profile, concentration, aerosol transfer, thermal behaviour, exposure frequency, product function and uncertainty within one defensible regulatory judgement. The central question is not whether an ingredient can ever cause harm, but whether its use in the specific formulation creates an avoidable or unacceptable risk when the product is manufactured, stored and used as intended and under reasonably foreseeable conditions.

The first requirement is complete identification. An ingredient cannot be assessed meaningfully if it is known only by a trade name, flavour description or commercial code. Each substance should be linked to a recognised chemical name, Chemical Abstracts Service number where available, molecular structure, function, concentration and supplier specification. For complex flavour mixtures, the responsible operator must obtain a full compositional breakdown, including carriers, solvents, process aids and known impurities. Commercial confidentiality can be protected through restricted access or direct disclosure arrangements, but it cannot justify ignorance. A manufacturer that does not know what is present cannot determine whether a restricted substance has been introduced, whether a sensitiser is present above a relevant threshold or whether a supplier reformulation has altered the toxicological profile.

Identity must also be linked to the actual material supplied. A chemical name alone does not describe grade, purity, stereochemistry, salt form, hydration state or impurity pattern. Nicotine of different origin or purification history may carry different impurity profiles. Flavour materials may use different carriers or stabilisers. Botanical extracts may vary according to plant source, harvest, extraction solvent and processing conditions. Two suppliers may sell materials under the same generic name while delivering meaningfully different products. The risk assessment should therefore be based on the approved specification and representative analytical data rather than on an abstract chemical identity detached from commercial reality.

Function should be documented because inclusion without a clear purpose is difficult to defend. Every ingredient should contribute something necessary to formulation, sensory performance, nicotine delivery, stability or manufacture. Nicotine provides pharmacological activity. Propylene glycol and glycerol control aerosol generation, viscosity and flavour delivery. Water may adjust fluidity and coil wetting. Acids influence nicotine protonation and sensory response. Flavour compounds provide aroma and taste, while antioxidants, sweeteners or other additives may be included for secondary technical effects.

The assessment should ask whether the function is legitimate, whether the concentration is proportionate and whether the same effect could be achieved using a better-characterised or lower-risk substance.

Unnecessary complexity should be treated as a risk factor. Every additional ingredient introduces another source of toxicological uncertainty, supplier variability, potential interaction and regulatory burden. Complex flavour systems may contain dozens or hundreds of substances, each present at a low level but collectively capable of altering aerosol chemistry, irritation potential and stability. The fact that each substance is individually below a concern threshold does not automatically establish that the mixture is acceptable. A disciplined formulation removes ingredients that do not provide a necessary function and avoids using excess flavour intensity to compensate for poor device performance or weak product design.

Concentration is central because toxicological significance is dose-dependent. The same ingredient may be acceptable at one level and difficult to justify at another. The assessment should use the actual target concentration and manufacturing tolerance, not a vague maximum or supplier recommendation. Where a proprietary flavour is used, the assessor must understand both the total flavour loading and the concentration of individual constituents. Broad categories such as "flavouring at 10 per cent" are inadequate because one formulation may contain mostly low-concern esters while another may contain aldehydes, diketones or sensitising compounds at materially different levels.

The assessment should also consider cumulative concentration where the same substance enters the formulation from multiple sources. Propylene glycol may be added as a base solvent and also arrive through flavour concentrates. Ethanol, water, acids or sweeteners may be present in more than one raw material. A compound that appears acceptable within each supplier blend may exceed the intended total when the full recipe is combined. The master formulation should therefore calculate aggregate concentration across all inputs, and the toxicological assessment should be based on the true finished-product level.

Purity and impurities can be as important as the main ingredient. A material may have an acceptable toxicological profile while carrying contaminants that create additional concern. Nicotine may contain tobacco alkaloids, degradation products, residual solvents or metals. Propylene glycol and glycerol may contain aldehydes or process-related impurities. Natural extracts may carry pesticides, allergens or microbiological contaminants. Device-contact materials may introduce leachables. The assessor should identify which impurities are plausible, whether supplier limits are adequate and whether verification testing is needed for critical materials.

Certificates of analysis should not be treated as complete evidence by default. They often report only a limited set of parameters and may omit contaminants that have not been tested. A statement of conformity to a pharmacopeial or food-grade specification may be useful, but the relevance of that grade to inhalation use should still be considered. The risk assessment should distinguish between confirmed absence, tested limits and unexamined possibilities. Where an impurity is toxicologically important, a specific analytical limit may be necessary within the raw-material specification.

The route of exposure must remain central throughout the assessment. Oral safety data can contribute to understanding systemic toxicity, metabolism and general hazard, but inhalation introduces different deposition, local effects and toxicokinetic pathways. A substance that is rapidly metabolised after ingestion may contact respiratory tissue directly before systemic processing. Local airway irritation, ciliary impairment, inflammatory signalling and sensitisation may occur at concentrations that would not produce significant oral toxicity. The risk assessment should therefore prioritise inhalation data where available and use route-to-route extrapolation cautiously where it is not.

Where only oral data exist, the assessor should consider absorption, metabolism, bioavailability and local effects before using them quantitatively. It may be possible to derive a conservative systemic estimate if the substance is well absorbed orally and inhalation is not expected to introduce a unique local hazard. This approach becomes weaker where the substance is reactive, poorly absorbed orally, rapidly metabolised in the liver or known to affect respiratory tissue directly. Route-to-route extrapolation should therefore be explained explicitly rather than hidden within a numerical calculation.

Dermal and ocular exposure may also be relevant because consumers can contact the liquid through leakage, refilling or accidental spillage. The ingredient assessment should identify substances capable of causing skin irritation, sensitisation or eye damage, particularly where the formulation is supplied in an open container. These hazards may not determine whether the ingredient can be inhaled, but they affect packaging, instructions, warnings and incident management. A complete product assessment therefore recognises that one ingredient may present different risks through different exposure routes.

Thermal behaviour distinguishes vaping ingredient assessment from conventional evaluation of an unheated consumer mixture. The product is intentionally heated, and the ingredient may decompose, react with other constituents or alter coil conditions. Aldehydes, esters, sugars, sweeteners, acids and terpenes may produce secondary compounds under elevated temperature. Some ingredients can increase residue formation, reduce wicking or contribute to overheating, thereby altering degradation of the carrier system as well as their own chemistry. The assessment should therefore consider both direct toxicity of the ingredient and indirect effects on aerosol generation.

Published thermal-decomposition information can support this review, but product-specific emissions data are often needed because behaviour depends on formulation and device conditions. An ingredient may appear stable under one laboratory method yet generate concerning products when used at higher power or with poor liquid supply. The assessor should understand the operating range of the intended device and identify whether normal use, upper-bound use and foreseeable stress conditions create different emission profiles. A substance should not be approved solely because it is stable in the bottle.

Aerosol transfer should be estimated or measured because liquid concentration does not equal inhaled dose. Highly volatile compounds may transfer efficiently, while less volatile substances may remain largely in the liquid or condense within the device. Some compounds may decompose before transfer. Others may be formed in the aerosol pathway despite being absent from the original formulation. Ingredient risk assessment should therefore use product-specific transfer data where available or conservative assumptions where it is not. The strength of the conclusion should reflect the quality of the transfer estimate.

Transfer efficiency may also vary with device power, puff duration, airflow and coil condition. A low-power pod and a high-power open system can produce different aerosol composition from the same liquid. Where a formulation is intended for use across several devices, the risk assessment should identify the range of plausible exposure and determine whether unrestricted compatibility can be justified. In some cases, product control may require limiting the formulation to specified hardware rather than assuming universal use.

Exposure assessment should consider realistic patterns of consumption. Daily liquid use, puff count, puff duration and frequency vary widely across consumers. Some users take occasional puffs, while others use the product continuously. Nicotine strength may influence compensatory behaviour, as users of lower-strength liquids can consume more liquid to achieve a similar pharmacological effect. A conservative upper-bound scenario is usually appropriate, but it should remain plausible. The risk assessment should distinguish between central estimates, high-use scenarios and extreme misuse rather than combining them into one opaque assumption.

Chronic exposure is particularly important for flavour ingredients because repeated use can continue for months or years. Acute irritation data may identify immediate effects but provide limited insight into long-term respiratory consequences. Where repeated-inhalation data are absent, the assessor should consider structural alerts, occupational experience, repeated-dose studies by other routes, mechanistic information and exposure magnitude. The absence of chronic evidence should increase uncertainty rather than automatically prevent use, but it may support lower concentration, substitution or additional monitoring.

Respiratory irritation should be evaluated carefully because it is a common but often poorly characterised endpoint. Some irritation is obvious through cough or throat discomfort, while subtler inflammatory effects may not produce immediate symptoms. Human sensory data can be useful, but tolerability does not equal absence of tissue effect. In vitro airway models, occupational limits and inhalation studies can provide additional evidence. The assessor should consider whether the ingredient contributes materially to the product's overall irritancy and whether the function can be achieved at a lower level.

Sensitisation presents a different challenge because no universally reliable threshold may exist for all substances, and susceptible individuals can respond at low exposure after sensitisation has occurred. Known respiratory sensitisers should be avoided where possible. Skin-sensitisation data, structural alerts and occupational reports may support concern even where direct respiratory evidence is absent. Where a substance has a credible sensitisation hazard and provides only a minor sensory benefit, exclusion is generally more defensible than attempting to justify continued use through uncertain exposure modelling.

Genotoxicity should be screened using available in vitro and in vivo data, structural alerts and authoritative evaluations. A positive genotoxic signal requires careful interpretation because assay conditions, cytotoxicity and metabolic activation can influence the result. However, credible genotoxic concern carries particular weight because DNA damage may not have a clearly safe threshold. Ingredients with unresolved genotoxicity should not be included casually, especially where alternatives exist. Where impurities rather than the parent substance create concern, specification limits and analytical control may provide an appropriate risk-management route.

Carcinogenicity, reproductive toxicity and developmental toxicity should be considered even where the expected consumer population is restricted to adults. The assessment should examine known classifications, study quality, mechanism and relevance to inhalation. Nicotine itself requires explicit consideration because of developmental and cardiovascular effects. Other ingredients may have only limited or route-specific evidence. The conclusion should state whether these endpoints are absent, inadequately studied or judged not relevant at the estimated exposure. Silence is not equivalent to assessment.

Systemic toxicity should be evaluated through available repeated-dose studies, toxicokinetics and points of departure. The assessor should determine whether exposure through vaping is likely to approach doses associated with liver, kidney, neurological, cardiovascular or haematological effects. Where only oral or dermal studies exist, route differences should be considered. Highly volatile substances may produce local respiratory exposure with limited systemic dose, while others may be readily absorbed into circulation. The risk assessment should separate local and systemic concerns rather than assuming that one controls the other.

Read-across becomes important where direct data are limited. A suitable analogue may provide evidence for metabolism, irritation, sensitisation or systemic toxicity, but the analogy must be justified chemically and biologically. Shared functional groups, similar physicochemical properties and common metabolic pathways can support read-across, while differences in reactivity, volatility or steric structure may weaken it. The assessment should identify the source substance, explain the relationship to the target and describe uncertainty. Choosing an analogue because it produces a convenient conclusion undermines the method.

Grouping may be useful for related flavour substances, particularly where a series of compounds shares a common metabolic pathway or toxicological mechanism. However, grouping should not conceal outliers. One member may be more reactive, more volatile or more potent than the rest. The assessor should identify whether the group can support a common conclusion and whether any member requires separate treatment. Conservative selection of a worst-case analogue may be appropriate where the scientific basis is strong.

Weight-of-evidence reasoning should integrate all available information. Human data, inhalation studies, oral studies, in vitro findings, computational predictions, structural alerts, emissions measurements and occupational limits may each contribute. Their relevance and reliability differ. Direct product-specific inhalation evidence generally carries greater weight than generic oral data, while well-conducted mechanistic studies may explain apparently conflicting results. The assessment should not count studies mechanically. It should explain why some evidence was considered more persuasive and how uncertainty influenced the conclusion.

Occupational exposure limits can be useful but require careful interpretation. They are designed for workplace conditions, often assuming adult workers, defined shift durations and different exposure patterns from consumer use. They may also include technical or socioeconomic considerations. An occupational limit can provide a screening benchmark or comparative context, but it should not be treated automatically as a consumer safe level. Continuous or repeated daily vaping may produce a different temporal pattern from an eight-hour workplace exposure.

Threshold-of-toxicological-concern approaches may be useful for substances present at very low exposure where direct data are sparse, provided the chemical falls within the applicability domain and does not belong to an excluded high-concern category. Structural class, genotoxic alerts and exposure magnitude must be considered. The approach is less suitable for reactive compounds, metals, proteins, persistent bioaccumulative substances or substances with specific respiratory hazards. It should therefore be used as part of a transparent tiered assessment rather than as a blanket waiver.

Margin-of-exposure calculations may support the ingredient conclusion where a suitable point of departure and credible exposure estimate are available. The margin separates estimated human exposure from the dose associated with a defined effect. Its interpretation depends on the endpoint, route, study duration and uncertainty factors. A large numerical margin derived from weak oral data may be less reassuring than a smaller margin based on a relevant inhalation study. The calculation should therefore be presented with its assumptions and limitations rather than used as a standalone pass criterion.

Mixture effects should be considered because the finished formulation may behave differently from its components assessed individually. Additive irritation, shared metabolic pathways, chemical reactions and cumulative exposure can alter the overall profile. Full mixture testing can provide useful evidence, particularly for cytotoxicity, irritation or emissions, but it does not identify which ingredient drives the effect. Ingredient-level and mixture-level assessments should therefore complement each other. A reassuring mixture result should not excuse the presence of a high-concern ingredient, while an adverse mixture result may require reformulation and targeted investigation.

Interactions between flavour compounds and nicotine form can also influence exposure. Acids alter nicotine protonation, pH and sensory harshness, which may change inhalation depth and use behaviour. Flavour intensity can mask irritation or encourage more frequent use. Sweeteners may increase residue formation and coil degradation. The risk assessment should recognise that ingredients affect not only chemical exposure but also product use and device performance.

Special attention should be given to poorly characterised natural extracts, essential oils and botanical preparations. These materials can contain large numbers of constituents, variable composition and biologically active compounds. Their natural origin does not reduce the need for toxicological control. Some may contain allergens, terpenes, phenolics or contaminants that are difficult to standardise. Where composition cannot be controlled adequately, the material may be unsuitable for use regardless of its marketing appeal.

Oils and lipid-rich materials require caution because inhalation of oil droplets can create respiratory concerns distinct from conventional water-miscible e-liquids. The formulation should therefore exclude unsuitable oils unless a specific inhalation justification exists. Similar caution applies to vitamins, colourants, proteins and other additives introduced for promotional rather than necessary technical reasons. The burden of justification increases where the ingredient provides little functional benefit and carries uncertain inhalation consequences.

The assessment should result in a clear regulatory decision for each ingredient. The substance may be accepted at the proposed concentration, accepted subject to a lower limit, accepted only from a specified supplier or grade, accepted with additional testing, or rejected. Conditional acceptance should identify the controls required, such as impurity limits, aerosol testing, stability monitoring or restricted device compatibility. A vague conclusion that the ingredient is "considered safe" is generally inadequate because safety is conditional on the assumptions and controls used.

The rationale should be documented in a standardised format so that assessments remain comparable across a product range. The record should include identity, function, concentration, source, purity, hazard profile, route-specific evidence, thermal behaviour, exposure estimate, read-across, uncertainty and conclusion. This structure supports quality review and makes it easier to identify inconsistent treatment of similar substances. It also allows the assessment to be updated when new evidence becomes available.

Uncertainty should be explicit. Data gaps may arise from missing inhalation studies, unknown aerosol transfer, uncertain impurities or limited chronic evidence. The assessment should state whether the uncertainty is low, moderate or substantial and explain how it was managed. Lower concentration, better supplier control, targeted testing or substitution may reduce uncertainty. In some cases, uncertainty may remain too great to support use. The decision should reflect both the seriousness of the potential hazard and the importance of the ingredient's function.

Change control must trigger reassessment. A new supplier, altered flavour composition, different nicotine source, revised concentration or new device can change the toxicological position. The ingredient name may remain the same while purity, carrier or aerosol transfer changes. The assessment should therefore be linked to the approved specification and version-controlled technical file. Historical assessments should be retained so that the basis for earlier product batches remains traceable.

Post-market information may also change the conclusion. Complaints involving irritation, allergic reaction, unusual flavour degradation or adverse effects should be reviewed against the ingredient profile. Emerging literature may identify a new hazard or challenge an earlier assumption. Regulatory restrictions may alter acceptability. Ingredient risk assessment is therefore not completed permanently at launch; it remains part of product stewardship for as long as the product is supplied.

The strongest assessments are neither reflexively permissive nor unnecessarily prohibitive. They recognise that complete inhalation datasets will not exist for every flavour compound and that scientific judgement is unavoidable. At the same time, they reject the idea that uncertainty can be managed by broad statements of food use, historical popularity or absence of reported harm. A defensible assessment uses the best available evidence, applies conservative reasoning where necessary and removes ingredients whose function does not justify their uncertainty.

Ingredient risk assessment ultimately determines whether formulation design is scientifically supportable rather than merely commercially successful. It forces the manufacturer to account for what each substance is, why it is present, how much reaches the user, what happens when it is heated and what evidence supports its continued inclusion. When performed properly, it reduces unnecessary complexity, strengthens supplier specifications, directs analytical testing and provides the foundation for exposure assessment and regulatory interpretation. The result is not a declaration that the formulation is free from all hazard, but a documented judgement that each ingredient has been identified, justified and controlled in relation to the product in which it is used.

Literature Reviews

Literature reviews are the principal mechanism through which existing toxicological knowledge is assembled, evaluated and converted into evidence capable of supporting regulatory decisions. Their importance is greatest where direct product-specific data are limited, fragmented or methodologically inconsistent, as is often the case for vaping ingredients, flavour compounds, aerosol constituents and device-related emissions. A literature review should therefore do more than gather published papers that mention a substance or product category. It must define the regulatory question, identify the evidence most relevant to that question, evaluate the quality and applicability of individual studies, reconcile conflicting findings and explain how the resulting body of evidence influences the assessment. When performed well, the review prevents unnecessary testing, reveals important hazards, identifies exposure thresholds and supports scientifically proportionate decisions. When performed poorly, it becomes a selective narrative capable of giving superficial authority to almost any conclusion.

The first requirement is a clearly framed question. A review of "the safety of an ingredient" is too broad to guide an efficient or defensible search because safety is conditional on route, dose, duration, product configuration and endpoint. The assessor should define whether the review concerns respiratory irritation, sensitisation, genotoxicity, repeated-dose toxicity, reproductive effects, thermal decomposition, aerosol transfer, occupational exposure or another specific issue. The question should also identify the substance or product form being assessed, the intended route of exposure and the regulatory purpose of the review. A search designed to determine whether cinnamaldehyde can impair airway cell function is different from one intended to estimate a tolerable daily inhalation exposure, and both differ from a review of whether the compound increases carbonyl formation during vaping. Clear framing prevents the review from expanding into a large but unfocused collection of information.

The review protocol should be established before the search begins. Even where a full systematic-review methodology is unnecessary, the assessor should record the databases, search terms, date limits, languages, inclusion criteria, exclusion criteria and evidence hierarchy used. This reduces the risk of selecting studies after their conclusions are known. Relevant databases may include biomedical, chemical, toxicological and regulatory sources, together with authoritative monographs, classification records and occupational-health publications. Search terms should account for chemical names, synonyms, trade names, CAS numbers, metabolites, structural groups and relevant endpoints. Where a substance has a common name used across several industries, the search may need to distinguish flavouring, occupational, pharmaceutical and environmental contexts.

Search breadth must be balanced against relevance. A narrow search may miss useful mechanistic or route-comparison evidence, while an excessively broad search can produce thousands of peripheral records. The most effective approach usually combines a precise substance-and-endpoint search with broader searches for structural analogues, metabolites, product emissions and route-specific effects. For vaping products, searches should include both the ingredient and its behaviour under heating, because some of the most relevant hazards arise from transformation products rather than the parent chemical. Searches may also need to include e-cigarette, electronic nicotine delivery system, aerosol, vapour, inhalation, pyrolysis, thermal degradation and occupational exposure terminology, as authors do not use one consistent vocabulary.

The search record should be reproducible. Dates, databases and complete search strings should be retained within the technical documentation. A future reviewer should be able to understand how the evidence base was assembled and why certain papers were included. This is particularly important because literature changes over time. A review may be current when the product is notified but become incomplete several years later as new studies emerge. Reproducible search documentation allows the review to be updated efficiently rather than repeated from the beginning.

Study selection should be based on predefined relevance and quality criteria. Direct inhalation studies using the exact substance are usually highly relevant, but they may not always be the most reliable evidence if exposure is poorly characterised or the study design is weak. Oral and dermal studies can contribute to systemic toxicity and metabolism, although their route relevance must be qualified. In vitro respiratory studies may provide useful mechanistic information, particularly for irritation, cytotoxicity, oxidative stress and inflammatory responses, but their concentrations and exposure systems must be compared with realistic product exposure. Occupational studies may reveal respiratory effects in exposed workers, yet the material, co-exposures and workplace conditions may differ from consumer vaping. Human case reports can identify possible signals but rarely establish causation by themselves.

The assessor should distinguish primary research from reviews, opinion pieces, conference abstracts and secondary reporting. Review articles can be useful for mapping the field and locating older studies, but conclusions should be checked against the underlying primary evidence where they materially influence the assessment. Conference abstracts may report important new findings, yet they often lack sufficient methodological detail for full evaluation. Regulatory opinions and authoritative monographs may carry substantial weight because they integrate multiple evidence streams, but their scope and date should be examined to determine whether they remain applicable to the product under review.

Publication quality cannot be inferred solely from the journal title or the presence of peer review. Each study should be assessed for methodological reliability. Important considerations include test-material identity, purity, exposure confirmation, dose selection, controls, sample size, statistical analysis, endpoint validity, blinding where relevant and completeness of reporting. A study using a commercially named flavour without compositional analysis may provide evidence about that particular product but little about the individual ingredients. A vaping emissions study that fails to report device power, coil resistance, puffing regime or liquid composition may be difficult to interpret. A cell study using concentrations that cause immediate non-specific cytotoxicity may exaggerate the importance of downstream inflammatory markers. The review should identify these limitations rather than treating every published result as equally informative.

Test-material identity is particularly important in vaping literature because products change rapidly and commercial names can conceal substantial formulation differences. Two studies may appear to examine the same flavour category while using liquids with different ingredients, nicotine strengths, carrier ratios and devices. Generic descriptions such as tobacco flavour, fruit flavour or disposable vape do not establish chemical comparability. Where the material is incompletely characterised, the study may support a broad hazard signal but should not be transferred directly to a defined product without caution.

Device conditions are equally important. Aerosol composition is affected by power, resistance, airflow, puff duration, interval, coil age and liquid supply. Studies conducted under dry-coil or overheating conditions may identify potential degradation hazards but may not represent normal use. Conversely, studies using very mild conditions may underestimate upper-bound consumer exposure. The literature review should therefore classify test conditions as representative, conservative, stress-based or poorly defined. A study should not be rejected merely because it uses severe conditions, but its conclusion should be restricted to what those conditions demonstrate.

Analytical method quality also affects interpretation. Detection of a compound depends on sampling efficiency, calibration, limits of detection, recovery and the distinction between aerosol and vapour phases. Some studies report concentrations below reliable quantification or compare results across methods with different sensitivities. Others may identify compounds tentatively without confirmation by reference standards. The review should consider whether the analytical evidence is robust enough to support quantitative exposure assessment or only qualitative hazard identification.

The route of exposure must remain visible throughout the review. Oral toxicity data are often more abundant than inhalation data, particularly for flavouring substances. These studies may provide useful information about systemic effects, repeated-dose toxicity and metabolism, but local respiratory effects can remain unaddressed. The assessor should identify which conclusions can reasonably be transferred and which cannot. A high oral no-effect level may be reassuring for systemic toxicity while offering little information about airway irritation. Conversely, a positive oral study may indicate a systemic hazard that remains relevant if inhaled absorption is expected.

Duration is another critical dimension. Acute studies can identify immediate irritation, toxicity or physiological changes, but they may not predict chronic effects. Repeated exposure over weeks or months may produce adaptation, accumulation, inflammation or tissue changes that are absent after a single exposure. For products used daily, chronic relevance is important even where direct long-term evidence is unavailable. The review should therefore distinguish acute, subacute, subchronic and chronic studies and avoid presenting short-term findings as complete evidence of long-term safety.

Dose selection and exposure relevance should be examined carefully. High-dose studies are often useful for identifying hazards and target organs, but they may produce effects that are not plausible at consumer exposure. Low-dose studies may be more relevant but less sensitive. In vitro studies frequently use concentrations expressed in micromolar, percentage or mass per culture surface, making direct comparison with inhaled dose difficult. The reviewer should resist simplistic statements that a study is irrelevant merely because the dose is high, since hazard identification often depends on high-dose testing, but should also avoid implying that any positive result predicts harm at much lower exposure.

The difference between statistical significance and biological significance should be preserved. A small change may be statistically significant in a large dataset but of uncertain toxicological importance. A larger effect in a small study may fail to reach statistical significance despite possible biological relevance. The review should examine magnitude, consistency, dose-response, reversibility and mechanistic plausibility rather than relying on p-values alone. Regulatory decisions require interpretation of the whole effect pattern, not mechanical extraction of whether a result crossed a statistical threshold.

Dose-response relationships strengthen causal interpretation. Effects that increase with exposure are generally more persuasive than isolated changes at one concentration, although non-linear responses can occur. The presence of a plausible threshold may support exposure-based risk assessment, while effects without a clear threshold may require more conservative treatment. The reviewer should identify whether the study design included sufficient dose levels to characterise the response and whether the highest dose was dominated by non-specific toxicity.

Consistency across studies is important but must be interpreted in context. Repeated findings in different laboratories, models and exposure systems increase confidence. Inconsistent results may reflect differences in material identity, dose, method sensitivity, species or exposure conditions rather than true contradiction. The review should explore these differences instead of selecting whichever study supports the preferred conclusion. Apparent disagreement can often be resolved once the test substance and conditions are examined closely.

Mechanistic evidence can help explain observed effects. Oxidative stress, electrophilic reactivity, mitochondrial disruption, inflammatory signalling, receptor activation and metabolic pathways may connect isolated findings into a coherent toxicological pattern. Mechanistic plausibility strengthens the interpretation of hazard, particularly where direct chronic evidence is limited. However, mechanistic biomarkers should not be confused automatically with adverse outcomes. An increase in a stress marker may indicate biological activity without demonstrating tissue injury or disease. The review should distinguish early molecular responses from apical toxicological effects.

Human evidence is highly relevant where available but frequently difficult to interpret. Controlled clinical studies may examine short-term physiological responses, while observational studies can address symptoms or disease associations. Confounding by prior smoking, dual use, product switching and underlying health conditions complicates interpretation. Cross-sectional studies may identify associations without establishing temporal sequence, and self-reported product use may be imprecise. The review should therefore assess study design, population, exposure classification and adjustment for confounding before drawing causal conclusions.

Case reports and poison-centre records can identify unusual or severe events, including accidental ingestion, battery injury, allergic reactions or respiratory illness. Their value lies primarily in signal detection. They often lack complete product information, exposure confirmation or alternative-cause assessment. A single report should not be dismissed, but neither should it be treated as proof of a general product effect. Repeated cases with a consistent pattern may justify further investigation and stronger controls.

Animal studies remain part of the literature base, although their relevance depends on species, route, dose and endpoint. Inhalation studies can provide information about respiratory and systemic effects, but interspecies differences in airway anatomy, metabolism and breathing patterns must be considered. Oral animal studies may support systemic hazard identification but require route extrapolation. The review should identify whether observed effects occurred at doses close to plausible human exposure or only at very high levels, and whether uncertainty factors would be needed for quantitative use.

Non-animal studies are increasingly important. Reconstructed human airway tissues, air–liquid interface models, organotypic cultures and computational tools can provide direct information about human-relevant mechanisms and comparative product effects. Their regulatory value depends on validation, reproducibility and exposure realism. A study using submerged cells exposed to undiluted liquid may be useful for screening but less representative than an air–liquid interface aerosol exposure. The review should classify the role of each model rather than treating all in vitro evidence as equivalent.

Read-across evidence may be included where the target substance is poorly studied. The literature review should identify analogues based on structure, physicochemical properties, metabolism and toxicological mechanism. Studies on related substances can fill important gaps, but the review must explain why they are relevant and where the analogy may fail. A source substance should not be selected solely because it has reassuring data. Equally, a hazardous analogue should not be transferred without considering differences that reduce applicability.

Authoritative assessments can provide efficient access to integrated evidence. Evaluations by regulatory agencies, scientific committees and international organisations may include hazard classifications, points of departure and critical study reviews. Their conclusions should be examined in relation to scope, route and date. An assessment prepared for food use may not resolve inhalation concerns. An occupational evaluation may be highly relevant to respiratory hazard but based on workplace exposures unlike consumer use. The literature review should use such sources as evidence, not as substitutes for independent relevance assessment.

Grey literature can be valuable where peer-reviewed evidence is limited. Government reports, standards documents, industry studies, regulatory submissions and laboratory reports may contain data unavailable elsewhere. Their inclusion should be transparent, and methodological quality should be assessed using the same principles applied to published studies. Industry sponsorship does not automatically invalidate a study, just as academic authorship does not guarantee independence. Funding source, conflicts of interest and access to underlying methods should be considered as part of credibility assessment.

The review should be alert to publication bias. Positive or novel findings are more likely to be published than negative studies, which can distort the apparent weight of evidence. Small studies with dramatic results may receive greater attention than larger negative datasets. The absence of published adverse findings should therefore not be treated as proof of safety, while a cluster of positive publications may reflect selective reporting. Regulatory submissions and unpublished reports can sometimes provide balance, although their quality must still be scrutinised.

Citation bias can also distort the field. A widely repeated statement may originate from one limited study and gain apparent authority through repetition. Secondary articles may cite each other rather than the primary source. The reviewer should trace important claims back to the original evidence and verify that the cited study actually supports the statement being made. This is especially important in contentious areas where scientific findings are often compressed into policy slogans.

The review should distinguish between product-category evidence and product-specific evidence. Studies comparing vaping with smoking may provide useful context for relative exposure, but they do not demonstrate the acceptability of every formulation. Broad findings that vaping aerosols contain fewer combustion-related toxicants than cigarette smoke do not remove the need to assess specific ingredients, devices and emissions. Conversely, a problem identified in one product should not automatically be generalised to the entire category. Regulatory toxicology requires both category context and product specificity.

Comparators should be chosen carefully. Cigarette smoke may be relevant for public-health context and relative exposure, but it is not always the correct benchmark for ingredient acceptability. Ambient air, occupational limits, medicinal inhalation products or toxicological thresholds may provide more appropriate comparisons depending on the question. A product should not be considered acceptable merely because it is less hazardous than smoking if avoidable hazards can still be removed. At the same time, comparisons that ignore the intended substitution of smoking may misrepresent the practical benefit–risk context.

Data extraction should be standardised. For each relevant study, the reviewer should record material identity, test system, route, dose, duration, endpoint, principal findings, study quality and relevance to the product. Structured tables can support consistency, although the final regulatory interpretation should not be reduced to tabulation. The purpose is to create a traceable connection between source evidence and conclusion. Important limitations should be recorded alongside results rather than mentioned only in a general disclaimer.

Evidence weighting should be explicit. Direct, well-conducted inhalation studies using the exact substance usually receive high relevance, while poorly characterised product studies may receive less. Human evidence may carry high relevance but still be weakened by confounding. Mechanistic studies may be reliable but insufficient on their own to establish adversity. The reviewer should explain why some findings were given greater weight than others. A conclusion based on several moderate-quality, consistent studies may be stronger than one resting on a single apparently definitive experiment.

The weight-of-evidence conclusion should address both what is known and what remains uncertain. It may identify a clear hazard, support a no-concern conclusion at the proposed exposure, justify a concentration limit, reveal the need for product-specific testing or conclude that the ingredient cannot be supported. The conclusion should not use vague language such as "appears safe" without explaining the evidence and conditions. Regulatory wording should reflect the strength of the database.

Conflicting evidence should be discussed directly. Suppressing unfavourable studies weakens the credibility of the review and may be exposed during regulatory scrutiny. The better approach is to explain why findings differ and whether one study is more applicable. Differences in dose, route, product composition, device condition, endpoint sensitivity or analytical method may account for disagreement. Where conflict cannot be resolved, uncertainty should be carried forward into a conservative assessment or additional testing.

The review should also identify data gaps systematically. Missing repeated-inhalation data, absence of chronic studies, uncertain aerosol transfer, limited information on metabolites or insufficient impurity data may each affect confidence. Data gaps should not be listed without consequence. The assessor should determine whether they can be addressed through read-across, computational methods, exposure analysis, targeted testing or ingredient substitution. Some gaps may be acceptable where exposure is very low and the hazard profile is otherwise reassuring; others may make the ingredient unsuitable.

Literature review and exposure assessment should interact continuously. A hazard reported at a particular concentration may be irrelevant if product exposure is orders of magnitude lower, while a modest hazard may become important if exposure is frequent and substantial. The reviewer should therefore extract quantitative points of departure where possible and identify whether the study can support margin-of-exposure calculations. Units, route and duration should be recorded carefully to avoid inappropriate comparison.

Thermal-decomposition literature requires particular care because experimental conditions vary widely. Studies may use isolated chemicals, bulk heating, pyrolysis systems or complete vaping devices. Results from high-temperature pyrolysis can identify possible degradation products but may not represent aerosol generation under normal conditions. Device studies may be more directly relevant but product-specific. The review should distinguish intrinsic thermal pathways from observed product emissions and explain how each informs the assessment.

Mixture literature presents additional complexity. Whole-aerosol studies may reveal combined effects that ingredient-by-ingredient assessment misses, but they are difficult to interpret mechanistically. Flavour mixtures can produce additive or interactive effects, and one dominant component may drive the response. The review should use mixture studies to assess overall product plausibility while retaining substance-specific analysis where possible. A positive mixture result should prompt reformulation or targeted investigation rather than a generic conclusion that all flavours are hazardous.

The date of the review should be clear because scientific evidence evolves rapidly. Vaping technology, formulations and analytical methods have changed considerably, and older studies may describe products no longer representative of current designs. Age alone does not make a study irrelevant, particularly for fundamental chemical or toxicological information, but product-specific applicability may decline. The reviewer should distinguish enduring evidence from technology-dependent findings.

Updates should be planned at intervals or triggered by specific events. New publications, supplier changes, formulation revisions, regulatory alerts or post-market complaints may require reassessment. A literature review should not remain frozen for the lifetime of a product. The review date, search end date and update history should be controlled within the technical file so that the evidence base remains traceable.

Automation and artificial intelligence may assist searching, screening and evidence extraction, but they do not replace scientific judgement. Automated systems can identify synonyms, cluster studies and accelerate review of large datasets, yet they may miss methodological nuance, misclassify relevance or reproduce bias from training data. Any machine-assisted process should be checked by a competent reviewer, particularly where the output influences a regulatory conclusion.

The final review should be readable as a scientific argument rather than a database dump. It should explain the regulatory question, search method, evidence base, study quality, consistent findings, conflicting findings, uncertainties and conclusion. Tables and appendices can hold detailed extraction data, allowing the main narrative to focus on interpretation. The reader should be able to follow how the evidence moved from individual studies to the final judgement.

A strong literature review can prevent both under-regulation and unnecessary testing. It identifies hazards that might otherwise be missed, while also showing where existing evidence is sufficient to avoid redundant experiments. It supports read-across, weight-of-evidence reasoning, exposure assessment and non-animal methods. It can also reveal that a proposed ingredient is difficult to defend before resources are spent on full product development.

The regulatory value of the review depends ultimately on intellectual discipline. The assessor must remain willing to revise an initial view when the evidence points elsewhere, separate product relevance from scientific interest and resist pressure to convert uncertainty into certainty for commercial convenience. Literature review is not a search for supportive quotations. It is the controlled examination of the available scientific record to determine what can reasonably be concluded, what cannot yet be concluded and what the product developer must do in response.

Within vaping regulation, where direct inhalation evidence is often incomplete and product configurations change quickly, literature review becomes one of the most important safeguards against arbitrary judgement. It connects established toxicology with emerging product science and ensures that regulatory decisions are informed by the full body of relevant evidence rather than isolated findings. Properly conducted, it does not eliminate uncertainty, but it defines that uncertainty, places it in context and turns it into practical choices concerning ingredient selection, concentration limits, testing, reformulation and market control.

Read-Across Methodologies

Read-across methodologies are used when direct toxicological data for a substance are incomplete, unavailable or insufficiently relevant to the exposure route under assessment, allowing information from one or more better-characterised substances to support evaluation of a related target chemical. In regulatory toxicology this is not an informal assumption that chemically similar substances behave in the same way, but a structured evidential approach requiring a clear scientific basis, transparent analogue selection and explicit consideration of uncertainty. The source substance must be shown to provide information that is meaningfully applicable to the target substance because the two share characteristics capable of driving comparable absorption, metabolism, reactivity or toxicological effects. When applied correctly, read-across can reduce unnecessary testing, make use of existing knowledge and support proportionate decisions where complete substance-specific datasets are unrealistic. When applied poorly, it can create false reassurance or exaggerate concern by transferring findings between substances whose apparent similarity does not extend to the biological properties that matter.

The need for read-across is particularly acute in the assessment of vaping products because flavour systems may contain numerous chemicals for which repeated-inhalation studies do not exist. Many flavouring substances have been studied through oral exposure, occupational handling or short-term in vitro systems, while direct respiratory evidence remains sparse. Conducting conventional animal inhalation studies for every constituent, concentration and combination would be scientifically inefficient, ethically difficult and practically impossible. The number of potential formulations, device combinations and thermal products would exceed the capacity of any realistic testing programme. Read-across therefore becomes one part of a tiered strategy through which known chemistry, existing toxicology, metabolism, exposure and mechanistic information are integrated before any new testing is considered.

The starting point is a precise definition of the target substance. Read-across cannot be reliable where the target is known only by a commercial name, flavour descriptor or incomplete supplier declaration. The exact chemical structure, molecular formula, stereochemistry, salt form, purity, impurities and physicochemical properties should be established. Where the target is a complex material, such as a natural extract or proprietary mixture, conventional single-substance read-across may be unsuitable unless the material can be characterised by its major constituents, marker compounds or defined compositional range. An undefined target cannot be compared coherently with a source substance because the assessor does not know which properties or components are actually being bridged.

The regulatory question must also be defined before analogues are selected. Read-across intended to address acute respiratory irritation may require different source information from read-across intended to support systemic repeated-dose toxicity, genotoxicity, sensitisation or reproductive effects. A substance may be a suitable analogue for one endpoint and unsuitable for another. Structural similarity may support common metabolism while offering little information about local airway reactivity. Comparable volatility may support inhalation exposure modelling without establishing comparable systemic toxicity. Read-across should therefore be endpoint-specific rather than presented as a universal declaration that one substance is toxicologically equivalent to another.

Analogue selection begins with chemistry, but chemical resemblance alone is not enough. Relevant similarities may include molecular size, functional groups, electronic structure, polarity, lipophilicity, volatility, water solubility, acid dissociation, vapour pressure and chemical reactivity. These properties influence how the substance partitions into aerosol, deposits in the respiratory tract, crosses biological membranes and undergoes metabolism. A difference that appears minor on paper can alter toxicological behaviour materially. Replacing one substituent may increase electrophilic reactivity, change metabolic stability or produce a more hazardous metabolite. The read-across justification must therefore identify the features believed to drive the endpoint and show that these features are shared sufficiently between source and target.

Functional groups require particular attention because they often influence reactivity and metabolism. Aldehydes may form adducts with proteins and nucleic acids. Esters may hydrolyse to corresponding acids and alcohols. Ketones may undergo reduction or oxidation. Terpenes can oxidise into products with different sensitisation profiles. Phenolic compounds may participate in redox reactions. Acids may alter local pH and tissue irritation.

The presence of the same broad functional group may suggest a common mechanism, but it does not establish equal potency. Chain length, branching, steric hindrance and neighbouring substituents can change how readily a molecule reacts or is metabolised. Read-across should therefore be based on the toxicologically relevant chemistry rather than simple category membership.

Metabolism is often one of the strongest bases for read-across because substances converted to the same intermediate or final metabolites may share systemic effects. If the source and target are both rapidly transformed through the same pathway and the metabolite drives toxicity, data from the source may be informative for the target. The assessor should examine likely phase I and phase II reactions, including oxidation, reduction, hydrolysis, conjugation and enzymatic specificity. Where metabolism has not been studied directly, computational prediction, in vitro metabolism data and information from structurally related substances may help. The argument is stronger where common metabolites are demonstrated than where they are merely assumed.

Metabolic differences can also defeat an otherwise attractive analogy. One substance may be rapidly detoxified while another is converted to a reactive intermediate. Stereoisomers may differ in enzyme affinity. Substitution can alter the balance between competing pathways. A source substance with extensive oral metabolism may not predict local respiratory effects if the target reacts directly with airway tissue before systemic processing. The read-across should therefore distinguish between local and systemic endpoints and should not rely on metabolism where the relevant hazard arises before metabolism occurs.

Physicochemical properties influence whether the source and target are likely to reach the same biological site. Volatility affects transfer into the gas phase and upper-airway deposition. Lipophilicity influences membrane penetration and tissue retention. Water solubility affects dissolution in airway surface fluid. Particle association can alter deposition deeper in the lung. A source analogue that is much less volatile or much more lipophilic may produce a different exposure distribution even if the molecules are structurally related. For vaping products, these differences are especially important because aerosol transfer and respiratory deposition determine the dose available at the target tissue.

The assessment should also compare the physical state and product context. A substance used in a liquid formulation and aerosolised through a heated device may behave differently from the same substance encountered as an occupational vapour, food ingredient or bulk chemical. The matrix can alter volatility, chemical reaction and deposition. Acids, nicotine, propylene glycol, glycerol and other flavour constituents may influence partitioning or thermal transformation. Read-across from an isolated chemical study should therefore be interpreted alongside product-specific exposure information rather than assumed to describe the finished aerosol directly.

There are several common read-across structures. The simplest is a one-to-one analogue approach in which one well-characterised source substance is used to support assessment of one target substance. This can be persuasive where the molecules are closely related, share a clear metabolic pathway and show comparable physicochemical behaviour. It is weaker where the source has been chosen from a broad class without sufficient justification. A single analogue may also create vulnerability because the conclusion depends heavily on one dataset and one assumption of similarity.

A category approach uses several related substances to identify a pattern across a chemical series. The target may fall within a group defined by common structure, mechanism, metabolism or physicochemical characteristics. Toxicity can then be interpolated where the target lies between well-characterised members or extrapolated where a defensible trend exists. Categories can be more robust than one-to-one analogues because they allow the assessor to examine consistency and identify outliers. They also require more work because the category must be defined clearly, and each member must be shown to belong for toxicologically meaningful reasons.

Trend analysis within a category can support quantitative prediction where toxicity changes systematically with molecular weight, chain length, substitution or another property. Such trends should be biologically plausible and supported by sufficient data. A neat numerical pattern based on a small number of substances may be misleading. The assessor should examine whether the target falls within the range of the source substances or whether the conclusion requires extrapolation beyond the evidence. Interpolation is generally more reliable because the target is bracketed by known data, while extrapolation carries greater uncertainty.

Worst-case analogue selection may be used where one source substance has properties expected to produce equal or greater toxicity than the target. This can provide a conservative basis for risk assessment if the reasoning is sound. The source may be more reactive, more bioavailable, more volatile or more potent for the endpoint of concern. The assessor should explain why the source can reasonably bound the target. Choosing the most hazardous member of a broad class without showing relevance can produce unnecessary conservatism, while choosing a reassuring source without comparing more hazardous analogues can create bias.

Read-across can be qualitative or quantitative. Qualitative read-across may support conclusions such as the absence of a specific structural alert, likely irritation potential or similarity of metabolic pathway. Quantitative read-across may use a source no-observed-adverse-effect level, benchmark dose or other point of departure to derive an exposure limit or margin of exposure for the target. Quantitative use requires greater confidence because numerical values are being transferred. Differences in potency, absorption, route and study design must be considered explicitly, and uncertainty factors may need to be increased where the analogy is imperfect.

Endpoint concordance strengthens the argument. If several source substances show similar effects on the same organ or biological pathway, and the target shares the properties believed to drive that effect, the read-across becomes more credible. Concordance across in vitro, animal and mechanistic evidence can be particularly useful. Conversely, inconsistent effects across close analogues may indicate that the category is too broad or that another property controls toxicity. Inconsistency should not be hidden; it should trigger refinement of the hypothesis.

The read-across hypothesis is the central scientific statement explaining why information from the source substance should apply to the target. It should identify the common property, pathway or mechanism and link this to the endpoint. A weak hypothesis states only that the substances have similar structures. A stronger hypothesis explains that both are rapidly hydrolysed to the same metabolite, share similar aerosol transfer and lack additional reactive groups, making comparable systemic toxicity plausible. Another strong hypothesis might show that a homologous series exhibits increasing irritation with volatility and that the target falls between two tested members. The quality of the hypothesis determines the quality of the entire methodology.

Analogue searching should be systematic enough to reduce selection bias. The assessor should consider structurally close substances, metabolites, precursors, homologues and category members rather than selecting the first convenient source. Search tools, chemical databases and computational similarity measures can assist, but they do not replace expert judgement. High numerical similarity does not guarantee toxicological similarity, and lower structural similarity may still be relevant where the mechanism or metabolite is shared. The search record should show which potential analogues were considered and why some were accepted or rejected.

Negative analogues are as important as supportive ones. A credible assessment should examine substances that resemble the target but show different toxicity and determine whether the difference can be explained. This process helps test the read-across hypothesis. If a close analogue is more hazardous because it contains an additional reactive group absent from the target, the difference may strengthen the argument. If no explanation can be found, confidence should fall. Ignoring inconvenient analogues creates an incomplete and potentially biased assessment.

Data quality remains critical because read-across cannot be stronger than the source evidence. A well-matched analogue with poor toxicological data may be less useful than a slightly less similar substance supported by robust studies. The source dataset should be evaluated for substance identity, purity, route, dose, duration, endpoint validity and reporting quality. Where the key study is old, incomplete or conducted by an irrelevant route, this should be reflected in the confidence assessment. Read-across does not repair weak source data; it adds another layer of inference to them.

Route relevance is particularly difficult in vaping toxicology because much of the available evidence is oral. Oral data may support systemic effects if absorption and metabolism are comparable, but they may fail to address local respiratory injury. Route-to-route read-across should therefore consider whether inhalation introduces higher local concentration, bypasses first-pass metabolism or changes the parent-to-metabolite ratio. A source substance with a high oral no-effect level may still irritate the airway at much lower inhaled doses. Where local respiratory endpoints are important, direct inhalation, occupational or respiratory in vitro evidence should be prioritised.

Occupational data can provide valuable respiratory information but must be interpreted carefully. Workplace exposure may involve vapour, dust or aerosol at concentrations and durations different from consumer use. Co-exposures and protective equipment can complicate interpretation. Occupational exposure limits may reflect technical feasibility or policy considerations in addition to toxicology. They can contribute to read-across, particularly for irritation and sensitisation, but should not be transferred mechanically as consumer limits.

Human evidence can strengthen a read-across where source and target share a plausible mechanism, but human observations often lack precise exposure characterisation. Case reports, workplace symptoms and clinical studies may indicate a hazard without defining a reliable dose-response. They can nevertheless identify endpoints requiring caution. Where human and animal evidence disagree, the assessor should examine whether route, metabolism, susceptibility or study design explains the difference.

In vitro methods can support biological similarity directly. Source and target substances can be tested side by side in the same respiratory model, allowing comparison of cytotoxicity, irritation, oxidative stress, inflammatory signalling or barrier function. Such bridging studies may be more informative than relying entirely on historical data because they test the read-across hypothesis experimentally. The models should be relevant and exposure concentrations should be interpreted carefully, but comparative testing can reduce uncertainty substantially.

Computational toxicology can also contribute. Quantitative structure–activity relationship models may predict mutagenicity, sensitisation, receptor binding, metabolism or physicochemical behaviour. Molecular descriptors can help define categories and identify outliers. Applicability domain is critical because predictions are less reliable where the target lies outside the chemical space used to build the model. Computational outputs should therefore support the read-across rather than replace empirical evidence.

New approach methodologies can strengthen read-across by providing mechanistic bridging information without conventional animal testing. Reconstructed airway tissues, organ-on-chip systems, high-throughput assays, transcriptomics and metabolomics may show whether source and target substances activate similar biological pathways. These data are especially useful where the read-across depends on a shared mode of action. Their interpretation requires caution because pathway activation does not always translate directly into an adverse outcome, but mechanistic concordance can increase confidence.

Adverse outcome pathways provide another framework by linking a molecular initiating event to cellular responses, tissue effects and final adverse outcomes. If source and target substances are expected to trigger the same initiating event and show comparable downstream activity, read-across may be justified more clearly. This approach is particularly valuable for reactive chemicals, sensitisers and substances producing oxidative stress. The pathway should be sufficiently established, and the evidence should show that the target genuinely enters the pathway rather than merely resembling a known source structurally.

Read-across should be connected to exposure. A moderate degree of uncertainty may be acceptable where consumer exposure is extremely low and the source data show effects only at much higher doses. The same uncertainty may be unacceptable where exposure approaches the source point of departure or where the endpoint is severe and potentially non-threshold. Exposure does not determine whether the read-across is scientifically valid, but it influences whether the remaining uncertainty is tolerable for regulatory decision-making.

The margin of exposure derived from read-across data should therefore be interpreted conservatively. The source point of departure may need adjustment for differences in molecular weight, absorption or potency. Additional uncertainty factors may be applied for analogue quality, route extrapolation, study duration or database limitations. These factors should be justified rather than multiplied automatically. Excessive stacking can produce an unusably conservative value, while insufficient adjustment can create false confidence.

High-concern endpoints require stronger evidence. Read-across for simple irritation may be acceptable with moderate confidence and conservative exposure control. Read-across intended to dismiss genotoxicity, carcinogenicity, reproductive toxicity or respiratory sensitisation generally requires a more robust justification because the consequences of error are greater. Structural alerts, conflicting analogues or positive computational predictions should be addressed directly. Where uncertainty remains substantial, exclusion or targeted testing may be more appropriate than reliance on inference.

Read-across should also consider impurities and degradation products. The target substance may be similar to the source in its pure form while differing in commercial impurity profile. Heating may produce products not generated by the source. A flavour aldehyde and its related alcohol may appear connected metabolically, yet their thermal behaviour in a vaping device may differ. The methodology should therefore compare the actual supplied material and relevant aerosol chemistry, not only idealised parent structures.

Mixtures create further difficulty because one constituent can influence the behaviour of another. Read-across between whole flavour mixtures is rarely straightforward unless composition is tightly controlled and similarities are demonstrated across major constituents and functional groups. A mixture bearing the same flavour description may contain different chemicals and cannot be treated as equivalent. Component-based assessment is usually stronger, supplemented by whole-mixture testing where interaction or combined irritancy is a concern.

Natural extracts present a similar challenge because compositional variability can undermine the stable target identity required for read-across. One batch may differ from another in major and minor constituents. Where a botanical material is used, the category may need to be based on a defined extraction process, marker profile and compositional range. Even then, read-across from the source plant or oral use may provide little information about inhalation of the extracted mixture. Poorly characterised materials may remain unsuitable despite extensive historical use.

The assessment should assign confidence to the read-across conclusion. Confidence may be high where structure, metabolism, physicochemical properties, biological activity and source data all align. It may be moderate where some differences exist but exposure is low and the endpoint is well understood. It may be low where analogue selection is uncertain, route relevance is weak or source data are limited. Confidence should be endpoint-specific and should influence risk-management decisions.

Uncertainty should be described by source. Analogue uncertainty concerns whether the source is sufficiently similar. Endpoint uncertainty concerns the quality and relevance of the toxicological data. Exposure uncertainty concerns aerosol transfer and consumer use. Metabolic uncertainty concerns whether source and target follow the same pathways. Product uncertainty concerns whether heating, formulation or device conditions alter behaviour. Separating these uncertainties prevents them from being hidden inside a single general statement.

The regulatory output should state what the read-across supports and what it does not. It may support absence of concern for a particular endpoint, provide a conservative point of departure, justify a concentration limit or identify the need for further testing. It should not be extended beyond the endpoints and conditions considered. A read-across supporting systemic repeated-dose toxicity does not automatically resolve respiratory sensitisation. A conclusion based on unheated material does not necessarily address thermal products.

Documentation should include the target identity, source substances, search strategy, analogue-selection criteria, similarity assessment, toxicokinetic comparison, endpoint data, contradictory evidence, uncertainty analysis and final conclusion. Structural diagrams, property tables and metabolic schemes can make the reasoning easier to review. The narrative should remain clear enough that another competent toxicologist can reconstruct the logic without relying on undocumented judgement.

Peer review or independent quality review is valuable because analogue selection can be influenced unconsciously by the desired regulatory outcome. A second reviewer may identify closer analogues, overlooked differences or unsupported assumptions. This is particularly important where read-across is being used to support a high-concern endpoint or avoid additional testing. The review should test the hypothesis rather than simply confirm that the document is complete.

Read-across is not static. New toxicological studies, improved computational models, new analytical data or post-market evidence may strengthen or weaken the original conclusion. Supplier changes can alter target identity or impurities. A formulation change may increase exposure. The assessment should therefore be version-controlled and reviewed when relevant new evidence emerges.

The greatest value of read-across lies in its ability to make scientific use of incomplete evidence without pretending that the missing study has somehow been performed. It recognises that chemicals exist within families of structure, metabolism and biological activity and that well-supported relationships can inform regulation. Its legitimacy depends on transparency. The assessor must show why the source substance is relevant, where the analogy is strong, where it is weak and how the remaining uncertainty affects the decision.

Within vaping regulation, read-across provides a practical bridge between the scale of the ingredient universe and the limited availability of inhalation data. It can identify substances that are likely to share irritation, sensitisation or systemic toxicity; support conservative exposure limits; reduce unnecessary animal testing; and direct experimental resources towards the uncertainties that matter most. It cannot convert a poorly characterised ingredient into a well-understood one, excuse incomplete supplier disclosure or replace product-specific emissions assessment where heating and device conditions control exposure.

A defensible read-across therefore remains conditional, endpoint-specific and integrated with the wider weight of evidence. It should be used when the biological and chemical basis is stronger than the uncertainty it introduces, and rejected where similarity is superficial or the consequences of error are too great. Applied with that discipline, it becomes one of the most useful tools in modern regulatory toxicology, allowing decisions to be made from existing science while preserving the distinction between evidence, inference and assumption.

Weight-of-Evidence Approaches

Weight-of-evidence approaches are used when the available toxicological information is too diverse, incomplete or contradictory to support a regulatory conclusion through any single study, method or dataset. This is the normal condition of modern vaping toxicology rather than an exceptional one. A formulation may contain ingredients supported by oral toxicity studies, occupational observations, limited inhalation evidence, in vitro respiratory assays, computational predictions, structural alerts and information from related substances, while the finished aerosol may have been characterised under only a small number of operating conditions. No single source provides a complete account of hazard or risk, yet the regulator and responsible manufacturer must still determine whether the product can be justified, whether additional controls are needed and whether uncertainty is too substantial to permit continued use. Weight of evidence provides the framework through which these different forms of information are evaluated together, giving greater influence to evidence that is reliable, relevant and biologically coherent while ensuring that weak, indirect or conflicting findings are not concealed.

The approach should not be confused with counting studies or taking a simple majority view. Ten weak studies do not necessarily outweigh one well-designed investigation, and several negative findings do not resolve a concern if the methods used were incapable of detecting the relevant effect. Evidence must be weighted according to its scientific value for the specific regulatory question. A direct repeated-inhalation study using a well-characterised substance may carry greater relevance than an oral study, but its reliability may still be limited by poor exposure confirmation or inadequate reporting. A human occupational study may provide highly relevant respiratory information but be weakened by co-exposures and uncertain dose. An in vitro airway model may offer mechanistic insight and direct respiratory relevance while remaining unable to predict chronic whole-body effects. Weight of evidence requires the assessor to separate reliability, relevance and sufficiency rather than compressing them into one general impression of study quality.

The first requirement is a clearly defined assessment question. Evidence cannot be weighted meaningfully in the abstract because the importance of each source depends on the endpoint and decision under consideration. An assessment of respiratory irritation requires different evidence from an assessment of genotoxicity, systemic repeated-dose toxicity, sensitisation or developmental effects. A dataset that is adequate for screening may be insufficient for setting a quantitative exposure limit. A study that supports identification of a hazard may not provide a suitable point of departure for margin-of-exposure analysis. The assessor should therefore define the substance or product, route of exposure, endpoint, intended use, exposure duration and regulatory decision before deciding which evidence deserves the greatest weight.

The product context must remain visible throughout the process. Evidence concerning an isolated ingredient may not describe its behaviour within a heated formulation, while whole-aerosol studies may identify an effect without revealing which constituent caused it. Device power, liquid composition, coil condition and puffing regime may determine whether a hazard becomes relevant. Weight-of-evidence reasoning should therefore integrate ingredient-level toxicology with product-specific chemistry, emissions and exposure. A formulation cannot be judged solely from the known properties of its raw materials if heating generates additional compounds, and an adverse whole-aerosol result cannot automatically be attributed to every ingredient in the mixture.

Evidence collection should be broad enough to identify both supportive and adverse findings. Relevant sources may include human observations, clinical studies, occupational reports, animal studies, in vitro assays, computational models, chemical reactivity data, physicochemical properties, toxicokinetics, read-across, regulatory classifications, analytical emissions studies, product complaints and post-market signals. The search should not stop when enough favourable evidence has been found to support a commercial decision. The credibility of the approach depends on active consideration of information capable of challenging the preferred conclusion.

Each evidence stream should first be evaluated independently. Human data should be examined for exposure definition, population selection, confounding, outcome measurement and temporal relationship. Animal studies should be assessed for species, route, duration, dose, study design and relevance to humans. In vitro studies should be reviewed for model validity, exposure realism, concentration, cytotoxicity and endpoint interpretation. Computational predictions should be checked for applicability domain and model confidence. Read-across should be assessed for analogue quality and mechanistic plausibility. Analytical studies should be reviewed for product identity, sampling, method sensitivity and operating conditions. Only after the strengths and weaknesses of each stream are understood should they be integrated.

Reliability describes whether a study was conducted and reported in a manner that supports confidence in its findings. It includes test-material identity, experimental controls, sample size, method validation, exposure confirmation, statistical analysis and completeness of reporting. A study can be highly relevant to inhalation but unreliable because the substance was not characterised or aerosol concentration was not measured. Conversely, a rigorously conducted oral study may be reliable but only indirectly relevant to respiratory exposure. Weight-of-evidence assessment should preserve this distinction because a single quality score can obscure whether the limitation lies in execution or applicability.

Relevance concerns the extent to which the evidence addresses the product, route, exposure and endpoint under consideration. Direct human inhalation evidence is often highly relevant, but such evidence may be rare or observational. Product-specific aerosol studies may be directly relevant to the marketed configuration but limited to short-term outcomes. Oral repeated-dose studies may provide useful systemic information while failing to address local airway effects. The assessor should identify precisely what each study can contribute rather than accepting or rejecting it as a whole. One study may be highly relevant to metabolism, moderately relevant to systemic toxicity and largely irrelevant to respiratory irritation.

Adequacy concerns whether the combined evidence is sufficient for the decision being made. A body of evidence may contain reliable and relevant studies yet remain inadequate because important endpoints or exposure periods are missing. Sufficiency is therefore a property of the evidence base as a whole, not of one study. The level of evidence required should be proportionate to the seriousness of the hazard, magnitude of exposure, intended duration of use and reversibility of the potential effect. More confidence is needed to dismiss a genotoxic or sensitisation concern than to manage mild, reversible irritation through concentration reduction.

Human evidence often receives substantial weight because it avoids uncertainty associated with species extrapolation, but it should not be treated as automatically decisive. Controlled human studies are generally limited in duration and cannot ethically investigate severe or irreversible endpoints. Observational studies may be confounded by prior smoking, dual use, occupational exposure, age, disease and socioeconomic factors. Self-reported vaping behaviour may not capture product composition, device conditions or actual dose. A finding in humans can be highly important, but the assessor must distinguish causation from association and consider whether alternative explanations have been addressed.

Absence of reported human harm should be interpreted cautiously. A flavour ingredient may have been used widely without obvious adverse reports, but surveillance may be weak, symptoms may be non-specific and product composition may not be traceable. Lack of case reports can contribute to the evidence base, particularly where exposure has been extensive and monitoring robust, but it rarely proves absence of risk. Severe or unusual effects are more likely to be recognised than chronic low-grade respiratory changes. Weight of evidence should therefore avoid giving excessive reassurance to passive absence of reporting.

Animal studies can provide information about repeated exposure, target organs, dose-response and systemic toxicity that cannot be obtained ethically in humans. Their weight depends on route, species, exposure characterisation and biological relevance. An inhalation study may be directly relevant to local respiratory effects, but species differences in nasal anatomy, breathing pattern and metabolism can influence the result. Oral studies may support systemic endpoints if absorption and metabolism are comparable, while offering limited evidence for local airway effects. The assessor should identify where interspecies and route extrapolation are required and reflect these uncertainties in the conclusion.

Positive animal findings should not be dismissed simply because exposure levels exceed consumer exposure. High-dose studies are designed to identify hazards and may reveal target organs or mechanisms. Their risk significance depends on dose-response and the distance between experimental exposure and anticipated human exposure. Conversely, negative studies conducted at inadequate doses or for insufficient duration may carry little weight. The absence of an effect is informative only where the study was capable of detecting the effect of concern.

In vitro evidence has become increasingly important because human-relevant respiratory models can compare ingredients, formulations and aerosols directly. Air–liquid interface systems, reconstructed airway tissues, epithelial cultures and immune-cell models can examine cytotoxicity, barrier integrity, oxidative stress, inflammatory signalling and ciliary function. These methods may offer strong mechanistic and comparative evidence, particularly where conventional inhalation studies are unavailable. Their limitations include incomplete metabolism, restricted exposure duration and uncertain translation from biomarker changes to clinical harm.

The concentration used in vitro requires careful interpretation. Direct application of undiluted e-liquid to submerged cells may identify intrinsic cytotoxicity but poorly represent inhalation exposure. Aerosol exposure at the air–liquid interface can be more realistic, although deposited dose must still be measured or estimated. Extremely high concentrations may trigger non-specific cell death, making secondary biomarkers difficult to interpret. Weight should be greater where exposure is characterised, effects are dose-related and the model is relevant to the endpoint.

Mechanistic evidence can strengthen causal interpretation when it connects chemical properties to observed biological effects. Electrophilic reactivity, oxidative stress, protein binding, mitochondrial disruption, receptor activation and metabolic formation of reactive intermediates may explain why an ingredient or emission produces a particular outcome. Consistency between structure, mechanism and apical effect increases confidence. Mechanistic plausibility is especially valuable where chronic outcome data are limited, although activation of a biological pathway does not necessarily establish an adverse effect at realistic exposure.

Physicochemical and chemical evidence can carry considerable weight in product assessment. Volatility, solubility, lipophilicity, pH, reactivity and thermal stability influence aerosol transfer, deposition and biological availability. A highly reactive aldehyde may justify concern even where direct repeated-inhalation evidence is limited. A non-volatile substance with negligible aerosol transfer may present less inhalation relevance despite hazardous properties by another route. The assessor should connect these properties to measured product behaviour rather than using chemical descriptors in isolation.

Analytical emissions data are essential because they determine whether identified hazards are actually present in the aerosol and at what level. The weight given to such data depends on the representativeness of the tested product and operating conditions. Results from the final formulation and intended device under justified puffing conditions carry more relevance than generic literature values. Stress testing can identify failure modes and upper-bound emissions, but should be distinguished from normal-use exposure. Multiple operating conditions may be necessary where the device permits variable power or where coil ageing alters performance.

Non-detection should not be interpreted as proof of absence without considering method sensitivity. A compound may fall below the analytical limit while still being relevant if the limit is too high relative to the toxicological threshold. Conversely, detection of trace quantities does not establish meaningful risk. The result must be considered alongside exposure, toxicological potency and uncertainty. Weight-of-evidence analysis should distinguish confirmed absence, non-detection under a defined limit and detection at levels of uncertain significance.

Computational predictions can contribute to endpoints such as mutagenicity, sensitisation, metabolism and receptor activity. Their weight depends on model validation, applicability domain and concordance with empirical evidence.

Several independent models producing the same prediction may strengthen confidence, particularly where structural features and known analogues support the result. Conflicting predictions should be investigated rather than averaged mechanically. A negative computational output should not override a credible positive experimental finding.

Read-across contributes inferred evidence where the source and target substances share relevant structure, metabolism or biological activity. Its weight depends on the strength of the read-across hypothesis, quality of the source data and degree of similarity. A well-supported analogue may provide a suitable point of departure, while a superficial structural match should carry little influence. Weight-of-evidence assessment should prevent read-across from becoming self-confirming: the analogue should be tested against contrary evidence, outliers and alternative candidates.

Regulatory classifications and authoritative evaluations can provide high-value evidence because they integrate multiple studies and expert review. Their applicability must still be considered. A classification developed for industrial exposure may identify an inherent hazard but not determine consumer risk. A food assessment may provide systemic information while leaving inhalation questions unresolved. The assessor should understand the scope, route, date and underlying evidence of each authoritative conclusion rather than treating it as a universal answer.

Occupational exposure limits can provide quantitative context, especially for respiratory irritation or systemic effects, but their weight should be moderated by the purpose for which they were developed. Worker populations, shift durations and workplace controls differ from consumer exposure. Some limits reflect feasibility and policy as well as toxicology. They may be valuable screening benchmarks or points of comparison, but they should not automatically become acceptable daily exposure limits for vaping.

Post-market evidence can alter the weighting of pre-market data. Complaints, adverse-event reports, poison-centre cases and product returns may reveal effects not predicted during development. Individual reports often lack complete exposure information and cannot establish causation, but repeated patterns can form a signal. A cluster of irritation complaints associated with one formulation, batch or device configuration may increase the weight given to earlier mechanistic or in vitro findings that previously appeared uncertain. Conversely, extensive controlled use without a signal may provide limited reassurance, particularly where monitoring is active and product identity is stable.

Temporal sequence strengthens interpretation. An effect that appears after exposure, diminishes after cessation and recurs after re-exposure is more persuasive than a symptom reported without timing information. Dose-response, biological plausibility, consistency and specificity also contribute to causal reasoning. These considerations should be applied flexibly rather than treated as a checklist, because many genuine toxic effects are not specific to one substance or do not show perfect dose-response in limited datasets.

Consistency across independent evidence streams increases confidence. If structural alerts, in vitro respiratory assays, occupational reports and animal inhalation studies all point towards airway irritation, the conclusion is stronger than any source alone. Concordance is particularly persuasive where different methods have different limitations, because the same finding is less likely to arise from one artefact. However, apparent consistency should not be manufactured by treating dependent evidence as independent. Several review papers based on the same primary study do not constitute multiple confirmations.

Inconsistency should be analysed rather than concealed. Conflicting results may arise from differences in test-material purity, dose, route, formulation, device settings, assay sensitivity or statistical power. One study may have examined the parent substance while another measured a thermal product. A negative result may reflect lower exposure rather than absence of hazard. The assessor should determine whether the evidence can be reconciled through these differences. Where inconsistency remains unexplained, confidence should be reduced and uncertainty carried forward.

Evidence should not be weighted according to whether it supports a preferred commercial or policy position. Confirmation bias is a major threat because vaping toxicology operates within a contested field. Evidence showing reduced exposure relative to smoking can be overextended into claims of product safety, while isolated adverse findings can be generalised across all products. Weight-of-evidence assessment must remain anchored to the specific regulatory question. Relative-risk context may be important for adult smokers, but it does not remove the need to identify and control avoidable product hazards.

The role of comparator selection should be made explicit. Cigarette smoke may be an appropriate comparator for evaluating potential harm reduction, but it is not always the correct benchmark for deciding whether an unnecessary ingredient should remain in a formulation. Ambient air, medicinal inhalation products, occupational limits or toxicological thresholds may be more relevant for particular questions. The same data can appear reassuring or concerning depending on the comparator, so the rationale should be transparent.

Quantitative integration may be possible where suitable data exist, but numerical scoring systems should be used cautiously. Assigning scores for reliability, relevance and consistency can improve transparency, especially across large datasets. However, scores can create false precision and may hide important qualitative differences. A study assigned seven points is not necessarily meaningfully stronger than one assigned six. Numerical tools should support expert judgement rather than substitute for it.

Formal evidence matrices can help organise the assessment. Each study or evidence stream can be recorded against identity, endpoint, route, reliability, relevance, direction of effect and uncertainty. This makes contradictions and data gaps visible. The final conclusion should still be expressed as a reasoned narrative because the significance of the evidence depends on relationships that tables cannot fully capture. A matrix is most useful as an audit trail, not as an automatic decision engine.

Bayesian or probabilistic approaches may be used in advanced assessments to update confidence as new evidence becomes available. Prior knowledge from chemical class or mechanism can be revised by product-specific analytical or biological data. These methods can make uncertainty explicit, but they require careful model definition and may not be practical for every ingredient. The underlying assumptions must remain understandable to regulators and decision-makers. Mathematical sophistication does not compensate for poor evidence selection.

Evidence weighting should consider direction and magnitude as well as presence or absence of an effect. A small, reversible change in a sensitive biomarker does not carry the same toxicological significance as persistent tissue injury. A statistically significant but biologically minor effect may receive limited weight, while a non-significant but large effect in an underpowered study may still warrant attention. Dose-response, persistence, reversibility and relation to known adverse pathways should guide interpretation.

Severity and reversibility influence the evidential threshold. Mild transient irritation may be manageable through concentration limits and user information, while evidence suggestive of sensitisation, genotoxicity or developmental toxicity demands greater caution. Where the potential outcome is severe or irreversible, the assessor may require stronger evidence before concluding that concern is adequately controlled. This does not mean every weak signal becomes decisive, but uncertainty should be handled asymmetrically where the consequences of a false-negative decision are substantial.

Exposure is the bridge between weight of evidence and regulatory risk assessment. Hazard evidence can be strong while product risk remains low if exposure is negligible, and moderate hazard evidence can become important where exposure is frequent or high. The assessor should therefore relate each evidence stream to measured or estimated consumer exposure. Studies conducted at concentrations far above realistic exposure may still identify a hazard, but their weight for risk characterisation depends on the available margin.

Exposure uncertainty should influence the final conclusion. Where aerosol transfer is measured reliably and use patterns are well characterised, the evidence can be interpreted with greater confidence. Where exposure depends on untested devices, variable power or poorly controlled consumer behaviour, a wider range should be considered. A favourable toxicological dataset cannot fully compensate for exposure that is undefined. Product restrictions, specified device compatibility or additional testing may be required.

Mixture effects present one of the most difficult areas for evidence integration. Ingredient-by-ingredient assessment may identify known hazards, while whole-aerosol testing captures combined biological activity. Additive irritation, shared mechanisms and chemical interactions can create effects not predicted from individual substances. Weight of evidence should therefore include both component and mixture information. A negative mixture test may provide reassurance for the endpoints and conditions examined, but it does not resolve all long-term or low-incidence hazards. A positive mixture result should trigger targeted investigation rather than immediate attribution to every component.

Thermal transformation should also be incorporated explicitly. Evidence about the parent ingredient may be reassuring while degradation products introduce different hazards. Literature on pyrolysis, product-specific emissions and device stress conditions should be integrated with the ingredient profile. If thermal products are identified only under severe dry-coil conditions, their weight for normal exposure may be lower but still relevant to foreseeable misuse. The conclusion should reflect the conditions under which the hazard emerges.

Data gaps are themselves part of the weight of evidence. Missing information does not count as adverse evidence, but it reduces confidence. The significance of the gap depends on the endpoint, exposure and surrounding evidence. Absence of chronic inhalation data may be tolerable for a low-exposure, well-characterised substance with no alerts and reassuring mechanistic evidence. The same gap may be unacceptable for a reactive ingredient used at high concentration. The assessor should explain why the available evidence is sufficient despite the gap or what additional action is required.

Uncertainty should be divided into identifiable categories. Substance uncertainty may arise from incomplete identity or impurities. Study uncertainty may arise from design limitations. Extrapolation uncertainty may arise from species, route or duration differences. Exposure uncertainty may arise from device variability and use patterns. Model uncertainty may arise from computational or in vitro assumptions. Separating these sources helps determine how uncertainty can be reduced and prevents a vague statement from concealing a critical weakness.

Risk-management measures can influence whether the overall evidence is sufficient. A substance with moderate uncertainty may be acceptable at a lower concentration, from a tightly controlled supplier or within a restricted device system. A concerning impurity may be managed through specification and release testing. An uncertain thermal pathway may be addressed through power limitation or formulation change. Weight of evidence therefore supports decisions about control as well as binary acceptance or rejection.

The final conclusion should reflect the strength of the evidence, not merely its direction. Terms such as strong, moderate, limited or insufficient support can be used if they are defined consistently. The assessment should state what is concluded, for which endpoint, under what exposure conditions and with what uncertainty. A conclusion that an ingredient is acceptable should identify the concentration, product configuration and controls on which that judgement depends. A conclusion of insufficient evidence should specify whether the appropriate response is additional testing, reformulation, restriction or rejection.

Documentation should allow the reasoning to be reconstructed. The assessor should identify the evidence streams considered, the criteria used to weight them, the principal supportive and contradictory findings, data gaps, exposure assumptions and final judgement. Important adverse evidence should be discussed directly. Merely citing a large reference list does not demonstrate weight-of-evidence analysis; the regulatory value lies in explaining how those references influenced the decision.

Independent review is particularly valuable because evidence weighting contains unavoidable expert judgement. A second toxicologist may identify overlooked studies, challenge relevance assumptions or give different weight to uncertainty. Disagreement should be resolved through scientific reasoning and recorded where material. The aim is not to eliminate judgement but to make it visible and robust enough to withstand external scrutiny.

Weight-of-evidence conclusions should be revisited when new information emerges. A new inhalation study, improved emissions dataset, supplier change or post-market signal can alter the balance. Evidence that was previously indirect may be replaced by product-specific data. A weak concern may become stronger through replication, while an early positive finding may be explained by methodological artefact. The assessment should therefore be version-controlled and maintained as part of lifecycle compliance.

The approach also supports reduction of animal testing because it requires existing evidence to be integrated before new studies are commissioned. In vitro models, read-across, computational predictions, human data and exposure information may collectively provide sufficient confidence without a conventional animal study. Where uncertainty remains, the weight-of-evidence analysis can identify the precise question that new testing must answer, avoiding broad programmes that duplicate existing knowledge.

This does not mean that every combination of alternative evidence will be sufficient. A large quantity of indirect information cannot always replace a critical missing dataset, particularly for severe endpoints or high exposure. The decision should depend on whether the combined evidence forms a coherent and biologically plausible account. Evidence integration is strongest when different methods converge on the same conclusion and each compensates for the limitations of the others.

Regulatory interpretation should remain proportionate to the product's intended context. For adult smokers replacing combustible cigarettes, comparative exposure and likely benefit may form part of the broader decision. This context does not change the intrinsic properties of an ingredient, but it can influence how residual risk is judged. A product may remain substantially less harmful than smoking while still containing an avoidable irritant that should be removed. Weight of evidence allows both realities to be recognised without reducing the assessment to either absolute safety or category rejection.

The greatest weakness of weight-of-evidence language is that it can be invoked without genuine analysis. Statements that the "totality of evidence supports safety" are meaningless unless the evidence, weighting and uncertainty are shown. The phrase should not function as a rhetorical shield for missing data or inconsistent findings. A defensible approach makes the path from evidence to decision explicit and allows another competent reviewer to disagree with particular judgements without being unable to see how they were reached.

Weight-of-evidence approaches are therefore not a relaxation of scientific standards but a disciplined response to the complexity of real regulatory evidence. They acknowledge that toxicological understanding rarely arrives through one decisive experiment and that different methods answer different parts of the question. Human observations provide direct relevance but limited control. Animal studies provide dose-response and chronic information but require extrapolation. In vitro methods provide mechanistic and respiratory relevance but limited whole-body prediction. Computational tools and read-across extend the evidence base but introduce model and analogue uncertainty. Analytical data define what the product emits, while exposure assessment determines whether identified hazards are likely to matter.

When these strands are evaluated transparently and integrated coherently, they can support decisions stronger than any individual dataset. They can identify where evidence converges, where uncertainty remains and which controls are necessary to maintain an acceptable product profile. The result is not certainty, because regulatory toxicology rarely offers it. The result is a reasoned conclusion proportionate to the quality of the evidence, the severity of the possible harm, the magnitude of exposure and the purpose of the product. Within vaping regulation, that is the standard required to move from fragmented scientific information to a decision capable of surviving both regulatory scrutiny and scientific challenge.

Exposure Assessment

Exposure assessment determines the amount of a substance that is likely to reach the consumer, the route by which it reaches them, the frequency and duration of contact and the degree of uncertainty surrounding those estimates. Within vaping regulation, this stage is essential because toxicological hazard cannot be interpreted meaningfully without knowing whether the user is exposed at a trivial, moderate or potentially concerning level. Ingredient concentration in the liquid is only the beginning of that calculation. The quantity ultimately inhaled depends on transfer into the aerosol, chemical transformation during heating, device design, power, airflow, puff duration, puff frequency, user behaviour, product consumption and respiratory deposition. A defensible exposure assessment must therefore connect the formulation, the hardware and the pattern of use rather than rely on nominal ingredient percentages or single-machine measurements. The central regulatory question is not simply how much of a substance is present in the product, but how much is available to the user under normal use, high-use conditions and reasonably foreseeable misuse.

The assessment should begin by defining the exposure scenario clearly. The product identity, formulation, device configuration, coil, power range, reservoir, nicotine strength, intended user and anticipated use pattern should all be specified. An exposure estimate derived from one device cannot automatically be transferred to another where heating power, aerosol mass and liquid consumption differ materially. A refill liquid intended for a restricted pod system may produce a relatively narrow exposure range, while the same liquid used in open systems with variable power can generate much greater uncertainty. The scenario should therefore state whether the assessment concerns one controlled product configuration, a family of variants or a wider range of compatible devices.

The route of exposure must be separated into inhalation, oral, dermal and ocular pathways where relevant. Inhalation is the intended route, but accidental ingestion, leakage onto the skin and splashes into the eyes may produce different risks and require separate calculations. A substance that is present at a low inhaled dose may still be relevant if a refill bottle contains a large total amount capable of causing acute harm when swallowed. Exposure assessment should therefore distinguish routine use from accidental events and avoid combining them into one average estimate.

For inhalation, the principal inputs are the concentration of the substance in the aerosol, the aerosol mass generated per puff, the number of puffs taken and the fraction deposited or absorbed. These variables can be expressed in several ways, including mass per puff, mass per litre of aerosol, mass per session, mass per millilitre of liquid consumed or estimated daily intake. The chosen metric should match the toxicological endpoint and allow comparison with the point of departure used later in risk characterisation. A per-puff result may be useful for analytical comparison, while a daily intake estimate is usually more appropriate for repeated-dose or margin-of-exposure calculations.

Liquid concentration alone is not a reliable exposure measure because transfer into aerosol varies by substance. Highly volatile flavour compounds may transfer efficiently, whereas less volatile compounds may remain in the reservoir or condense within the device. Some substances may decompose before they are inhaled, while others may be formed during heating despite being absent from the original liquid. The assessment should therefore use measured aerosol data where available and avoid assuming one hundred per cent transfer unless the intention is to create an explicitly conservative screening estimate.

Transfer efficiency can be calculated by comparing the amount of a substance in the aerosol with the amount consumed from the liquid over the same test period. This requires accurate measurement of liquid mass loss, aerosol collection and analytical recovery. The result should be interpreted cautiously because apparent transfer can be affected by sampling losses, condensation, degradation and the distinction between vapour and particulate phases. For volatile compounds, collection systems that capture only the particulate fraction may underestimate total emissions. The analytical method should therefore be appropriate to the physicochemical properties of the substance.

Device conditions have a major influence on exposure. Power, resistance, coil design, wick saturation, airflow and temperature determine aerosol yield and chemical transformation. A product tested at low power may produce a lower mass of aerosol and fewer degradation products than the same system operated at its upper limit. The exposure assessment should identify the intended operating range and include conditions that reflect ordinary use and credible upper-bound use. Stress conditions may be evaluated separately to determine whether a sharp increase in emissions occurs under poor wicking, low liquid level or excessive power.

The puffing regime is equally important. Puff duration, interval, volume and flow rate affect coil temperature, aerosol generation and total emissions. Standardised machine regimes improve comparability, but they may not represent all users. Some consumers take longer or more frequent puffs, particularly with low-power products or lower nicotine concentrations. The assessment should explain why the selected regime is appropriate and whether a second, more intensive regime is needed to characterise upper-bound exposure.

Machine-generated exposure should not be treated as identical to human exposure. Laboratory puffing provides repeatable aerosol generation, but users vary in topography, maintenance and product handling. They may alter puff duration, inhale more deeply, chain-vape or continue using a coil after performance has degraded. Human-use studies, observational data or realistic consumption surveys can help refine machine estimates. Where such data are unavailable, conservative but plausible assumptions should be used rather than extreme scenarios that bear little resemblance to actual behaviour.

Daily liquid consumption is one of the strongest determinants of total exposure. Users of low-strength liquids may consume greater volumes than users of higher-strength products, while experienced users may adopt different puffing patterns from new users. Product format also matters. A small closed pod may limit daily volume, whereas a high-power open system can aerosolise several millilitres. The assessment should consider central tendency and high-percentile use rather than one average value. A realistic upper-bound estimate is often more appropriate for regulatory screening.

Nicotine concentration can alter behaviour through compensation. When nicotine delivery is low, users may puff more frequently or inhale larger aerosol volumes to achieve the desired effect. Conversely, higher nicotine concentration may reduce liquid consumption but increase acute dose per puff. Exposure assessment should therefore avoid assuming that liquid consumption is independent of nicotine strength. Where several strengths are marketed, each may require separate or adjusted use assumptions.

Aerosol mass should be measured accurately because it provides the link between machine output and constituent exposure. Gravimetric collection can estimate total particulate matter or collected aerosol mass, but volatile losses and collection efficiency should be considered. The product may also produce a variable yield as the coil ages or the reservoir empties. Repeated measurements across units and time points can identify whether exposure remains stable or drifts during use.

Coil age can materially change exposure. New coils may release manufacturing residues or metals, while aged coils can accumulate deposits, alter resistance and generate higher thermal degradation. A product tested only with a fresh coil may underestimate later-life emissions. The assessment should consider the intended service period and include aged or stressed components where they are relevant to the product. The same principle applies to prefilled pods that remain in contact with liquid during storage.

Batch and unit variability should be incorporated. Identical nominal products may differ in fill volume, resistance, airflow or material quality. Exposure testing should use enough replicates to characterise this variation. Reporting only the mean can conceal high-emitting units, particularly where variability is wide. Upper confidence bounds or high-percentile results may provide a better basis for conservative regulatory assessment.

Analytical uncertainty should be documented. Limits of detection, limits of quantification, recovery, calibration, matrix effects and sampling efficiency all influence the result. A reported non-detect does not mean zero exposure. Where the detection limit is higher than the toxicologically relevant level, the method may be inadequate for risk assessment. In those cases, a conservative substitution value or improved method may be necessary.

For compounds formed during heating, exposure assessment should identify the relationship between the precursor, device conditions and emitted product. Carbonyls such as formaldehyde, acetaldehyde and acrolein can increase under overheating or poor liquid supply. The assessment should distinguish normal-use emissions from those associated with obvious dry-puff conditions. Severe conditions may still be relevant to misuse assessment, but they should not be presented as representative of routine exposure without qualification.

Metals require a different approach because their presence may arise from coils, solder, connectors or manufacturing contamination. Exposure can change with device age, acidity of the liquid and power. Measurements should distinguish metal concentration in the unused liquid from that in the aerosol. The assessment should also consider whether metals are present as dissolved ions, particles or nanoparticles, because form can influence deposition and toxicological behaviour.

Particle size influences where aerosol deposits in the respiratory tract. Smaller particles can penetrate more deeply, while larger droplets may deposit in the mouth and upper airways. Vaping aerosols are dynamic and can change through evaporation, condensation and hygroscopic growth after inhalation. A detailed dosimetry model may not be necessary for every product, but the assessor should recognise that emitted mass is not identical to deposited dose. Where local respiratory effects are central, deposition assumptions may materially affect the conclusion.

Deposition fraction can be estimated using respiratory models or empirical data, but the selected assumptions should match the particle and vapour characteristics of the aerosol. Volatile compounds may be absorbed in the upper airways or exhaled, while particle-bound substances may deposit according to size distribution. Systemic exposure can then depend on dissolution, absorption and clearance. The assessment should state whether it is estimating inhaled, deposited or absorbed dose because these are not interchangeable.

Body weight normalisation may be appropriate for systemic toxicity comparisons. Daily intake can be expressed as milligrams per kilogram of body weight where the point of departure is reported in the same form. The chosen body weight should be justified. A standard adult value may be suitable for general assessment, while lower body weight may be used for a conservative scenario. The calculation should not imply protection of children if the product is restricted to adults, but accidental exposure scenarios may require separate consideration of lower body weight.

Exposure duration should align with the toxicological study used for comparison. Acute exposure should be compared with acute endpoints, while chronic daily use requires repeated-dose or chronic points of departure where available. Extrapolating from a short-term study to long-term use introduces uncertainty. The assessment should record whether exposure is intermittent, daily, continuous or episodic and whether accumulation is plausible.

Frequency of use may vary by substance where exposure is tied to one flavour or product variant. A user may rotate products rather than use one formulation exclusively. The assessment may use a conservative assumption of exclusive use if this is plausible and protective. Where the product is likely to be used intermittently, a lower frequency may be appropriate, but the rationale should be explicit. Market assumptions should not be adjusted simply to create a more favourable result.

Co-exposure should be considered where several ingredients share the same endpoint or mechanism. Multiple irritants may contribute additively to airway effects, and several aldehydes may act through related pathways. A substance-by-substance calculation may underestimate combined exposure. Where common assessment groups can be defined, cumulative exposure or hazard-index approaches may be considered. This is more difficult for complex mixtures but should not be ignored where the formulation contains several known contributors to the same effect.

Background exposure can also matter. Consumers may encounter the same substance through food, air, occupation or other products. For local respiratory effects, product-specific inhalation may dominate, but for systemic endpoints total exposure may be relevant. The assessment should consider background sources where they are substantial and where the toxicological benchmark was intended to cover aggregate exposure.

Exposure to impurities and degradation products should be estimated separately where they have distinct hazards. A raw-material specification may limit an impurity in the liquid, but heating can increase or transform it. The finished-product aerosol should therefore be the preferred basis where feasible. For storage-related degradation, end-of-shelf-life samples may provide a more conservative and realistic estimate than freshly manufactured product.

The stability programme and exposure assessment should be connected. Changes in nicotine concentration, pH, viscosity or packaging interaction can alter aerosol yield and constituent transfer. A formulation that becomes thinner may leak more or aerosolise differently. Aged liquid may produce different emissions from fresh liquid. Where stability data show material change, exposure testing may need to include aged product.

Dermal exposure assessment should consider the concentration in the liquid, area of contact, duration, absorption and likelihood of repeated leakage. For many substances, a qualitative assessment may be sufficient, particularly where the principal concern is irritation. Nicotine may require a more quantitative approach because dermal absorption can contribute to systemic dose. Packaging integrity and user instructions should be treated as exposure controls.

Ocular exposure is usually accidental and episodic, but liquids containing nicotine, acids or irritants can cause pain or injury. The assessment should consider splash potential during filling and whether the container design reduces this. Quantitative ocular dose is rarely necessary, but hazard classification and concentration can inform warnings and first-aid instructions.

Accidental ingestion requires scenario-based assessment. The total nicotine content of the container or pod, concentration, closure performance and likelihood of child access are central. The assessment may consider the amount available from one unit and the consequences of partial or complete ingestion. Child-resistant packaging reduces likelihood but does not eliminate the hazard. For nicotine-free products, flavouring ingredients and solvents may still require consideration if large quantities are accessible.

Reasonably foreseeable misuse should be described separately from intentional abuse. Overfilling, using an incompatible charger, operating at the maximum setting, continuing to use a burnt coil or storing the product in heat are plausible behaviours. Extreme laboratory conditions that no consumer would tolerate may have limited exposure relevance. The assessment should therefore rank misuse scenarios by plausibility and consequence rather than treating every possible condition equally.

Uncertainty analysis is a core part of exposure assessment. Uncertainty may arise from product variability, consumer behaviour, analytical limitations, transfer assumptions, deposition models, study duration and market scope. These sources should be identified individually. Some can be reduced through additional testing, while others are inherent to consumer use. The final exposure estimate should reflect the direction of uncertainty. Where a parameter is uncertain and could increase exposure, conservative assumptions may be justified.

Sensitivity analysis can identify which inputs drive the result. Daily liquid consumption, aerosol transfer and puff count may have a greater influence than body weight or minor analytical variation. Understanding this helps direct further data collection. If the conclusion changes substantially with a small change in one assumption, confidence is low. If the conclusion remains stable across a realistic range, the assessment is more robust.

Tiered exposure assessment is often appropriate. An initial screening estimate may assume complete transfer and high daily consumption. If the resulting exposure remains far below the toxicological point of departure, no further refinement may be necessary. If the screening estimate approaches concern, product-specific aerosol measurements, realistic use data and deposition modelling can refine the result. This avoids unnecessary analytical complexity while ensuring that borderline substances receive more detailed assessment.

Conservatism should be deliberate and transparent. Combining the highest possible value for every parameter can produce an implausible scenario and may distort the regulatory conclusion. A more defensible approach uses high but realistic values and explains where conservative assumptions have been applied. Central and upper-bound estimates can be presented together to show the range of plausible exposure.

The output should be expressed in units appropriate for later risk characterisation. These may include micrograms per puff, micrograms per day, milligrams per kilogram body weight per day or concentration in inhaled air. Conversion steps should be traceable. Units should not be mixed or transformed without explanation, as small errors in volume, mass or time can materially alter the margin of exposure.

Where a point of departure is route-specific, the exposure estimate should match that route. An inhalation concentration in milligrams per cubic metre may be compared with an inhalation benchmark, while a systemic dose may require conversion to absorbed mass per kilogram. Route-to-route comparison should be avoided unless toxicokinetics and local effects have been considered. A mathematically neat comparison can still be biologically invalid.

For local respiratory effects, average daily systemic dose may be the wrong metric. Peak concentration, per-puff exposure or deposited dose to airway tissue may be more relevant. Irritation can depend on concentration at the contact site rather than total daily mass. The assessment should therefore select metrics according to the mechanism. One exposure estimate may not serve every endpoint.

For chronic systemic effects, average daily intake may be appropriate, especially where the substance is absorbed and does not produce a strong local effect. For acute toxicity, short-term dose and maximum single-event exposure are more relevant. For sensitisation, repeated low-level exposure and susceptible populations may matter more than average dose. Exposure assessment should therefore be endpoint-specific rather than a single universal calculation.

The relationship between nicotine delivery and use behaviour should be considered in interpreting product exposure. A product that delivers nicotine efficiently may reduce total aerosol consumption, while a weak product may encourage more intensive use. This does not mean high nicotine delivery is automatically preferable, because dependence and acute dose remain relevant. It does mean that aerosol exposure cannot be understood solely from liquid strength or device output without considering behavioural compensation.

Comparative exposure can provide useful context. Emissions may be compared with cigarette smoke, occupational benchmarks, medicinal inhalers or background air, depending on the regulatory question. Comparisons should use equivalent units and conditions. A lower level than cigarette smoke may support harm-reduction context, but it does not establish that the exposure is negligible or that an avoidable ingredient should remain. The comparator should illuminate the decision rather than determine it automatically.

Product-family assessment can reduce duplication where variants share a common platform, but grouping must be justified. The highest flavour loading, greatest transfer efficiency, highest power or worst-case emissions may be used to represent a family if the selected product genuinely bounds the others. Different flavour chemistries can alter aerosol behaviour significantly, so one representative product may not cover all variants. The assessment should state which features are shared and where separate testing remains necessary.

Exposure assessment should also support change control. A new supplier, reformulated flavour, different coil or altered power range can change transfer and emissions. The original estimate may no longer apply. Changes should therefore be screened for exposure impact before implementation, with bridging data or new testing where required.

Post-market data can refine exposure assumptions. Sales, pod consumption, refill frequency, complaint patterns and human-use studies may provide information on actual use. These data can reveal whether pre-market assumptions were conservative or whether certain groups use the product more intensively than expected. Exposure assessment should be updated where real-world evidence materially changes the scenario.

The final document should include the product and scenario definition, analytical methods, use assumptions, transfer data, calculations, uncertainty analysis and conclusions. It should identify whether the estimate represents typical, high-end or worst-case use and whether it is suitable for acute, chronic, local or systemic endpoints. The supporting data should be traceable to the correct product version and batch.

A strong exposure assessment avoids both extremes of underestimation and artificial worst-case inflation. It does not assume that nominal liquid concentration equals inhaled dose, and it does not rely on unrealistic laboratory abuse as though it describes normal use. It integrates measured emissions, plausible consumer behaviour and endpoint-relevant dosimetry to produce an estimate that is scientifically defensible and regulatorily useful.

Within the wider toxicological process, exposure assessment is the stage that turns hazard information into a product-specific question of relevance. It determines whether a respiratory irritant is present at a level likely to matter, whether a degradation product requires reformulation, whether a read-across point of departure provides an adequate margin and whether uncertainty can be controlled through design or specification. Without exposure assessment, toxicology remains a catalogue of chemical properties. With it, those properties can be translated into decisions about concentration limits, testing priorities, product configuration and market acceptability.

Margin of Exposure

Margin of exposure provides a structured way of comparing the level at which a toxicological effect has been observed with the level of exposure expected from the product under assessment. It is not a direct measurement of safety, nor is it a universal threshold that can be applied mechanically across all substances and endpoints. It is a comparative tool that expresses the distance between an experimental point of departure and the estimated human exposure arising from use of the product. In its simplest form, the point of departure is divided by the estimated exposure, producing a numerical margin. A larger margin generally indicates greater separation between the dose associated with an adverse effect and the dose expected in the consumer, while a smaller margin indicates less separation and therefore a greater need for scrutiny, refinement or control. The apparent simplicity of that calculation can be misleading because every element depends on scientific judgement. The point of departure may come from an oral rather than inhalation study, from an animal rather than a human population, from a short-duration rather than chronic exposure, or from an endpoint that does not correspond precisely to the effect of concern in the respiratory tract. The exposure estimate may depend on aerosol transfer, liquid consumption, body weight, puffing behaviour, deposition and analytical sensitivity. Margin-of-exposure analysis is therefore only as reliable as the evidence placed on both sides of the equation.

The first requirement is selection of an appropriate point of departure. This may be a no-observed-adverse-effect level, lowest-observed-adverse-effect level, benchmark dose, benchmark concentration or another scientifically justified value derived from the toxicological literature. The selected point should relate as closely as possible to the route, duration and endpoint under assessment. A repeated-inhalation benchmark for respiratory irritation is generally more relevant to vaping exposure than an oral repeated-dose value, while a systemic oral study may still be informative where the substance is well absorbed and the principal concern is liver, kidney or neurological toxicity rather than local airway injury. The assessor should resist the temptation to select the largest available value simply because it produces a more favourable margin. The critical study should be the one that best reflects the most sensitive relevant effect, not the one that offers the greatest numerical separation. Where several credible studies exist, their design, route, duration, dose-response and study quality should be compared before one is selected.

A no-observed-adverse-effect level is often used because it appears to define a dose below which no adverse effect was seen, but its interpretation depends heavily on study design. A study with widely spaced dose groups may report a high no-effect level simply because no intermediate dose was tested. The true threshold may lie anywhere between the no-effect and lowest-effect doses. Sample size, endpoint sensitivity and duration also matter. A negative result from a short study may not exclude chronic effects, and a no-effect level based on gross pathology may miss subtle functional or biochemical changes. The value should therefore be regarded as an experimental boundary rather than a precise biological threshold.

Benchmark-dose methods can provide a stronger basis where suitable data are available because they model the dose-response curve rather than relying on one experimental dose group. A benchmark dose lower confidence limit is often preferred because it incorporates uncertainty around the estimate. The chosen benchmark response should be toxicologically meaningful and appropriate to the endpoint. A small statistical change may not represent an adverse effect, while a larger benchmark response may miss an early but important biological signal. The quality of the model fit, data range and biological plausibility should all be considered. A mathematically derived value should not be treated as superior merely because it appears more precise.

Where only a lowest-observed-adverse-effect level is available, additional caution is required because an adverse effect was already present at the selected dose. The margin calculated from such a point may need to be interpreted more conservatively or adjusted to estimate a plausible no-effect level. This should not be done automatically by applying arbitrary factors without considering the steepness of the dose-response and severity of the effect. A mild, reversible change observed only at the highest dose is different from severe tissue injury occurring across several dose groups. The nature of the effect is central to determining how much separation is needed.

Route relevance is one of the most important limitations in vaping toxicology. Many flavouring ingredients have oral toxicity data but little or no inhalation evidence. Converting an oral point of departure into an inhalation margin assumes that systemic dose is the main determinant and that local respiratory effects are not more sensitive. That assumption may be reasonable for some well-characterised, non-reactive substances with high oral bioavailability and no respiratory alerts. It is much weaker for volatile, reactive or irritant chemicals capable of interacting directly with airway tissue. A substance may be rapidly detoxified after oral absorption but cause local respiratory damage before systemic metabolism can occur. Where local inhalation toxicity is plausible, an oral margin should not be used as if it resolves the respiratory question.

Route-to-route extrapolation also requires consideration of bioavailability. An oral dose expressed in milligrams per kilogram does not necessarily equal an inhaled dose of the same numerical value because absorption may differ. First-pass metabolism may reduce systemic exposure after ingestion, while inhalation can deliver the parent compound directly into circulation. Conversely, a substance may be poorly absorbed through the lung or largely exhaled. Where toxicokinetic data are available, they can support adjustment. Where they are not, the uncertainty should be recorded and the margin interpreted conservatively. The numerical result should not conceal the fact that the comparison may rest on imperfect route equivalence.

Duration must also be aligned. A point of departure from an acute study cannot support chronic daily exposure without substantial uncertainty. A 28-day study may identify short-term repeated-dose effects but remain insufficient for a product used over years. Subchronic and chronic studies generally provide a stronger basis for long-term exposure, although they may still use a different route or species. Where only shorter studies exist, the assessor should consider whether the effect is likely to accumulate, whether the substance is persistent, whether adaptation occurs and whether the endpoint is reversible. Additional uncertainty may be needed, but this should be explained scientifically rather than applied as a routine multiplier detached from the substance.

Species extrapolation is another source of uncertainty. Animal studies can provide dose-response information unavailable in humans, but differences in metabolism, respiratory anatomy, breathing pattern and tissue sensitivity may affect relevance. Rodents often receive higher dose rates relative to body weight and may metabolise substances differently. In inhalation studies, nasal deposition and obligate nose breathing can produce effects not directly comparable with human exposure. The margin should therefore be interpreted in the context of the species and endpoint, and uncertainty factors may be used where appropriate to account for interspecies differences. These factors are not evidence that the animal response will occur in humans; they are protective tools used when precise cross-species relationships are unknown.

Human variability creates a separate challenge. Consumer populations include individuals with different age, body weight, metabolic capacity, respiratory health and susceptibility. People with asthma, chronic obstructive pulmonary disease or cardiovascular disease may respond differently from healthy adults. A point of departure based on healthy experimental animals or adult workers may not protect all users equally. In conventional risk assessment, uncertainty factors are often applied for interindividual variability, but the relevance of a standard factor depends on the endpoint and quality of the database. Margin-of-exposure interpretation should recognise that the intended user population is not biologically uniform, even where the product is restricted to adults.

The exposure side of the calculation requires equal discipline. The estimated daily dose should be based on product-specific aerosol data wherever possible, together with realistic assumptions about consumption and use. Liquid concentration should not be equated automatically with inhaled exposure because transfer efficiency varies and some ingredients may degrade during aerosolisation. Measured mass per puff or per unit of liquid consumed can be combined with a typical and high-use scenario to estimate daily intake. Where only screening data are available, conservative assumptions may be used, but the assessment should state that the margin is provisional and may require refinement.

Exposure estimates should match the point of departure in both units and biological meaning. A systemic point expressed in milligrams per kilogram per day should be compared with an absorbed or plausibly systemic daily dose, not simply with the concentration in the liquid. An inhalation concentration expressed in milligrams per cubic metre should be compared with an equivalent inhaled-air concentration or suitably adjusted product exposure. Local respiratory effects may be better related to deposited airway concentration, per-puff dose or peak exposure than to average daily systemic intake. A margin can be numerically correct and biologically meaningless if the units are aligned mathematically but the exposure metric does not correspond to the mechanism.

Daily exposure assumptions should be transparent. The assessor may calculate a central estimate using average consumption and an upper-bound estimate using high-percentile use. Exclusive use of one product may be assumed for conservatism, but the plausibility of that assumption should be stated. Nicotine concentration may alter liquid consumption through behavioural compensation, and device power can change aerosol yield substantially. A low-strength liquid used heavily may produce greater exposure to non-nicotine constituents than a higher-strength product used less frequently. The margin should therefore be calculated for the actual product configuration and use pattern rather than borrowed from a generic vaping scenario.

Body weight normalisation can influence the result materially. A standard adult body weight may be suitable for systemic exposure estimates, but a lower value may provide a conservative assumption. The selected value should reflect the intended population and regulatory convention. Accidental exposure by children requires a separate scenario and should not be folded into routine adult inhalation assessment. Margin-of-exposure analysis for normal use is not a substitute for acute poisoning risk assessment.

Non-detect results also require careful handling. If an ingredient or degradation product is not detected in aerosol, the exposure should not automatically be assigned a value of zero. The analytical limit may still exceed the toxicologically relevant concentration. A conservative estimate may use the limit of detection or quantification, depending on the context. If the resulting margin remains large, the conclusion may be reassuring. If the margin is narrow, a more sensitive method is needed. Analytical absence is only as meaningful as the method's ability to detect the substance at a level relevant to risk.

The numerical size of an acceptable margin cannot be determined by one universal rule. Conventional toxicology sometimes uses reference values such as one hundred-fold separation to account broadly for interspecies and human variability, while larger margins may be expected where the evidence is weak, the endpoint is severe or the point of departure is poorly matched to exposure. These conventions can be useful, but they should not be applied as though every substance and dataset carry the same uncertainty. A margin of one thousand based on a high-quality inhalation study may be more reassuring than a margin of ten thousand derived from a weak oral analogue with uncertain transfer. The number must be interpreted in relation to data quality, route, duration, severity and uncertainty.

High-concern endpoints require particular caution. For genotoxic carcinogens, a threshold may not be assumed, and margin-of-exposure analysis may be used primarily for prioritisation rather than to declare a safe level. A large margin can indicate lower concern relative to another exposure, but it does not necessarily justify deliberate inclusion of an avoidable genotoxic substance. Where credible genotoxicity exists, removal or reduction to the lowest reasonably achievable level is generally preferable. The same caution applies to respiratory sensitisers, where susceptible individuals may react at low exposures and reliable thresholds may be absent.

For threshold effects such as systemic toxicity or some forms of irritation, margin-of-exposure analysis can be more directly useful. If a robust point of departure exists and product exposure is well below it, the margin can support acceptance. Even here, local concentration and peak exposure may matter. An average daily dose can obscure brief high concentrations that cause irritation during each puff. The assessor should determine whether the toxicological effect is driven by cumulative dose, peak concentration or repeated local contact before relying on one margin.

Multiple margins may be needed for the same ingredient. One may address systemic repeated-dose toxicity, another respiratory irritation, another reproductive effects and another a specific metabolite. The most critical margin is not always the smallest numerically because the evidence quality and severity differ. The assessment should identify which endpoint drives the regulatory conclusion and why. A favourable systemic margin does not resolve a narrow respiratory margin, and a reassuring irritation assessment does not dismiss an unresolved genotoxicity concern.

Mixture effects complicate interpretation because each ingredient may have an acceptable individual margin while several compounds contribute to the same toxicological endpoint. Where substances share a mechanism or target organ, combined exposure may need to be considered. A hazard index or grouped assessment can sum exposure relative to each reference point, although the scientific basis must be appropriate. Additivity should not be assumed for unrelated effects, but ignoring several irritants merely because each one passes separately may underestimate total respiratory burden.

Thermal degradation products should be assessed independently where they have distinct hazards. A parent flavour ingredient may have a wide margin, while a carbonyl formed during heating may have a much narrower one. Product-specific emissions under normal and upper-bound conditions are therefore essential. If the margin collapses under foreseeable high-power or low-liquid conditions, the product may require engineering controls, formulation change or restricted compatibility. It is not enough to show that the margin is acceptable under ideal operation.

Margin-of-exposure analysis can also support comparison between formulation options. If two ingredients perform the same sensory function but one produces a substantially larger margin and has a better inhalation dataset, the safer choice becomes clearer. The method can help prioritise reformulation by identifying substances contributing most strongly to the toxicological burden. It can also support concentration limits, showing how much reduction is needed to reach an acceptable level of separation.

The method is particularly useful as part of a tiered assessment. An initial conservative calculation may assume high consumption and complete transfer. If the resulting margin is very large, further refinement may be unnecessary. If the margin is borderline, product-specific transfer data, realistic use information and improved toxicological analysis can refine the estimate. If the margin remains narrow after refinement, the ingredient concentration should be reduced, the product restricted or the substance removed. This staged approach directs resources towards substances that actually influence the regulatory decision.

Sensitivity analysis improves confidence by showing which assumptions drive the result. Daily liquid consumption, transfer efficiency, body weight or study selection may each affect the margin. If a small change in one input causes the margin to shift from reassuring to concerning, the conclusion is unstable and further data are needed. If the margin remains large across a wide range of plausible assumptions, the assessment is more robust. Sensitivity analysis also prevents false precision by demonstrating that the reported figure is one estimate within a range.

Uncertainty should be presented explicitly rather than hidden behind the final number. The assessor should identify uncertainties in the point of departure, route extrapolation, species, duration, exposure measurement, consumer behaviour and product variability. These should be discussed in terms of their likely direction and magnitude. Some uncertainties may increase the margin, while others may decrease it. A qualitative confidence rating can accompany the numerical result, provided the basis is clear.

The calculation itself should be fully traceable. The source study, selected endpoint, point of departure, exposure estimate, unit conversions, body weight and assumptions should all be documented. The product version and analytical method should be identified. Another competent reviewer should be able to reproduce the margin without reconstructing missing steps. Spreadsheet errors, unit mistakes and mismatched time bases can change results by orders of magnitude, so independent verification is valuable.

The margin should remain linked to the product specification. Acceptance may depend on a maximum ingredient concentration, a defined supplier purity, a restricted power range or a particular device. If any of those conditions change, the assessment may no longer apply. Change control should therefore trigger review when the formulation, hardware, supplier, manufacturing process or use instructions change. A margin calculated for one product should not be transferred automatically to another that shares only the ingredient name.

Post-market data may also influence interpretation. Complaints of irritation or adverse effects can challenge an apparently favourable margin, particularly where the original exposure estimate was uncertain. Conversely, long-term controlled use without a signal may provide some reassurance, although absence of reporting remains weak evidence on its own. Emerging toxicological studies can alter the selected point of departure and should trigger reassessment where relevant.

Comparative-risk context may be considered, particularly for products intended to replace smoking. A vaping product may produce exposure far below that associated with cigarette smoke while still containing an ingredient with a narrow margin relative to its own toxicological benchmark. Reduced exposure compared with smoking does not remove the need to address avoidable hazards. Margin-of-exposure analysis helps separate those questions by evaluating the product on its own toxicological terms while allowing broader public-health context to be considered later.

The method should not be used to manufacture reassurance from weak data. A very large margin obtained by dividing a poorly relevant oral no-effect level by a low estimated aerosol dose can appear impressive while offering limited confidence. Equally, a small margin based on extreme laboratory conditions may overstate routine risk. The scientific strength lies not in the magnitude alone but in the relevance and quality of the inputs. The number should summarise the evidence, not replace it.

Margin of exposure is therefore best understood as a disciplined framework for proportionate judgement. It translates hazard and exposure into a common quantitative relationship, supports comparison between substances and identifies where additional control is needed. It can reveal that a hazardous substance is present at a level unlikely to be materially relevant, or that an apparently minor ingredient is being used too close to an effect level. It can help regulators and manufacturers decide whether existing evidence is sufficient, whether concentration reduction is required or whether uncertainty remains too great to support use.

Within vaping regulation, the method is especially valuable because direct inhalation data are often incomplete and products vary in the way they generate aerosol. It cannot overcome missing evidence by itself, but it forces the assessor to show how the chosen toxicological point relates to the measured product exposure. A defensible margin is one derived from the most relevant available evidence, tested against realistic upper-bound use, adjusted transparently for uncertainty and tied to the exact formulation and device assessed. The final conclusion should therefore state not merely that the margin is large or small, but what it means, which assumptions control it and what regulatory action follows from it.

Missing Inhalation Data

Missing inhalation data represent one of the most persistent and consequential weaknesses in the regulatory assessment of vaping products because the route by which these products are used is often the route for which the least direct toxicological evidence exists. Many ingredients have long histories of use in food, fragrance, cosmetics or pharmaceuticals, and some are supported by extensive oral or dermal datasets, yet relatively few have been studied through repeated inhalation under conditions capable of informing chronic consumer exposure. This mismatch creates a structural problem. The product is designed to deliver an aerosol to the respiratory tract, but the evidence available for individual ingredients frequently originates from ingestion, occupational handling, acute irritation studies or general chemical classifications. The absence of inhalation data does not prove that an ingredient is harmful, but it removes the most direct basis for determining how it behaves in the airway, whether it causes local effects at realistic concentrations and whether repeated use introduces risks that would not be apparent from another route. Regulatory toxicology must therefore decide how far existing evidence can be extended, when uncertainty can be managed and when the data gap is too important to ignore.

The scale of the problem is partly a consequence of the number and diversity of substances used in flavour systems. A single formulation may contain dozens of compounds, while a commercial flavour concentrate can include far more. Across the market, the potential ingredient universe runs into the thousands, many with limited inhalation histories and some with no repeated-dose data by any route. Even if one were to consider conventional animal inhalation studies acceptable in every case, the practical burden of testing each substance individually, at multiple concentrations and in relevant combinations, would be impossible to sustain. The difficulty increases further because heating can alter the substance, meaning that inhalation testing of the parent ingredient may still fail to capture the degradation products actually reaching the user. The data gap is therefore not a temporary administrative omission that can be corrected simply by commissioning enough studies. It is an inherent feature of complex consumer-product toxicology and must be managed through a combination of evidence integration, exposure control, prioritisation and alternative methods.

The respiratory tract presents specific biological conditions that make route extrapolation uncertain. Inhaled substances first encounter airway surface liquid, mucus, epithelial cells, cilia and immune defences before reaching deeper regions of the lung. Highly water-soluble compounds may deposit predominantly in the upper airways, while less soluble or particle-associated substances may penetrate further. Reactive chemicals can bind locally before systemic metabolism occurs, producing irritation or tissue injury that would not be predicted from oral data. Some compounds are rapidly detoxified in the liver after ingestion but may interact directly with respiratory tissue when inhaled. Others may be absorbed efficiently across the lung and reach systemic circulation with reduced first-pass metabolism. The same external dose can therefore produce different internal distributions and biological effects depending on route. Missing inhalation data matter because they leave these local and kinetic differences unresolved.

Oral toxicity studies remain useful, but their role should be defined carefully. They can provide information about systemic target organs, general dose-response, metabolism and repeated-dose effects, particularly where the substance is well absorbed and local respiratory toxicity is not strongly suspected. A high oral no-effect level may suggest that systemic toxicity is unlikely at the much lower doses expected from vaping. However, this does not establish the absence of local airway irritation, sensitisation or direct chemical reactivity. The assessor should therefore separate the systemic question from the respiratory question. Oral data may support one while leaving the other largely unanswered. The weakness arises when a reassuring oral point of departure is treated as though it resolves inhalation safety in full.

Dermal evidence is even more limited in route relevance, though it may still identify irritation, sensitisation or corrosivity. A substance positive in a skin-sensitisation assay may possess electrophilic properties that justify concern about immune reactivity, but the relationship between skin and respiratory sensitisation is not straightforward. Conversely, a negative dermal result does not prove the absence of respiratory effects. Such data can contribute to the hazard profile but should not be overextended. Missing inhalation data demand route-specific reasoning rather than the simple accumulation of whatever studies happen to exist.

Occupational evidence can be particularly valuable because it sometimes provides the only human inhalation information available for flavouring agents, volatile chemicals and industrial intermediates. Workplace studies may identify respiratory symptoms, asthma, changes in lung function or disease associated with repeated exposure. They can also support the development of occupational exposure limits. Yet their interpretation is difficult. Workers may be exposed to higher concentrations, complex mixtures, dusts or vapours different from vaping aerosols. Co-exposures may be substantial, and historical workplace controls may have been poor. Exposure estimates are often uncertain, and affected workers may represent only a small proportion of the population. Occupational data can therefore identify credible respiratory hazards and potential mechanisms, but they do not provide a direct consumer-risk answer without careful comparison of dose, duration and form.

The absence of direct inhalation studies is most problematic where the substance possesses properties that make local respiratory effects plausible. Volatile aldehydes, reactive carbonyls, known irritants, sensitising compounds and substances with strong electrophilic character should be treated more cautiously than inert, well-characterised molecules with low aerosol transfer. A data gap is not equally important for every ingredient. The significance depends on inherent hazard, concentration, physicochemical behaviour, expected transfer and severity of the potential endpoint. A low-level, non-reactive substance with extensive oral data and no structural alerts may be supportable despite missing inhalation studies, while a reactive flavour aldehyde used at high concentration may not be.

This distinction is central to a tiered approach. The first stage should screen for known respiratory hazards, structural alerts, authoritative classifications, occupational evidence, volatility, reactivity and expected exposure. Substances with no concerning features and very low estimated dose may be provisionally placed at lower priority. Those with evidence of irritation, sensitisation, genotoxicity, thermal instability or high transfer should move to more detailed assessment. The aim is not to declare low-priority substances safe, but to direct analytical and toxicological resources towards the uncertainties most likely to affect the regulatory decision.

Exposure becomes the principal means of contextualising the data gap. Where a substance is present at a very low concentration, transfers poorly to aerosol and yields a wide margin relative to an appropriate point of departure, missing inhalation data may be less consequential. Where exposure is high or uncertain, the same absence becomes more serious. This is why product-specific aerosol measurement is so important. Without it, the assessor may know that the ingredient lacks inhalation data but have no reliable way to determine whether the gap matters. Screening assumptions can be conservative, but they should be refined when the initial estimate approaches concern.

A threshold-of-toxicological-concern framework may sometimes support low-exposure substances, particularly where the chemical falls within a defined structural class and does not belong to an excluded high-concern category. This method uses broad toxicological distributions to establish exposure levels below which appreciable risk is considered unlikely. It can be useful for flavour constituents present at trace levels where direct data are sparse. Its limitations are significant. It is not appropriate for genotoxic substances, metals, proteins, persistent chemicals, highly potent compounds or substances with specific respiratory hazards. It also does not resolve local airway effects automatically. Used carefully, it can reduce unnecessary testing; used indiscriminately, it can disguise important route-specific uncertainty.

Read-across provides another route through the data gap. If the target ingredient is closely related to substances with inhalation or repeated-dose information, the assessor may infer likely behaviour from shared structure, metabolism, physicochemical properties and mechanism. This is stronger where the analogue is well characterised and the basis of similarity is biologically meaningful. It is weaker where the comparison rests only on broad structural resemblance. Missing inhalation data do not justify casual analogue selection. The source substance should be at least as relevant and preferably capable of bounding the target for the endpoint of concern. Differences in volatility, reactivity and metabolism should be addressed directly.

Category approaches can be useful where several related substances show a coherent toxicological pattern. A homologous series may reveal increasing irritation with chain length, volatility or reactivity. The target can then be positioned within that trend. Such approaches are more persuasive than one-to-one analogies when the category is well defined and outliers are understood. They also allow the assessor to use existing data more efficiently across multiple ingredients. However, flavour chemistry often contains substances that appear related but behave differently due to subtle structural features. Category logic must therefore remain endpoint-specific.

Weight-of-evidence analysis is the broader framework through which missing inhalation data are judged. Oral studies, in vitro respiratory models, occupational reports, computational predictions, emissions measurements, read-across and mechanistic information may collectively provide enough confidence even though no conventional inhalation study exists. The strength lies in convergence. If structural analysis shows low reactivity, computational models show no major alerts, in vitro airway testing is negative at relevant concentrations, aerosol transfer is minimal and oral repeated-dose data are reassuring, the absence of an animal inhalation study may be of limited regulatory importance. If several lines of evidence point towards airway irritation or reactive chemistry, the same absence becomes a major uncertainty rather than a neutral gap.

In vitro respiratory systems are especially valuable because they allow direct investigation of airway-relevant effects without requiring whole-animal exposure. Reconstructed human bronchial tissues, epithelial cultures, air–liquid interface models and co-culture systems can examine cytotoxicity, barrier integrity, ciliary function, oxidative stress and inflammatory signalling. These methods can compare the target ingredient with known irritants, assess concentration-response and test the complete aerosol rather than only the liquid. Their principal limitation is that they do not reproduce the full complexity of chronic human exposure, including systemic metabolism, immune interactions, repair mechanisms and disease progression. Nevertheless, they can provide highly relevant mechanistic evidence and are often more informative for local respiratory effects than oral animal studies.

Air–liquid interface exposure is particularly important because it allows cells or tissues to encounter aerosol in a form closer to actual inhalation. Submerged exposure to e-liquid can be useful for screening intrinsic cytotoxicity, but it may deliver unrealistically high and poorly comparable doses. Aerosol exposure systems can characterise deposited mass and compare device conditions, though method standardisation remains challenging. The deposited dose should be quantified where possible, because nominal chamber concentration alone does not establish what reached the tissue. A negative result is more meaningful when the model was exposed to levels at or above realistic consumer exposure and demonstrated adequate assay sensitivity.

Organoid and organ-on-chip technologies offer further potential by incorporating multiple cell types, dynamic airflow, mechanical stretch or fluid interfaces. These systems may improve the study of chronic irritation, barrier disruption and tissue-level responses. They remain technically demanding and are not yet universally accepted as replacements for all inhalation endpoints, but they can provide important bridging evidence. Their regulatory value will increase as validation, reproducibility and interlaboratory comparability improve.

Computational toxicology can identify structural alerts, likely metabolites, receptor interactions and chemical reactivity. Quantitative structure–activity relationship models can support mutagenicity, sensitisation and systemic toxicity screening. Physiologically based kinetic models may help compare oral and inhaled exposure by estimating tissue concentrations. These methods are useful where empirical data are absent, but they depend on applicability domain and model quality. A prediction outside the model's chemical space should carry little weight, and a negative result should not override strong experimental evidence. Missing inhalation data cannot be replaced simply by generating multiple computer outputs that all depend on similar assumptions.

Adverse outcome pathways provide a way to organise mechanistic evidence. If a substance is expected to trigger a known molecular initiating event, such as protein binding or oxidative stress, and the downstream sequence towards respiratory injury is well established, non-animal evidence can be interpreted more coherently. This can help determine which assays are most informative and whether observed biomarker changes are plausibly linked to harm. The framework is especially useful for irritation and sensitisation, though many chronic respiratory outcomes remain incompletely mapped.

Whole-aerosol testing adds another essential layer because it captures interactions, thermal transformation and device effects that ingredient-level analysis cannot. A product may contain ingredients with limited inhalation data but produce an aerosol that shows low cytotoxicity and limited inflammatory activity under representative conditions. This does not prove long-term safety, but it can reduce concern for the endpoints tested. Conversely, a positive whole-aerosol result may reveal combined effects or degradation products not predicted from the individual ingredient list. Missing inhalation data for one ingredient may therefore be managed partly through product-level testing, provided the limitations are understood.

The same applies to analytical emissions assessment. If a poorly studied ingredient transfers minimally to aerosol and does not generate concerning degradation products, the respiratory data gap may be less important. If it transfers efficiently or alters carbonyl formation, concern increases. Product-specific data are particularly valuable because generic literature cannot always predict the behaviour of one formulation-device combination. The absence of ingredient inhalation studies should therefore drive stronger analytical characterisation rather than passive acceptance.

Chronicity remains one of the hardest unresolved issues. Many alternative methods are best suited to acute or short-term responses, while vaping products may be used repeatedly for years. Short-term negative findings do not exclude cumulative effects, tissue remodelling or chronic inflammation. Repeated-exposure in vitro systems can improve relevance, but they still cannot reproduce every long-term process. Missing chronic inhalation data should therefore be acknowledged explicitly. The absence may be acceptable where exposure is low and the wider evidence is strongly reassuring, but it should not disappear behind short-term assay results.

The interpretation of no evidence is often distorted in regulatory debate. One side may treat the lack of inhalation studies as proof that the ingredient is unsafe, while another may treat long commercial use without obvious reports as proof that it is acceptable. Both positions exceed the evidence. Missing data create uncertainty, not a predetermined answer. The regulatory task is to determine whether the uncertainty can be bounded sufficiently through other evidence and exposure control. In some cases it can. In others, the appropriate response is concentration reduction, reformulation or exclusion.

Precaution should be proportionate rather than absolute. A strict rule that every ingredient requires a complete inhalation dataset would eliminate most flavour chemistry and make product development impossible. A permissive rule that any food-approved substance can be inhaled would ignore fundamental route differences. The defensible position lies between those extremes. High-concern, reactive or poorly characterised ingredients should face a high evidential burden. Low-exposure, well-characterised substances may be supported through integrated non-animal evidence. The level of precaution should reflect the potential severity of error.

The intended function of the ingredient also matters. A substance that is essential to product performance may justify more effort to resolve uncertainty than one included for a marginal sensory effect. If a poorly characterised additive provides little functional benefit, removal is often the most efficient risk-management action. This principle is important because missing inhalation data are not distributed randomly. Some of the most uncertain substances are optional flavour embellishments rather than necessary formulation components. Product design should therefore reduce the toxicological burden before relying on increasingly complex assessment methods.

Concentration limits provide another practical control. Where an ingredient can be justified only at low exposure, the approved specification should reflect that condition. The assessment should state the maximum concentration, supplier grade and device configuration on which the conclusion depends. Broad approval of the ingredient without these controls invites later use at levels unsupported by the evidence. Change control should trigger reassessment when concentration, supplier or formulation changes.

Supplier transparency is critical. Missing inhalation data are difficult enough to manage when the substance is known; they become almost impossible where the composition itself is uncertain. Proprietary mixtures, natural extracts and variable botanical materials may contain constituents with their own unrecognised respiratory hazards. Confidentiality mechanisms can protect intellectual property, but complete compositional access is necessary for assessment. Unknown composition cannot be compensated for by generic statements that the mixture is food-grade.

Natural origin provides no solution to missing data. Essential oils, extracts and botanical preparations may contain complex and variable mixtures of terpenes, phenolics, allergens and oxidation products. Some have strong biological activity and limited inhalation evidence. Historical oral or traditional use does not establish suitability for aerosol delivery. Where the material cannot be standardised and its constituents cannot be assessed individually, exclusion may be more defensible than attempting broad read-across from the source plant.

Post-market surveillance plays a supplementary role because some effects may become apparent only after wider use. Complaints of irritation, wheeze, allergic response or unusual respiratory symptoms should be trended by formulation and ingredient. Individual reports rarely establish causation, but repeated signals can strengthen concern where pre-market evidence was uncertain. Post-market experience cannot replace inhalation studies, particularly for chronic effects, but it can reveal whether assumptions made at launch remain reasonable.

Real-world absence of a signal should be treated cautiously. Under-reporting is common, symptoms may be attributed to smoking history or other causes, and consumers may switch products without notifying the manufacturer. A product can therefore remain on the market for years without generating a clear adverse-event pattern even if low-grade effects occur. Active surveillance, retailer feedback and structured complaint coding provide more value than passive reliance on the absence of reports.

Regulatory inconsistency is common because different authorities may interpret the same data gap differently. One may accept read-across and low exposure, while another may require direct inhalation information or reject the ingredient. These differences can reflect legal frameworks, institutional precedent, risk tolerance and political context as much as toxicology. The manufacturer should therefore understand the evidential expectations of each market and avoid assuming that one assessment will be accepted universally.

The scientific reality remains that inhalation toxicology is expensive, technically difficult and imperfect. Even a conventional study may not answer every relevant question. Species differences, exposure method, aerosol generation and study duration all influence interpretation. The existence of an inhalation study should not be mistaken for certainty, just as its absence should not be mistaken for impossibility. The quality and relevance of the evidence matter more than the label attached to the method.

A robust assessment of missing inhalation data should therefore document the gap precisely. It should state which endpoints lack direct evidence, which alternative data are available, how route differences were considered, what exposure is expected, what uncertainties remain and why the proposed controls are judged sufficient. Generic wording that "no inhalation data were identified" is not enough. The regulatory decision depends on what was done in response.

The outcome may differ by endpoint. Systemic toxicity may be supported through oral studies and toxicokinetic reasoning, while respiratory irritation remains uncertain. Genotoxicity may be addressed through a strong in vitro battery and structural assessment, while sensitisation remains unresolved. The ingredient should not receive one blanket conclusion. Each endpoint should be considered on its own evidence and linked to the relevant exposure.

Where uncertainty remains high and the endpoint is severe, the appropriate action may be exclusion. This is particularly true for unresolved genotoxicity, credible respiratory sensitisation, strong electrophilic reactivity or significant thermal degradation. Where uncertainty is moderate and exposure is low, additional non-animal testing or tighter concentration limits may be sufficient. Where uncertainty is low and multiple evidence streams are reassuring, continued use may be justified despite the absence of direct inhalation studies.

Missing inhalation data should also influence research priorities. Not every gap deserves the same investment. Priority should be given to high-use ingredients, substances with strong aerosol transfer, compounds carrying structural alerts, constituents repeatedly found in multiple products and substances associated with signals from occupational or mechanistic evidence. Coordinated research on these categories can support many products more effectively than isolated studies on low-priority ingredients.

Shared data frameworks could reduce duplication across industry. Toxicological profiles, read-across justifications, respiratory in vitro results and emissions data for common ingredients could be developed collaboratively, provided quality and transparency are maintained. This would allow resources to focus on poorly characterised and high-concern substances rather than repeating the same basic assessments commercially. Regulatory acceptance would depend on access to methods, raw data and clear substance identity.

The movement towards non-animal science is likely to make missing inhalation data more manageable, but it will not remove the need for judgement. New approach methodologies can provide mechanistic and human-relevant evidence at greater speed, yet they still require validation and integration. The goal should not be to replace one rigid testing requirement with another. The strongest framework is flexible enough to use the most informative methods for the question while demanding transparency about uncertainty.

Missing inhalation data are therefore not merely a weakness in the evidence base; they are a test of the quality of regulatory reasoning. A poor assessment either ignores the gap or treats it as an automatic prohibition. A strong assessment asks whether the substance is known well enough, whether exposure is controlled sufficiently, whether alternative evidence converges and whether the residual uncertainty is proportionate to the product's function and public-health context. It accepts that certainty will often remain incomplete while refusing to let uncertainty become an excuse for unsupported use.

Within vaping regulation, this issue sits at the boundary between scientific realism and regulatory expectation. The market cannot wait for exhaustive inhalation datasets on every constituent, but it cannot be built responsibly on food-use assumptions and supplier assurances alone. The practical answer lies in tiered assessment, rigorous product characterisation, conservative exposure analysis, read-across, weight of evidence, non-animal methods, post-market review and willingness to remove ingredients that remain unjustifiable. Missing inhalation data should not end the assessment, but they should shape it. They determine where greater caution is needed, where alternative science must be strongest and where commercial preference must give way to evidential restraint.

Animal Testing Alternatives

Animal testing alternatives have become central to modern regulatory toxicology because the scientific, ethical and practical limitations of conventional animal studies are increasingly difficult to ignore, particularly for products containing large numbers of ingredients, rapidly changing formulations and exposure conditions that are difficult to reproduce faithfully in laboratory animals. Vaping products expose this problem with unusual clarity. A single formulation may contain dozens of flavour constituents, each with different physicochemical properties, toxicological histories and aerosol-transfer behaviours, while the device itself alters exposure through power, coil design, airflow, wick saturation and heating profile. Testing every ingredient, mixture, concentration and device combination through repeated animal inhalation would be impossible in scale, slow in delivery and of uncertain relevance to actual human use. The purpose of alternative methods is therefore not merely to reduce the number of animals used while preserving the same decision structure. It is to develop a more efficient and human-relevant system for identifying hazards, comparing products, understanding mechanisms and directing regulatory attention towards the uncertainties most capable of affecting consumer safety.

The term alternative should not imply that every non-animal method is a weaker substitute for an animal study. In many cases, the opposite may be true. Human respiratory cells, reconstructed airway tissues and organotypic models can examine biological responses in human-derived systems without requiring uncertain translation across species. Computational methods can screen large chemical inventories for structural alerts, probable metabolites and mechanisms before a formulation is finalised. Product-specific aerosol testing can measure the substances actually emitted under defined conditions rather than infer exposure from the liquid recipe. Read-across and weight-of-evidence approaches can make systematic use of existing knowledge instead of repeating studies whose likely result is already understood. These methods can answer questions that conventional animal studies address only indirectly, although none should be accepted uncritically merely because it is newer, faster or animal-free. Regulatory value still depends on method validity, exposure relevance, reproducibility and a clear relationship to the endpoint under assessment.

The scientific case for alternatives begins with the limitations of animal models themselves. Laboratory animals differ from humans in airway anatomy, breathing patterns, metabolic capacity, immune response and susceptibility to respiratory injury. Rodents are obligate nose breathers, which can alter deposition of soluble and reactive chemicals within the nasal passages and reduce delivery to deeper lung regions. Their airway branching, clearance mechanisms and metabolic enzymes may not reproduce human exposure accurately. A substance producing marked nasal effects in a rat may affect humans differently, while another may be detoxified efficiently in the animal yet remain more reactive in human tissue. These differences do not make animal studies useless, but they limit the certainty with which findings can be transferred across species. The need for uncertainty factors is itself evidence that the model is an approximation rather than a direct representation of human biology.

Exposure generation creates further difficulty. Vaping aerosols are dynamic mixtures of droplets, vapours, thermal products and sometimes particles released from device materials. Their composition can change over seconds through evaporation, condensation and interaction with collection systems. Delivering a stable and representative aerosol concentration to animals over prolonged periods requires specialised equipment and careful analytical control. The device may need to be operated repeatedly under machine conditions that differ from consumer use. The animal may inhale through the nose only, while human users inhale through the mouth and often draw aerosol intermittently rather than continuously. Stress from restraint or exposure chambers can introduce additional biological effects. A conventional inhalation study may therefore appear route-relevant while still differing substantially from the way the product is actually used.

The problem becomes more pronounced when whole-product testing is attempted. A formulation assessed in one device and at one power setting may produce a different emissions profile in another. A study can consume months and substantial resources, only for the commercial product to change before completion. A new flavour, coil, battery or supplier can make the original evidence only partially applicable. This lack of agility is poorly matched to a product category in which technical specifications and market offerings change quickly. Alternative methods are valuable partly because they can be deployed earlier and repeated more readily when the product changes.

Ethical considerations remain important but should not be separated from scientific efficiency. The use of animals is difficult to justify where the question can be answered through existing evidence, human-relevant in vitro methods or analytical measurement. A study that duplicates known information or uses an insensitive model does not become scientifically valuable simply because it follows a traditional protocol. The ethical principle is strongest when linked to better study design: unnecessary testing should be avoided, the most informative methods should be selected first and any remaining animal work should address a clearly defined uncertainty that cannot reasonably be resolved otherwise.

This logic is often expressed through the principles of replacement, reduction and refinement. Replacement seeks to use non-animal methods wherever they can answer the regulatory question. Reduction limits animal numbers by improving experimental design, sharing control groups, using existing data and avoiding duplication. Refinement modifies procedures to minimise pain, distress and unnecessary exposure severity. In vaping toxicology, replacement has the greatest long-term potential because the scale of ingredient assessment makes conventional one-substance-at-a-time testing unsustainable. Reduction and refinement remain relevant where animal data are still considered necessary, but the broader objective should be to restructure the evidence pathway so that animal studies are no longer treated as the default starting point.

The most immediate alternative is better use of existing information. Many substances already have data from pharmaceuticals, occupational exposure, food chemistry, environmental toxicology or related industrial uses. A disciplined literature review can identify systemic toxicity, metabolism, irritation, genotoxicity and structural concerns without generating new data. The challenge is to determine route relevance and avoid overextending evidence derived from ingestion or skin contact. Existing evidence should therefore be organised by endpoint and exposure route, with direct inhalation data given appropriate priority and route-to-route extrapolation explained. The purpose is not to claim that all missing information has been filled, but to establish which questions genuinely remain unanswered.

Read-across is one of the most powerful alternatives when direct data are limited. Information from a well-characterised source substance can support assessment of a related target where structure, physicochemical properties, metabolism and biological activity are sufficiently similar. This can reduce the need for new testing across groups of related flavour compounds. The method is strongest where a common metabolic pathway or reactive functional group explains the endpoint and where the target falls within a well-defined chemical category. It becomes weaker where similarity is superficial or where volatility, reactivity or metabolism differ materially. Read-across is therefore not a waiver from evidence but a formal use of existing evidence through a transparent scientific hypothesis.

Grouping and category approaches can extend this efficiency further. Instead of assessing every substance independently, chemicals can be organised into families based on common structure, metabolic transformation or toxicological mechanism. Trends across chain length, substitution or reactivity may then support interpolation for untested members. This can be particularly useful for esters, alcohols, acids and related flavour compounds. The category must be defined carefully, and outliers should be examined rather than forced into the group. A successful category reduces duplication while preserving substance-specific control where the chemistry indicates that one member may behave differently.

Computational toxicology can screen large ingredient inventories rapidly. Quantitative structure–activity relationship models can predict mutagenicity, sensitisation, receptor interaction, physicochemical properties and potential metabolites. Structural-alert systems can identify electrophilic groups, DNA-reactive motifs or other features associated with concern. These tools are particularly useful at the formulation-design stage because problematic ingredients can be excluded before commercial development progresses. Their limitations lie in model applicability and training data. A prediction is reliable only where the target falls within the model's chemical domain and where the endpoint is represented adequately. Computational outputs should therefore support evidence integration rather than replace empirical data automatically.

Physiologically based kinetic modelling can help translate external exposure into tissue dose. By combining physicochemical properties, breathing rates, absorption and metabolism, these models can compare oral and inhalation routes or estimate concentrations reaching the respiratory tract and systemic circulation. They may be useful where oral toxicity data exist but inhalation exposure must be interpreted. The quality of the result depends on parameter accuracy and biological assumptions. Where data are limited, the model can still identify which parameters drive uncertainty and which measurements would provide the greatest improvement.

Threshold-based approaches can also reduce testing where exposure is very low. The threshold of toxicological concern uses distributions of toxicity data to identify exposure levels below which appreciable risk is considered unlikely for defined structural classes. This can be useful for trace flavour constituents with no high-concern alerts and low aerosol transfer. It is not appropriate for every substance. Genotoxic compounds, metals, proteins, persistent chemicals and known respiratory hazards may fall outside the framework. The method should therefore be applied as a screening tool within a broader assessment, not as a universal exemption from evidence.

In vitro respiratory models provide one of the most direct alternatives to animal inhalation studies. Human bronchial and alveolar epithelial cells can be exposed to ingredients or aerosols and examined for cytotoxicity, oxidative stress, inflammatory signalling, barrier disruption and changes in ciliary function. These models can compare formulations rapidly and identify concentrations at which biological responses emerge. Their relevance depends heavily on how exposure is delivered. Applying concentrated liquid directly to submerged cells may be useful for initial screening but can produce conditions far removed from inhalation. Air–liquid interface exposure is generally more representative because aerosol contacts the apical surface while the cells receive nutrients from below.

Reconstructed human airway tissues improve biological relevance by incorporating differentiated epithelial layers, mucus production and ciliated cells. These tissues can be used to examine irritation, tissue viability, inflammatory markers and structural changes after repeated exposure. They allow comparison of complete aerosols from different devices and formulations under controlled conditions. The model still lacks full systemic metabolism, vascular interaction and long-term immune complexity, but it provides a direct view of human respiratory-tissue response that may be more relevant than observations from another species.

Repeated-exposure protocols are particularly important because vaping products are used chronically. A single exposure may reveal acute irritation but miss adaptation, accumulation or progressive tissue effects. In vitro systems can be exposed over several days or weeks, with recovery periods and repeated measurement of function. These protocols are technically more demanding because tissue viability, aerosol dose and exposure consistency must be maintained, yet they offer a route towards addressing chronicity without conventional long-duration animal studies.

Co-culture models can add immune cells, fibroblasts or endothelial cells to epithelial systems, allowing more complex interactions to be studied. Macrophage responses may reveal effects on innate immunity and particle clearance. Endothelial components can provide information about vascular signalling, while fibroblasts may help investigate tissue remodelling. These systems do not reproduce the entire organism, but they can examine pathways that single-cell models overlook. Their value lies in targeted mechanistic understanding rather than in claiming to represent every possible clinical outcome.

Organoids and organ-on-chip systems extend this complexity. Three-dimensional respiratory organoids can reproduce aspects of tissue architecture and cellular diversity, while microfluidic chips can introduce airflow, mechanical movement and fluid interfaces. Some systems simulate breathing-related stretch or permit interaction between airway and vascular compartments. These technologies can provide insight into barrier function, inflammation and tissue-level responses under repeated exposure. They remain less standardised and may require substantial technical expertise, but they are developing rapidly and may eventually support endpoints that conventional cell cultures cannot address adequately.

High-content imaging and omics technologies can extract more information from these models. Transcriptomics, proteomics, metabolomics and epigenetic analysis can reveal pathway-level responses before overt toxicity occurs. A formulation may alter oxidative-stress pathways, lipid metabolism or inflammatory signalling even where cell viability remains high. These findings can support mechanistic interpretation and identify early biological changes. The challenge is distinguishing adaptive responses from adverse ones. Large datasets can create an appearance of precision while remaining difficult to interpret regulatorily. Omics evidence is strongest when connected to an established adverse outcome pathway and supported by functional changes.

Adverse outcome pathways provide a framework for linking molecular events to tissue effects and eventual harm. A chemical may initiate protein binding, oxidative stress or receptor activation, leading through a sequence of cellular and tissue responses towards irritation, sensitisation or another adverse outcome. Alternative tests can then be selected to examine key events within that pathway. This is more rational than using one general cytotoxicity assay for every question. The framework also helps explain why different evidence streams belong together and where uncertainty remains.

For respiratory sensitisation, no single alternative method currently resolves every question, but integrated approaches can combine chemical reactivity, structural alerts, in vitro immune responses and occupational evidence. For genotoxicity, established in vitro batteries can assess mutation, chromosomal damage and DNA effects, although positive findings require careful interpretation and may need follow-up. For irritation, reconstructed tissues and cytokine responses can provide direct evidence. For systemic toxicity, computational kinetics and non-respiratory data may be integrated. The objective is to build endpoint-specific testing strategies rather than search for one replacement assay capable of answering all toxicological questions.

Whole-aerosol testing is essential because the product is used as an aerosol rather than as a set of isolated ingredients. Alternative methods can expose human respiratory tissues to emissions generated from the final formulation and device. This captures thermal degradation, component interactions and the complete mixture. Product comparisons can identify whether a formulation change reduces or increases biological activity. Whole-aerosol studies also allow testing under normal and upper-bound operating conditions. They remain limited by exposure duration and model scope, but they provide evidence directly linked to the marketed product.

Chemical emissions analysis should sit alongside biological testing. Measuring carbonyls, volatile organic compounds, metals, nicotine and other relevant constituents identifies what is present and supports quantitative exposure assessment. Biological assays then examine whether the complete aerosol produces a response. The two approaches are complementary. Analytical chemistry without biological context may detect substances of uncertain significance, while biological testing without chemistry may identify an effect without explaining its cause. Integrated evaluation is stronger than either alone.

Benchmarking improves interpretation. Test aerosols can be compared with clean-air controls, carrier-only formulations, known irritants, cigarette smoke or reference products, depending on the question. The comparator should be chosen carefully. Cigarette smoke may provide relative-risk context but should not become the only standard of acceptability. A product can be much less biologically active than smoke while still containing an avoidable irritant. Carrier controls help identify the contribution of flavours or nicotine, while known positive controls demonstrate that the assay is capable of detecting a response.

Dose characterisation remains fundamental. An alternative method is not informative if the amount reaching the tissue is unknown. Aerosol concentration in the exposure chamber may differ from deposited dose on the cells. Filters, quartz-crystal microbalances or chemical markers can help quantify delivery. Results should be related to realistic consumer exposure where possible. Testing only extreme concentrations can identify intrinsic hazard but may provide limited support for risk assessment. A useful programme includes a concentration range spanning realistic and conservative exposures.

Method validation is often presented as the main barrier to regulatory acceptance, but validation should be understood properly. A method does not need to reproduce an animal study exactly to be valuable. It must demonstrate reliability, reproducibility and relevance to the biological process or regulatory question. Interlaboratory comparison, standard operating procedures, reference controls and defined acceptance criteria help establish confidence. Some methods may be ready for routine screening before they are accepted as complete replacements for a traditional endpoint. Regulatory systems should allow evidence to be used proportionately rather than treating methods as either fully validated or worthless.

The danger of requiring every alternative method to predict animal-study outcomes is that the animal model becomes the assumed truth even where its human relevance is uncertain. A human airway model should be judged partly on its ability to represent human biology, not only on whether it reproduces findings from rats or mice. Validation against human data, known irritants and mechanistic pathways may be more meaningful. This requires regulators to move from protocol-based acceptance towards question-based evaluation.

Integrated approaches to testing and assessment provide the most realistic regulatory pathway. No single alternative method is expected to resolve identity, hazard, exposure, metabolism and chronic risk. Instead, evidence can be assembled in stages. The substance is first characterised chemically. Existing literature and authoritative assessments are reviewed. Structural alerts and computational predictions are examined. Exposure is estimated from formulation and aerosol data. Read-across is considered. Relevant in vitro methods are selected. Whole-aerosol testing is used where mixture or thermal effects matter. The resulting evidence is integrated through weight-of-evidence reasoning. Only if a critical uncertainty remains should higher-tier testing be considered.

This tiered structure improves efficiency because low-concern substances can be resolved early, while resources are concentrated on high-exposure, reactive or poorly characterised ingredients. It also supports better product design. Screening can identify problematic flavours before they are built into a commercial range. Comparative assays can guide concentration reduction or substitution. Device changes can be assessed rapidly for their effect on emissions and biological response. Toxicology becomes part of development rather than a retrospective barrier at the point of submission.

Alternative methods also support change control. When a supplier changes a flavour composition or a new coil is introduced, repeating a full animal programme would be unrealistic. Targeted chemical and in vitro testing can determine whether the change materially alters exposure or biological activity. Bridging studies can compare old and new versions directly. This makes lifecycle compliance more responsive and prevents regulatory evidence from becoming obsolete after minor product evolution.

Mixture assessment remains difficult, but alternatives are particularly useful here. Conventional toxicology often evaluates single substances, while consumers inhale complex aerosols. Whole-mixture in vitro testing can detect additive or interactive effects, even where every ingredient appears acceptable individually. Fractionation or targeted reformulation can then help identify the driver. The process is not simple, but it is more directly connected to the actual product than testing one ingredient at a time in animals.

Chronic disease prediction remains the hardest challenge. Short-term models cannot reproduce years of exposure, ageing, comorbidity and systemic interaction. This limitation should be acknowledged rather than disguised. The answer is not necessarily to return automatically to long animal studies. Repeated-exposure human tissue models, mechanistic pathways, epidemiology, biomonitoring and post-market surveillance can contribute progressively. Long-term confidence will often come from several evidence streams accumulated over time rather than one definitive pre-market test.

Human biomonitoring may eventually strengthen this framework by measuring biomarkers of exposure or effect in users under real-world conditions. Such studies can examine nicotine metabolites, selected toxicant biomarkers, inflammation and physiological responses. Their interpretation is complicated by previous smoking, dual use and background exposure, but they can provide direct evidence of actual human dose. They should be designed carefully and should not be used to claim absence of long-term risk from short-term biomarker reduction alone.

Clinical and observational studies remain important complements. Controlled switching studies can compare exposure and short-term physiological outcomes when smokers move to vaping products. Cohort studies can examine longer-term patterns, though confounding remains substantial. These human data do not replace product-specific toxicology, but they help test whether mechanistic and exposure predictions align with real use. Alternative testing is strongest when laboratory and human evidence inform each other.

Post-market surveillance is another component of the alternative framework. Complaints, adverse-event reports and product failures can reveal issues not identified pre-market. Active surveillance is more informative than passive absence of reports. Standardised coding, product traceability and trend analysis are required. Post-market evidence cannot justify releasing a poorly assessed product, but it can refine risk estimates and identify where additional testing or reformulation is needed.

Regulatory acceptance remains uneven. Some authorities continue to favour traditional datasets because they are familiar and embedded in guidance, while others increasingly recognise new approach methodologies and integrated evidence. This creates uncertainty for manufacturers developing products across multiple jurisdictions. A scientifically strong alternative programme should therefore document methods, exposure conditions, controls, limitations and links to the regulatory question in exceptional detail. The objective is to make the evidence understandable and auditable even where the specific method is not yet standard practice.

The burden should not fall entirely on individual manufacturers. Shared reference methods, validated protocols, ingredient databases and common aerosol-generation standards would improve consistency. Industry consortia, academic laboratories and regulators can cooperate on common ingredients and endpoints. Repeated confidential testing of the same substances wastes resources and slows progress. Data sharing must preserve quality and intellectual property appropriately, but common toxicological problems benefit from collective solutions.

Competence remains essential. Alternative methods are not easier simply because they avoid animals. They require expertise in chemistry, exposure science, cell biology, toxicology, statistics and regulatory interpretation. A visually impressive assay can produce misleading conclusions if the exposure is unrealistic or the endpoint is misunderstood. The programme should be designed by people capable of connecting the method to the product and the regulatory decision. Outsourcing the test does not outsource responsibility for interpretation.

Quality systems should apply to alternative evidence in the same way they apply to conventional testing. Test materials should be characterised, protocols controlled, equipment calibrated, raw data retained and deviations recorded. Biological systems require defined passage number, tissue condition and acceptance criteria. Computational analyses should record software version, model and applicability domain. Reproducibility depends on these details, and regulators cannot evaluate evidence that exists only as a summary conclusion.

The strongest alternative-testing strategy is one that begins with product restraint. No methodology can make an unnecessary, poorly characterised ingredient easier to justify than simply removing it. Formulations should minimise complexity, avoid known respiratory hazards and use the lowest effective concentrations. Suppliers should provide complete composition and change notification. Devices should operate within controlled thermal conditions. Alternatives then evaluate a product already designed to reduce uncertainty rather than being used to defend avoidable complexity.

The approach should also be endpoint-driven. Respiratory irritation, genotoxicity, sensitisation, systemic toxicity and developmental effects require different evidence. A negative cytotoxicity result does not resolve mutagenicity. A reassuring computational model does not exclude local irritation. A whole-aerosol assay may not identify an individual high-concern impurity. Integrated testing should therefore map each regulatory question to the evidence capable of addressing it and identify where no adequate method currently exists.

Uncertainty remains unavoidable and should be stated directly. An alternative programme may provide strong evidence for acute respiratory tolerance and low genotoxic concern while leaving chronic immune effects less certain. That does not invalidate the entire assessment. It defines the conditions under which the product can be justified and the areas requiring monitoring or further research. The credibility of the conclusion depends on not overstating what the methods have shown.

Animal testing alternatives are therefore not a shortcut around toxicology. They demand more integration, not less. Traditional studies often produce one large report that appears self-contained. Alternative programmes distribute evidence across chemistry, modelling, human tissues, exposure assessment and product testing. The assessor must bring these strands together coherently. This can be more intellectually demanding, but it also creates a richer and more product-relevant understanding.

Within vaping regulation, the most defensible position is neither automatic rejection of animal studies nor automatic reliance on them. The method should follow the question. Where existing evidence, human-relevant models and product-specific exposure data can support a decision, additional animal testing is difficult to justify. Where a severe and unresolved endpoint remains, further evidence may still be necessary, but the study should be targeted and scientifically essential. The aim is not to preserve traditional testing by default or to declare every new method sufficient. It is to use the best available evidence in the form most capable of predicting human risk.

The future of regulatory toxicology will depend increasingly on this shift. Product categories are becoming too complex, chemical inventories too large and innovation cycles too fast for conventional testing programmes to remain the sole foundation of decision-making. Human-relevant systems, computational science, analytical chemistry and structured evidence integration offer a way to improve both speed and relevance while reducing unnecessary animal use. Their success will depend on rigorous validation, transparent limitations and willingness from regulators and industry to move beyond procedural familiarity.

For vaping products, the case is particularly strong because the central questions are often product-specific and exposure-dependent. What is emitted, at what level, under which device conditions and with what biological effect matters more than whether a generic ingredient once produced an effect in a distant model at an unrelated dose. Alternative methods allow those questions to be asked earlier, more directly and across more product variants than conventional animal testing could support. Used without discipline, they can produce fragmented evidence and false reassurance. Used properly, they provide a scientifically credible pathway through the scale and uncertainty of modern inhalation-product regulation.

The regulatory objective should therefore be to replace routine animal testing with a structured sequence of chemical characterisation, literature review, read-across, computational screening, human-relevant respiratory models, product-specific emissions analysis, exposure assessment and weight-of-evidence interpretation. That sequence does not promise absolute certainty, because no toxicological method can. It provides something more useful: a transparent and proportionate account of what is known, what remains uncertain and why the available evidence is sufficient or insufficient for the product decision. Animal testing alternatives become meaningful not when they imitate every feature of the old system, but when they produce better evidence for the actual human exposure being regulated.

Regulatory Interpretation Versus Scientific Reality

Regulatory interpretation and scientific reality do not always move at the same speed, use the same language or require the same degree of certainty. Science develops through revision, qualification and the gradual accumulation of evidence, while regulation must convert that evolving evidence into decisions that can be applied consistently across products, companies and markets. The scientist may conclude that an ingredient presents low concern under a defined exposure scenario but that important uncertainty remains around chronic inhalation. The regulator may still need to decide whether the product can be notified, whether additional information is required, whether the ingredient should be restricted or whether the uncertainty is too great to support market placement. This difference is not necessarily evidence that one side is wrong. It reflects two systems performing different functions. Scientific reality is often conditional, probabilistic and dependent on product configuration, whereas regulation requires categories, thresholds, documentary standards and enforceable outcomes. The difficulty arises when these systems are treated as though they were interchangeable, because scientific nuance can be compressed into administrative rules and regulatory caution can be mistaken for proof of toxicological danger.

The first tension concerns certainty. Scientific conclusions are rarely absolute, particularly in inhalation toxicology where direct data may be limited, products vary in design and consumer exposure is difficult to define precisely. A toxicologist may be able to state that no significant hazard has been identified at the expected dose, that several evidence streams are reassuring and that the remaining uncertainty is manageable through specification and monitoring. That is a scientifically meaningful conclusion, but it is not the same as proving that the product is safe under every condition, for every user and over every possible period of use. Regulation often struggles with this distinction because legal and administrative systems prefer clear outcomes. A product is accepted, rejected, notified, authorised, restricted or removed. Scientific evidence, by contrast, may support a range of confidence rather than a binary answer. The regulatory process must therefore decide how much uncertainty is tolerable and what level of evidence is sufficient for the particular legal pathway.

This issue becomes especially visible in vaping because the scientific question is not whether the product is harmless. No inhaled consumer product containing nicotine and complex aerosol constituents can be described credibly in those terms. The relevant questions concern the magnitude and character of risk, the comparison with combustible tobacco, the avoidability of particular hazards and the adequacy of controls. A product can be materially less harmful than smoking and still require reformulation. An ingredient can have a wide margin of exposure and still remain poorly characterised by inhalation. A device can reduce exposure to many combustion toxicants while generating its own avoidable carbonyl or metal emissions. Scientific reality allows these statements to coexist. Regulatory interpretation often seeks a simpler conclusion and may emphasise one part of the evidence at the expense of another.

The treatment of hazard provides a clear example. Regulatory systems often begin with classification of intrinsic hazardous properties. This is necessary because carcinogenicity, mutagenicity, sensitisation, reproductive toxicity and severe respiratory effects deserve attention regardless of the product in which a substance is used. The danger arises when hazard classification is presented as if it determines product risk without regard to concentration, transfer, exposure and route. A substance may carry a severe hazard classification based on industrial exposure or high-dose animal studies while being present in a product at a level producing negligible consumer exposure. Conversely, an unclassified substance may remain poorly studied and capable of causing local respiratory effects. Scientific interpretation must consider both hazard and exposure, while regulatory communication sometimes collapses the two because hazard categories are easier to administer and explain.

The opposite error also occurs when exposure is used to dismiss hazard too readily. A manufacturer may argue that a compound is present at a low level and therefore cannot be relevant, yet the exposure estimate may be based on the liquid concentration rather than measured aerosol transfer, or may ignore peak local deposition and repeated use. A narrow numerical margin can be made to appear reassuring through favourable assumptions, just as a wide margin can be made to appear concerning through unrealistic worst-case conditions. Scientific reality requires examination of the assumptions, whereas regulatory records may preserve only the final number. The quality of interpretation therefore depends on whether the evidence pathway remains visible from the source study and analytical method through to the regulatory conclusion.

Legal frameworks also influence how toxicological evidence is interpreted. Different jurisdictions may apply different product definitions, notification systems, ingredient restrictions, warning requirements and evidential thresholds even when they are considering similar scientific information. A product accepted under one framework may face additional questions or rejection under another. This can occur because the legislation differs, because guidance has evolved unevenly or because competent authorities have adopted different levels of precaution. It does not necessarily mean that the toxicology changed at the border. The scientific reality may be the same, while the legal tolerance for uncertainty is different.

This variation creates practical difficulty for manufacturers operating across multiple markets. One authority may accept read-across supported by low exposure and in vitro evidence, while another may expect direct inhalation data. One may treat a flavour ingredient as supportable below a defined concentration, while another may regard the data gap as unacceptable. A company may therefore need to maintain regional formulations or evidential packages even where the underlying product concept is unchanged. Regulatory interpretation becomes part of product architecture, and the formulation may be shaped as much by institutional expectations as by toxicological necessity.

The precautionary principle is often central to this divide. Properly applied, precaution allows regulatory action where there is credible potential for serious harm and scientific uncertainty prevents complete risk characterisation. It is not a rule that uncertainty must always lead to prohibition, nor is it a substitute for exposure assessment and evidence weighting. Precaution should be proportionate to the severity of the possible harm, the plausibility of the mechanism, the magnitude of exposure and the availability of lower-risk alternatives. In practice, however, the principle can be applied inconsistently. One regulator may use uncertainty to justify a concentration limit or additional monitoring, while another may use the same uncertainty to reject the ingredient entirely.

The problem is not precaution itself but the absence of a transparent account of how it was used. If a substance is restricted because direct inhalation data are missing, the decision should explain why read-across, exposure analysis and alternative methods were considered insufficient. If a product is accepted despite uncertainty, the record should identify the controls that make the residual uncertainty tolerable. Without that explanation, precaution becomes indistinguishable from institutional preference. Scientific reality is then replaced by an administrative position that may be difficult to challenge because the underlying reasoning is not visible.

Regulation also tends to standardise evidence through guidance and templates. This improves consistency and allows authorities to process large numbers of submissions, but it can encourage a checklist mentality. A technical file may contain the expected sections, studies and declarations while still failing to address the actual toxicological weakness of the product. Another product may be supported by a strong integrated evidence package that does not fit neatly within the preferred format. The existence of a required document should not be confused with the quality of the science within it. A toxicological assessment is not robust because it contains a literature review, exposure calculation and margin-of-exposure table; it is robust only if those elements relate accurately to the product and support the conclusion.

Standardisation can also create false equivalence between very different products. A low-power closed pod, a high-power open device and a prefilled disposable may all pass through a similar notification structure even though their exposure profiles, failure modes and degree of user control differ substantially. Regulation may require common fields for ingredient identity, emissions and device characteristics, but the scientific interpretation should remain product-specific. Treating every product in a category as though one test regime or exposure assumption is sufficient can obscure important variation.

Puffing regimes illustrate this problem. Standard machine conditions are necessary for comparability and routine testing, yet no single regime reproduces the diversity of consumer use. A regulator may require testing under a defined method, and the resulting data may be administratively complete, but scientific reality demands attention to the product's operating range, power control, coil ageing and foreseeable use. A product that performs well under the standard condition may generate higher emissions at another setting available to consumers. Conversely, a stress test designed to provoke failure may produce results that are irrelevant to normal use if presented without context. Regulation needs standardisation, but toxicology needs interpretive boundaries around what standardised data can and cannot prove.

The same tension applies to ingredient lists. Regulatory systems often require complete chemical disclosure, and this is essential. Yet the presence of an ingredient name does not establish its toxicological significance. Concentration, purity, carrier, aerosol transfer and thermal transformation all matter. A database may contain thousands of declared substances without providing a coherent account of which are high priority or why. Scientific reality requires prioritisation. Regulation may collect information successfully while failing to distinguish between a trace low-concern constituent and a reactive substance used at a high level.

This can lead to an administrative illusion of knowledge. The product is fully notified, all fields are completed and the ingredient list is technically comprehensive, yet the regulator and manufacturer may still lack a meaningful inhalation assessment for key constituents. Submission completeness is not equivalent to scientific adequacy. The opposite is also possible: a strong assessment may exist internally, but a condensed portal entry may make the product appear less well supported because the system cannot capture the reasoning. The technical file must therefore remain the primary scientific record, with the notification acting as a regulatory summary rather than the complete evidence base.

Regulatory interpretation is also influenced by precedent. Once an authority has accepted or rejected a particular form of evidence, that decision can shape later assessments. Precedent supports consistency, but it can preserve outdated assumptions. A method considered experimental several years ago may become well validated, while an older default animal study may remain embedded in guidance despite limited human relevance. Regulatory systems change slowly because revisions require consultation, legal review and institutional agreement. Scientific methods can advance more quickly, creating periods in which the most relevant evidence is not yet the most familiar to the regulator.

Animal testing alternatives expose this gap sharply. Human-relevant respiratory models, computational methods and integrated testing strategies may provide strong evidence, yet an authority may hesitate because the method is not formally recognised for the exact endpoint. The result can be a preference for conventional animal data despite known species limitations. From an administrative perspective, the traditional method is easier to accept because the procedure and precedent are familiar. From a scientific perspective, the newer method may be more directly relevant to human airway exposure. The challenge is to evaluate methods according to the question they answer rather than according to institutional familiarity.

Validation should support this transition, but validation itself can become restrictive if alternative methods are required to reproduce animal outcomes rather than predict human biology. An in vitro human airway model may disagree with a rodent study because the species respond differently, not because the model is defective. If the animal result is treated automatically as the reference truth, human relevance becomes secondary. Scientific reality requires a broader evaluation involving known human irritants, mechanistic pathways, reproducibility and exposure realism. Regulation must evolve from protocol recognition towards evidence-function recognition.

Commercial pressure introduces another layer of distortion. Manufacturers may present uncertainty as insignificant because a product is close to launch, while regulators may interpret the same uncertainty conservatively because they carry responsibility for population protection. Consultants may be asked to convert incomplete evidence into a favourable conclusion, and laboratories may generate standard datasets that answer contractual requirements without resolving the critical scientific question. The integrity of toxicological interpretation depends on resisting these pressures. A conclusion should not become more certain because a commercial deadline is approaching, and a data gap should not become unacceptable merely because a category is politically contentious.

Political context can influence regulatory interpretation even when the formal process is scientific. Vaping sits within debates about youth use, smoking cessation, industry conduct, environmental waste and nicotine dependence.

These issues are legitimate, but they can shape how toxicological findings are framed. A modest adverse effect may receive heightened attention because the product category is controversial, while evidence of reduced exposure relative to smoking may be discounted because it conflicts with a broader prevention message. Conversely, harm-reduction advocates may minimise emerging concerns because they fear that acknowledging them will be used to justify prohibition. Scientific reality requires the evidence to remain separate from the strategic use others may make of it.

This does not mean toxicology should ignore public-health context. A product used by adult smokers cannot be interpreted in exactly the same way as a product intended for a nicotine-naive population. The comparator matters. If a smoker replaces cigarettes with a well-controlled vaping product, substantial reduction in exposure to combustion-derived toxicants may produce a favourable overall health effect even though residual risks remain. If the same product is adopted by a young person who would not otherwise use nicotine, there is no displaced smoking exposure and the risk-benefit balance is different. Regulation must account for both scenarios, but toxicological evidence alone cannot determine population behaviour.

The scientific assessment should therefore remain clear about its scope. It can describe the hazards, exposure and likely product-specific risks. It can compare emissions and biological activity with relevant comparators. It cannot determine by itself how the product will affect smoking prevalence, youth initiation, cessation behaviour or illicit markets. Those are broader policy questions requiring epidemiology, behavioural science and economics. Problems arise when toxicology is used to support claims beyond its evidential reach, whether to declare a product harmless or to justify category-wide prohibition.

Relative risk is particularly vulnerable to misinterpretation. A product can be much less harmful than smoking without being safe, and those statements are not contradictory. Regulation often struggles to communicate this because warnings and public messages seek simplicity. Overstating safety can encourage uptake among non-smokers, while overstating danger can deter smokers from switching. Scientific reality is comparative and conditional. Regulatory communication must preserve enough nuance to support informed choice without becoming so qualified that the message loses meaning.

The same challenge appears in language such as safe, toxic, harmful and compliant. Safe is often interpreted as absence of risk, which is rarely scientifically defensible. Toxic describes the capacity to cause adverse effects but says little about dose. Harmful may refer to intrinsic hazard, measured exposure or observed outcome, depending on context. Compliant means that legal requirements have been met; it does not prove scientific optimality. A compliant product can still contain avoidable hazards, just as a non-compliant product may fail administratively without presenting a major toxicological threat. Precision in language is essential because regulatory terms can acquire scientific meaning they were never intended to carry.

Regulatory databases and notifications can also create misunderstanding. Publication of a product in a regulatory list may be interpreted by manufacturers, retailers or consumers as approval. In many systems, notification confirms that information has been submitted and that certain administrative conditions have been met, but it does not mean that the authority has conducted a complete pre-market toxicological evaluation or endorsed the product as safe. Scientific responsibility therefore remains with the manufacturer or responsible operator. The technical file, specification and post-market system must continue to support the product after notification.

This distinction is crucial because regulation cannot inspect or test every product continuously. Authorities rely heavily on producer declarations, documentary evidence and market surveillance. A company that treats notification as the transfer of responsibility has misunderstood the system. Scientific reality remains tied to the formulation, device and manufacturing process, all of which are controlled by the producer. If a supplier changes a flavour composition or a coil is substituted, the regulator may not know unless the company's change-control system identifies and reports it. Compliance is therefore maintained operationally before it is enforced externally.

The interpretation of absence is another recurring problem. No detected compound does not mean no exposure, because the analytical method may lack sensitivity. No reported adverse events do not mean no harm, because surveillance may be weak. No published inhalation studies do not mean the substance is unsafe, but they also do not mean it is safe. No regulatory restriction does not establish acceptance. Scientific reality distinguishes these different forms of absence, while regulatory and commercial narratives often treat them selectively.

Data quality is equally vulnerable to compression. A positive result from a poorly characterised product may become a headline, while a negative result from an insensitive method may become reassurance. Regulators must evaluate methodology rather than outcome alone. The test material, device settings, exposure concentration, controls and analytical confirmation determine what the study can support. Scientific interpretation requires examination of the complete evidence chain. Regulatory summaries that extract only the conclusion can lose the limitations that make the conclusion meaningful.

The reproducibility crisis affecting several areas of biomedical science is relevant here. Small studies, flexible analysis and incomplete reporting can produce findings that fail to replicate. Vaping research is especially exposed because products are variable and methods are not always standardised. A single striking study should therefore rarely determine a major regulatory decision without consideration of replication, method quality and product relevance. At the same time, waiting for perfect replication can delay action where the potential harm is serious. Weight-of-evidence reasoning is needed to balance these concerns.

Regulatory decision-making is often asymmetric because the consequences of error differ. Accepting a harmful product may expose consumers, while rejecting a low-risk product may reduce consumer choice or impede switching from smoking. Authorities may focus more heavily on the first error because it is visible within their protective mandate. Harm-reduction policy requires consideration of the second error as well. Excessive evidential demands can preserve the market position of cigarettes by making lower-risk alternatives harder to develop or sustain. Scientific reality therefore includes counterfactual harm: what happens if the product is unavailable, unaffordable or replaced by an illicit alternative.

This does not justify lowering standards indiscriminately. A harm-reduction product should still be well characterised, manufactured consistently and stripped of avoidable hazards. The public-health context affects proportionality, not the obligation to control quality. A poor-quality product should not be accepted merely because smoking is worse. The correct comparison is between the product as it could reasonably be designed and the product actually presented. Avoidable toxicants, unsupported ingredients and uncontrolled devices remain legitimate regulatory concerns.

Regulatory interpretation should therefore distinguish minimum legal compliance from best scientific practice. Legislation may specify maximum nicotine concentration, reservoir capacity, warnings and notification fields, but it cannot anticipate every formulation or device risk. A product can meet each explicit requirement while relying on weak supplier data, broad tolerances or limited stability evidence. Best practice goes further by applying toxicological judgement, conservative formulation, robust specifications and active stewardship. The law sets the floor; scientific responsibility determines how far above it the product should be controlled.

The relationship between regulation and innovation is equally complex. Prescriptive rules can reduce uncertainty and prevent recurrent failures, but they can also freeze technology around existing formats. Performance-based requirements may allow better designs but demand more sophisticated assessment. If the rule specifies one refill mechanism, manufacturers know what to build, yet a novel system that achieves better leak control may struggle for acceptance. Scientific reality may support the new design, while regulatory interpretation remains anchored to the recognised standard. Authorities need mechanisms for justified equivalence and emerging evidence if regulation is to remain responsive.

Product evolution also challenges the assumption that a regulatory decision remains valid indefinitely. A notified product may change through supplier substitution, software revision, new coil materials or altered manufacturing scale. Each change may seem minor in isolation, yet collectively they can create a materially different product. Scientific reality changes as the product changes. Regulation often relies on the manufacturer to recognise when the threshold for a new submission has been crossed. Weak change control can therefore create a gap between the product in the regulatory record and the product on the market.

Lifecycle evidence should be capable of correcting that gap. Stability studies, complaints, emissions testing, supplier reviews and periodic risk assessment can reveal whether the original conclusion remains valid. Regulation should not treat the pre-market dossier as permanent truth. Scientific reality is dynamic, and the evidence base should evolve with real-world use. A product that appeared acceptable at launch may require reformulation after a new respiratory hazard is identified. Another may prove more stable and consistent than initial conservative assumptions suggested.

Post-market signals must also be interpreted proportionately. A small number of adverse reports may justify investigation without proving causation. A dramatic incident may be linked to misuse, counterfeit product or incompatible components rather than the notified design. Regulatory response should distinguish signal detection from causal conclusion. Immediate containment may be necessary where severity is high, but the investigation should remain scientifically open. Public communication issued before causality is established can shape perception long after the evidence becomes clearer.

Transparency is the most effective means of managing these tensions. Manufacturers should state assumptions, data gaps and limitations rather than presenting every conclusion as definitive. Regulators should explain why evidence was accepted or rejected and how precaution influenced the decision. Researchers should describe product identity and method conditions sufficiently for studies to be interpreted. Transparency does not weaken authority. It allows uncertainty to be understood and makes decisions easier to revise when new evidence emerges.

Scientific advisory processes can improve regulatory interpretation where they include expertise in chemistry, inhalation toxicology, exposure science, engineering, behavioural science and public health. No single discipline can resolve the entire product. A toxicologist may understand hazard and dose but not device failure. An engineer may understand power control but not sensitisation. A policy specialist may understand legal objectives but not analytical uncertainty. Integrated review reduces the risk that one perspective becomes the whole decision.

Conflicts of interest should be managed without assuming that affiliation determines validity. Industry-funded studies may have access to detailed product information and high-quality laboratories, while academic studies may provide independence but use poorly characterised commercial products. Regulatory work should evaluate methods, transparency and reproducibility. Declaring funding and interests is necessary, but scientific evidence should rise or fall on its quality rather than on institutional identity alone.

The role of expertise itself must be preserved. Regulatory templates, algorithms and automated review can improve consistency, but they cannot replace judgement in areas where evidence is incomplete and product-specific. Artificial intelligence may assist literature searching, data extraction and structural analysis, yet it can reproduce errors or miss context. The final interpretation requires a competent person who understands both the toxicology and the regulatory consequences. Expertise is not the authority to assert a conclusion without explanation; it is the ability to make the reasoning explicit.

Regulatory science is strongest when it accepts that not every decision can be reduced to one number. Margins of exposure, hazard scores and model predictions are useful, but they are tools within a broader judgement. A product may have a wide margin for systemic toxicity and a narrower but manageable irritation concern. Another may produce low emissions under normal use but show unstable performance under ageing. The decision may therefore depend on concentration limits, device restrictions and post-market monitoring rather than a universal pass or fail.

The final regulatory interpretation should answer several questions directly. It should state what is known about the product, which hazards are relevant, what exposure is expected, where the evidence is weak, how uncertainty has been managed and what controls are necessary. It should identify whether the conclusion applies to one formulation, one supplier, one device or a wider product family. It should also explain what would invalidate the conclusion, such as a supplier change, new hazard information or altered power range. This makes the decision scientifically bounded rather than rhetorically absolute.

Where evidence is insufficient, the response should also be specific. The assessment should identify whether the deficiency concerns identity, exposure, chronicity, inhalation relevance, analytical sensitivity or product variability. Additional work can then target the real gap. Requests for more data without a clear scientific question waste resources and may encourage indiscriminate testing. A regulator should be able to explain what uncertainty the requested evidence is intended to reduce and how the result would affect the decision.

Where evidence is sufficient, the conclusion should still avoid overstatement. Acceptance means that the available evidence, exposure and controls support the proposed use within the applicable framework. It does not establish absence of all risk or guarantee that future evidence will not change the assessment. This conditionality is not weakness. It is an accurate description of scientific knowledge.

Regulatory interpretation and scientific reality will never align perfectly because they serve different purposes. Regulation must act, while science can continue questioning. The objective is not to eliminate that difference but to prevent it from becoming distortion. Regulation should remain scientifically literate enough to preserve route, dose, uncertainty and product specificity. Science should remain practically engaged enough to support real decisions rather than retreating into perpetual uncertainty. Both should recognise that vaping products exist within a comparative public-health landscape in which the consequences of action and inaction matter.

The strongest regulatory system is therefore neither permissive nor reflexively restrictive. It demands complete product identity, relevant evidence, controlled exposure, transparent uncertainty and continuing stewardship. It accepts alternative methods when they answer the question credibly and rejects them when they do not. It uses precaution proportionately, distinguishes notification from approval and allows decisions to evolve with the evidence. It also recognises that a scientifically imperfect but well-controlled lower-risk product may have a different public-health value from a combustible product whose harms are already established.

Scientific reality does not offer the comfort of absolute certainty, and regulation should not pretend that it does. What it can offer is a disciplined account of probability, exposure, mechanism, uncertainty and control. Regulatory interpretation becomes defensible when it preserves that account instead of reducing it to a slogan, a database entry or a single threshold. Toxicology within regulation reaches its proper conclusion when the decision reflects both the limits of the evidence and the consequences of the product as it will actually be used.

CHAPTER 4

Analytical Science and Laboratory Testing

Toxicology determines which substances and exposures may matter; analytical science determines whether they can be measured reliably. Regulation cannot control a chemical merely because it might be present, nor can a manufacturer demonstrate compliance through an unsupported laboratory value. Every reported concentration depends on a sequence of choices involving sampling, aerosol generation, collection efficiency, calibration, extraction, instrumentation, data processing and interpretation. A result may appear precise to several decimal places while carrying substantial uncertainty arising from the method used to produce it. Analytical science therefore occupies a critical position between the physical product and the regulatory decision made about it.

A vaping product presents an unusually complex analytical system. It combines a liquid formulation, an electrical device, a heating element, a reservoir, airflow and user-controlled operating conditions. The liquid may contain nicotine, solvents, acids, water and numerous flavour constituents. During use, these materials are heated, transferred into an aerosol, partially transformed and delivered as a mixture of droplets, vapours, gases and particles. The composition measured in the unheated liquid cannot be assumed to represent the composition inhaled by the consumer. Compounds may transfer with different efficiencies, react with one another, degrade thermally, adsorb onto internal surfaces or remain within the device. Metals may arise from coils, solder, contacts or manufacturing residues rather than from the formulation itself. Analytical testing must therefore describe both what was placed into the product and what the operating product produced.

Emissions testing is the principal mechanism through which this transition is examined. A laboratory generates aerosol under defined conditions, captures selected constituents and measures them using appropriate analytical techniques. The apparent simplicity of this process conceals a large number of variables. Puff duration, puff volume, interval, airflow, device orientation, battery charge, power setting, coil age, liquid level and preconditioning can all alter the result. The number of puffs collected may affect overheating, condensation and analyte recovery. The collection system may retain one class of compounds efficiently while allowing another to pass through. A test result therefore describes the product under the conditions of the method; it does not automatically describe every possible pattern of consumer use.

Regulatory testing requires those conditions to be scientifically justified and recorded in sufficient detail for the work to be repeated. Standardised puffing regimes provide consistency between laboratories and products, but no single regime can represent the full range of human behaviour. A fixed laboratory protocol is a controlled model rather than a complete simulation of use. It becomes useful when its limitations are understood, when comparative products are tested under equivalent conditions and when additional stress or misuse testing is separated clearly from measurements intended to represent routine operation. The analytical report should state whether the purpose was regulatory characterisation, comparative assessment, batch release, failure investigation or identification of worst-case emissions. Combining these purposes without distinction produces numbers that are difficult to interpret.

Method validation establishes whether an analytical procedure is suitable for its intended purpose. A sophisticated instrument does not make an unsuitable method reliable. The laboratory must demonstrate that the procedure measures the intended analyte with adequate specificity, sensitivity, accuracy and precision within the relevant matrix and concentration range. Parameters such as linearity, recovery, repeatability, intermediate precision, limit of detection, limit of quantification, robustness and measurement uncertainty determine whether the final result can support a regulatory conclusion. Validation should reflect the actual sample. A method developed for a simple aqueous solution may not perform equivalently in a viscous e-liquid, condensed aerosol extract or filter containing complex flavour constituents.

Matrix effects are particularly important in vaping analysis. Propylene glycol, glycerol, acids, flavour compounds and aerosol condensate can alter extraction efficiency, chromatographic behaviour, ionisation and detector response. Analytes may co-elute, degrade during preparation or react after collection. Calibration standards prepared in clean solvent may produce a different response from the same concentration within the sample matrix. Internal standards, matrix-matched calibration, recovery studies, blanks and spiked samples help identify and control these effects. Without such measures, a laboratory may report an apparently valid concentration that reflects analytical interference rather than the true composition of the product.

Laboratory accreditation provides an organisational framework for controlling these processes. Accreditation to ISO/IEC 17025 demonstrates that a laboratory has systems governing technical competence, equipment, calibration, personnel, methods, records, quality control and the reporting of results within its accredited scope. It does not mean that every method used by the laboratory is equally suitable or that every result is beyond challenge. The scope of accreditation must be examined carefully. A laboratory may be accredited for nicotine analysis in liquid but not for aerosol emissions, carbonyl collection or elemental analysis of device-generated aerosol. Accreditation strengthens confidence where the relevant method and matrix are covered, but it cannot replace scientific examination of the protocol itself.

Repeatability and reproducibility reveal whether a measurement can be relied upon beyond one analytical run. Repeatability concerns results obtained under the same conditions, commonly using the same method, analyst, equipment and laboratory over a short period. Reproducibility considers variation when testing is performed under changed conditions, particularly between laboratories. Vaping products can challenge both because variation may arise from the analytical method and from the product. Two nominally identical devices may have different coil resistance, liquid supply or heating behaviour. The same device may change during a puff sequence as the coil warms, the wick dries or the battery voltage falls. A meaningful study design must distinguish product variability from analytical variability rather than attributing all disagreement to laboratory error.

Replicate testing is therefore not a procedural formality. A single result provides little information about the distribution of product performance. Multiple devices, batches and analytical replicates may be required to understand whether an elevated emission is an isolated event, a recurring product characteristic or a method artefact. The number of replicates should reflect the purpose and expected variability of the measurement. Averaging can summarise central performance, but it can also conceal intermittent failures. A product that usually produces low emissions but occasionally overheats may present a different regulatory concern from one that performs consistently at a moderately higher level. The raw results, variability and circumstances of unusual values should remain visible.

Carbonyl testing demonstrates many of these difficulties. Formaldehyde, acetaldehyde and acrolein can arise through thermal degradation of propylene glycol, glycerol and other formulation constituents. Their formation is highly sensitive to temperature, liquid supply, coil condition and puffing intensity. Laboratories commonly derivatise carbonyl compounds during collection and quantify the derivatives chromatographically. Collection efficiency, derivatisation conditions, blank contamination, reagent purity and storage stability can materially influence the result. Carbonyl measurements generated under liquid-starved or overheated conditions may be useful for identifying product failure, but they should not be presented as representative of normal use unless the operating state is shown to be realistic and reasonably foreseeable.

Heavy metal analysis presents a different set of analytical challenges. Nickel, chromium, lead, copper, tin and other elements may arise from heating coils, solder, connectors, reservoirs, pigments, raw materials or environmental contamination. Their presence in the liquid does not necessarily predict their concentration in aerosol because device operation can release metals through corrosion, erosion, heating and repeated use. Inductively coupled plasma techniques can measure very low elemental concentrations, but the result depends on sample digestion, collection efficiency, contamination control and the distinction between dissolved material and particles. Sampling equipment, laboratory glassware and collection media can themselves introduce trace metals. Rigorous blanks and controlled handling are indispensable where measurements are made close to instrumental detection limits.

Nicotine verification appears more straightforward because the target compound is known and usually present at comparatively high concentration, yet it remains analytically important. The declared strength influences labelling, formulation control, taxation, product classification and consumer exposure. Verification must account for nicotine form, assay basis, density, dilution, extraction and possible degradation. Nicotine salts require particular care because the analytical method may quantify total nicotine while product presentation refers to a salt or equivalent concentration. Laboratories and manufacturers must use consistent conventions so that the result, formulation record and label describe the same quantity.

Nicotine analysis also provides an important measure of manufacturing consistency. A formulation designed at a specified concentration can vary because of raw-material assay, weighing error, mixing inefficiency, evaporation, filling variation or degradation during storage. Testing one development sample does not establish that later commercial batches remain equivalent. Batch-to-batch consistency requires defined specifications, representative sampling and trend analysis. Results should be examined over time rather than treated as isolated pass-or-fail events. A gradual movement towards a specification limit may reveal deterioration in raw materials, equipment calibration or process control before a formal failure occurs.

The same principle applies to emissions and other product attributes. Regulatory evidence is commonly generated from a limited number of samples during development, but the product continues to be manufactured long after the original report has been completed. Changes in flavour supply, coil material, resistance, wick construction, battery output or manufacturing site may alter analytical performance. Periodic verification, change-triggered testing and investigation of complaints connect the original dossier to the product actually sold. Analytical science becomes part of lifecycle control rather than a one-time requirement completed for notification.

Laboratory uncertainty must be reported and understood rather than hidden behind numerical precision. Every measurement is an estimate influenced by sampling variation, calibration, recovery, instrumental response, environmental conditions and data treatment. Measurement uncertainty describes the range within which the true value is reasonably expected to lie under the defined method. This becomes especially important when a result is close to a regulatory limit or product specification. A reported nicotine concentration of 20.0 milligrams per millilitre does not mean that the true concentration is known without uncertainty. Decisions made at regulatory boundaries should consider method performance, rounding conventions, specification tolerances and the consequences of false compliance or false non-compliance.

Limits of detection and quantification require similar discipline. A result below the detection limit does not prove that the substance is absent. It means that the method could not detect it reliably below a stated concentration. A detected signal below the validated quantification limit may indicate presence without supporting an accurate numerical value. Terms such as "not detected", "below quantification" and "zero" are not interchangeable. Regulatory reports should identify the relevant limits and avoid converting analytical limitations into claims of chemical absence or safety.

The final stage is the conversion of analytical data into a regulatory decision. Numbers do not interpret themselves. A measured compound must be considered in relation to product use, aerosol yield, likely exposure, toxicological relevance, method uncertainty, product variability and appropriate comparators. Comparison with cigarette smoke may demonstrate a substantial reduction in exposure to particular toxicants, but it does not establish that the residual exposure is irrelevant. Comparison with ambient air or non-use may identify additional exposure, but it does not show whether that exposure outweighs the benefit of replacing smoking. Analytical science supplies the evidence needed for these comparisons; regulatory judgement determines what action follows.

This chapter examines that evidential chain from emissions requirements and method validation through accreditation, repeatability, carbonyls, metals, nicotine verification and batch consistency to laboratory uncertainty and regulatory interpretation. These subjects are inseparable. A result cannot support a defensible decision unless the sample represents the product, the method measures the analyte correctly, the laboratory controls the procedure, variability is understood and uncertainty is communicated honestly. Analytical testing becomes regulatory science only when the measurement remains connected to the product, the exposure and the decision it is intended to support.

Figure 4.1. Analytical Science and Laboratory Testing: From Product to Regulatory Decision.

The analytical evidence pathway begins with a defined product, representative sample and clearly stated testing purpose. Device conditioning and a justified puffing regime generate emissions that are collected using media appropriate to the target analytes. Validated methods then measure nicotine, carbonyls, metals and other constituents through controlled calibration, recovery, quality-control samples and blank correction. Replicate testing separates analytical variation from device and batch variability, while laboratory accreditation and documented competence support confidence in the procedure. Measurement uncertainty, detection limits and method limitations remain attached to the reported result as it progresses into exposure assessment, toxicological interpretation, specification review and regulatory decision-making. The pathway emphasises that no analytical number should be considered independently of the method, product conditions and uncertainty through which it was produced.

CHAPTER 4 – ANALYTICAL SCIENCE AND LABORATORY TESTING

Lab-to-regulator data pathway

How emissions testing becomes regulatory evidence

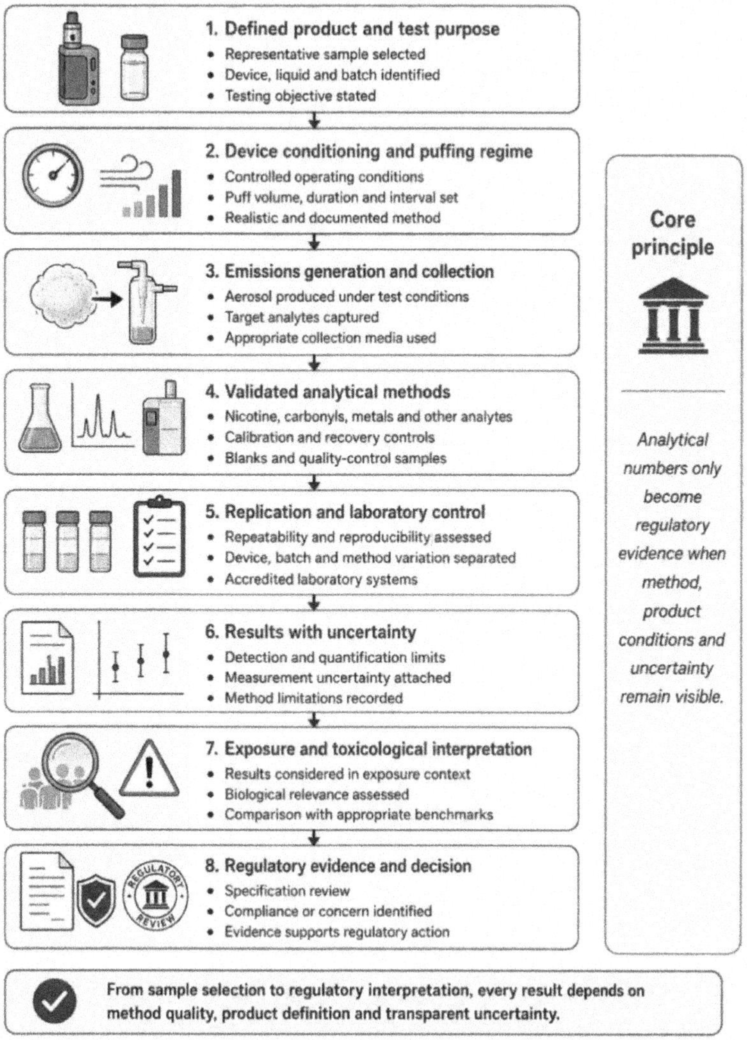

Emissions Testing Requirements

Emissions testing begins from a regulatory recognition that the composition of a vaping liquid does not, by itself, describe the exposure created when the product is used. A formulation may be fully characterised before heating, with each ingredient identified and quantified, yet the aerosol produced by the finished device can contain transferred ingredients, thermal degradation products, volatile compounds, particles and trace materials originating from the heating system. The regulatory object is therefore not only the liquid placed into the reservoir but the complete product as operated. Emissions testing provides the analytical bridge between formulation composition, device performance and the substances potentially inhaled by the consumer.

This distinction is fundamental to the control of electronic cigarettes. A conventional chemical analysis can determine whether a liquid contains the declared nicotine concentration, solvents, flavour constituents and identifiable impurities. It cannot establish how efficiently those constituents enter the aerosol, whether heating changes their chemical structure or whether the device introduces additional substances during operation. Propylene glycol, glycerol and flavour compounds do not transfer uniformly. Some compounds volatilise readily, some condense within the device, some remain within the liquid and others undergo oxidation, dehydration, fragmentation or reaction with surrounding constituents. Heating elements, solder, electrical contacts, reservoirs and wicking materials can also contribute substances that were not present in the original formulation. The aerosol must therefore be measured directly where the regulatory question concerns inhalation exposure.

Within European and United Kingdom consumer-product frameworks, manufacturers and importers are required to provide information concerning product emissions as part of the notification process. This requirement creates a formal expectation that the product will be assessed under defined operating conditions before it is placed on the market. It does not prescribe one universal test programme capable of answering every analytical or toxicological question. The producer must determine which emissions are relevant, how they will be generated, how they will be collected and whether the resulting data describe the intended product adequately. The legal obligation may be expressed in relatively concise terms, but satisfying it competently requires a detailed scientific strategy.

The first requirement is to define the product being tested. A vaping product cannot be represented adequately by a brand name or flavour description alone. The test item should be connected to a specific formulation, nicotine strength, device configuration, coil or atomiser, power setting, reservoir, airflow arrangement and production batch. Where a liquid is intended for use only within a closed system, testing the specified device and liquid together is relatively straightforward. Where a refill liquid may be used in numerous open-system devices, the selection of a representative configuration becomes more difficult. A laboratory result generated using one coil resistance and power level cannot be assumed to describe every device into which the liquid might later be placed.

Closed systems reduce some analytical uncertainty because the manufacturer controls more of the exposure system. The device, liquid, heating element and operating parameters can be defined as one product. Open systems create a wider range of foreseeable use conditions because consumers may combine liquids and devices from different manufacturers, alter power, replace coils or use components outside the circumstances originally considered. The regulatory testing strategy must therefore reflect the product's intended use and the degree of control retained by the producer. It should not imply a level of universality that the study design cannot support.

Sample identity must be preserved from receipt through testing and reporting. The laboratory should record batch or lot number, manufacture date where available, nicotine strength, flavour, product identifier, device version, coil specification and any relevant storage history. Photographs, packaging details and component identifiers may be necessary where products change rapidly or where several visually similar variants exist. A report that describes only a generic product category may be impossible to connect reliably to the notified or marketed item. Regulatory evidence loses value when the tested sample cannot be distinguished from later variants, modified devices or products carrying similar branding.

Representative sampling is equally important. One device or bottle selected without a documented rationale cannot establish the performance of an entire product family. Manufacturing variation can arise from coil resistance, wick placement, filling volume, battery output, component tolerances, liquid composition and storage. The sampling plan should therefore reflect the purpose of the testing and the expected variability of the product. Developmental screening may use a limited number of samples to identify obvious concerns. Regulatory characterisation normally requires sufficient independent units or batches to show that the result is not dependent on one unusually favourable specimen. Investigation of a suspected defect may require targeted sampling of the affected batch rather than general market stock.

The purpose of the test must be defined before aerosol is generated. Regulatory characterisation, product development, comparative assessment, routine quality control, complaint investigation and failure analysis are not interchangeable objectives. A method designed to examine emissions during intended use may differ from one used to identify emissions under stressed or abnormal conditions. A screening study may cover a broad range of possible analytes with comparatively limited quantification. A compliance study may focus on a defined set of compounds using fully controlled procedures and specified reporting limits. Without a clear purpose, the laboratory may generate technically competent measurements that do not answer the regulatory question.

Emissions testing commonly considers several classes of constituent. Nicotine is measured to assess aerosol delivery and consistency. Carbonyl compounds may be examined because thermal degradation of solvents and other formulation constituents can generate formaldehyde, acetaldehyde, acrolein and related substances. Volatile and semi-volatile compounds may include flavour constituents, residual solvents, degradation products and environmental contaminants. Elemental analysis may identify nickel, chromium, lead, copper, tin or other metals associated with raw materials, heating components or manufacturing residues. Other testing may address tobacco-specific nitrosamines, selected organic compounds, particulate characteristics or substances identified through formulation review and toxicological assessment.

The correct analyte list should arise from knowledge of the product rather than from an unchanged laboratory package applied to every formulation and device. A standard panel provides useful consistency and may address substances commonly associated with regulatory concern, but it cannot identify every relevant emission from every product. Ingredient composition, flavour chemistry, device materials, heating conditions and previous analytical findings should inform the programme. A formulation containing a substance with a known thermal degradation pathway may justify targeted testing for the resulting products. A device using particular alloys may require attention to corresponding metals. Product-specific reasoning strengthens the evidential value of the standard analytical panel rather than replacing it.

The aerosol-generation regime is one of the most influential parts of the test. Puff volume, duration, interval, number of puffs, airflow, device orientation, power and activation sequence all affect heating and aerosol production. Small changes in these variables can alter liquid consumption, coil temperature, transfer efficiency and degradation. A result cannot therefore be interpreted independently of the regime that produced it. The conditions should be stated clearly enough for another competent laboratory to reproduce the work and understand how they relate to foreseeable use.

Standardised puffing regimes are necessary because unrestricted laboratory operation would make comparisons almost meaningless. If one product were tested using short, widely spaced puffs and another using longer, closely spaced puffs, differences in emissions could reflect the method rather than the products. Standardisation creates a common analytical reference point. It does not turn a laboratory regime into a universal model of consumer behaviour. Real users vary substantially in puff duration, interval, depth, device maintenance and frequency of use. The regulatory value of a standard regime lies in control and comparability, not in the claim that it recreates every consumer.

The selected regime should be technically compatible with the product. A puffing condition developed around one generation of electronic cigarette may not operate a later product realistically. Devices differ in draw activation, airflow resistance, power control, heating lag and aerosol output. A machine must trigger the device consistently and maintain the intended flow without creating pressure conditions that would not arise during use. Where power is adjustable, the selected setting requires justification. Testing only at the lowest available power may understate reasonably foreseeable emissions, while operating continuously at the highest possible setting may create failure conditions that consumers would reject immediately.

Normal-use testing and stress testing should be separated. Normal-use testing aims to characterise the product under conditions that reflect its intended operation. Stress testing examines performance near operational limits, under repeated puffing, reduced liquid supply or other foreseeable challenges. Both can provide important evidence. Problems arise when emissions generated during deliberate overstressing are presented as though they represent ordinary use, or when a benign normal-use regime is used to imply that the product cannot produce elevated emissions under any circumstances. The report should identify what each condition was intended to demonstrate and avoid combining unlike results into one general conclusion.

Dry-puff or liquid-starved conditions illustrate the importance of this distinction. Where the wick fails to supply sufficient liquid, coil temperature can rise and carbonyl formation may increase sharply. Such conditions may reveal weaknesses in liquid delivery, coil design or product protection. They may also produce an unpleasant sensory response that causes users to stop puffing. The regulatory significance depends on whether the state is readily detectable, how often it may occur and whether the device includes effective controls. A stress-condition result is not irrelevant merely because it is unpleasant, but neither should it be treated automatically as typical exposure.

Device conditioning must be controlled before formal collection begins. New coils and wicks may contain residues, behave differently during initial saturation or require several activation cycles before performance stabilises. Conversely, ageing may change surface condition, resistance, metal release, liquid supply and aerosol generation. The test plan should state whether the device was new, preconditioned or aged and how the conditioning procedure was performed. Discarded conditioning puffs, rest periods, filling procedures and time allowed for liquid saturation can all influence subsequent results.

Battery condition is another source of variation. Rechargeable devices may produce different power as the battery discharges unless output is regulated effectively. Disposable or closed products may change during their operational life. Testing only from a fully charged state may not represent later performance, while collecting across an uncontrolled discharge cycle can introduce variability that is difficult to interpret. Battery charge, voltage or device status should therefore be controlled or recorded in accordance with the design of the product.

The number of puffs included in each collection affects both analytical sensitivity and product behaviour. Collecting more puffs may increase the mass of analyte available for measurement and improve quantification at low concentrations. It may also increase condensation, saturate collection media, change device temperature or deplete the reservoir. Where several collection blocks are combined, the result may conceal changes that occur during the sequence. Dividing the test into defined puff blocks can show whether emissions remain stable or increase as the device warms, ages or approaches liquid depletion.

Collection efficiency must be appropriate to the chemical properties of the target substance. Vaping aerosol contains droplets, gases and vapours with different behaviour. One collection medium may retain particulate-phase material effectively while allowing volatile compounds to pass through. Reactive compounds may need to be trapped or derivatised immediately to prevent loss or transformation. Tubing, filters, impingers and connectors can adsorb analytes or create condensation. The design of the collection train is therefore part of the analytical method rather than a neutral route between the device and the instrument.

Blank controls are necessary to distinguish product-derived emissions from laboratory contamination. Reagents, collection media, tubing, ambient air and analytical equipment may contribute background signals. This is particularly important where the target compounds are present widely in laboratory environments or are being measured at trace concentrations. Machine blanks, reagent blanks, field blanks and procedural blanks may each be appropriate depending on the method. A low result cannot be considered reliable unless the laboratory has demonstrated that the background is understood and controlled.

The test requirement should also account for product mass balance and consumption. Recording the amount of liquid consumed during aerosol generation helps interpret emissions on a per-puff, per-mass-consumed or concentration basis. Two devices may produce the same measured mass of a compound per puff while generating very different quantities of aerosol. Without liquid-consumption or aerosol-mass information, comparisons can be misleading. The denominator used in reporting should be selected according to the regulatory purpose and stated clearly.

Reporting units require consistency. Emissions may be expressed per puff, per collection block, per gram of liquid consumed, per unit of aerosol mass or through another defined basis. Each presentation answers a different question. Per-puff reporting supports estimation based on puff frequency but depends on a standardised puff. Reporting relative to liquid consumed can help compare degradation efficiency but may be less intuitive for consumer exposure. Results should not be converted between bases without the underlying consumption and collection data. Regulatory submissions should preserve sufficient information for the calculation to be reviewed.

The relationship between emissions testing and toxicological assessment must remain explicit. A laboratory can establish that a substance was detected and quantify it within the capabilities of the method. It cannot determine the full health significance of the result without exposure context and toxicological interpretation. The number of puffs used in the test, estimated daily consumption, frequency of use and relevant reference values all influence the assessment. A trace detection may be analytically real but toxicologically minor. A compound present below the reporting limit may still require attention if the method is insufficiently sensitive for the applicable exposure benchmark.

Comparative testing can be valuable where products are assessed against previous versions, reference devices or combustible cigarettes. Equivalent conditions are essential. Comparing data generated by different laboratories, puffing regimes, collection systems or reporting units can create an impression of difference unsupported by the methods. Cigarette smoke and vaping aerosol also require different analytical treatment because their physical and chemical compositions are not identical. The value of comparison lies in a controlled examination of relative emissions, not in forcing dissimilar products into an analytical framework that obscures their mechanisms.

Regulatory requirements should not encourage testing solely as a documentary exercise. A report commissioned after development may provide the fields needed for a notification while contributing little to product improvement. Testing is more valuable when the findings feed back into formulation, device design and quality control. Elevated carbonyls may indicate excessive power, inadequate liquid supply or formulation instability. Unexpected metals may point towards component materials, manufacturing contamination or corrosion. Variable nicotine delivery may reveal inconsistency in aerosol generation. The producer should be able to explain how significant findings were investigated and what action followed.

A compliant result is not permanent. The tested product can change through reformulation, supplier substitution, coil revision, battery modification, manufacturing transfer or component obsolescence. Any change capable of altering aerosol generation should be assessed for its effect on the original emissions evidence. Some modifications may be supported through technical justification; others require partial or complete retesting. The decision should form part of formal change control rather than being left to commercial judgement alone.

Continued emissions testing may also be triggered by complaints, adverse-event reports, market surveillance or emerging scientific concern. A product that performed acceptably during initial development may later show leakage, overheating, unusual taste, coil failure or batch variability. Targeted testing can determine whether the concern reflects misuse, isolated defect, manufacturing drift or a systematic product problem. Regulatory evidence therefore extends beyond the pre-market dossier into the period during which the product remains available.

The central emissions-testing requirement is not the production of a laboratory certificate. It is the generation of traceable, product-specific and exposure-relevant evidence. The sample must represent the product. The operating conditions must be defined. The collection system must suit the target analytes. Controls must distinguish emissions from contamination. Results must retain their units, limits and context. Significant findings must connect to toxicological assessment, product development and regulatory responsibility.

Emissions testing becomes meaningful regulation only when the analytical pathway remains visible from the marketed product to the reported value. Without that connection, the result is simply a number produced from a device under laboratory conditions. With it, emissions data can demonstrate how the formulation and device behave together, identify avoidable sources of exposure and provide regulators with evidence capable of supporting proportionate decisions.

Method Validation

Method validation establishes whether an analytical procedure is capable of producing results that are sufficiently reliable for its intended regulatory purpose. It is not a ceremonial exercise completed after an instrument has generated acceptable-looking data, nor is it satisfied merely because a recognised laboratory technique has been used. High-performance liquid chromatography, gas chromatography, mass spectrometry and inductively coupled plasma methods are powerful analytical tools, but the instrument does not validate the measurement. The complete procedure must be shown to perform adequately within the relevant sample matrix, concentration range, collection system and product conditions.

This distinction is particularly important in vaping analysis because the products generate several different analytical matrices. Nicotine may be measured directly in an e-liquid, in diluted aerosol condensate or on a collection medium. Carbonyls may be trapped through derivatisation and measured as reaction products rather than as the original compounds. Metals may be present in liquid, dissolved aerosol extract, suspended particles or residues released from device components. Volatile flavour constituents may partition between aerosol droplets, vapour, tubing and collection media. A method that performs well in a clean calibration solution may behave differently when applied to glycerol-rich liquids, complex flavour mixtures or condensed aerosol containing numerous co-extracted substances.

Validation must therefore begin with a defined analytical purpose. The laboratory should specify what is being measured, in which matrix, over what concentration range and for what decision. A method intended to confirm nicotine concentration in a finished liquid has a different purpose from one intended to quantify trace carbonyl emissions across a puff block. A screening method designed to identify possible substances does not require the same performance characteristics as a quantitative method used to determine whether a product complies with a specification or regulatory limit. The validation criteria must reflect the consequence of the result.

The intended use also determines the required level of validation. A developmental method used to compare early prototypes may initially be qualified sufficiently to support formulation or device decisions. A method used for formal regulatory submission requires more comprehensive evidence. A procedure used routinely for batch release, market surveillance or enforcement must remain controlled over time and across analysts, instruments and sample sets. Treating all methods as though they serve the same purpose either creates unnecessary work or, more seriously, produces insufficient evidence for high-consequence decisions.

The first requirement is analytical specificity, sometimes described as selectivity. The method must distinguish the target analyte from other substances present in the sample. In a complex e-liquid, compounds with similar chemical properties may produce overlapping chromatographic peaks or detector responses. Flavour constituents, acids, solvents, degradation products and impurities can interfere with nicotine or carbonyl measurements. In elemental analysis, spectral or polyatomic interferences may affect the apparent concentration of a target metal. The laboratory must demonstrate that the signal attributed to the analyte is not materially distorted by the matrix.

Specificity may be assessed through blank matrices, individual standards, spiked samples, peak-purity evaluation, alternative detection wavelengths, mass transitions or confirmatory techniques. The appropriate approach depends on the instrument and analyte. A chromatographic peak at the expected retention time is not necessarily sufficient evidence of identity where co-elution is possible. A mass-spectrometric transition can improve selectivity, but it can still be affected by matrix suppression, fragmentation behaviour or interfering species. Validation should establish that the method measures the intended compound rather than merely producing a response in the expected region.

The calibration model defines the relationship between analytical response and analyte concentration. Laboratories often assume that this relationship is linear, but linearity must be demonstrated across the range in which samples will be measured. The selected calibration range should include the concentrations expected in actual samples and provide suitable performance near any regulatory or specification boundary. A method validated only at high concentration may be unsuitable for trace emissions, while a method optimised for low-level detection may require dilution or a separate range for concentrated samples.

The number and distribution of calibration levels matter. A small number of standards clustered in one part of the range can produce an apparently strong correlation while providing weak control elsewhere. The correlation coefficient alone is not an adequate demonstration of calibration performance. Residuals, back-calculated concentrations, weighting and behaviour at the upper and lower ends of the range should also be examined. Where variance increases with concentration, an unweighted regression may give disproportionate influence to high-level standards and reduce accuracy at the low end. The selected model should be justified by the data rather than chosen automatically.

Calibration standards should be traceable, appropriately prepared and stable under the conditions of use. Errors in stock-solution preparation, purity correction, dilution or storage can affect every sample result while remaining invisible within a well-fitted calibration curve. Certified reference materials or well-characterised analytical standards strengthen traceability, but they must still be handled correctly. Preparation records, balances, volumetric equipment, storage conditions and expiry periods are part of the method-control system.

Accuracy concerns how closely the measured result agrees with the accepted or reference value. In many vaping matrices, a true value cannot be observed directly. Accuracy is therefore assessed through recovery experiments, certified materials, independently prepared samples or comparison with an established reference method. A nicotine method may be challenged using formulations prepared gravimetrically at known concentrations. An emissions method may be assessed by spiking known quantities of analytes onto the collection medium or into the extraction matrix.

Recovery is useful but must be interpreted carefully. Adding a standard after aerosol collection demonstrates part of the analytical procedure, particularly extraction and instrumental measurement. It does not necessarily assess losses during aerosol generation, transport, condensation or trapping. A carbonyl method may recover a derivatised standard efficiently while still losing reactive analytes before derivatisation. A metal method may recover a soluble spike without representing the digestion of particles or residues released from a device. Validation should identify which stages of the process are covered by the recovery experiment and which remain outside it.

Where possible, whole-process recovery should be considered. This may involve introducing a known quantity of analyte before collection or using a controlled generation system that challenges the trapping and analytical stages together. Whole-process experiments are more difficult because they require realistic and stable analyte delivery, but they provide stronger evidence that the complete measurement system performs as intended. Where they are not practical, the limitations should be stated explicitly.

Precision describes the closeness of repeated results under specified conditions. Repeatability is usually assessed over a short period using the same method, analyst, instrument and laboratory. Intermediate precision introduces deliberate variation, such as different days, analysts, instruments, reagent preparations or calibration sets. Reproducibility refers more broadly to performance between laboratories. These levels answer different questions and should not be treated as interchangeable.

Repeatability may show that one analyst can generate consistent results from replicate preparations. It does not establish that the method will remain reliable when used routinely over several months or transferred to another laboratory. Intermediate precision is especially important for regulatory methods because normal operation involves changes in analyst, equipment condition, reagent lots and environmental conditions. A method that performs only when one experienced scientist controls every step is not robust enough for routine use.

Vaping-product variability complicates precision assessment. Replicate measurements may differ because of analytical error, sample-preparation variation, device-to-device variability or changes during aerosol generation. The validation design should separate these sources where possible. Instrumental precision can be examined through repeated injections of the same preparation. Preparation precision can be evaluated through independent extraction or dilution of the same sample. Product precision requires separate devices, coils, bottles or batches. Combining all these levels into one relative standard deviation may conceal the source of variability.

The distinction becomes particularly important in emissions testing. A laboratory may observe wide variation between aerosol collections even though the analytical instrument performs precisely. The cause may lie in coil resistance, wick saturation, device activation, battery output or liquid consumption. It would be incorrect to conclude that the analytical method is imprecise merely because the product itself is variable. Equally, product variability should not be used to excuse poor analytical control. Validation should demonstrate the performance of the analytical procedure independently, while the wider study characterises the variability of the test item.

Limits of detection and quantification define the lower end of method performance. The limit of detection represents the concentration or amount at which a signal can be distinguished reliably from background noise. The limit of quantification is higher and represents the level at which the analyte can be measured with acceptable accuracy and precision. These limits should be established through an approach appropriate to the method and verified experimentally rather than calculated mechanically from ideal calibration data.

For regulatory emissions testing, the quantification limit should be considered against toxicological and exposure needs. A method may be technically valid but insufficiently sensitive if its reporting limit exceeds the concentration relevant to the assessment. Reporting a substance as not detected offers little reassurance where the method could not have detected it at a biologically meaningful level. Method development and validation should therefore be connected to the expected exposure range and the decision the result will support.

Detection limits are also affected by sample size and collection design. Collecting more puffs can increase the total analyte captured and improve apparent sensitivity, but it may change the operating state of the product or the stability of the trapped material. Concentrating an extract may lower the instrumental reporting limit while increasing matrix effects. Sensitivity cannot be improved in isolation from the wider method. The selected approach must preserve product relevance as well as analytical performance.

Matrix effects occur when other substances in the sample change the response to the target analyte. They are common in mass spectrometry, where co-eluting compounds may suppress or enhance ionisation. They can also affect extraction, derivatisation, chromatography and detector behaviour. E-liquids with high concentrations of propylene glycol, glycerol, acids and flavours can behave differently from simple solvent standards. Aerosol extracts may contain a broader and less predictable range of compounds than the original formulation.

Matrix-matched calibration, internal standards and standard addition can help control these effects. Isotopically labelled internal standards are especially valuable where available because they can compensate for variation in extraction, injection and ionisation. Their performance is not automatic, however. The internal standard must behave sufficiently like the analyte and be added at a stage that allows it to correct the relevant sources of loss. Adding it immediately before instrumental analysis cannot compensate for analyte lost during aerosol collection or earlier sample preparation.

Sample and standard stability must also be validated. An analyte may degrade, evaporate, adsorb onto container surfaces or react within the sample after collection. Carbonyl derivatives may have limited stability under certain storage conditions. Nicotine can oxidise, while volatile flavour compounds may be lost during prolonged handling or repeated opening. Metals may precipitate or adsorb if extraction conditions are unsuitable. The laboratory should establish acceptable storage temperature, container type, holding time and number of permitted freeze–thaw or reanalysis cycles where relevant.

Stability testing should cover the stages through which samples actually pass. This may include the collected aerosol before extraction, the prepared extract awaiting analysis, the autosampler period and stored standards. A method cannot be considered controlled if results depend strongly on whether the sample was analysed immediately or left overnight without a defined stability period. Where instability is unavoidable, the procedure should impose time limits and sequence controls that keep samples within the validated window.

Carryover is another potential source of error, particularly when high-concentration liquids and low-level emissions samples are analysed using the same instrument. Residual analyte from one injection can appear in the next and produce a false positive or inflated result. Validation should examine carryover after high standards and representative samples and establish wash procedures, blank requirements or injection sequences capable of controlling it. Carryover becomes especially significant near the detection limit, where a small residual signal can materially affect interpretation.

Robustness examines the effect of small deliberate changes in method conditions. These may include extraction time, reagent concentration, pH, column temperature, flow rate, derivatisation period or storage interval. A robust method continues to perform acceptably when minor variations occur within normal laboratory practice. A method that fails when a parameter shifts slightly may be technically capable under tightly controlled development conditions but unsuitable for routine regulatory use.

Ruggedness considers broader changes, often involving analysts, instruments or laboratories. In practice, the terms robustness and ruggedness are sometimes used differently, but the underlying question is whether the method remains reliable outside one idealised set of circumstances. Deliberate evaluation of sensitive parameters helps identify which steps require the strongest procedural control. If carbonyl recovery is highly dependent on derivatisation time, that time should be specified precisely and monitored. If elemental recovery changes with digestion temperature, the digestion programme becomes a critical method parameter.

System suitability tests provide a continuing check that the instrument and analytical system are functioning adequately before or during sample analysis. Parameters may include retention-time stability, peak resolution, signal response, calibration performance, sensitivity, blank acceptance and replicate injection precision. System suitability does not replace validation. It confirms that the validated method is operating within its expected performance on a particular day.

Quality-control samples extend this control through the analytical run. Blanks identify contamination. Low, medium and high control samples assess performance across the range. Duplicate samples provide information on preparation precision. Spikes can monitor recovery within representative matrices. Acceptance criteria should be defined before the run is interpreted. Repeating or excluding a result because it appears inconvenient, without reference to predetermined criteria, introduces analytical bias.

Out-of-specification and atypical results require structured investigation. The laboratory should not assume that an unexpected result is caused by analytical error, nor should the producer accept it automatically as proof of product failure. Instrument performance, calibration, standards, sample preparation, collection records and product behaviour must be examined systematically. Retesting should be justified and documented. Repeated analysis until a favourable result appears is not a defensible investigation strategy.

Measurement uncertainty connects validation data to the interpretation of the reported result. Precision, calibration, recovery, sample preparation and other contributors create a range around the measured value. Validation provides much of the information needed to estimate that uncertainty. The estimate should be relevant to the actual method and matrix rather than copied from a general laboratory capability statement. Where a result lies close to a specification or legal boundary, uncertainty may influence whether the evidence supports compliance, non-compliance or further investigation.

Validation documentation should permit an independent reviewer to understand what was done and why. The protocol should define the method purpose, analytes, matrices, range, performance characteristics, experiments and acceptance criteria. The report should present the data, deviations, calculations, conclusions and limitations. A statement that the method was validated is insufficient without evidence supporting the claim. Raw data, chromatograms, calibration records, preparation details and statistical treatment should remain traceable to the final report.

Validation is not permanent. A method may need partial or complete revalidation when the instrument changes, the matrix becomes materially different, the analytical range is extended, the collection system is modified or a critical reagent is replaced. A method validated for one type of aerosol extract cannot automatically be assumed suitable for a substantially different product category. The extent of revalidation should reflect the effect of the change rather than requiring every experiment to be repeated without consideration.

Method transfer requires similar discipline. When an established method moves to another laboratory, the receiving laboratory must demonstrate that it can perform the procedure successfully. This is sometimes described as verification rather than full validation. Verification confirms performance under the receiving laboratory's equipment, personnel and operating conditions. Comparative samples, predefined acceptance criteria and investigation of systematic differences are essential. A written method alone cannot guarantee equivalent implementation.

The distinction between validation and verification should remain clear. Validation establishes that the procedure is suitable for its intended purpose. Verification demonstrates that a laboratory can achieve the expected performance when using an already validated method. Where the receiving laboratory changes critical parameters, equipment or sample preparation substantially, verification may no longer be sufficient and additional validation may be required.

Method validation ultimately protects the integrity of the regulatory decision. Without it, a numerical result may reflect interference, poor recovery, unstable samples, unsuitable calibration or uncontrolled variability. A method may produce precise-looking values while systematically underestimating or exaggerating exposure. The appearance of scientific measurement can then conceal a weak evidential foundation.

A validated method does not guarantee that the product is safe, compliant or consistently manufactured. It establishes something more limited but indispensable: that the analytical result is sufficiently trustworthy for the purpose for which it was generated. When specificity, calibration, accuracy, precision, sensitivity, robustness, stability and uncertainty have been demonstrated in the relevant matrix, the reported value can move from instrument output into regulatory evidence. Without that foundation, analytical precision is largely cosmetic.

Laboratory Accreditation

Laboratory accreditation provides independent assurance that a testing organisation has the technical competence, management systems and controlled procedures needed to produce reliable results within a defined scope. In vaping regulation, this matters because analytical data often sit at the centre of product notifications, toxicological assessments, specification decisions, complaint investigations and enforcement action. A regulator may rely on a laboratory report to determine whether a nicotine concentration is accurate, whether carbonyl emissions are elevated, whether metals are present in aerosol or whether a product differs materially from its declared composition. The credibility of those decisions depends not only on the analytical instrument but on the competence and control of the organisation operating it.

Accreditation is commonly associated with ISO/IEC 17025, the principal international framework for testing and calibration laboratories. The standard addresses both management requirements and technical competence. It requires laboratories to control personnel, equipment, methods, environmental conditions, measurement traceability, sampling, handling of test items, quality assurance, reporting and corrective action. It also places emphasis on impartiality, confidentiality, risk-based thinking and the laboratory's ability to demonstrate the validity of its results. Accreditation against this framework does not guarantee that every result is correct, but it provides evidence that the laboratory operates within a structured system capable of identifying, controlling and investigating analytical error.

The distinction between accreditation and certification is important. Certification generally confirms that an organisation's management system conforms to a specified standard. Accreditation goes further by assessing whether the laboratory is technically competent to perform particular tests. A laboratory may hold a certified quality-management system without being accredited for analytical work. Conversely, an accredited laboratory must demonstrate competence for the specific activities listed within its scope. The relevant question is therefore not merely whether the laboratory is accredited, but whether the actual method, analyte and matrix used for the vaping product fall within the accredited scope.

Scope defines the limits of the assurance provided. A laboratory may be accredited to measure nicotine in e-liquids but not nicotine in aerosol emissions. It may be accredited for elemental analysis in water or food but not for metals collected from vaping aerosol. It may perform carbonyl testing competently as a developmental method while that method remains outside the formal scope. The accreditation certificate alone cannot establish suitability. The scope must be examined in sufficient detail to determine which methods, matrices, analytes and measurement ranges have been assessed by the accreditation body.

This distinction is easily overlooked where commercial reports display an accreditation symbol prominently. Clients may assume that every test performed by the laboratory is accredited. In reality, laboratories often conduct a mixture of accredited and non-accredited work. Non-accredited testing is not automatically unreliable. A newly developed method may be scientifically sound but not yet added to the formal scope. Specialist research work may fall outside routine accreditation. The report should nevertheless state clearly whether the specific result was generated under the accredited scope. Ambiguity risks converting a general organisational credential into an unsupported claim about a particular measurement.

The assessment process examines whether the laboratory has the resources and systems needed to conduct the work competently. This includes the education, training, experience and authorisation of personnel. Analytical methods can contain numerous judgement-dependent steps, particularly in aerosol generation, sample preparation, chromatographic integration and interpretation of atypical results. Competence therefore involves more than reading a written procedure. Analysts must understand the principles of the method, recognise abnormal instrument behaviour, identify contamination and distinguish product variability from analytical failure.

Personnel competence should be demonstrated through training records, supervised practice, witnessed assessments, successful analysis of known samples and continuing review of performance. Authorisation should be method-specific. An analyst competent in nicotine assay by liquid chromatography is not necessarily competent to operate an aerosol-generation system or interpret elemental analysis. Laboratories should define which staff may prepare samples, operate particular instruments, review calculations, approve results and sign reports. Clear authorisation reduces the risk that complex work is performed by staff whose general laboratory experience does not extend to the method concerned.

Training must remain current as methods, software and equipment change. A laboratory may introduce a new instrument, revise a derivatisation procedure or modify its collection system. Staff who were competent under the previous arrangement may require additional training before performing the revised method independently. Competence is therefore a continuing condition rather than a qualification obtained once and retained indefinitely.

Impartiality is equally important. Commercial laboratories depend on clients, and those clients may have a direct financial interest in favourable results. Accreditation requires the laboratory to identify and manage risks to impartiality. This does not imply that client-funded testing is inherently compromised. Most regulatory testing is paid for by the manufacturer or responsible economic operator. The risk arises when commercial pressure influences sample selection, test conditions, reporting, investigation of failures or decisions about whether results are released.

A laboratory should not alter a method, exclude an atypical result or repeat testing solely because the initial outcome is inconvenient to the client. Where retesting is justified, the reason should be scientifically documented. Where a sample fails or produces an unexpected result, the laboratory should report the finding in accordance with the agreed procedure rather than providing only the most favourable replicate. Commercial confidentiality must be respected, but it should not be confused with selective reporting.

The management of test items begins before analysis. Samples should be received, identified, logged, stored and handled in a manner that preserves their integrity. Vaping products may be affected by temperature, light, evaporation, oxidation, leakage, battery discharge and physical damage. Nicotine concentration can change through degradation or solvent loss. Volatile compounds may be lost if containers are opened repeatedly. Devices may arrive partially charged, damaged or previously used. The laboratory must record the condition of the item and determine whether any departure could affect the result.

Chain of custody becomes especially important in enforcement or dispute work. The laboratory should be able to show where the sample originated, who handled it, when it was opened, how it was stored and which portion was tested. Tamper-evident seals, unique identifiers, photographs and controlled access may be required where the result could support legal action. Even in routine manufacturer testing, traceability between the sample, batch, test request, raw data and final report is essential. A scientifically sound result loses regulatory value if the tested item cannot be connected reliably to the product placed on the market.

Equipment control is another central element. Analytical instruments, balances, pipettes, flow meters, puffing machines, temperature probes and volumetric devices all influence the final result. Each item must be suitable for its intended use, maintained appropriately and calibrated or verified at defined intervals. Calibration establishes the relationship between the indicated value and a traceable reference. Verification confirms that the equipment continues to perform within specified limits between formal calibrations.

Aerosol-generation equipment deserves particular attention because it defines the conditions under which emissions are produced. Puff volume, duration, interval and flow must remain within controlled tolerances. Device activation must be consistent, and leaks within the collection system must be detected. A chromatograph may measure a collected analyte accurately while the puffing machine generates an incorrect volume or fails to activate the device properly. Accreditation requires the laboratory to consider the complete measurement process rather than concentrating only on the final instrument.

Measurement traceability links the result to recognised references through an unbroken chain of calibrations, each contributing to uncertainty. In practical terms, this means that balances, volumetric equipment, calibration standards and other critical measurements should be connected to suitable national or international references where available. Chemical standards should have documented identity, purity and handling conditions. Standard solutions should be prepared through controlled procedures with appropriate corrections for purity and concentration.

Traceability does not make the result automatically meaningful. A calibration standard can be traceable while the extraction recovery is poor or the matrix interferes with the detector. It does, however, ensure that the numerical scale used by the laboratory is connected to a recognised basis rather than depending on an uncontrolled local reference. This is essential where results from different laboratories or jurisdictions are compared.

Environmental conditions can also affect analytical performance. Temperature and humidity influence balances, solvents, aerosol condensation, flow measurement and instrument stability. Airborne contamination can affect trace-metal and volatile-compound analysis. Laboratories should identify which environmental parameters matter for each method and monitor them accordingly. Clean areas, controlled ventilation, segregated preparation spaces or specialist materials may be needed for low-level elemental work. The required controls should reflect the sensitivity of the measurement rather than being applied as general decoration.

Method selection remains the responsibility of the laboratory even where the client specifies the test. Standardised or published methods should be used where they are suitable, but vaping analysis frequently requires adaptation because products, devices and matrices differ. A method written for one product format may not operate correctly with another. The laboratory must review whether the requested procedure is capable of answering the stated question. It should not accept a method unquestioningly merely because it has been used previously or requested by a commercial customer.

Where a standard method is modified, the effect of the modification must be assessed. Changes in collection medium, extraction solvent, puffing regime, instrument, calibration range or reporting basis may alter performance. The laboratory should validate the modified elements to the extent necessary. Minor administrative changes may require little additional work, whereas a change in matrix or collection principle may require substantial revalidation.

Accreditation assessments examine whether methods are documented clearly enough to support consistent implementation. Controlled procedures should describe sample preparation, instrument settings, calibration, system suitability, acceptance criteria, calculations and reporting. They should also identify critical steps and permissible tolerances. Informal knowledge held by one experienced analyst is not an adequate substitute for a controlled method. If performance depends on unwritten judgement, the procedure is vulnerable when staff change or work is transferred.

Control of documents and records ensures that laboratories use the correct method version and retain evidence of what occurred. Historical results must remain linked to the procedure in force at the time. If a method is revised, the laboratory should be able to determine which samples were analysed under the earlier version. Records should include instrument output, calibration data, chromatograms, integration decisions, preparation details, deviations, quality-control results and calculations. The final report is only the visible summary of a much larger evidential record.

Data integrity has become increasingly important as laboratories rely on electronic systems. Instrument software can allow peaks to be reintegrated, files to be overwritten or results to be recalculated. Access controls, audit trails, secure storage and review procedures are needed to ensure that data remain complete and attributable. The reviewer should be able to determine who generated the data, who changed them, why changes were made and which version supported the reported result.

Manual data treatment requires equal control. Chromatographic integration can be particularly sensitive to analyst judgement. Reprocessing may be justified where automatic integration fails, but the rationale and original result should remain visible. Unexplained manual adjustment creates a risk that the reported concentration reflects preference rather than a defined rule. Laboratories should establish integration procedures and require independent review where intervention affects the result materially.

Ensuring the validity of results is one of the most important elements of laboratory accreditation. Internal quality-control samples, blanks, duplicates, spikes, control charts and reference materials provide continuing evidence that the method remains under control. Validation demonstrates capability under defined conditions; ongoing quality assurance demonstrates that this capability is being maintained during routine work.

Control charts can identify gradual drift before a formal failure occurs. A quality-control sample may remain within its acceptance range while moving steadily towards one limit over successive runs. This pattern can indicate deterioration in calibration standards, instrument response, column performance or sample preparation. Trend review allows preventive action rather than waiting for an out-of-control event.

Proficiency testing provides external comparison. The laboratory receives a sample or dataset whose assigned value is not known to the participating analysts and reports its result for comparison with other laboratories or a reference value. Successful performance provides evidence that the method operates effectively outside the laboratory's internal quality system. Poor performance requires investigation and corrective action.

Proficiency testing in vaping analysis can be difficult because suitable schemes may not exist for every matrix and analyte. E-liquids can be prepared and distributed comparatively easily, but aerosol emissions depend on device operation, puffing systems and collection procedures. Where formal schemes are unavailable, interlaboratory comparison, split-sample testing or alternative external checks may be used. The absence of a convenient proficiency scheme does not remove the obligation to obtain independent evidence of performance.

Interlaboratory disagreement requires careful analysis. Different results may arise from calibration, extraction, collection efficiency, puffing conditions, product variability or reporting conventions. Accreditation does not guarantee identical numbers from all laboratories. It does require each laboratory to understand its method and investigate differences that exceed the expected uncertainty. Comparability improves when methods, units and product conditions are harmonised, but the result must still retain its uncertainty and context.

Measurement uncertainty is central to accredited work because it describes the range associated with the result. The laboratory should identify significant contributors and estimate their combined effect where relevant. These contributors may include calibration, weighing, volumetric preparation, recovery, repeatability, flow, puff number and sample variability. The uncertainty estimate should correspond to the reported method and matrix rather than being adopted from a generic instrument specification.

Uncertainty becomes especially important near regulatory limits. A nicotine result close to a legal maximum or specification boundary may not support a simple binary conclusion without considering the method's uncertainty. The same applies to low-level metals, carbonyls or impurities assessed against an internal action limit. Accreditation promotes transparent reporting of uncertainty, but the laboratory and regulator must still decide how it should be applied to compliance decisions.

Decision rules should therefore be agreed where results will be judged against a limit. A decision rule explains how measurement uncertainty is considered when declaring conformity or non-conformity. Different rules allocate the risk of false acceptance and false rejection differently. The report should not imply certainty greater than the method provides. Where no decision rule has been agreed, the laboratory may report the result and uncertainty without making a conformity statement.

Reporting must be accurate, clear and unambiguous. The test report should identify the laboratory, client, sample, method, dates, results, units and any deviations or limitations. Where testing falls within the accredited scope, the report should indicate this in accordance with the accreditation body's rules. Results outside the scope should be distinguished clearly. The report should not display an accreditation mark in a way that suggests broader coverage than actually exists.

For vaping emissions, the report should also describe the device and aerosol-generation conditions. A concentration value without puff volume, duration, interval, number of puffs, power setting, coil identity and collection basis cannot be interpreted reliably. The laboratory may be accredited for the analytical measurement yet produce a report that is of limited regulatory value because the product conditions are insufficiently described. Accreditation supports good reporting, but the client and regulator must still ensure that the requested information answers the relevant question.

Opinions and interpretations should be separated from measured results unless the laboratory is competent and authorised to provide them. A laboratory can state that a sample contains a measured concentration or that a result exceeds an agreed specification. Broader claims concerning consumer safety, toxicological acceptability or population risk may require expertise outside the analytical scope. Accreditation in chemical testing does not automatically confer competence in toxicology or regulatory policy.

Subcontracting requires transparency. A laboratory may send part of the work to another organisation because it lacks the relevant equipment or expertise. The client should be informed, and the subcontractor should be competent for the work. Where accredited status is required, the subcontracted activity should fall within an appropriate accredited scope. The primary laboratory remains responsible for ensuring that the final report identifies the source and status of the result correctly.

Complaints, non-conforming work and corrective action provide evidence of whether the quality system operates in practice. No competent laboratory is entirely free from errors, instrument failures or disputed results. The important question is how these events are detected and managed. Non-conforming work may include failed quality controls, incorrect sample preparation, equipment malfunction, use of an obsolete method or reporting error. The laboratory should assess the effect on previous and current results, notify affected clients where necessary and prevent recurrence.

Corrective action should address root cause rather than only the immediate symptom. Recalibrating an instrument may restore performance, but it does not explain why the calibration failed. Retraining an analyst may be appropriate, but it should not be used automatically where the underlying problem lies in an ambiguous procedure or unsuitable equipment. Accreditation assessment tests whether the laboratory learns from failures and improves its controls.

Internal audits and management review examine the system as a whole. Internal audits determine whether procedures are being followed and whether the laboratory conforms to its own requirements. Management review considers broader performance, including audit findings, complaints, proficiency testing, quality trends, resource needs and opportunities for improvement. These activities prevent accreditation from becoming a collection of procedures maintained solely for an external visit.

External assessment by the accreditation body provides independent scrutiny. Assessors review documents, observe methods, examine records, question staff and evaluate technical performance. Nonconformities must be corrected before accreditation is granted or maintained. Surveillance and reassessment continue after the initial decision. The process therefore creates an ongoing relationship between the laboratory's claimed competence and external evidence supporting it.

The accreditation body's assessment is itself limited to the defined scope and sampled evidence. Assessors cannot observe every test, analyst or result. Accreditation should therefore be understood as structured assurance rather than an absolute guarantee. A laboratory can remain accredited and still make an error. The value lies in the presence of systems capable of preventing, detecting and correcting error, together with independent evaluation that those systems are functioning.

For manufacturers, accreditation does not remove responsibility for selecting and overseeing the laboratory. The producer should define the testing need, review the scope, confirm method suitability and examine the report critically. Choosing a laboratory solely because it offers an accredited certificate at the lowest cost is not a sufficient scientific strategy. The laboratory may perform the requested method correctly while the method itself does not represent the product or answer the regulatory question.

Technical agreements can clarify responsibilities. They may define sample selection, storage, methods, reporting limits, uncertainty, retesting, data access, deviations, subcontracting and retention of records. Such agreements are particularly valuable where repeated regulatory testing is performed across several products. They ensure that the laboratory and client share the same understanding of what the test is intended to establish.

Regulators and enforcement authorities should apply the same scrutiny. An accredited report deserves greater confidence than unsupported testing, but it should not be accepted without examining scope, method, product conditions and limitations. Accreditation strengthens the evidence; it does not replace interpretation. A report generated under an accredited nicotine method does not prove that the full product is compliant, nor does an accredited emissions panel establish the absence of every relevant hazard.

The strongest role of accreditation is therefore to create confidence in the process through which evidence is generated. It establishes expectations for competence, impartiality, traceability, validation, equipment, quality control, uncertainty and reporting. It gives manufacturers and regulators a basis for distinguishing laboratories that merely possess instruments from those that can demonstrate controlled analytical capability.

Its limitation is equally important. Accreditation cannot transform an irrelevant test into a relevant one, an unrepresentative sample into a representative product or an unsuitable puffing regime into realistic exposure evidence. It cannot compensate for a poorly defined regulatory question. The laboratory must be competent, but the study must also be scientifically appropriate.

Accredited laboratory evidence is most valuable when organisational assurance and technical relevance coincide. The method falls within the scope, the analysts are competent, the sample is traceable, the equipment is controlled, the measurement is validated, uncertainty is understood and the report describes the product conditions fully. Under those circumstances, the result becomes a credible element of regulatory decision-making rather than a number supported only by institutional appearance.

Repeatability and Reproducibility

Repeatability and reproducibility determine whether an analytical result represents a stable property of the product or only the circumstances of one test. A laboratory can generate a precise numerical value from a single run, but that value has limited regulatory meaning unless comparable results can be obtained when the measurement is repeated. The central question is not simply whether the instrument produced a result. It is whether the result remains sufficiently consistent when the same sample is tested again, when another analyst performs the work, when another device or batch is examined, and when the method is applied by a different laboratory.

The distinction between repeatability and reproducibility is important because each describes a different level of analytical confidence. Repeatability concerns agreement between results obtained under closely controlled conditions, normally within the same laboratory, over a short period, using the same method, equipment, analyst and test material. Reproducibility considers agreement under changed conditions, particularly between laboratories, analysts, instruments, locations or method implementations. Intermediate precision occupies the space between them, examining variation within one laboratory across different days, analysts, instruments, reagent preparations or environmental conditions.

These terms are sometimes used loosely, but their regulatory implications differ. Good repeatability shows that the immediate analytical procedure is controlled. It does not prove that the method will perform similarly elsewhere or over time. Good reproducibility provides stronger evidence that the measurement is not dependent on one laboratory's equipment, interpretation or local practice. A method may be highly repeatable within one laboratory yet produce systematically different results when transferred. Conversely, apparently poor repeatability may reflect genuine product variability rather than analytical weakness. The study design must therefore distinguish the behaviour of the method from the behaviour of the product.

This distinction is particularly difficult in vaping analysis because the test system contains several independent sources of variation. The analytical instrument may vary in response. Sample preparation may introduce error. Aerosol generation may differ between runs. Devices may differ in battery output, resistance, airflow or liquid supply. Coils may be wound or positioned slightly differently. Wicks may saturate unevenly. Formulations may vary between batches. The same device may also change during use as the coil heats, the liquid level falls, the wick ages or deposits accumulate. A repeated result therefore reflects both measurement variability and product variability unless the experiment separates them deliberately.

Instrumental repeatability is usually the most controlled level. The same prepared sample may be injected several times into a chromatograph or analysed repeatedly by another instrument. Agreement between these measurements shows that the detector, injection system, calibration and immediate analytical conditions are stable. Poor instrumental repeatability suggests an equipment, integration, calibration or sample-stability problem. Strong instrumental repeatability does not establish that the complete method is reliable, because it excludes sample preparation, extraction, aerosol generation and product operation.

Preparation repeatability expands the assessment by requiring the same test material to be prepared independently several times. Separate dilutions, extractions, derivatisations or digestions are performed and analysed. This introduces variability from weighing, pipetting, mixing, extraction and analyst technique. It is often more informative than replicate injections because many analytical errors occur before the sample reaches the instrument. A method that produces consistent injections from one vial but inconsistent results across independently prepared samples is not sufficiently controlled for routine regulatory use.

Whole-method repeatability includes aerosol generation and collection as well as analysis. Separate aerosol collections are produced under nominally identical conditions and taken through the complete procedure. This is the most relevant level for emissions testing, but it is also the most difficult to interpret. Differences between results may arise from the analytical method, the collection system or the product itself. Replicate aerosol collections should therefore be accompanied by information capable of identifying where the variation arose, including liquid consumption, puff count, device resistance, power, battery status, airflow, collection efficiency and visible abnormalities during the run.

The number of replicates must be sufficient to characterise the expected variation. Duplicate testing can identify gross disagreement, but it provides limited information about the distribution of results. Three replicates are common in analytical work because they provide an initial estimate of central tendency and spread, but even three may be insufficient where devices are highly variable or failure occurs intermittently. The appropriate number depends on the intended decision, the expected magnitude of variability and the cost and complexity of the test.

A developmental screening study may use a small number of replicates to identify obvious formulation or device problems. A regulatory characterisation study should provide enough data to demonstrate that the result is not dependent on one favourable unit. A batch-release method may rely on fewer measurements if the manufacturing process is well controlled and the method has a strong historical performance record. An enforcement investigation may require broader sampling because the result could support legal action or market withdrawal.

Statistical treatment should reflect the size and structure of the dataset. The mean summarises the central result, while the standard deviation or relative standard deviation describes dispersion. Relative standard deviation is useful when comparing variability across concentration levels because it expresses variation as a proportion of the mean. It can become misleading near zero, where a small absolute difference produces a large percentage. Confidence intervals may provide a more useful indication of the uncertainty surrounding the estimated mean, particularly when comparing products or laboratories.

Acceptance criteria for repeatability should be defined before the results are reviewed. Selecting criteria after seeing the data encourages subjective interpretation. The limits should reflect method capability, concentration, matrix, regulatory purpose and product variability. A criterion appropriate for nicotine assay at milligram-per-millilitre concentrations may be unsuitable for trace metals measured close to the quantification limit. Low-level emissions generally show greater relative variation because small changes in blank contribution, recovery or product performance have a larger proportional effect.

The use of a single universal percentage criterion across all analytes and matrices is rarely defensible. Precision expectations should be tighter where the analyte is abundant, the method is mature and the matrix is simple. Wider limits may be scientifically justified for trace constituents, complex aerosols or products with inherent variability. Wider criteria should not become a convenient means of accepting poor control. They should be supported by validation data, historical performance and the consequences of the decision.

Repeatability should also be assessed across the analytical range. A method may perform well at medium and high concentrations but poorly near its lower limit of quantification. If regulatory samples are expected near that lower limit, the precision observed there is more relevant than performance at higher levels. Validation should therefore include low, medium and high concentrations representative of actual use. Results below the validated precision range should not be reported with the same confidence as values generated within it.

Intermediate precision examines whether the method remains reliable under ordinary laboratory variation. Different analysts may prepare and analyse the samples on different days using different instruments, reagent lots or calibration standards. These changes reflect routine operation more accurately than same-day repeatability. A method that performs only under one tightly controlled arrangement may be suitable for research but fragile for regulatory testing.

Analyst variation can be significant where the procedure contains manual or interpretive steps. Aerosol-collection apparatus may be assembled differently. Derivatisation timing may vary. Chromatographic peaks may be integrated manually. Samples may be mixed, diluted or extracted with slightly different technique. A well-written method should reduce dependence on individual judgement, but it cannot eliminate it entirely. Intermediate-precision studies reveal which stages require tighter instruction, training or automation.

Instrument variation can also expose weaknesses. Two chromatographs may have different detector response, dwell volume, column condition or software behaviour. Different aerosol-generation machines may control flow or activation differently. A method transferred between instruments should produce results that remain within predefined performance criteria after appropriate calibration. Systematic differences require investigation rather than being absorbed automatically into a wider acceptance range.

Day-to-day variation may arise from environmental conditions, reagent preparation, equipment drift and sample stability. A method assessed only within one analytical sequence may appear more stable than it is during routine work. Running replicate preparations across several days provides a more realistic estimate of laboratory precision. It also helps identify whether standards, derivatives or extracts remain stable over the periods required by the procedure.

Reproducibility extends the assessment beyond one laboratory. The same or equivalent samples are tested independently by different laboratories using the agreed method. The objective is not necessarily to obtain identical values, because every measurement carries uncertainty. It is to determine whether the laboratories reach sufficiently comparable results for the method to support regulatory interpretation across organisations and jurisdictions.

Interlaboratory reproducibility is one of the most demanding tests of an analytical procedure. Laboratories may interpret apparently simple instructions differently. One may condition a device for five puffs and another for ten. One may define the puff start from valve opening and another from device activation. Tubing length, filter placement, extraction time, reagent preparation and peak integration may differ. These variations can produce systematic differences even where each laboratory follows its own procedure consistently.

Detailed method standardisation reduces such variation but cannot remove it entirely. Written procedures should define critical conditions precisely, including sample handling, device conditioning, puffing parameters, collection arrangement, extraction, calibration, integration and reporting. Illustrations, equipment specifications and reference materials may be necessary where textual description is insufficient. Method transfer should also include training, demonstration and comparison samples rather than relying only on document exchange.

Round-robin studies are useful for examining reproducibility. Multiple laboratories receive the same or carefully prepared test items and analyse them under a common protocol. The combined results reveal interlaboratory variation, systematic bias and ambiguous parts of the method. The design must account for the stability and homogeneity of the distributed samples. E-liquids can usually be subdivided and distributed with reasonable control, but devices and coils may be less uniform. Emissions studies add the complication that each laboratory may operate a different physical unit.

Where product variability is substantial, a round-robin study may need reference devices, pooled materials or carefully characterised samples. Otherwise, differences between laboratories may be confused with differences between the units received. One approach is to separate the study into stages. Laboratories may first analyse a common liquid or aerosol extract to assess the analytical method. They may then generate aerosol from specified products to assess the combined generation and analytical system. This layered design helps identify whether disagreement arises from aerosol production or chemical measurement.

Proficiency-testing schemes provide a formal form of interlaboratory comparison. Participating laboratories analyse blinded samples and compare their results with an assigned value or the consensus of competent participants. Performance may be evaluated through statistical scores that consider deviation from the assigned value and expected variation. Successful participation provides continuing evidence of competence, while poor performance triggers investigation and corrective action.

Proficiency testing is more straightforward for nicotine concentration in liquids than for whole-product emissions. Stable liquids can be prepared at known concentrations, distributed and analysed without operating a device. Aerosol emissions depend on the interaction between product, machine and collection method. Suitable proficiency materials may therefore be difficult to produce. Interlaboratory comparison using common extracts or standard generation systems can provide partial assurance where full schemes are unavailable.

Between-laboratory disagreement should not be resolved simply by choosing the result from the preferred laboratory. The difference should be examined systematically. Calibration standards, traceability, collection efficiency, blanks, recovery, sample preparation, puffing parameters, reporting units and uncertainty may all contribute. A laboratory may be internally repeatable but systematically biased because of incomplete extraction or calibration. Another may generate greater within-run variability but a mean closer to the reference value. Precision and accuracy must therefore be considered together.

A repeatable method can be wrong. If the same interference, calibration error or incomplete recovery occurs in every run, the results may agree closely while remaining inaccurate. This is why repeatability alone cannot demonstrate validity. Reproducibility does not guarantee accuracy either, because several laboratories may share the same flawed method. Agreement strengthens confidence only when the procedure is also specific, calibrated, recovered adequately and linked to suitable reference materials.

The use of standard methods can improve reproducibility by providing common procedures, terminology and performance expectations. Standardisation is particularly valuable where laboratories need to compare products, support notifications or conduct enforcement. It reduces the number of methodological differences that must be considered when results conflict. Standard methods should still be verified for the specific product and matrix.

A method can be standardised yet unsuitable for a new device format, high-viscosity liquid or unusual analyte.

Vaping products present a special challenge because technological change can outpace standard development. A method developed around early refillable devices may not trigger, condition or collect emissions from compact pod systems in the same way. Standardisation should therefore control the measurement without preventing justified adaptation. Any adaptation must be documented and assessed for its effect on precision and comparability. Otherwise, laboratories may all claim to use the same standard while applying materially different procedures.

Product repeatability is distinct from method repeatability and deserves separate assessment. A product should perform consistently enough that nominally identical units do not generate widely different results under the same conditions. Device-to-device variation may arise from component tolerances, coil manufacture, wick placement, battery output, assembly and filling. Liquid batch variation may arise from raw-material assay, mixing, flavour composition, nicotine concentration or storage.

Replicate testing across independent product units provides information about this manufacturing consistency. Repeated aerosol collections from one device may underestimate the variation experienced across the market. Conversely, testing a new device for every replicate may combine device variation with analytical variation. Both approaches can be useful when their purposes are stated. Repeated testing of one unit examines within-device stability, while testing multiple units examines between-device consistency.

Within-device performance may change over the product's life. Early puffs may differ from later puffs because the coil and wick are new. Performance may stabilise after conditioning and then deteriorate as deposits accumulate or liquid supply changes. Testing only one short period can miss this evolution. A longitudinal design that examines defined stages of product use may reveal whether emissions remain stable or whether particular constituents increase with age.

Battery discharge and reservoir depletion may introduce additional variation. A regulated device may maintain power until the battery approaches its lower limit, while an unregulated system may decline progressively. A closed pod may deliver differently as the liquid level falls. The test plan should control or record these states so that variation is interpreted correctly. A result generated at full charge and full reservoir cannot necessarily describe the complete use cycle.

Outliers require careful handling. An extreme result may reflect analytical error, contamination, product failure or genuine intermittent behaviour. Automatically excluding it because it increases variability can remove the most important safety signal in the dataset. Equally, treating every isolated extreme value as representative can exaggerate risk. The correct approach is investigation.

The laboratory should examine the raw data, collection records, device behaviour, calibration, quality controls and sample handling. If a clear analytical failure is identified, exclusion may be justified and documented. If no analytical cause is found, the result remains evidence of product variability or potential failure. Additional testing may be needed to determine its frequency and significance. The regulatory question is not only what the average product does but whether foreseeable units can behave materially differently.

Averaging should therefore be used with caution. Mean values support comparison and exposure estimation, but they can conceal intermittent high emissions, unstable nicotine delivery or occasional metal release. The distribution, range and individual results should remain available. Where a product has a low average but a wide spread, the variability itself may be a quality concern. Consistency is not merely a statistical preference; it affects whether consumers receive the product described in the technical dossier.

Trend analysis provides a broader view of repeatability over time. Results from routine batch testing, stability work, complaint investigations and periodic verification can be examined collectively. A slow increase in mean emissions or widening variability may indicate equipment wear, supplier change, raw-material drift or weakening process control. Individual batches may remain within specification while the trend shows deterioration. Regulatory quality systems should therefore retain and review data rather than treating each report as an isolated certificate.

Specification setting should reflect demonstrated repeatability and reproducibility. A specification narrower than the combined capability of the manufacturing process and analytical method will generate repeated apparent failures even when the product has not changed materially. A specification that is excessively wide may accept poor consistency or elevated exposure. The limit should consider product risk, process capability, method uncertainty and the consequences of non-conformity.

Measurement uncertainty incorporates elements of repeatability and reproducibility into the reported result. The within-laboratory precision observed during validation contributes to the uncertainty budget. Where results are intended to be compared across laboratories, interlaboratory variation may also be relevant. Uncertainty does not excuse poor reproducibility, but it provides the range within which differences may be expected.

Two results should not be described as contradictory merely because their reported central values differ. Their uncertainties, sample identities and test conditions must be considered. Results may be statistically compatible even where the numbers are not identical. Conversely, overlapping ranges do not automatically establish equivalence where the study design, method or product differs substantially. Scientific comparison requires examination of the complete evidential context.

Regulatory authorities depend on reproducible methods because decisions should not vary arbitrarily according to which laboratory performed the analysis. A product should not appear compliant in one jurisdiction and non-compliant in another solely because laboratories use incompatible collection systems, calibration conventions or reporting units. Complete uniformity may be unattainable, but the sources of variation should be controlled sufficiently that differences larger than the expected uncertainty can be investigated meaningfully.

Manufacturers also depend on reproducibility when commissioning work from different laboratories over the product lifecycle. Development testing may be performed by one organisation, notification testing by another and complaint investigation by a third. If methods are not comparable, changes in results may be attributed incorrectly to the product. Technical agreements should define methods, units, sample conditioning and acceptance criteria so that later testing remains connected to the original evidence.

Repeatability and reproducibility ultimately determine how much confidence can be placed in an analytical conclusion. Repeatability shows whether the measurement can be produced consistently under controlled conditions. Intermediate precision shows whether it survives ordinary laboratory variation. Reproducibility shows whether the procedure can be applied elsewhere without losing its meaning. Product replication reveals whether nominally identical units behave as one controlled product or as a collection of variable devices.

The strongest evidence separates these components rather than combining them into one general measure of variation. Instrument response, sample preparation, aerosol generation, device behaviour and batch consistency should each be examined at the level appropriate to the regulatory question. A single precise result may be technically correct, but repeated and reproducible evidence is what establishes that the result can support product assessment, comparison and regulatory action.

Carbonyl Testing

Carbonyl testing examines one of the most important classes of compounds formed during the thermal operation of vaping products. Carbonyl compounds include aldehydes and ketones generated through oxidation, dehydration, fragmentation and other reactions involving propylene glycol, glycerol, flavour constituents and minor formulation components. Formaldehyde, acetaldehyde and acrolein receive the greatest regulatory attention because of their recognised toxicological significance, but analytical programmes may also include acetone, propionaldehyde, crotonaldehyde, butyraldehyde, glyoxal and methylglyoxal. Their presence and concentration depend not only on the liquid formulation but on the interaction between formulation, device design, heating conditions and consumer behaviour.

The importance of carbonyl testing arises from the difference between an unheated liquid and the aerosol generated from it. Formaldehyde or acetaldehyde may be present initially as impurities or flavour-related constituents, but they can also form during heating. Acrolein is associated particularly with thermal degradation pathways involving glycerol, although its formation depends strongly on local temperature and liquid supply. The analytical question is therefore not simply whether a carbonyl compound exists somewhere within the product. It is whether the complete product generates that compound under defined and relevant conditions of use, at what level, with what variability and through which mechanism.

Carbonyl formation is highly sensitive to temperature. Vaping devices do not normally measure the exact temperature of every part of the heating coil, and a single reported power setting does not translate directly into one uniform thermal condition. Local temperature depends on coil resistance, applied voltage, surface area, wick contact, liquid viscosity, airflow, reservoir level and the rate at which liquid replaces material evaporated during each puff. A coil that remains adequately wetted can operate differently from the same coil when liquid supply becomes restricted. Carbonyl emissions can consequently change substantially without any alteration to the nominal device setting.

Power is nevertheless an important variable. Increasing electrical power generally increases the rate of aerosol generation and may increase carbonyl formation, particularly when the rate of evaporation begins to exceed the capacity of the wick to supply liquid. The relationship is not always linear. A moderate increase in power may increase aerosol mass without producing a proportionate increase in carbonyl concentration, while a relatively small additional increase may move the system into partial liquid starvation and generate a sharp rise. Testing at only one setting may therefore describe one operational point while failing to reveal the conditions under which emissions increase rapidly.

Adjustable devices present a particular regulatory challenge because consumers can select different power levels. Testing only at the lowest recommended setting may produce favourable results but fail to represent foreseeable use. Testing only at the maximum possible setting may create conditions that are technically available but immediately unpleasant or unsustainable. The test plan should identify the manufacturer's recommended range, the settings likely to be used in practice and the point at which the device begins to show abnormal operation. Where several conditions are tested, normal-use and stress-test results should be distinguished clearly.

Wick saturation is one of the principal determinants of carbonyl production. During each puff, liquid evaporates from the region surrounding the coil. The wick must transport replacement liquid rapidly enough to keep the surface wet. High-viscosity formulations, narrow liquid channels, compressed wick material, low reservoir levels and rapid sequential puffing can all impair replenishment. When the coil becomes insufficiently wetted, its temperature may rise and solvent degradation can accelerate.

This condition is commonly described as a dry puff, although the transition from normal wet operation to complete dryness is not necessarily abrupt. Partial liquid starvation may occur before the consumer experiences the unmistakable harshness associated with a severe dry puff. A product may therefore generate elevated carbonyls during a developing supply problem without reaching the most extreme sensory state. Testing should examine whether increases occur gradually, intermittently or only after a clear product failure.

Sensory rejection is relevant but should not be used as the sole basis for dismissing elevated results. An experienced user may stop puffing when a burnt or acrid taste develops, limiting exposure. A less experienced user may not identify the change immediately. Device design, flavour intensity and cooling can also affect how readily overheating is detected. The scientifically useful question is whether the test condition represents normal operation, reasonably foreseeable degradation or an artificial failure state that the user would not sustain.

Device conditioning influences this assessment. New coils may contain manufacturing residues, oils, fibres or surface contaminants and may behave differently during their first activations. Wicks require sufficient time to saturate fully. Some systems stabilise after a number of preliminary puffs, while others show increasing emissions as deposits accumulate during extended use. A carbonyl study should state whether the device was new, conditioned, aged or used through a defined portion of its expected life.

The number of conditioning puffs should be justified rather than selected only from laboratory habit. Too few may cause the formal collection to include unstable early behaviour. Too many may exclude a period that consumers would encounter when first using the product. Where early performance is materially different, it may be more informative to characterise it separately rather than discard it. The same principle applies to late-life operation, when coil deposits, wick deterioration or reduced reservoir supply may change emissions.

Puff volume, duration and interval all influence carbonyl formation. Longer puffs apply power for a greater period and can increase both aerosol production and heat accumulation. Short intervals allow less time for the coil to cool and the wick to resaturate. High airflow may cool the coil but can also alter evaporation and aerosol transport. A laboratory regime must therefore describe the sequence precisely enough that another laboratory can reproduce not only the number of puffs but the thermal burden imposed on the device.

Standardised puffing regimes improve comparability, but they remain controlled models. Human puffing varies according to device, nicotine strength, airflow resistance and individual preference. A regime appropriate for a low-powered closed system may not operate a high-powered open system realistically. Carbonyl testing should therefore combine standardisation with product relevance. The method should not be changed casually for every device, but neither should one historical regime be applied to all products irrespective of design.

The formulation itself can alter carbonyl emissions. Propylene glycol and glycerol have different physical properties and degradation pathways. Their ratio affects viscosity, heat transfer, wick supply, aerosol production and the distribution of thermal products. A high-glycerol liquid may create dense aerosol but may also move more slowly through some wicking systems. A high-propylene-glycol liquid may supply the wick more readily but produce different sensory and chemical behaviour. The resulting carbonyl profile depends on the complete device–liquid system rather than on solvent ratio alone.

Water content can influence viscosity, aerosol formation and thermal behaviour. Even modest changes may alter liquid transport and evaporative cooling. Water may arise intentionally through formulation or indirectly through hygroscopic absorption during storage. A carbonyl result should therefore remain linked to the actual product composition and condition tested. Results obtained from freshly prepared development samples may not describe aged commercial liquids whose water content or oxidation state has changed.

Flavour compounds can contribute directly or indirectly. Some carbonyls are used as flavouring substances or may be present within flavour mixtures. Others form through degradation of flavour constituents during heating. Acids, sweeteners and reactive aromatic compounds can alter local chemistry or deposit formation. Certain formulations may reduce carbonyl production by improving wetting or lowering effective thermal stress, while others may increase emissions under the same nominal device setting.

This makes product-specific testing essential. A device tested with an unflavoured reference liquid cannot establish the carbonyl profile of every commercial formulation intended for that device. The reference liquid may be useful for understanding baseline solvent degradation, but flavour systems should be assessed where they are capable of changing thermal behaviour or contributing target compounds. Product grouping may be possible where formulations are genuinely comparable and a scientifically justified worst case is selected. Grouping should not become a means of avoiding testing of chemically distinct products.

The most common analytical approach for carbonyls involves derivatisation with 2,4-dinitrophenylhydrazine, usually abbreviated to DNPH. Carbonyl compounds react with DNPH to form more stable hydrazone derivatives, which can then be separated and quantified by high-performance liquid chromatography with ultraviolet or diode-array detection. The approach is widely used because it converts reactive and volatile compounds into derivatives suitable for controlled chromatographic analysis.

The apparent simplicity of derivatisation conceals several critical variables. The carbonyl must first be transferred from the aerosol into the collection medium, react efficiently with the reagent and remain stable until analysis. Reaction conditions, acidity, solvent composition, reagent concentration, temperature and contact time can affect derivative formation. Different carbonyl compounds do not necessarily react at the same rate or with equal efficiency. A procedure optimised for formaldehyde may not perform identically for acrolein, glyoxal or other reactive species.

Collection can be performed using DNPH-coated cartridges, impingers containing derivatisation solution or combinations of trapping devices. Each arrangement has advantages and limitations. Cartridges are convenient and can reduce handling, but their capacity and breakthrough performance must be understood. Impingers provide direct contact with liquid reagent but can create losses through incomplete trapping, evaporation or transfer between vessels. Tubing and connectors may retain condensate before it reaches the reagent.

The collection system must be validated as part of the complete method. A highly accurate chromatographic analysis of the derivative does not correct for carbonyl material that never reached the collection medium. Recovery studies performed by adding standards directly to the final extract assess only the analytical stages after collection. Whole-process recovery or challenge experiments are needed where practical to evaluate transport, trapping and derivatisation together.

Breakthrough occurs when the first trap does not retain the complete analyte load and material passes into the downstream system. This may occur because the cartridge or reagent becomes saturated, because flow is too high or because the compound is trapped inefficiently. A second trap placed in series can be used during validation or routine testing to determine whether breakthrough is occurring. The result from the first trap should not be assumed complete without evidence supporting collection capacity under the chosen puff number and product output.

High aerosol mass can create particular difficulties. Condensed propylene glycol and glycerol may coat the collection medium, alter reagent contact or physically obstruct flow. Extended puff blocks may load the system more heavily than the validation conditions. Increasing the number of puffs to improve sensitivity can therefore reduce collection efficiency or derivatisation performance. The selected puff block should balance analytical sensitivity with the capacity and stability of the collection system.

Blank contamination is a major concern because formaldehyde and acetaldehyde are common in laboratory environments, reagents, solvents, packaging and air. DNPH materials can contain background derivatives before use. Tubing, filters and collection vessels may contribute contamination. Reagent blanks, cartridge blanks, machine blanks and full procedural blanks are required to identify the background associated with each stage.

Blank correction should follow a defined procedure. Subtracting a variable or unusually high blank can create uncertainty greater than the reported sample concentration. Where background is substantial relative to the sample signal, the method may not be suitable at that level. The laboratory should establish blank acceptance criteria and investigate contamination rather than relying automatically on numerical subtraction.

Ozone and other environmental oxidants can interfere with some DNPH methods by degrading derivatives or generating artefacts. Laboratories may need to control air exposure, use appropriate scrubbers or minimise storage before analysis. The importance of such measures depends on the collection arrangement and laboratory environment. Environmental monitoring and method-specific validation are more reliable than assuming that general laboratory conditions are adequate.

Carbonyl derivative stability must be demonstrated. Some derivatives remain stable for extended periods under controlled refrigeration, while others may degrade, isomerise or change in response during storage. Acrolein analysis can be particularly demanding because of its reactivity and the complexity of derivative behaviour. The laboratory should establish a holding time between collection, extraction and analysis and should not rely on generic stability claims where the actual matrix differs.

Calibration standards should represent the derivative being measured. Pre-prepared hydrazone standards can improve control but require documented purity and stability. Alternatively, standards may be generated through derivatisation of known carbonyl solutions. In either case, the calibration procedure should reflect the chemistry of the samples and account for derivative isomers or multiple chromatographic peaks where they occur.

Some carbonyl derivatives can appear as more than one chromatographic form. If the method integrates only one peak without accounting for relevant isomers, the result may be underestimated. Peak identification and integration rules should therefore be defined during validation. Co-elution with flavour-derived compounds or other derivatives may also occur, especially in complex aerosols. Retention time alone may be insufficient where interference is plausible.

Liquid chromatography with ultraviolet detection provides a robust and accessible platform, but its selectivity is limited compared with mass-spectrometric confirmation. Complex samples may require additional chromatographic resolution, alternative columns or mass-spectrometric detection to confirm identity. The appropriate level of selectivity depends on the matrix, target concentration and consequence of the decision. Enforcement or disputed results may justify confirmatory analysis beyond that required for routine screening.

Alternative derivatisation reagents and analytical techniques may be used where they offer better performance for particular carbonyls. Oxime formation followed by gas chromatography and mass spectrometry is one example. Direct spectroscopic or real-time techniques may also provide information about dynamic formation during individual puffs. These approaches can reveal temporal behaviour that is lost when several puffs are combined into one collection, although they may present their own calibration and matrix challenges.

No analytical technique should be selected only because it generates a broad list of compounds. The method must be capable of measuring the target analytes quantitatively, at relevant concentrations, with demonstrated specificity and recovery. A screening technique may identify unexpected compounds but may not provide the validated numerical evidence required for regulatory interpretation. Screening and quantitative confirmation serve different purposes and can be used together.

A further analytical question concerns the chemical form in which formaldehyde exists within aerosol. Formaldehyde can participate in reversible reactions with aerosol constituents, including the formation of hemiacetal-type species. Different collection and derivatisation approaches may measure free formaldehyde, formaldehyde released during sample treatment or a broader pool of formaldehyde-related species. Reports should state what the method is designed to quantify and avoid treating values from different chemical definitions as directly interchangeable.

This distinction has contributed to disagreement between studies. A method that measures immediately reactive gaseous formaldehyde may produce a different result from one that converts formaldehyde-releasing species during collection or extraction. Neither value is necessarily invalid, but each describes a different analytical fraction. Toxicological interpretation requires knowledge of which forms are bioavailable, how they behave in the respiratory tract and whether the analytical treatment reflects likely exposure.

Carbonyl results can be expressed per puff, per collection block, per mass of liquid consumed or per mass of aerosol generated. Each basis has a legitimate use. Per-puff values support estimation of exposure under a defined puff frequency. Normalisation to liquid consumed helps compare the proportion of formulation converted into a carbonyl. Normalisation to aerosol mass can distinguish concentration within the emitted aerosol from total yield. Reporting only one basis may conceal an important difference between products.

For example, a device producing more aerosol may emit a higher mass of formaldehyde per puff while producing a similar or lower concentration relative to aerosol mass. From an exposure perspective, total inhaled mass matters. From a product-efficiency perspective, emission relative to liquid consumption may be informative. The report should therefore retain the raw puff count, liquid consumption and aerosol yield where available so that alternative calculations can be examined.

Liquid consumption should be measured carefully. Weighing the device or reservoir before and after the puff block is common, but evaporation, leakage, handling and balance resolution can affect the result. A change in total device mass may include losses unrelated to aerosol generation. The approach should be validated sufficiently for the intended normalisation. Where liquid consumption is very small, measurement uncertainty may become large relative to the difference observed.

Results should also preserve individual replicate values. Carbonyl emissions can be highly variable, particularly near the transition to liquid starvation. Averaging several low results with one very high result may produce a moderate mean that represents no actual puff block. The elevated replicate may indicate an analytical error, a defective device or intermittent overheating. It requires investigation rather than automatic exclusion or unqualified averaging.

Time-resolved collection can provide valuable insight. Separating the first, middle and later puff blocks can show whether emissions remain stable, decline after conditioning or increase as the device warms and liquid supply changes. A pooled collection across a long sequence may obscure these patterns. The appropriate design depends on whether the purpose is average product characterisation, identification of failure or estimation of exposure over a typical use period.

Product age should be incorporated where relevant. Coil deposits can alter heat transfer, create catalytic surfaces or restrict liquid movement. Metals and carbonyls may therefore change together as the device ages. A study based entirely on unused devices may underestimate later-life performance, while testing only heavily aged products may not describe most use. Defined lifecycle points provide a more complete picture.

Carbonyl testing should also consider storage and ageing of the liquid. Oxidised or degraded formulations may contain different precursors from fresh liquids. Changes in colour, pH, nicotine oxidation or flavour composition can indicate chemical evolution that affects heating behaviour. Stability programmes and emissions programmes should therefore inform one another where shelf life may alter the aerosol profile.

The analytical result must then be interpreted toxicologically. Detection of formaldehyde, acetaldehyde or acrolein establishes exposure potential but does not by itself define risk. The measured mass must be connected to realistic consumption, exposure frequency, uncertainty and relevant toxicological reference points. Acute irritation, chronic inhalation effects and carcinogenic potential may require different interpretive approaches.

Comparisons with occupational exposure limits require caution. Workplace limits are generally designed for adult workers exposed under defined conditions and may not translate directly to consumer use or short aerosol peaks. They can provide context but should not be treated automatically as regulatory pass–fail limits for vaping. Similar care is needed when comparing per-puff emissions with concentration limits expressed over an eight-hour working day.

Comparison with cigarette smoke is also informative but incomplete. Carbonyl emissions from a vaping product may be substantially lower than those from combustible cigarettes under matched reporting conventions. This supports comparative exposure assessment and harm-reduction analysis. It does not establish that the remaining emissions are negligible or that avoidable product-generated carbonyls should be accepted without control.

The appropriate regulatory objective is to minimise unnecessary carbonyl generation while preserving product performance sufficient to replace smoking. This requires examination of whether emissions arise during normal operation, whether they increase under foreseeable conditions and whether design changes could reduce them. A product that generates low carbonyls under one narrow test condition but overheats readily outside it may require improvement. A product that remains stable across a realistic operating range provides stronger evidence of control.

Action limits or internal specifications may be useful where they are scientifically justified. These can support development, supplier comparison and batch or design control. They should account for method uncertainty, product variability and the basis of reporting. A limit expressed per puff cannot be compared directly with a result normalised to liquid consumption. A specification derived from one method may not remain valid after the collection or analytical procedure changes.

Carbonyl testing is particularly vulnerable to false precision. A chromatographic system may report several decimal places, while the larger uncertainties lie in aerosol generation, trapping efficiency, device variability and blank correction. The final report should present results at a level of precision consistent with the complete method. Measurement uncertainty should accompany values used near a specification or decision boundary.

Interlaboratory reproducibility remains a substantial challenge. Laboratories may use similar DNPH chemistry while differing in puffing conditions, cartridge type, impinger arrangement, extraction volume, calibration standards, blank correction, peak integration and reporting units. Results described generally as formaldehyde emissions may therefore not be directly comparable. Method details must be reviewed before combining datasets or ranking products.

Round-robin studies and common standards can improve comparability. Their value lies not only in generating consensus values but in exposing ambiguous method steps. Differences in device conditioning, activation timing and collection capacity may become visible only when several laboratories attempt the same protocol. Harmonisation should focus on the variables that materially affect results rather than producing procedural uniformity for its own sake.

Carbonyl testing should ultimately function as an investigative and preventive tool. Elevated results can reveal inadequate wick supply, excessive power, unsuitable solvent ratio, device ageing, flavour-related instability or manufacturing variation. The correct response is not simply to place the value in a regulatory dossier. The producer should determine why it occurred, whether it is reproducible and whether formulation or engineering changes can reduce it.

Where the cause is product design, corrective action may include changing the power range, coil geometry, wick material, liquid channels, firmware, formulation viscosity or user instructions. Where the cause is analytical, the method may require improved collection, cleaner blanks, better derivatisation control or increased selectivity. Where the result arises only under severe misuse, that finding should still be documented, but its relevance should be explained rather than generalised.

The strongest carbonyl evidence therefore combines realistic aerosol generation, validated collection, controlled derivatisation, suitable chromatography, transparent blanks, replicate product testing and toxicological interpretation. It distinguishes normal use from failure conditions, free carbonyls from broader releasable forms and analytical detection from regulatory significance. It retains enough information for another scientist to understand how the number was produced and what it represents.

Carbonyl testing is not simply a search for formaldehyde, acetaldehyde and acrolein. It is an examination of thermal control within the complete vaping system. Properly designed testing shows whether the formulation and device remain stable during operation, whether emissions rise as conditions change and whether avoidable degradation has been reduced. Poorly designed testing can produce dramatic or reassuring numbers that reflect the laboratory regime more than the marketed product. The regulatory value lies in distinguishing between those possibilities.

Heavy Metal Analysis

Heavy metal analysis examines whether vaping products release metallic elements from the formulation, device components, manufacturing process or aerosol-generation system. The term "heavy metal" is widely used, although it is chemically imprecise. Regulatory and analytical programmes generally focus on elements with toxicological relevance or plausible origins within the product, including lead, cadmium, nickel, chromium, copper, tin, zinc, iron, aluminium, manganese, cobalt and antimony. Some may be present as impurities in raw materials, while others originate from coils, solder, electrical contacts, reservoirs, pigments, alloys, plating, machining residues or corrosion. Their regulatory importance depends not simply on detection, but on chemical form, concentration, particle characteristics, exposure and the conditions under which they are released.

Metal analysis presents a different problem from the analysis of volatile organic compounds or carbonyls. Metals do not arise through thermal decomposition in the same manner. They are introduced physically or chemically from materials already present within the product. Heating, repeated wetting, electrical current, mechanical abrasion and contact with acidic or complex flavour formulations can mobilise material from device surfaces. Some elements may dissolve into the liquid before use. Others may be released only during aerosol generation as dissolved ions, ultrafine particles, fragments of oxide or alloy, or residues carried from the heating system. Analysis of the unheated liquid alone therefore cannot describe the complete inhalation exposure.

The distinction between liquid composition and aerosol composition is central. A refill liquid may contain very low concentrations of metals when tested directly, yet the aerosol generated through a particular device may contain higher levels because the coil or other components contribute additional material. Conversely, a liquid containing trace metal impurities may transfer only a proportion of those elements into the aerosol. The relationship is influenced by solubility, chemical form, deposition, aerosol transport and the interaction between the liquid and device materials. A complete assessment should therefore consider both the formulation and the operating product where the source and exposure pathway remain uncertain.

Potential sources should be identified before the analytical programme is designed. Heating coils commonly use alloys containing nickel, chromium, iron, aluminium or combinations of these elements. Stainless steel may contribute iron, chromium and nickel. Nickel–chromium alloys contain the elements indicated by their name, while iron–chromium–aluminium materials can contribute a different pattern. Copper may arise from wiring, contacts or brass components. Tin and lead may be associated with solder, although modern manufacturing should control the use of lead-containing materials. Zinc may originate from brass, plating or environmental contamination. Antimony can be associated with plastics or manufacturing processes. The observed elemental profile should therefore be interpreted alongside the bill of materials and component specifications.

A result becomes more meaningful when the detected elements correspond to a plausible source. Elevated nickel and chromium in aerosol from a nickel–chromium coil may suggest release from the heating element, particularly if the liquid itself contains little of either metal. Tin detected inconsistently may indicate solder, contamination or component-specific variation. Lead requires particular scrutiny because its presence may indicate raw-material contamination, unsuitable solder, pigment, environmental exposure or poor manufacturing control. The analytical result should direct investigation towards the product rather than being treated only as an isolated numerical finding.

Raw materials remain relevant. Nicotine, propylene glycol, glycerol, water, acids and flavour preparations can contain elemental impurities arising from manufacture, catalysts, processing equipment, water quality or storage. These impurities may be present at low concentrations that are difficult to measure reliably without strict contamination control. Supplier specifications and certificates of analysis can provide useful information, but they should not be accepted uncritically where metals are a material concern. The reporting limit, analytical method and batch represented by the certificate must be understood. A statement that a metal "passes" or is "not detected" is of limited value without the associated method capability.

Water quality deserves specific attention because water can introduce metals directly into formulations or cleaning processes. Purified water systems, storage vessels, transfer lines and production equipment may contribute trace contamination if they are inadequately controlled. The same applies to mixing tanks, filling machinery and metallic utensils. Where an element appears across several unrelated formulations, the source may lie in shared manufacturing equipment rather than the individual flavour or device.

The device can contribute metals at several stages of its life. New components may carry machining debris, surface residues or incompletely removed manufacturing contamination. Early puffs may therefore show a different profile from later operation. Repeated heating can change oxide layers, produce corrosion, loosen particles or alter the contact between coil and wick. Deposits formed from the liquid may retain metals or modify local heating. A product tested only when new may not describe the exposure generated after extended use.

Ageing studies can reveal whether emissions remain stable across the expected product life. Aerosol may be collected at defined intervals, such as initial use, mid-life and near the end of the intended coil or device duration. The design should avoid creating artificial degradation through an excessively severe puffing regime, but it should also examine reasonably foreseeable use. A product that releases little metal initially but shows a progressive increase as the coil ages raises a different regulatory concern from one that remains consistently low.

The number of devices tested is important because metallic emissions may be highly variable. Small differences in coil construction, welds, soldering, wick placement, surface finish and assembly can produce large differences between nominally identical units. One product may generate undetectable levels while another from the same batch produces an elevated result. This variability can be more informative than the mean alone because it reflects manufacturing consistency and the possibility of intermittent high exposure.

Replicate design should distinguish between analytical replication and product replication. Repeated instrumental analysis of one aerosol extract provides information about the measurement system. Separate aerosol collections from the same device assess within-device variability. Testing several devices from the same batch examines unit-to-unit consistency. Testing several batches introduces manufacturing variation over time. Combining these levels into one average can conceal where the variability originates.

Sampling strategy should reflect the regulatory question. Developmental work may focus on comparing materials or identifying the source of a specific element. Notification or product-characterisation testing should examine representative marketed configurations. Complaint investigations may require targeted sampling of affected batches, used devices or products returned by consumers. Enforcement work requires strict chain of custody and confidence that the sample represents the product found in commerce.

Aerosol collection must capture the metallic fraction efficiently. Metals may be present in droplets, dissolved material or particles spanning a range of sizes. Filters are commonly used to collect particulate matter, while additional traps may be needed where transport beyond the primary filter is plausible. Collection tubing and connectors can retain particles or contribute contamination. The choice of materials within the sampling train is therefore critical. Stainless steel components, metal fittings or contaminated glassware may introduce the same elements being measured.

High-purity, low-background materials should be used wherever possible. Acid-washed vessels, metal-free tubing, clean filters and controlled handling reduce contamination. Sampling assemblies should be evaluated through blanks before product testing begins. A laboratory cannot interpret low-level nickel, chromium or lead confidently if the collection system contributes comparable amounts.

Blank control is one of the most demanding aspects of trace-metal analysis. Reagent blanks identify contamination from acids and water. Filter blanks assess the collection medium. Machine blanks examine the aerosol-generation system without the test product. Procedural blanks pass through the complete preparation and analytical sequence. Environmental blanks may be necessary where airborne dust or laboratory surfaces create a risk. Each type answers a different question, and the required combination depends on the method.

Blank results should be monitored over time rather than treated as a one-off validation exercise. A laboratory environment can change through maintenance, new equipment, construction, sample load or contamination from previous work. Trace-metal methods are particularly vulnerable to background drift. A low-level sample result becomes unreliable where the blank is unstable or constitutes a substantial proportion of the measured signal.

Blank correction requires restraint. Subtracting the average blank from each sample may be appropriate where the background is small and consistent. Where the blank varies widely or approaches the sample concentration, numerical subtraction can create an apparently precise result from uncertain data. The laboratory should define acceptance limits and reject or investigate runs in which blank contamination compromises interpretation.

Sample digestion converts collected material into a form suitable for instrumental analysis. Filters, aerosol condensate and device residues may contain metals within organic material, particles or insoluble oxides. Acid digestion is commonly used to dissolve the sample, often with nitric acid and additional reagents depending on the matrix. Microwave-assisted digestion can improve control of temperature, pressure and recovery. The digestion procedure must be capable of releasing the target elements without introducing contamination or losing volatile species.

Incomplete digestion can produce systematic underestimation. A soluble spike may recover well even when metallic particles or refractory oxides remain undissolved. Recovery experiments should therefore reflect the forms likely to be present. Certified reference materials with a similar matrix are valuable where available, although truly representative vaping-aerosol materials are limited. Alternative checks may include spiking filters before digestion, analysing known alloy particles or comparing digestion procedures.

Different elements require different digestion and stabilisation conditions. Some may adsorb onto container surfaces or precipitate if the acid concentration is inadequate. Others can be affected by chloride, organic residue or high dissolved solids. The procedure should be validated for the target panel rather than assuming that one generic acid treatment performs equally for every element.

Inductively coupled plasma mass spectrometry, commonly abbreviated to ICP-MS, is widely used because it offers high sensitivity across a broad range of elements. Samples are introduced into a plasma, ionised and separated according to mass-to-charge ratio. The technique can detect metals at very low concentrations, making it suitable for trace aerosol analysis. Its sensitivity is also a source of vulnerability because contamination or spectral interference that would be negligible in a less sensitive method can become significant.

Inductively coupled plasma optical emission spectrometry, or ICP-OES, provides another approach. It measures light emitted by excited atoms and ions within the plasma. It is generally less sensitive than ICP-MS but can be robust for higher-concentration samples and may be less affected by some forms of interference. The choice depends on expected concentrations, matrix, analytes and required reporting limits. Graphite furnace atomic absorption and other techniques may also be used for specific elements, although multi-element plasma methods are often more efficient for broad regulatory panels.

ICP-MS methods require careful management of spectral interferences. Polyatomic ions formed from plasma gases, acids, water and matrix components can overlap with the mass of a target element. Isobaric interference can arise where different isotopes share the same nominal mass. Collision or reaction cells, alternative isotopes, mathematical corrections and suitable internal standards can reduce these effects. The laboratory should demonstrate that the selected approach is effective in the actual sample matrix.

Matrix effects can suppress or enhance signal. High concentrations of dissolved propylene glycol, glycerol, salts or digestion residues may alter nebulisation, plasma behaviour or ion transmission. Dilution can reduce the matrix burden but may raise reporting limits. Internal standards help correct variation where they behave similarly to the target analytes, but they cannot compensate for every form of interference. Matrix-matched calibration, standard addition or controlled digestion may be required where suppression is substantial.

Calibration should cover the expected range without sacrificing performance near the low end. A broad calibration curve may fit statistically while producing poor accuracy close to the reporting limit. Low-level regulatory samples require standards and quality controls positioned appropriately around the concentrations of interest. Calibration blanks, continuing calibration verification and independent check standards help confirm that the instrument remains stable through the run.

The purity and traceability of calibration standards are fundamental. Multi-element standards are convenient but must be compatible, stable and free from precipitation. Standards and samples should have comparable acid composition where practical. Errors in standard preparation affect every reported value, while the calibration curve may still appear linear. Independent preparation or second-source verification can identify such errors.

Internal standards should be selected according to mass, ionisation behaviour and matrix response. They are added at known concentrations to standards and samples so that changes in signal can be corrected. An unsuitable internal standard may fail to reflect the behaviour of the target element. The method should demonstrate that the correction improves accuracy rather than applying it automatically.

Detection limits and quantification limits must be established in the complete analytical context. Instrumental sensitivity measured in clean acid does not represent the method capability after collection, blank contribution, digestion and dilution. The method detection limit should account for the full procedure. The practical reporting limit should also reflect blank variability and acceptable precision. A nominally impressive instrumental limit has little regulatory value if the collection medium contributes a larger background.

Results close to the quantification limit should be reported with appropriate caution. A detected signal may indicate presence without supporting a reliable numerical value. "Not detected" should mean that the signal did not exceed the validated detection criterion, not that the element is absent. "Below quantification" indicates that the signal may be distinguishable from background but cannot be measured with the precision and accuracy required for a numerical result.

Speciation introduces an additional layer of complexity. Toxicity can depend strongly on oxidation state and chemical form. Hexavalent chromium, for example, differs toxicologically from trivalent chromium. Nickel may be present as dissolved ions, oxides or metallic particles. Total elemental analysis measures the amount of the element after digestion but usually does not identify the form in which it was emitted. A total chromium result cannot therefore establish the amount of hexavalent chromium without a separate speciation method.

Speciation methods are more demanding because chemical forms can change during collection, storage and extraction. Acid digestion intentionally destroys much of the original chemical information. Where a specific species is toxicologically important, the sampling and analytical strategy must preserve it. This may require selective extraction, chromatographic separation or surface analysis. Total-element screening remains valuable, but its limitations should be stated clearly.

Particle size and morphology may also influence biological behaviour. A metal present as dissolved ions may deposit and distribute differently from a larger particle. Ultrafine particles may reach deeper regions of the respiratory tract and have greater surface area relative to mass. Conventional ICP methods quantify total elemental content after digestion but do not describe particle number, size or shape.

Additional techniques may be needed where particulate form is relevant. Electron microscopy can visualise particles and provide elemental information through energy-dispersive spectroscopy. Single-particle ICP-MS can offer information on particle size and number for selected materials, although method development is complex. Such techniques are generally investigative rather than routine regulatory tools, but they can help determine whether an elevated total-metal result arises from dissolved contamination or discrete material released from a component.

Normalisation affects interpretation. Results may be reported per puff, per collection block, per mass of liquid consumed or per mass of aerosol generated. Per-puff data support exposure estimation under a defined use pattern. Normalisation to aerosol mass describes the concentration within the emitted aerosol. Normalisation to liquid consumption can help compare release efficiency between products. The selected basis should match the regulatory question and remain accompanied by the underlying data.

A product generating more aerosol may emit a greater metal mass per puff while having a lower concentration relative to aerosol mass. From the user's perspective, inhaled mass matters. From a materials or process perspective, release per unit of liquid may help identify abnormal corrosion or erosion. Reporting several bases can provide a fuller understanding, provided calculations are transparent.

The aerosol-generation regime can materially affect metal release. Longer puffs, higher power, shorter intervals and extended use may increase coil temperature, electrical stress and material degradation. Metal emissions may not respond in the same way as carbonyls, but severe or repeated operation can alter component surfaces. Tests should therefore define whether they represent routine use, extended life or stress conditions.

Device orientation can matter where liquid supply changes with position. Poor wetting may expose parts of the coil more directly to heat and air, potentially affecting oxidation and release. Repeated thermal cycling may loosen particles or alter oxide layers. The design should consider how the product is used realistically rather than assuming that one fixed laboratory orientation captures every relevant state.

Cleaning and reuse can also affect refillable systems. Consumers may rinse, wipe or replace components, introduce tools or use incompatible liquids. These behaviours can damage surfaces or increase corrosion. Regulatory testing cannot reproduce every form of misuse, but foreseeable maintenance should inform design and instructions. Where a product is intended to be reused, component durability becomes part of the materials assessment.

Acidified formulations deserve particular attention because pH and ligand chemistry can influence metal solubility. Organic acids used in nicotine-salt products may interact with metallic surfaces differently from neutral formulations. Flavour compounds can also chelate metals or alter corrosion. A device that performs acceptably with one liquid may release more metal with another. Testing the device and formulation as a defined system is therefore stronger than treating either in isolation.

Grouping products for metal testing requires caution. Products sharing the same device may still contain formulations with different acidity, water content or complexing agents. Products sharing the same liquid may use different coils, contacts or reservoirs. A worst-case selection should be based on plausible materials and formulation interactions rather than on the highest nicotine concentration or strongest flavour alone. The justification should identify why the chosen configuration is expected to represent equal or greater release.

Manufacturing controls are often more effective than end-product testing alone. Material specifications should define alloy composition, prohibited substances, solder requirements, surface finish, cleanliness and corrosion resistance. Supplier qualification should confirm that components match the declared materials. Incoming inspection, certificates, elemental screening and change control can prevent unsuitable components from entering production. Testing finished aerosol remains necessary where exposure depends on operation, but it should sit within a broader materials-control system.

Component substitution is a significant risk. A manufacturer may change coil wire, plating, solder or supplier without altering the external appearance or brand name. The product can remain commercially identical while its elemental profile changes. Formal change control should assess whether retesting is needed. A bill of materials that does not reflect actual production undermines both analytical interpretation and regulatory notification.

Heavy metal findings should be investigated through source analysis. Testing the liquid, unused components, used components, aerosol and manufacturing materials can help locate the origin. Elemental mapping or surface analysis may be useful where one component is suspected. The pattern across samples can distinguish a formulation impurity from device-generated release. For example, a metal present in aerosol but absent from liquid and strongly represented in the coil alloy points towards the heating system.

The investigation should also examine whether the result is batch-specific or systemic. A high value from one device may indicate contamination, damaged solder or manufacturing debris. Repeated elevation across batches suggests a design or materials problem. Both require attention, but the corrective action differs. Batch-specific contamination may be managed through process correction and recall, while a systemic source may require redesign or material replacement.

Toxicological interpretation should consider the measured dose, frequency of exposure, route, chemical form and relevant reference values. Metals with no safe exposure threshold or known cumulative toxicity require particular caution. Lead and cadmium are examples where avoidable exposure should be minimised. Nickel and chromium may raise concerns involving respiratory sensitisation, irritation, carcinogenicity or systemic effects depending on form and exposure.

Occupational exposure limits can provide context but should not be applied mechanically. They are designed for workplace conditions, defined durations and adult worker populations. Vaping exposure occurs through intermittent inhalation and may involve different particle forms and concentration peaks. Translating a per-puff mass into an airborne concentration requires assumptions about inhaled volume, frequency and distribution. Such comparisons can be informative but should not be presented as direct consumer-product pass–fail criteria without justification.

Comparison with cigarette smoke may demonstrate substantial differences in exposure to certain metals, but the comparator depends on the element and product. A vaping product may emit less of one metal while introducing another associated with its device materials. Reduced exposure relative to smoking supports harm-reduction analysis, but it does not remove the obligation to control avoidable metallic emissions. The appropriate objective is not merely to remain below cigarette smoke, but to reduce release as far as reasonably achievable through competent design and manufacture.

Measurement uncertainty is especially important because metal results can vary across devices and sit close to analytical limits. The uncertainty estimate should include significant contributions from collection, blank correction, digestion, calibration and repeatability. Where product variation dominates, this should be reported separately rather than hidden within the analytical uncertainty. A precise instrument cannot compensate for an inconsistent product population.

Interlaboratory comparison requires close examination of method details. Laboratories may differ in filters, digestion acids, puffing regimes, blank treatment, isotopes, collision-cell settings and reporting units. Two reports may both describe nickel in aerosol while measuring under materially different conditions. Reproducibility improves when the complete method is harmonised, but apparent disagreement should be investigated before one result is dismissed.

The strongest heavy metal analysis combines product knowledge, contamination control, representative sampling, validated collection and digestion, sensitive instrumentation and source-focused interpretation. It identifies what was measured, where it may have originated and whether the result is consistent across units and product life. It distinguishes total elemental content from chemical form and analytical detection from toxicological significance.

Heavy metal analysis is therefore not simply a multi-element scan appended to an emissions report. It is an examination of material integrity within the complete vaping system. Properly designed testing can reveal unsuitable alloys, manufacturing residues, corrosion, component wear, raw-material contamination and uncontrolled product variation. Poorly controlled testing can measure the laboratory, sampling train or one anomalous device more readily than the product itself. Its regulatory value depends on preserving the connection between the detected element, the source, the emitted aerosol and the exposure decision that follows.

Nicotine Verification

Nicotine verification confirms whether a vaping product contains and delivers the nicotine concentration declared by the manufacturer. It appears, at first, to be one of the simpler analytical requirements within product regulation. Nicotine is normally present at concentrations far above trace contaminants, established chromatographic methods are available and the declared value is printed clearly on the label. In practice, however, verification involves several distinct questions. The laboratory must determine what form of nicotine is present, how the labelled strength has been defined, whether the manufactured liquid matches the formulation record, whether concentration remains stable during storage and whether the device delivers nicotine consistently in the generated aerosol. A single numerical assay can answer only part of that wider regulatory problem.

The first distinction is between formulation concentration and delivered nicotine. Liquid analysis measures the amount of nicotine present in the e-liquid before use. Aerosol analysis measures the amount transferred from the liquid and emitted by the operating product under defined conditions. These values are related but not interchangeable. A liquid containing 20 milligrams of nicotine per millilitre does not deliver 20 milligrams during one millilitre of apparent consumption with complete efficiency. Some liquid remains within the device, some nicotine may condense on internal surfaces or collection tubing, and the amount emitted per puff depends on aerosol generation, power, airflow, puff duration and formulation behaviour. Verification should therefore identify whether the regulatory question concerns the labelled liquid strength, the consistency of aerosol delivery or both.

Liquid concentration remains the principal control because it connects the formulation, manufacturing process, label declaration and applicable legal limit. In the European and United Kingdom consumer-product framework, nicotine-containing liquids are subject to a maximum concentration, making accurate assay a direct compliance issue. The manufacturer must demonstrate that the nominal value is supported by the measured product and that ordinary manufacturing variation does not place lawful batches above the permitted boundary. A product labelled at the maximum concentration leaves less room for uncertainty and process variation than one formulated comfortably below it.

The declared strength must be defined unambiguously. Nicotine may be reported as milligrams per millilitre, as a percentage, as nicotine by mass or as nicotine equivalent within a nicotine salt. These conventions can produce confusion when they are used inconsistently. A percentage may mean mass per volume, mass per mass or an informal conversion from milligrams per millilitre. The formulation record, analytical specification, notification and consumer label should all refer to the same basis. An apparently minor difference in convention can produce a material discrepancy between the amount formulated, the amount measured and the amount communicated to the consumer.

Nicotine salts require particular care. A nicotine salt consists of nicotine combined with an acid, commonly through protonation of the nicotine molecule. The resulting material has a greater total molecular mass than nicotine alone because the acid contributes to the salt. A product may therefore be described according to the mass of the complete salt or according to the equivalent mass of nicotine contained within it. These are not the same quantity. Regulatory limits and most consumer declarations are generally concerned with nicotine concentration rather than the total mass of nicotine salt. The laboratory must know which basis is required before interpreting the result.

The acid and stoichiometric relationship should be documented. Benzoic, lactic, levulinic, malic and other acids may be used, and the proportion added influences protonation, pH, sensory character and the mass balance of the formulation. In practice, the system may contain protonated and unprotonated nicotine rather than one perfectly defined crystalline salt. Analytical methods often quantify total nicotine after sample preparation, without distinguishing the fraction present in each chemical form. This can be entirely appropriate for concentration verification, provided the report states that total nicotine is being measured and does not imply that nicotine speciation has been determined.

The nicotine raw material provides the starting point for accuracy. Its assay, water content, impurity profile, source and storage history should be known. Commercial nicotine is not necessarily 100 per cent active material, and its certified assay may need to be incorporated into formulation calculations. A nominal mass of raw nicotine does not equal the same mass of pure nicotine where the material contains water, residual solvent or other impurities. Failure to correct for assay can produce systematic under- or over-strength formulations even when weighing is performed accurately.

Raw nicotine can also change during storage. Exposure to oxygen, light, heat and reactive contaminants may cause oxidation, colour development and the formation of degradation products. Containers should therefore be suitable, tightly closed and stored under defined conditions. Repeated opening can introduce air and moisture, while poor stock rotation may result in older material being used after its original quality assumptions are no longer justified. Verification of finished-product strength cannot compensate for inadequate control of the active raw material.

Formulation calculations should be independently checked before manufacture. Errors can arise through incorrect units, density assumptions, nicotine assay corrections, batch scaling or confusion between nicotine and salt mass. Spreadsheet-based calculations are efficient but can reproduce an embedded error across many products and batches. Controlled formulas, locked fields, version control and independent review reduce the likelihood that a simple calculation mistake becomes a commercial-scale compliance failure.

The method of addition also matters. Nicotine may be introduced as concentrated freebase nicotine, as a diluted stock solution or as part of a pre-prepared salt system. Concentrated material reduces the volume added but increases the consequence of a weighing or transfer error. Diluted stocks may improve handling and dosing accuracy but require their own preparation, assay, homogeneity and stability controls. The manufacturing record should identify the actual material and concentration used rather than relying only on the intended formulation.

Gravimetric preparation generally offers stronger control than informal volumetric addition, particularly where temperature-dependent density and viscous liquids are involved. Calibrated balances allow each component to be recorded by mass and linked directly to the batch record. Volumetric methods can also be suitable where equipment, density and temperature are controlled, but a marked container or nominal pump stroke should not be assumed accurate without verification. The method selected should be capable of achieving the required tolerance at the batch scale concerned.

Density becomes important when a product is formulated by mass but labelled by volume. Propylene glycol, glycerol, water, nicotine, acids and flavours all contribute to the density of the finished liquid. Density can vary with composition and temperature. Converting a mass fraction into milligrams per millilitre using a generic density can therefore produce an inaccurate label value. Product-specific or composition-appropriate density information should be used, and the measurement temperature should be controlled where precision matters.

Mixing is another source of variability. Nicotine must be distributed uniformly throughout the batch before filling begins. Inadequate mixing time, unsuitable impeller design, dead zones, viscosity differences or premature filling can create concentration gradients. A bulk sample taken from the top of the vessel may pass while early or late filled units differ. Process validation and stratified sampling from different locations or stages of filling provide stronger evidence of homogeneity than one conveniently selected sample.

Homogeneity testing is particularly important when concentrated nicotine or acid is added to a viscous base. The system may appear visually uniform before chemical distribution is complete. Temperature can improve mixing by lowering viscosity, but excessive heat may accelerate oxidation or flavour loss. The manufacturing process should therefore define mixing order, time, speed, temperature and hold period rather than leaving these conditions to operator judgement.

Sampling determines whether the laboratory result represents the manufactured batch. A retained bulk sample may not reflect filling variation, container interaction or line sequencing. Finished-unit samples selected from the beginning, middle and end of the filling run can reveal segregation, dosing drift or labelling error. Where several nicotine strengths are filled on the same equipment, line clearance and sample identity become critical because a low-strength product contaminated by residue from a stronger batch may still appear plausible by visual inspection.

Sample preparation for analysis should be simple enough to control but capable of handling the formulation matrix. E-liquids are commonly diluted in a suitable solvent before chromatographic analysis. The dilution factor may be substantial because nicotine is present at relatively high concentration compared with trace analytes. Each weighing, pipetting and volumetric step contributes to uncertainty. Gravimetric dilution can reduce dependence on density and meniscus reading, provided balances and calculations are controlled appropriately.

Viscosity can affect sample transfer. Glycerol-rich liquids may adhere to pipette tips, vessel walls and closures. Air bubbles can produce volumetric error, while incomplete mixing before subsampling can affect representativeness. The method should define how the sample is equilibrated, mixed and transferred. Disposable equipment should be shown to be compatible with nicotine and the solvent system, and rinse or transfer losses should be understood where they are significant.

High-performance liquid chromatography is widely used for nicotine verification. Nicotine can be separated from formulation constituents and quantified using ultraviolet detection, diode-array detection or mass-spectrometric detection. The method should demonstrate sufficient specificity in the presence of acids, flavours, oxidation products and other components. A retention-time match alone may not be adequate where co-elution is plausible, particularly in complex flavour systems.

Gas chromatography can also be used, often with flame-ionisation, nitrogen-selective or mass-spectrometric detection. The technique may offer good separation and sensitivity, but sample preparation and injector conditions must prevent degradation or inconsistent transfer. Nicotine can interact with active surfaces and may show tailing where the chromatographic system is not properly controlled. The choice between liquid and gas chromatography should be based on validated performance rather than laboratory familiarity alone.

Titration and spectroscopic techniques may provide rapid estimates in simpler systems, but they can lack specificity where other basic or absorbing compounds are present. Acids used in nicotine-salt products can complicate acid–base titration, while flavour components may interfere with ultraviolet measurements. Such methods may be suitable for process monitoring where the matrix is controlled and correlation with a reference method has been demonstrated. They require greater caution when used as the sole basis for regulatory verification.

Calibration standards must be traceable and prepared accurately. The purity and concentration of the reference nicotine should be known, with correction for assay where necessary. Calibration should cover the expected sample range after dilution and should include controls close to the specification or legal boundary. A wide curve that extends far beyond the working concentration may produce an acceptable correlation coefficient while providing weaker accuracy near the value that determines compliance.

Internal standards can improve precision by correcting for injection and preparation variation. Structurally similar or isotopically labelled compounds may be used where appropriate. The internal standard should not be present naturally in the sample and should behave predictably within the method. Its addition stage determines which sources of variation it can correct. Added immediately before injection, it cannot compensate for earlier dilution or extraction errors.

Specificity should include consideration of nicotine-related substances. Nicotine-N-oxide, cotinine, nornicotine, anatabine, anabasine and other impurities or degradation products may be present at lower concentrations. A nicotine assay should separate the principal analyte sufficiently from compounds that could inflate or distort its response. Where the method is also used for impurity profiling, the sensitivity and calibration requirements become more demanding than those required for total strength alone.

Accuracy can be assessed through recovery from representative formulations, analysis of prepared reference liquids and comparison with an independent method. Recovery experiments should include different solvent ratios, acid systems and flavour matrices where these may affect response. A method validated only with unflavoured propylene glycol may not perform equivalently in a heavily flavoured, glycerol-rich nicotine-salt product.

Precision should be examined at several levels. Repeated injections assess instrumental stability. Independent sample preparations assess dilution and handling. Multiple units assess filling and product variation. Several batches assess manufacturing consistency over time. A laboratory may show excellent analytical precision while the manufactured product remains variable. Nicotine verification should identify which source of variation is being measured rather than presenting one combined percentage as though it describes the whole system.

The result should be compared with a predefined specification. The nominal label value is not itself a complete specification because no manufacturing or analytical process produces an infinitely exact concentration. An appropriate tolerance should reflect formulation capability, analytical uncertainty, stability and legal requirements. The tolerance should not be so broad that materially mislabelled products are accepted, nor so narrow that normal analytical variation creates repeated apparent failures.

Where a legal maximum applies, the internal target should normally provide sufficient margin to account for process variation and uncertainty. Formulating exactly at the legal ceiling creates a substantial risk that some batches or units will measure above it. A result slightly above the declared value may appear minor from a sensory perspective but can be significant where it crosses a statutory threshold. Regulatory design should therefore include a control margin rather than treating the maximum as the routine manufacturing target.

Measurement uncertainty should be considered when a result lies near a decision boundary. The reported concentration is an estimate influenced by calibration, reference-standard purity, weighing, dilution, repeatability and sample variation. A value printed to several decimal places does not imply equivalent knowledge of the true concentration. The laboratory should report at a precision consistent with the validated method and should make clear how uncertainty is handled in conformity decisions.

Decision rules are especially important where laboratories are asked to declare a product compliant or non-compliant. One rule may require the measured result, including uncertainty, to remain below the limit before compliance is stated. Another may use the central estimate. These approaches allocate the risk of false acceptance and false rejection differently. The manufacturer, laboratory and regulator should understand which rule is being applied rather than assuming that all laboratories interpret marginal results identically.

Stability testing connects initial verification to shelf life. Nicotine concentration may decrease through oxidation, reaction, adsorption or loss associated with the packaging system. The change may be modest, but it can affect label accuracy and product performance over time. Samples should be tested at appropriate intervals under defined storage conditions, using the same concentration basis and a method capable of separating nicotine from degradation products.

A falling assay does not necessarily mean that nicotine has simply disappeared. It may have converted into related compounds that require separate toxicological and quality consideration. Colour darkening, odour change and pH movement can accompany oxidation. The analytical programme should therefore consider both nicotine strength and relevant degradation indicators rather than treating a reduced assay as the only stability concern.

Container closure can influence concentration. Poor seals may allow solvent evaporation, increasing the apparent nicotine concentration even where the total amount of nicotine has not increased. Repeated opening can introduce oxygen and alter water content. Plastic materials may adsorb constituents or allow limited permeation. Stability results should be interpreted alongside changes in fill mass, water content and packaging integrity where these mechanisms are plausible.

Nicotine verification also supports investigation of consumer complaints. Reports of unexpected harshness, weak effect, dizziness or product inconsistency may justify testing of retained and market samples, although such reports do not establish that nicotine concentration is the cause. Incorrect strength, mislabelling, mixing failure or cross-contamination can be examined analytically. The investigation should compare the complaint unit with batch records, retained samples and other units from the same production run.

Mislabelling may be more serious than a small assay deviation. A product manufactured correctly at one strength but packaged as another creates direct consumer and regulatory risk. Analytical verification can identify the discrepancy, but label reconciliation, line clearance, barcode control and packaging inspection are the preventive mechanisms. Finished-product release should confirm both chemical strength and label identity.

Aerosol nicotine testing provides a further measure of product performance. It determines the nicotine mass emitted under a defined puffing regime and can be expressed per puff, per collection block, per mass of aerosol or per mass of liquid consumed. The result reflects liquid concentration and device efficiency together. Two products containing the same nicotine strength may produce very different aerosol yields because of power, coil design, airflow and formulation.

Consistent nicotine delivery is relevant because consumers rely on predictable product performance. Wide variation between puffs or devices may indicate unstable aerosol generation, poor liquid supply or manufacturing inconsistency. It can also affect comparative exposure assessment. The test should distinguish emitted nicotine from absorbed dose. Aerosol measurement establishes what leaves the product under laboratory conditions; it does not determine how much is retained in the respiratory tract or enters systemic circulation.

Collection efficiency must be demonstrated. Nicotine can exist within aerosol droplets and vapour and may deposit in tubing, filters or traps. The collection system should recover the emitted mass adequately under the chosen flow and puff count. Breakthrough, adsorption and condensation can produce underestimation. Whole-system recovery and mass-balance studies are more informative than recovery from the final extract alone.

Nicotine transfer efficiency can be estimated by comparing the amount emitted with the amount removed from the liquid, although both measurements carry uncertainty. Such analysis can help identify internal retention, leakage or changes across device life. It should not be simplified into a universal delivery percentage because the result depends on the method and product state.

Puff-by-puff or block analysis may reveal dynamic variation. The first puffs after activation may differ from later puffs as the coil reaches a stable thermal state. Delivery may decline as the battery discharges or the reservoir empties. It may increase temporarily after rest periods as the wick resaturates. Pooling a large number of puffs into one average can conceal these patterns.

Device-to-device testing is therefore essential where delivery consistency forms part of the product claim or regulatory assessment. Repeated analysis of one well-performing device cannot represent the manufactured population. Coil resistance, airflow, battery output and fill volume should be recorded where possible so that anomalous results can be investigated rather than treated as unexplained statistical noise.

Comparison with labelled nicotine concentration should remain conceptually clear. Liquid assay verifies the product strength. Aerosol yield characterises the operating system. A product may pass the liquid specification while delivering nicotine inconsistently because of device variation. Conversely, a highly consistent device cannot correct a liquid manufactured at the wrong concentration. Both controls are needed where the finished product consists of a defined liquid–device combination.

Trend analysis strengthens ongoing control. Batch results can be plotted over time to identify gradual movement in mean concentration or increasing variability. A process may remain within specification while drifting steadily towards one limit. This can indicate raw-material assay changes, balance calibration issues, formulation error, solvent loss or mixing deterioration. Reviewing trends allows intervention before a formal failure occurs.

Change control should determine when re-verification is required. Changes in nicotine supplier, raw-material assay, acid type, formulation ratio, batch scale, mixing equipment, filling line, container or manufacturing site can affect concentration or stability. Device changes may affect aerosol delivery even where the liquid remains unchanged. The original data should not be assumed to cover a materially altered product without technical justification.

Regulatory verification is strongest when laboratory data remain connected to the quality system. The measured value should trace back to the raw nicotine certificate, formulation calculation, batch record, mixing process, fill sequence, finished-unit sample and label. Where the result falls outside expectation, the manufacturer should be able to investigate each stage rather than treating the laboratory report as an isolated pass-or-fail certificate.

Nicotine verification is therefore more than confirmation that a chromatographic peak corresponds approximately with the number printed on the bottle. It establishes whether the nicotine basis is defined correctly, the formulation calculation is accurate, the batch is homogeneous, the label is truthful, the concentration remains stable and the operating product delivers nicotine consistently. It also provides one of the clearest tests of whether regulatory documentation reflects the physical product.

The strongest verification programme combines raw-material control, validated assay, representative sampling, manufacturing trend analysis, stability assessment and, where relevant, aerosol-delivery testing. Each part answers a different question. Together they show that nicotine has been formulated deliberately, measured accurately and controlled throughout the product lifecycle. Without that chain, a label declaration remains an intention rather than demonstrated evidence.

Batch-to-Batch Consistency

Batch-to-batch consistency determines whether successive production lots correspond to the product that was originally designed, assessed, tested and notified. A regulatory dossier describes a defined formulation, device configuration, manufacturing process and expected analytical profile. Consumers, however, do not receive the development sample used to generate that dossier. They receive commercial batches manufactured over months or years using changing raw-material lots, equipment, operators, component suppliers and production conditions. The credibility of the regulatory record therefore depends on the manufacturer's ability to show that later batches remain materially equivalent to the product represented by the original evidence.

Consistency does not mean that every batch will produce numerically identical results. All manufacturing and analytical systems contain variation. Raw materials differ within approved specifications, equipment operates within tolerances, environmental conditions change and laboratory measurements carry uncertainty. The purpose of batch control is to keep that variation within scientifically justified limits so that product identity, performance and exposure remain predictable. A batch may differ slightly from the nominal target while remaining acceptable, but the process should not drift in a way that changes nicotine strength, emissions, flavour composition, device function or consumer exposure without detection.

For e-liquids, the principal sources of batch variation include nicotine assay, solvent composition, flavour concentration, acid addition, water content, mixing efficiency and filling accuracy. Each component contributes to the final product, and small errors can accumulate. A nicotine raw material with a slightly lower assay than the previous lot may reduce finished concentration unless the formulation calculation is corrected. A flavour supplied at a different strength may alter sensory performance and emissions. Variation in glycerol, propylene glycol or water content can change viscosity, aerosol generation and wick supply. An acid added outside its intended ratio may alter pH, nicotine protonation and product harshness.

Device batches introduce a different but equally important set of variables. Coil resistance, wire composition, wick density, airflow, battery output, firmware, reservoir dimensions, seals and assembly tolerances can all change product performance. Two devices carrying the same external design and brand name may deliver different aerosol mass, nicotine yield, carbonyl emissions or metal release if internal components vary. The regulatory product is therefore not represented adequately by one visually approved design. Its critical materials and performance attributes must be controlled through specifications that remain connected to actual production.

The finished vaping system combines both forms of variation. A liquid that performs acceptably with one coil batch may behave differently with another. A change in wick compression can affect liquid supply, which in turn affects thermal conditions and carbonyl formation. A change in battery output can alter aerosol mass and nicotine delivery even though liquid concentration remains constant. Batch-to-batch consistency must therefore consider the interaction between formulation and device rather than treating each as independent where they are marketed as a defined combination.

Raw-material control is the first line of defence. Every critical ingredient and component should be purchased against an approved specification that identifies the characteristics necessary for product performance and safety. For liquids, this may include identity, assay, purity, water content, density, impurity profile and microbiological or elemental limits where relevant. For device components, specifications may include dimensions, resistance, alloy composition, surface finish, electrical performance, material declarations and compatibility requirements.

Supplier certificates of analysis can support release decisions, but they do not replace supplier qualification or verification. Certificates may differ in analytical method, reporting limit and interpretation. One supplier may report a metal as not detected using a highly sensitive method, while another uses a method incapable of detecting the concentration relevant to the product. A stated pass therefore has meaning only when the underlying specification and method are understood. Manufacturers should verify critical attributes periodically and increase testing where supplier performance is uncertain or a material has a direct effect on exposure.

Supplier changes are a frequent source of hidden inconsistency. A flavour house may reformulate a concentrate while retaining the same trade name. A coil supplier may change alloy, wire diameter or manufacturing location. A plastic component may be produced from a different resin grade. These changes can occur without altering the commercial identity of the finished product. Formal change-notification agreements with suppliers are therefore essential, particularly for proprietary mixtures and high-risk components.

Incoming inspection should be proportionate to the criticality of the material. Visual examination may be sufficient for non-critical packaging attributes, but it cannot confirm nicotine assay, flavour composition or coil alloy. Identity testing, dimensional checks, resistance measurement, density, pH or selected chemical analysis may be appropriate depending on the material. The frequency can be adjusted according to supplier history, process capability and risk, but it should not be abandoned merely because several previous lots were acceptable.

Sampling of incoming materials must also be representative. A single container from a large shipment may not reveal segregation, contamination or inconsistent blending. The sampling plan should consider the number of containers, batch size, supplier process and potential consequence of failure. Where materials are supplied in multiple drums or intermediate containers, composite sampling may provide an overall assessment, while individual-container testing may be necessary where variability is expected or the material is highly critical.

Manufacturing instructions translate approved formulations and designs into controlled production. These instructions should define component quantities, order of addition, equipment, mixing conditions, temperatures, process times and acceptance checks. Leaving critical parameters to operator preference creates unnecessary batch variation. Operators may compensate informally for viscosity, flavour intensity or equipment behaviour, producing a product that appears acceptable but no longer matches the documented process.

Batch records provide the evidence that the approved instructions were followed. They should identify raw-material lot numbers, quantities added, equipment used, process conditions, start and completion times, operator and reviewer identities, yields, in-process results and any deviations. For devices, records may also include component lots, assembly lines, software versions, resistance checks, battery tests and functional inspection. The record should make it possible to reconstruct how the batch was produced and which materials entered it.

Yield reconciliation can reveal hidden errors. The expected finished quantity should be compared with the actual bulk and filled yield, accounting for normal process loss. A discrepancy may indicate incorrect addition, leakage, evaporation, transfer loss or recording error. A batch can appear analytically acceptable in one sample while the yield suggests that the manufacturing process did not occur as intended. Reconciliation should therefore form part of release review rather than being treated only as an inventory exercise.

In-process testing provides an opportunity to correct problems before the batch is completed. For e-liquids, this may include appearance, density, pH, nicotine concentration or homogeneity. For devices, resistance, battery voltage, airflow, leak performance and activation may be checked during assembly. In-process tests should target attributes that can vary materially and that can still be corrected at that stage. Testing every measurable parameter is unnecessary if it does not inform process control.

Bulk homogeneity is particularly important. Nicotine, acids and concentrated flavours must be distributed uniformly before filling begins. Sampling only from one location may not detect stratification or incomplete mixing. Samples from the upper, middle and lower parts of the vessel, or from different stages of the filling run, can show whether the batch is uniform. The required design depends on vessel size, mixing system, viscosity and process validation.

Filling can introduce variation even after the bulk has been mixed correctly. Pumps may drift, nozzles may clog, product temperature may change and containers may be filled at different rates. Net content, nicotine amount per unit and headspace can therefore vary across the run. Sampling from the beginning, middle and end of filling helps identify process drift. Where several strengths or flavours are produced on shared equipment, line clearance and cleaning become critical to preventing cross-contamination or mislabelling.

Finished-product testing confirms whether the commercial batch meets its defined specification. The release panel should include attributes that establish identity, strength, quality and performance. For liquids, this may include nicotine concentration, appearance, density, pH and selected impurity or compositional checks. For closed-system products, fill volume, device function, leak resistance and aerosol performance may also be relevant. The test programme should reflect product risk rather than relying on an unchanged checklist for every formulation.

The specification must distinguish between nominal targets and acceptable limits. A nominal nicotine concentration may be 10 milligrams per millilitre, while the release specification allows a defined range around that value. The range should account for manufacturing capability, analytical uncertainty, stability and legal requirements. It should be narrow enough to ensure truthful labelling and consistent consumer experience, but not so narrow that normal measurement variation creates repeated false failures.

Specifications should be derived from development data, validation batches, method performance, toxicological assessment and process capability. Arbitrary tolerances can create either false assurance or unnecessary rejection. A wide range may conceal weak manufacturing control, while an unrealistically narrow range may encourage repeated retesting until a favourable result appears. The specification should represent what the process can achieve consistently and what the product requires scientifically.

Acceptance criteria for emissions are more difficult than those for liquid concentration because emissions may show greater product and method variability. A single fixed limit may be appropriate where a specific regulatory threshold exists, but many emissions are interpreted through exposure and toxicological relevance rather than direct legal maxima. Internal alert and action levels can nevertheless help identify drift. These may be based on historical data, worst-case development results, toxicological evaluation and known product performance.

Alert limits and action limits serve different purposes. An alert limit indicates that the process may be moving away from its normal state and warrants review. An action limit indicates that the result is no longer acceptable or requires formal investigation. A product can remain within its release specification while showing a trend towards an action boundary. Detecting that movement early allows preventive action before batches fail or consumer exposure changes materially.

Statistical process control provides a structured means of monitoring such trends. Individual results can be plotted over time and compared with the established process mean and control limits. Control charts can reveal gradual drift, sudden shifts, cyclical behaviour or increasing variability that would not be obvious from isolated pass-or-fail decisions. The objective is to determine whether the process remains stable, not merely whether each batch falls within a broad specification.

A process can be within specification but statistically out of control. For example, nicotine results may remain inside the permitted range while increasing steadily across several batches. This pattern could reflect changes in raw-material assay, balance calibration, evaporation or operator practice. Waiting until the legal limit is exceeded would miss the opportunity to identify the cause earlier. Statistical control therefore complements specification testing rather than replacing it.

Process capability analysis examines whether a stable process can operate comfortably within the specification. A capable process produces most batches near the target with variation small relative to the permitted range. A process operating close to one limit may generate frequent failures even if its short-term mean remains acceptable. Capability should be assessed only after stability has been demonstrated; calculating capability from a drifting process can provide misleading reassurance.

The analytical method contributes to observed batch variation. Where method precision is poor, genuine manufacturing trends may be concealed by measurement noise. Conversely, highly precise methods can reveal small differences that are not toxicologically or operationally important. The manufacturer must therefore understand how much of the observed spread comes from the product and how much from the laboratory. Replicate preparations, quality controls and method uncertainty support this distinction.

The same laboratory and method should be used consistently where long-term trending is intended, unless comparability has been demonstrated after change. Switching laboratory, instrument or method can create an apparent batch shift even where the product has not changed. Where a change is necessary, bridging studies should compare old and new procedures using shared samples. The trend record should identify the transition so that later reviewers do not interpret a methodological difference as manufacturing drift.

Out-of-specification results require formal investigation. A result outside an approved limit may arise from product failure, analytical error, sampling error or record discrepancy. The laboratory should first examine instrument performance, standards, calculations, sample preparation, quality controls and method execution. The manufacturer should examine raw materials, batch records, equipment, process conditions, labelling and related batches. The investigation should identify evidence rather than assume a preferred explanation.

Retesting must be controlled. Repeating the analysis can be justified where an assignable laboratory cause is suspected or additional information is required.

It should not be used to replace an unfavourable result simply because later replicates fall within specification. The original result remains part of the evidence until a documented investigation establishes why it is invalid. Repeated testing until a passing value appears undermines both the quality system and the credibility of the release decision.

Resampling requires similar justification. A second sample may be appropriate where the first was damaged, unrepresentative or taken incorrectly. It should not be used automatically when the initial sample fails. A new sample may differ because the batch is non-homogeneous, which is itself a product problem. The investigation should therefore determine whether resampling addresses a sampling failure or conceals genuine variability.

Out-of-trend results may be more informative than formal failures. A batch can meet every specification while differing substantially from its historical pattern. An unexpected shift in pH, density, nicotine concentration, aerosol yield or metal emission may indicate a change in raw materials or process. Out-of-trend criteria should be defined sufficiently to trigger review without generating excessive investigation of normal variation.

Deviations occurring during manufacture should be assessed before release. A shortened mixing time, temporary temperature excursion, substituted component or equipment malfunction may or may not affect the finished product. The decision should be supported by scientific reasoning, testing and process knowledge. The absence of a failed release result does not automatically prove that the deviation had no effect, particularly where the tested attribute does not capture the risk introduced.

Batch release should be performed by an authorised person who is independent enough to review the evidence objectively. Release involves more than signing the laboratory certificate. The reviewer should confirm that materials were approved, the process followed, yields reconciled, deviations investigated, results met specification and the correct labels and packaging were used. A batch that passes chemical testing but has incomplete traceability or labelling errors is not adequately controlled.

Contract manufacturing can complicate this responsibility. The brand owner or regulatory submitter may not operate the production site directly, but the legal and regulatory obligations remain. Technical agreements should define who approves suppliers, controls specifications, performs testing, investigates deviations, releases batches and communicates changes. Both parties should have access to the records needed to assess consistency.

A contract manufacturer may produce similar products for several clients on shared equipment. This creates risks involving cross-contamination, line clearance, component mix-up and confidentiality. The brand owner should not assume that the existence of a quality certificate guarantees product-specific control. Audits, performance review and data trending should confirm that the contracted process remains capable of reproducing the notified product.

Device suppliers and assemblers require the same oversight. Components may be produced through several subcontracting tiers, making actual material control difficult. A coil assembly sold under one part number may be sourced from different factories or alloys. Approved supplier lists, component testing and change-notification obligations help maintain consistency. Where product performance depends strongly on a component, reliance on external appearance or catalogue description is insufficient.

Reference or retention samples provide an important link between released batches and later investigations. Representative units from each batch should be retained under controlled conditions for an appropriate period. If a complaint, adverse event or analytical concern arises, the retained sample can be compared with the market unit and original release data. Retention conditions should preserve the product sufficiently for meaningful analysis and should reflect the intended shelf life.

Retained samples cannot always reproduce the condition of a product after distribution. Market samples may have experienced heat, light, vibration, repeated opening or poor storage. Comparing market and retained samples can nevertheless help distinguish manufacturing defects from distribution or consumer-related changes. Where both show the same abnormality, a batch issue becomes more likely. Where only the market sample differs, storage, tampering, counterfeiting or use conditions may require investigation.

Stability testing extends batch consistency across time. A batch that meets specification at release may change during storage. Nicotine may oxidise, volatile constituents may be lost, pH may move and packaging interaction may occur. Device components may corrode or seals may deteriorate. Stability studies should therefore use representative production batches rather than only specially prepared development samples.

Several batches are generally more informative than one because they incorporate normal manufacturing variation. If all stability work is performed on an unusually favourable batch, the claimed shelf life may not represent later production. Batches chosen for stability should reflect the commercial process, formulation, packaging and manufacturing site. Significant changes may require new or bridging stability evidence.

Annual product review or periodic quality review can bring the separate batch records together. The review may examine production volumes, failures, deviations, complaints, returns, stability results, supplier performance, analytical trends and changes. Its value lies in identifying patterns that are not visible within individual batch files. Repeated minor deviations may reveal a systemic weakness even where no single event appears critical.

Complaint trends provide another measure of consistency. Reports of leaking, harshness, weak nicotine effect, burnt taste, device failure or colour variation may indicate batch or component differences. Complaints should be coded by product, batch, manufacturing date and failure type so that clusters can be identified. A low overall complaint rate can still conceal a serious issue concentrated in one production lot.

Counterfeit and diverted products complicate batch analysis. A consumer may report a product carrying the correct brand but manufactured outside the approved supply chain. Genuine batch coding, tamper evidence and authentication systems help distinguish authorised goods from copies. Analytical differences between market samples and retained batches may indicate counterfeiting, but the conclusion requires evidence from packaging, supply-chain records and product construction as well as chemistry.

Change control is one of the principal safeguards against gradual loss of consistency. Any proposed change to raw material, supplier, equipment, process, formulation, component, software, packaging or manufacturing site should be assessed before implementation. The assessment should consider product identity, analytical performance, emissions, stability, toxicology, labelling and regulatory status. Some changes can be managed through documentation and limited verification; others require substantial retesting or notification.

Minor changes can become significant cumulatively. A flavour supplier changes one carrier, a coil supplier adjusts resistance tolerance and the filling site introduces a different storage condition. Each change may appear negligible in isolation, while together they alter aerosol behaviour. Periodic review should therefore consider the cumulative history of modifications rather than evaluating each event as though the product remained otherwise static.

Comparability studies support change decisions. Pre-change and post-change batches can be tested side by side using the same methods and conditions. The comparison should focus on attributes most likely to be affected rather than attempting to reproduce every historical test without purpose. Equivalent nicotine concentration may not establish equivalent emissions where the device or formulation has changed. The study design should follow the mechanism through which the change could influence exposure.

Regulatory implications depend on the extent of the difference. A small adjustment remaining within the approved product definition may require internal documentation only. A substantial modification affecting composition, delivery or emissions may require updated notification or other regulatory action. The manufacturer should not redefine a material change as minor merely to avoid administrative burden. The technical assessment should determine the regulatory conclusion.

Batch-to-batch consistency also underpins toxicological assessment. Exposure estimates, margins of exposure and ingredient justifications normally rely on expected product composition and emissions. If commercial batches vary widely, those calculations no longer describe the product population reliably. A toxicological conclusion based on one low-emitting development sample cannot support batches that operate differently in the market.

The same applies to claims of relative performance. A manufacturer may state that a product delivers nicotine consistently or produces reduced emissions under defined conditions. Such claims require evidence that the performance is reproducible across production batches, not merely achievable by selected samples. Consistency therefore converts product-development findings into commercially meaningful characteristics.

The appropriate level of testing should remain risk-based. It is neither necessary nor efficient to repeat the complete emissions and toxicology programme on every batch. Routine release testing should focus on critical attributes that provide confidence in product identity and process control. More extensive periodic verification, rotating panels and change-triggered testing can examine attributes that are expensive or slow to measure. The strategy should be justified by process understanding and historical data.

Reduced testing may be appropriate where the process has demonstrated strong capability and suppliers remain reliable. Such reduction should follow evidence of control rather than precede it. Testing frequency should increase when failures, supplier changes, complaints or process drift occur. A fixed programme that never responds to performance is less effective than one that adapts according to risk.

Batch-to-batch consistency is ultimately demonstrated through a combination of design control, supplier management, validated manufacturing, representative sampling, analytical testing and statistical review. No single laboratory result can establish it. Consistency is visible when successive batches cluster around the intended target, when variability remains understood, when changes are controlled and when unusual results trigger investigation rather than concealment.

The regulatory significance is straightforward. The product placed on the market should remain the product described in the technical file. Its nicotine concentration, formulation, materials, emissions and performance should not vary unpredictably according to production date or component lot. Where variability is unavoidable, it should remain within limits that preserve safety, quality and truthful presentation.

A manufacturer that can produce one compliant batch has demonstrated a development achievement. A manufacturer that can reproduce that product reliably over time has demonstrated control. Batch-to-batch consistency is the evidence that compliance is part of the manufacturing system rather than a favourable result obtained once for regulatory submission.

Laboratory Uncertainty

Laboratory uncertainty describes the extent to which an analytical result remains an estimate rather than an exact statement of the true value. Every reported concentration, emission rate, nicotine strength or elemental measurement is affected by variation arising from sampling, preparation, calibration, recovery, equipment, environmental conditions, product behaviour and data interpretation. The purpose of uncertainty analysis is not to weaken confidence in laboratory evidence, but to define that confidence honestly. A numerical result becomes more useful when the limits of the measurement are understood.

This is especially important in vaping analysis because the measurement system extends beyond the analytical instrument. A laboratory may use highly sensitive chromatography or mass spectrometry, yet the largest sources of uncertainty may arise before the sample reaches the instrument. The device may generate different aerosol masses between puffs. Coil resistance may vary between units. The wick may supply liquid inconsistently. Collection efficiency may change as aerosol condenses within the sampling system. Reactive compounds may be lost before derivatisation. Trace metals may be introduced through the collection apparatus or laboratory environment. A precise instrumental signal does not remove uncertainty created by the product, sampling process or preparation method.

The distinction between error and uncertainty should remain clear. An error is a difference between a measured value and the true value, although the true value is often unknown. Errors may arise systematically, such as through incorrect calibration, incomplete recovery or a biased puffing machine, or randomly through short-term variation in instrument response, sample preparation or product performance. Uncertainty is the quantified doubt associated with the result after known sources of variation and bias have been considered. It does not identify one specific mistake. It expresses the range within which the value being measured is reasonably expected to lie under the stated conditions.

A result can be highly precise but inaccurate. Repeated measurements may agree closely because the same systematic error affects every run. A nicotine method may produce almost identical results while using an incorrectly prepared calibration standard. A metal analysis may show excellent replicate agreement while incomplete digestion causes consistent under-recovery. A carbonyl method may be instrumentally stable while the collection system loses a substantial fraction of the analyte before analysis. Precision describes agreement; accuracy describes closeness to an accepted value. Uncertainty must consider both.

The true value itself may be difficult to define in a vaping product. For a homogeneous reference solution, the measurand can be described relatively simply as the nicotine concentration at a stated temperature and basis. For aerosol emissions, the measurand is more conditional. It may be the mass of formaldehyde emitted during a specified number of puffs under a stated regime, from a particular device and liquid configuration. Altering the puff duration, device power, coil age or liquid level changes the measurand rather than merely changing the measurement. Uncertainty analysis begins by defining precisely what is being measured.

A poorly defined measurand cannot be rescued through sophisticated statistics. A result described only as "formaldehyde emissions" leaves important questions unanswered. It does not identify the product state, puffing conditions, collection period, normalisation basis or chemical fraction measured. The laboratory may have quantified the captured DNPH derivative accurately, but the regulatory meaning remains uncertain because the object of measurement has not been described adequately. Defining the measurand is therefore both a scientific and regulatory requirement.

Uncertainty is commonly evaluated through a combination of observed statistical variation and other information. Type A evaluation uses repeated measurements to estimate variation statistically. Repeatability data, replicate preparations, repeated aerosol collections and control-sample results can all contribute. Type B evaluation uses information from calibration certificates, reference-material values, equipment specifications, recovery studies, method validation, published data and scientific judgement. The labels do not indicate that one form is superior to the other. They describe how the contribution was estimated.

A balance calibration uncertainty may be obtained from a calibration certificate rather than repeated weighing and therefore enter as a Type B contribution. The variation between independently prepared nicotine samples may be estimated statistically and enter as a Type A contribution. The uncertainty associated with a reference standard's certified purity may come from the supplier documentation. Recovery variation may be estimated through validation studies. The complete uncertainty estimate combines these components according to how they influence the final calculation.

The first practical step is to construct an uncertainty budget. This identifies the significant stages of the measurement and estimates the contribution from each. For nicotine assay, relevant components may include reference-standard purity, weighing, dilution volume, density conversion, calibration model, recovery and repeatability. For metal analysis, the budget may include blank correction, filter variability, digestion recovery, standard preparation, instrumental calibration and aerosol collection. For carbonyl testing, puffing volume, collection efficiency, derivatisation, blank response, calibration, extraction and product variability may all be relevant.

Not every conceivable factor needs to be included separately. The aim is to capture contributions that affect the result materially. Some sources are already represented within repeatability or intermediate-precision data. Counting them again can inflate the estimate. Others may be correlated. For example, several volumetric preparation steps may depend on the same temperature or calibration system. A sound uncertainty budget reflects the structure of the actual method rather than producing a long list of components for appearance.

Individual uncertainty contributions are usually converted into standard uncertainties so that they can be combined consistently. The combined standard uncertainty represents the estimated standard deviation associated with the result. An expanded uncertainty is then calculated by applying a coverage factor, commonly chosen to provide a level of confidence close to 95 per cent under appropriate assumptions. The report may therefore express a result as a measured value plus or minus an expanded uncertainty.

The coverage factor and confidence interpretation should be stated. A result of 19.8 milligrams per millilitre with an expanded uncertainty of 0.6 milligrams per millilitre communicates more than a result of 19.800 alone. It indicates that the method cannot establish the true concentration to three decimal places and that the plausible range may cross an important regulatory boundary. The expanded uncertainty does not mean that every value within the interval is equally likely, nor does it guarantee that the true value lies within it. It expresses the degree of confidence supported by the measurement model and available evidence.

False precision is a recurring weakness in laboratory reporting. Analytical software may calculate concentrations to many decimal places because the calibration equation produces them mathematically. Those digits may have no scientific meaning. A result reported as 0.003847 micrograms per puff may imply a level of knowledge unsupported by aerosol-generation variability, blank correction and recovery. Significant figures should reflect the uncertainty of the complete method, not the display capacity of the instrument.

Rounding becomes important near specifications and statutory limits. A laboratory should establish a consistent rounding convention and apply it only after the calculation has been completed. Rounding intermediate figures can create additional error, while selective rounding can alter the apparent compliance conclusion. A value should not be rounded down merely because doing so produces a pass. The result, uncertainty and decision rule should be evaluated before the final conformity statement is made.

The uncertainty associated with sampling is often larger than the uncertainty associated with analysis. A laboratory may measure one bottle or one device very precisely, but the selected unit may not represent the batch or product population. Sampling uncertainty arises from variation between containers, batches, coils, devices, filling stages and storage histories. It is conceptually different from analytical uncertainty, although both affect the confidence placed in the final conclusion.

Where one bottle is tested from a batch of thousands, the laboratory result describes that bottle unless the sampling design supports a broader inference. A low analytical uncertainty cannot establish batch uniformity. Similarly, repeated injections of one aerosol extract do not establish that other devices generate the same emissions. The report should distinguish uncertainty in measuring the test item from uncertainty in generalising the result to the marketed product.

This distinction matters particularly in batch-to-batch assessment. A manufacturer may observe variation between production lots that is far greater than the method uncertainty. In that case, the process rather than the laboratory is the dominant source of inconsistency. Conversely, a highly variable analytical method may conceal genuine manufacturing trends. Process capability and analytical capability should therefore be considered separately before conclusions are drawn about product consistency.

Device-generated aerosol introduces dynamic uncertainty that does not occur to the same degree in conventional solution analysis. The product changes during testing. The battery discharges, the coil heats and cools, the liquid level falls and deposits accumulate. Each puff is generated from a slightly different physical state. A collected puff block therefore represents an integrated sequence rather than repeated measurement of one perfectly stable object.

Puff volume, duration and interval contribute directly to uncertainty where they affect emissions. The aerosol-generation machine must control these parameters within known tolerances. Flow meters, timers, valves and activation systems should be calibrated or verified. A small variation may have little effect on a stable product but a large effect near the onset of liquid starvation or overheating. The influence of each parameter should be examined during robustness or validation work rather than assumed to be negligible.

The device itself may amplify minor method variation. A small change in puff interval can reduce wick recovery time. A modest increase in power can move the coil into a different thermal regime. A slight difference in liquid viscosity can change replenishment. Uncertainty is therefore not always additive in a simple way. Interacting factors can produce non-linear effects, particularly in carbonyl formation and aerosol yield. The measurement model should remain scientifically realistic even where a complete mathematical representation is impossible.

Collection efficiency is another major source. The laboratory measures what reaches and remains within the collection medium, not necessarily everything emitted at the mouthpiece. Aerosol can deposit in tubing, connectors and chambers. Volatile compounds can pass through filters. Reactive substances can degrade or react before capture. Particles can be lost according to size, charge and flow conditions. A method may include recovery corrections, but the correction itself carries uncertainty.

Whole-process recovery is preferable where it can be established, because it challenges the generation, transport, collection and analytical stages together. In practice, introducing a known aerosol-phase amount of a reactive or particulate analyte may be difficult. Laboratories may therefore use partial recovery experiments and estimate the remaining contribution from other evidence. The report should identify where the uncertainty estimate is based on direct data and where it relies on assumptions or scientific judgement.

Blank uncertainty is particularly important for trace analysis. A sample concentration may be calculated by subtracting a blank value from the observed response. Both values carry uncertainty, and their difference can be much less certain than either result appears. When the sample signal is only slightly above the blank, the relative uncertainty may become very large. Reporting a low numerical value without explaining the influence of the blank can create false confidence.

An unstable blank is more serious than a consistently low one. If blank results vary across the analytical run or between days, subtraction cannot correct the problem reliably. The laboratory should establish blank acceptance criteria and investigate excessive background. A method whose blank contribution approaches the expected sample level may require improved materials, cleaner preparation, different reagents or a higher reporting limit.

Detection and quantification limits are themselves associated with uncertainty. Below the limit of detection, the method cannot distinguish the analyte signal reliably from background. Between the detection and quantification limits, presence may be indicated without supporting accurate numerical measurement. Above the quantification limit, uncertainty generally decreases as the signal becomes larger relative to noise, although matrix effects and other sources remain.

The phrase "not detected" should therefore not be interpreted as zero exposure. It means that the method did not detect the analyte above its established capability under the stated conditions. Two laboratories may report different conclusions simply because their reporting limits differ. A more sensitive method may detect a substance that another reports as absent, even when both products contain the same amount. Regulatory comparison should consider method capability before treating detection frequency as evidence of product difference.

Uncertainty is not necessarily symmetrical at very low concentrations. A corrected result close to zero cannot extend meaningfully into negative physical concentration, even if a conventional statistical interval would do so. Censoring, reporting-limit conventions and non-normal distributions may require alternative treatment. Substituting zero or half the detection limit into exposure calculations can be convenient but introduces model assumptions that should be acknowledged.

Calibration contributes uncertainty through standard purity, preparation, regression and instrument response. A calibration curve is an estimated relationship rather than a perfect conversion. The uncertainty may vary across the range, usually becoming more important near the lower and upper limits. A method validated across a broad range should not assume one constant percentage uncertainty without evidence. Samples should be diluted or prepared so that measurements occur within the part of the curve where performance is established.

Matrix effects introduce further uncertainty where sample composition changes detector response. Matrix-matched standards, internal standards and standard addition can reduce the problem, but none eliminates it automatically. A method validated in one representative formulation may not perform identically in another containing different acids, flavours or solvent ratios. Product grouping should therefore consider whether the analytical matrix remains sufficiently comparable.

Recovery corrections deserve particular caution. If a method consistently recovers 80 per cent of an analyte, the laboratory may correct the measured result mathematically. The corrected value will carry uncertainty from the recovery estimate as well as from the original measurement. A correction based on a small number of experiments can create an appearance of accuracy unsupported by the evidence. Where recovery varies substantially between matrices or concentration levels, improving the method may be preferable to applying a broad correction.

Intermediate precision often provides a practical estimate of combined laboratory variation. Results generated across different days, analysts, instruments and reagent preparations capture several routine sources simultaneously. This can reduce the need to estimate every minor contribution separately. It does not necessarily include sampling, device variability or long-term product changes, and those components should remain visible where relevant.

Interlaboratory reproducibility provides an even wider perspective. A method may produce a small uncertainty estimate within one laboratory but show much greater variation when applied elsewhere. Differences in implementation, calibration standards, collection systems and data treatment may reveal sources not captured during internal validation. Proficiency testing and round-robin studies can therefore inform whether the laboratory's uncertainty estimate is realistic.

A laboratory should review its uncertainty estimate when interlaboratory performance falls outside expectation. The solution is not simply to enlarge the stated uncertainty until every result becomes compatible. The discrepancy may expose a systematic difference requiring method harmonisation or corrective action. Uncertainty should reflect known measurement capability, not serve as a defence against investigating disagreement.

Product variability should not be absorbed indiscriminately into analytical uncertainty. The laboratory may report the variation observed across several devices, but this is a characteristic of the tested product population rather than solely the measurement. Combining it with instrumental and method uncertainty can be useful for some exposure assessments, but it can obscure whether the manufacturer or laboratory controls are responsible. Separate reporting of analytical uncertainty and product variability is often more informative.

The same applies to between-batch variation. If nicotine concentration differs across batches, the variation belongs to the manufacturing process. The laboratory's uncertainty describes confidence in each measurement. The manufacturer may then use the batch results to estimate process variability and determine whether the product remains within specification. Treating all variation as laboratory uncertainty would weaken accountability for manufacturing control.

Decision-making near regulatory limits requires an explicit conformity rule. A result can fall below a limit while its uncertainty interval extends above it. Alternatively, the measured value can sit slightly above the limit while the interval includes compliant values. The laboratory and regulator must decide how the risk of false acceptance and false rejection will be managed.

A guard band creates a zone between the legal limit and the internal acceptance threshold. For example, a manufacturer may set its formulation target and release specification below the statutory maximum so that ordinary process and analytical variation do not create marginal batches. This is generally stronger than routinely manufacturing at the legal ceiling and relying on uncertainty arguments after testing.

Decision rules can be designed to favour consumer protection, producer protection or a balance between them. A stringent rule may declare conformity only where the upper uncertainty bound remains below the limit. This reduces the risk of accepting a non-compliant product but increases the possibility of rejecting a compliant one. A rule based solely on the measured value carries different risks. The chosen approach should be stated transparently rather than hidden within the laboratory's internal practice.

Enforcement testing raises additional considerations. A regulatory authority may test a market sample and obtain a result close to the legal boundary. The manufacturer may hold a different result from another laboratory. Before concluding that one side is wrong, the samples, methods, uncertainty estimates and decision rules should be compared. The products may come from different batches, or the methods may measure on different bases. A legal dispute can arise from methodological incompatibility as readily as from actual product non-compliance.

Uncertainty should not be used to avoid action where evidence of non-compliance is clear. A result well beyond the limit does not become acceptable merely because the method carries uncertainty. Nor should a broad uncertainty estimate be used to excuse an inadequately controlled method. The function of uncertainty is to clarify borderline and comparative interpretation, not to make every result inconclusive.

Toxicological interpretation contains a further layer of uncertainty beyond the analytical measurement. The laboratory may quantify an emission with reasonable confidence, but translating that value into consumer exposure requires assumptions about puff frequency, daily consumption, product use, inhaled fraction and duration. Reference values may themselves contain uncertainty factors. The overall risk assessment therefore combines measurement uncertainty with exposure-model and toxicological uncertainty.

These layers should not be collapsed into one undifferentiated range. Analytical uncertainty concerns the measured emission under defined conditions. Exposure uncertainty concerns how laboratory output relates to consumer behaviour. Toxicological uncertainty concerns the relationship between dose and biological effect. Separating them allows the reviewer to understand whether the dominant limitation lies in the measurement, the behavioural assumptions or the available health evidence.

Comparative-risk analysis is also affected. When vaping emissions are compared with cigarette smoke, both datasets carry uncertainty and may have been generated under different regimes. A large difference may remain meaningful despite these limitations. A small difference may not. The comparison should consider methodological equivalence, product variability and reporting basis before presenting a precise reduction percentage.

The same discipline applies when comparing products. Ranking several devices from lowest to highest emission can imply real differences where their uncertainty intervals overlap substantially. The apparent order may change if the test is repeated. Product comparison should therefore consider effect size, variability and method capability rather than relying only on central values.

Uncertainty can be expressed visually as well as numerically. Error bars, ranges and individual replicate values often communicate the evidence more effectively than a table of means. They show whether the product behaves consistently, whether groups overlap and whether one extreme result drives the average. Visual presentation should remain faithful to the type of uncertainty shown; analytical error bars, confidence intervals and product ranges are not interchangeable.

Laboratory reports should state the measurement result, units, uncertainty where relevant, coverage factor, confidence basis, method and significant limitations. Where uncertainty is not reported numerically, the laboratory should be able to explain why it is not required or how method capability is otherwise controlled. Qualitative statements such as "results may vary" are insufficient where the value supports a conformity decision.

The uncertainty estimate should be reviewed when the method, matrix, equipment or laboratory process changes. A new instrument may improve sensitivity but alter calibration behaviour. A revised collection system may reduce losses but introduce different flow uncertainty. A new flavour matrix may increase interference. Historical uncertainty cannot be transferred automatically to a materially changed procedure.

Long-term quality-control data should also be used to confirm whether the original estimate remains realistic. Control charts, replicate performance, proficiency testing and corrective-action records may show that routine variation is wider or narrower than predicted during validation. Updating the uncertainty model is part of maintaining the method rather than evidence that the original validation failed.

The strongest uncertainty analysis is proportionate. It does not create unnecessary mathematical complexity where the measurement is far from any decision boundary and the method is demonstrably stable. Nor does it reduce a complex emissions measurement to the instrument manufacturer's stated accuracy. It identifies the components that matter and communicates their combined effect at the level required for the regulatory use.

Laboratory uncertainty is sometimes presented as though it diminishes scientific evidence. In reality, the opposite is true. Evidence becomes less credible when a result is reported without acknowledging how it was produced and how much confidence it deserves. A transparent uncertainty estimate allows manufacturers, toxicologists and regulators to distinguish clear findings from marginal ones, genuine product differences from analytical noise and meaningful compliance failures from unresolved boundary cases.

The laboratory's responsibility is not to produce certainty where none exists. It is to reduce avoidable variation, quantify the remaining doubt and prevent numerical precision from exceeding scientific knowledge. When uncertainty remains attached to the result, the measurement can support proportionate judgement. When it is ignored, a laboratory value may appear decisive while concealing limitations that materially affect the regulatory conclusion.

Turning Analytical Data into Regulatory Decisions

Analytical data become regulatory evidence only when the measurement is connected to a defined product, a validated method, an appropriate exposure model and a clear decision criterion. A chromatographic peak, elemental concentration or nicotine assay is not, by itself, a regulatory conclusion. It is one component within a chain of reasoning that begins with product identity and ends with an action: acceptance, rejection, reformulation, further investigation, notification, market restriction, corrective action or withdrawal. The quality of that action depends on whether each stage of the chain remains visible and scientifically defensible.

The first task is to establish what the result represents. An analytical value cannot be interpreted properly without knowing which product was tested, which batch and formulation were involved, which device configuration was used, how the sample was stored and whether the test conditions reflected intended use, foreseeable use or deliberate stress. A result generated from a development prototype may not describe the later commercial product. Data from one nicotine strength cannot automatically support another. Emissions produced using one coil, power setting or puffing regime may not apply to a device that differs materially in design or operation.

Product identity is therefore the foundation of regulatory interpretation. The analytical report should connect the result to the same formulation, materials, components and manufacturing specification described within the technical file. Where grouping or read-across is used, the rationale must explain why the tested configuration represents the wider product family. A nominal similarity in brand, flavour or device appearance is not enough. The relevant question is whether the differences could affect composition, aerosol generation, thermal behaviour, nicotine delivery, metal release or another attribute connected to exposure.

Once identity is established, the regulator or responsible manufacturer must determine whether the method was capable of answering the intended question. A measured value is only as strong as the procedure used to obtain it. The method must possess adequate specificity, accuracy, precision, sensitivity and robustness in the relevant matrix. Collection efficiency, recovery, blank contribution, calibration and sample stability should be understood. Accreditation can increase confidence that the laboratory operates within a controlled system, but the accredited status of the organisation does not make every result automatically relevant or correct.

A conformity decision should therefore never be based solely on the presence of an accreditation mark or a statement that a recognised instrument was used. The scope of accreditation, method validation and study design must still be examined. A laboratory may be accredited for nicotine analysis in liquids but not for aerosol collection. It may quantify metals accurately in the final digest while using a sampling system that loses particles or introduces contamination. It may apply a validated carbonyl method under puffing conditions that do not represent the product. Organisational competence and scientific relevance must coincide.

The next distinction is between measurement and interpretation. The laboratory measures a defined characteristic. Toxicologists, regulatory scientists and product specialists determine what that characteristic means. A formaldehyde result may be analytically valid but require interpretation through aerosol yield, daily use, exposure frequency, method uncertainty and toxicological reference points. A nickel result may require examination of alloy composition, chemical form, particle size and product age. A nicotine result may indicate a labelling or formulation failure even where the toxicological implications of the deviation are modest. Different analytical findings therefore enter different regulatory pathways.

Some results can be compared directly with a statutory requirement. Nicotine concentration, liquid volume or specified product dimensions may be subject to explicit legal limits. Where the measurand and limit are aligned, the regulatory decision can appear comparatively straightforward. Even then, sampling, method uncertainty, reporting basis and decision rules must be considered. A measured value just below a limit does not provide the same level of confidence as one comfortably within it, particularly where the uncertainty interval or manufacturing variation extends beyond the boundary.

Other analytical results do not have direct legal maxima. Carbonyls, metals, volatile compounds and many impurities may need to be interpreted through general safety obligations, toxicological assessment, product-comparison data or internal specifications. The absence of a statutory number does not mean that any concentration is acceptable. It means that the decision requires a more explicit scientific argument. The responsible operator must identify the hazard, estimate exposure, consider avoidability and determine whether the product presents an unacceptable risk under intended and reasonably foreseeable conditions.

This difference between direct compliance and scientific acceptability should remain clear. A product may comply with every numerical limit explicitly stated in legislation while still presenting a problem through excessive emissions, poor manufacturing or unstable performance. Conversely, detection of a hazardous substance does not establish non-compliance automatically where the concentration is low, exposure is limited and the product remains substantially less hazardous than the relevant alternative. Regulation requires both adherence to prescribed rules and competent assessment of risks that are not captured fully by those rules.

Hazard identification is the beginning of that assessment rather than its end. Analytical techniques can detect substances at extremely low concentrations. The presence of a compound with a hazardous classification is therefore not sufficient to determine regulatory action. The decision must consider how much is present, how often exposure occurs, whether the substance is transferred efficiently, whether it accumulates and what biological effect is plausible at the measured dose. Detection without exposure context can exaggerate significance, while comparison only with a higher-emitting product can understate avoidable risk.

Dose remains central. Carbonyls, metals and nicotine all have effects that depend on concentration and exposure. The same substance may be of little significance at one level and require urgent action at another. Analytical reports should therefore provide units and normalisation that support exposure estimation. Values expressed per puff, per collection block, per gram of liquid consumed or per mass of aerosol answer different questions. Regulators should be able to trace the conversion from the laboratory result to the daily or lifetime exposure assumption used in the risk assessment.

This conversion should be transparent. If a laboratory reports an emission per ten puffs, the exposure calculation should state how many puffs per day are assumed and whether that assumption represents an average, upper percentile or conservative scenario. If the result is normalised to aerosol mass, the calculation should explain how daily aerosol consumption was estimated. If the device delivers inconsistently, a single average exposure may not capture the range experienced by consumers. The purpose is not to create one apparently exact number, but to describe the plausible exposure distribution.

Consumer behaviour introduces uncertainty that laboratory testing cannot remove. Users differ in puff duration, frequency, device setting, maintenance and liquid consumption. Some use products lightly; others compensate for lower nicotine delivery by increasing puffing. Adjustable devices create additional variability. Exposure assessment should therefore use scenarios rather than pretending that one puffing regime represents every individual. A central estimate may describe typical use, while higher-use and foreseeable stress scenarios reveal whether the conclusion remains robust.

The comparator also shapes the regulatory interpretation. For a person who does not use nicotine, vaping introduces an avoidable exposure. For a smoker who switches completely, the relevant comparison is often continued inhalation of tobacco smoke. The same analytical result can therefore carry different public health meaning depending on the population and alternative behaviour considered. Regulation should protect non-users and children without ignoring the reduction in toxicant exposure that may occur when vaping replaces smoking.

Comparative risk should not become an excuse for weak product control. Producing fewer toxicants than a cigarette does not establish that every emission is acceptable or unavoidable. Manufacturers should still reduce carbonyl formation, metallic release and contamination where feasible. The correct comparison operates at two levels. First, the product should be evaluated against its own reasonable standard of design and manufacture. Secondly, its residual risk should be considered within the broader nicotine and tobacco market. A product can be materially less harmful than smoking while still requiring improvement or restriction.

Risk thresholds are not always available or directly transferable. Occupational exposure limits, environmental standards and pharmaceutical impurity limits may provide context, but they were developed for different populations, durations, routes or exposure patterns. Applying them mechanically can create false precision. An eight-hour workplace concentration cannot simply be treated as a consumer-product limit without considering inhaled volume, intermittent peaks, particle form and repeated daily use. Reference values must be selected and adapted with their original purpose in mind.

Where toxicological reference points are absent, approaches such as read-across, threshold concepts, margin-of-exposure analysis and weight-of-evidence reasoning may be used. Each contains assumptions. Read-across depends on the relevance of the analogue. Threshold approaches may not apply equally to all endpoints. A margin of exposure depends on both the selected toxicological point of departure and the estimated consumer dose. Regulatory decisions should make these assumptions explicit rather than presenting the final number as though it were observed directly.

Analytical uncertainty must remain attached to this interpretation. A reported result is an estimate, and the uncertainty may matter greatly where the value lies near a decision boundary. The regulator should know whether the dominant uncertainty arises from the analytical method, the product population, the exposure scenario or the toxicological reference point. Combining these sources into one opaque range makes it difficult to understand how the decision might change if better evidence became available.

A result far below a relevant concern level may remain reassuring despite moderate uncertainty. A result close to the boundary requires greater care. Further replication, improved sensitivity, additional product sampling or confirmation by another laboratory may be justified. A value far above the action threshold should not be rendered inconclusive through an artificially broad uncertainty argument. Uncertainty should guide proportionality, not protect every result from decision.

Decision rules provide the formal mechanism through which uncertainty is incorporated into conformity assessment. Where a legal or internal limit exists, the rule should state whether the central measured value, uncertainty interval or guard-banded threshold determines acceptance. A rule designed to minimise false acceptance may require strong confidence that the true value remains below the limit. A less conservative rule may accept the product where the measured value alone falls within specification. Each approach distributes the risk of error differently.

The rule should be agreed before the result is known. Selecting an interpretation after seeing whether the product passes creates bias. Manufacturers, laboratories and regulators should understand how marginal values will be handled, how rounding is applied and whether repeat analysis is permitted. The same evidence should not produce a pass when commissioned by the producer and a failure when generated by an authority merely because each side uses a different unstated convention.

Guard bands are often a practical solution. An internal release limit can be set below the statutory maximum so that normal process and measurement variation do not place commercial batches at risk of non-compliance. This approach is particularly important for nicotine concentration. Manufacturing routinely at the legal ceiling leaves no meaningful margin for raw-material variation, filling error, solvent evaporation or analytical uncertainty. The internal target should preserve compliance under foreseeable variation rather than treating the statutory boundary as the desired formulation value.

The same principle can be applied to product emissions even where statutory maxima are absent. Internal alert and action levels can identify deteriorating performance before a serious or legally actionable failure occurs. These limits may be derived from development data, toxicological assessment, historical batch performance and achievable design control. Their purpose is to detect change, not to create arbitrary pass–fail numbers for every analyte.

Trend analysis is therefore as important as the interpretation of individual results. A batch can meet specification while showing a gradual movement away from the established process mean. Nicotine concentration may drift upwards, carbonyl emissions may increase as a component supplier changes, or metal results may become more variable across successive coil batches. Regulatory quality systems should detect these patterns before consumers are exposed to a formally failing product.

An isolated elevated result requires investigation, but it should not be dismissed automatically as an outlier. Intermittent failures may reveal a product characteristic that an average conceals. One device with unusually high metal release may represent contamination, defective solder or manufacturing debris. One puff block with sharply increased carbonyls may indicate intermittent liquid starvation. The investigation must determine whether the result reflects analytical error, a defective unit or a wider process problem.

The decision to exclude data should be supported by an assignable cause. A failed calibration, documented contamination event or instrument malfunction may invalidate the result. The fact that a value is inconvenient or inconsistent with the remaining replicates is not enough. If no analytical cause is identified, the result remains evidence of product variability and may justify additional sampling or manufacturing review. Regulatory decisions should be based on the behaviour of the product population, not only on the most favourable average.

Replication strengthens the evidential base. Additional devices, batches and analytical runs can show whether the finding is reproducible. Replication should be targeted at the uncertainty that matters. Reinjecting the same extract will not resolve device-to-device variability. Testing more devices will not correct an interfering analytical method. The follow-up design should identify whether the question concerns instrument precision, sample preparation, aerosol collection, batch consistency or product failure.

Independent laboratory confirmation may be appropriate where the finding has major consequences or the original result remains disputed. The second laboratory should receive a well-defined protocol, representative samples and sufficient product information. Differences should be examined through methods, calibration, collection and uncertainty rather than resolved through simple majority. Two laboratories agreeing does not make a flawed method correct, but independent reproducibility increases confidence where the procedures are suitable.

Regulatory decisions should draw on the totality of evidence rather than one analytical number. Formulation records, supplier specifications, materials data, stability results, emissions testing, toxicological review, complaints, adverse-event reports and manufacturing history may all contribute. A high nickel result becomes more significant where the coil supplier has changed, complaints describe metallic taste and later batches show the same pattern. The same isolated value may carry less weight where repeat testing, component analysis and market surveillance provide no supporting evidence.

Weight-of-evidence reasoning should not become a means of diluting strong analytical findings among large quantities of weak information. The evidence should be weighted according to relevance, reliability and consistency. A validated, replicated product-specific result deserves more weight than a general literature report involving a different device. A documented manufacturing change may be more informative than a broad assurance from the supplier. The process should explain why particular evidence was considered decisive.

Data quality and decision significance should be matched. A preliminary screening result may justify further investigation but not immediate public claims about product danger. A fully validated and replicated result showing substantial non-compliance may justify withdrawal or enforcement. The regulatory response should be proportionate to the strength of the evidence, magnitude of the risk, number of products affected and availability of corrective measures.

Not every analytical deviation requires product removal. Some can be managed through investigation, process correction, additional monitoring or revised specifications. A minor nicotine deviation within a non-critical internal tolerance may require process adjustment. A systematic concentration above the legal maximum requires stronger action. Low-level detection of an unexpected flavour impurity may justify supplier review and confirmatory testing. Repeated lead release from device components may require immediate cessation of supply and recall.

The available actions form a regulatory ladder. At the lowest level, the producer may record the finding and continue routine monitoring. Greater concern may require enhanced testing, supplier investigation, additional toxicological assessment or change control. Confirmed non-conformity may require batch quarantine, reformulation, component replacement or suspension of release. Products already distributed may require market withdrawal, consumer communication or formal recall. Regulatory authorities may impose sales restrictions, penalties or wider enforcement where the responsible operator fails to act.

The choice should reflect both severity and reversibility. Where the risk is uncertain but potentially significant, temporary suspension may be more proportionate than either unrestricted sale or permanent prohibition. Where a defect can be corrected through a component change, targeted action may protect consumers without removing the entire product family. Where the analytical evidence shows a systemic and serious hazard, broad action may be necessary.

The number of exposed consumers and duration of market availability also matter. A modest individual risk can become important when millions of units are sold. Conversely, an extreme result confined to one defective unit may require a focused manufacturing response rather than a conclusion about the whole category. Population exposure, distribution records and traceability therefore connect laboratory evidence to the scale of regulatory intervention.

Traceability determines whether action can be targeted effectively. The regulator should be able to identify the affected batches, component lots, production dates, importers and retail channels. Without that information, a batch-specific failure may force a broader withdrawal because the affected units cannot be distinguished. Strong batch coding and supply-chain records therefore reduce both consumer risk and unnecessary commercial disruption.

Analytical findings can also reveal that the original technical file is no longer accurate. A formulation may have changed, a component may have been substituted or the commercial product may perform differently from the notified version. In such cases, the issue is not only whether the measured value is acceptable. It is whether the product retains the regulatory identity under which it entered the market. An undocumented substantial change can invalidate earlier evidence even where the new version does not appear immediately hazardous.

Change control should therefore follow every significant finding. Where the investigation identifies a material or process cause, corrective action must be assessed for its effect on composition, emissions, stability, product performance and notification status. Replacing a coil alloy may reduce one metal but alter resistance and thermal behaviour. Changing the formulation viscosity may improve wick supply but affect aerosol yield and nicotine delivery. Corrective action should solve the identified problem without creating another that remains untested.

The effectiveness of corrective action must be verified analytically. A revised process or component should not be considered successful merely because the proposed mechanism appears reasonable. Pre-change and post-change products should be compared using appropriate methods and representative samples. The evidence should show that the undesirable result has been reduced and that critical performance attributes remain controlled.

Post-market data should remain linked to the analytical programme. Complaints, adverse events, returns and enforcement samples can reveal conditions not anticipated during pre-market testing. A laboratory result obtained during development reflects a limited set of products and operating states. Real-world use introduces ageing, storage, misuse, incompatible components and variable consumer behaviour. Regulation becomes more credible when analytical testing responds to these signals rather than remaining a one-time dossier exercise.

A cluster of complaints may trigger targeted testing even where routine release results remain acceptable. Burnt taste may justify investigation of carbonyl formation and liquid supply. Metallic taste may lead to component and aerosol elemental analysis. Reports of unusually strong effects may justify nicotine verification and device-delivery testing. The analytical response should be guided by the nature of the signal rather than applying the same standard panel indiscriminately.

Absence of complaints does not prove absence of risk. Consumers may not recognise a chemical exposure or may not report it. Some effects are chronic rather than immediately perceptible. Market surveillance, periodic verification and scientific literature therefore remain necessary even where post-market reporting is quiet. The balance lies between signal-driven investigation and planned monitoring of risks unlikely to generate obvious consumer complaints.

Regulators must also consider whether a laboratory finding is product-specific or category-wide. One formulation generating elevated carbonyls under a particular device condition does not prove that all vaping products behave similarly. A repeated pattern across several products using the same design or material may justify broader investigation. General regulatory measures should be based on evidence that the problem is sufficiently widespread and not merely a feature of one defective product.

This distinction is important because category-wide conclusions can shape legislation, public communication and consumer behaviour. A dramatic result from an obsolete or poorly operated device may be cited as though it represents the current market. Conversely, favourable data from a carefully controlled product may be used to imply that all products are equally well managed. Regulatory decisions should describe the scope of the evidence accurately.

Public communication forms part of the decision process. Analytical results can be difficult to explain without either exaggerating or minimising them. Statements that a substance has been detected may cause concern even where the concentration is very low. Statements that emissions are lower than cigarette smoke may be interpreted as proof of safety. Regulators and manufacturers should communicate both absolute and comparative information, together with the relevant uncertainty.

The language should distinguish detection from risk, non-compliance from danger and lower exposure from harmlessness. A product may be withdrawn because it fails a legal nicotine limit even where the immediate toxicological consequence is limited. Another may comply formally but require action because of a serious unregulated emission. Public explanation should make clear whether the issue concerns labelling, quality, acute safety, chronic exposure or legal status.

Transparency also requires explanation of what remains unknown. Analytical methods do not measure every compound, every operating condition or every consumer behaviour. A standard emissions panel can identify important constituents without proving that no other concern exists. Regulators should avoid presenting a tested product as comprehensively safe merely because the selected analytes met expectations.

The same caution applies to "not detected" results. The reporting limit should be visible, particularly where different products or laboratories are compared. A substance may be absent, present below the detection capability or lost through the method. The regulatory conclusion should reflect which of these statements the evidence actually supports.

Documentation is essential because decisions must be reviewable. The technical record should show the product tested, sample selection, method, accreditation status, validation, raw results, quality controls, uncertainty, exposure assumptions, toxicological reasoning, decision rule and final action. Where judgement was required, the basis should be recorded. A later reviewer should be able to reconstruct how the analytical value became a regulatory conclusion.

This record protects both the public and the responsible operator. It demonstrates that action was not arbitrary and that favourable results were not accepted without scrutiny. It also allows decisions to be revisited when new evidence emerges. A product restricted under an earlier assumption may warrant reassessment if later data reduce the concern. A product accepted initially may require stronger control if post-market evidence changes the risk estimate.

Regulatory decisions should therefore be capable of revision. Scientific evidence develops, products evolve and analytical methods improve. A result once reported as not detected may become measurable using a more sensitive technique. A toxicological reference point may be revised. A device design previously considered representative may be replaced. Adaptive regulation requires mechanisms for reviewing earlier conclusions without treating every change as institutional failure.

The strongest regulatory systems use analytical evidence to learn. They identify which product attributes predict undesirable emissions, which suppliers or processes create variation and which test conditions reveal meaningful failure. This knowledge can then refine standards, notification requirements, market surveillance and future product design. Analytical data become more valuable when they inform the system rather than remaining stored within individual reports.

Data architecture will increasingly influence this process. Standardised product identifiers, electronic submission fields, laboratory metadata and linked batch records can allow regulators to compare products and detect patterns across the market. A database containing concentrations without method details or product conditions has limited scientific value. The data structure should preserve units, reporting limits, puffing regimes, uncertainty and product configuration so that apparent differences can be interpreted properly.

Automated screening may help identify unusual values, repeated ingredients or product families requiring review. Artificial intelligence and statistical tools can assist with pattern recognition, but they cannot determine relevance without sound data and expert oversight. Poorly harmonised data can produce false signals or conceal real ones. Automation should support regulatory judgement rather than creating an appearance of objectivity around inconsistent information.

Decision-making also requires institutional competence. Regulators need expertise in analytical chemistry, aerosol science, toxicology, statistics, engineering and product manufacture. Without this internal capacity, authorities become dependent on the laboratory's summary, the manufacturer's interpretation or advocacy from external groups. Competent review means being able to question the method, understand uncertainty and distinguish analytical significance from political visibility.

Manufacturers require similar capability. Outsourcing testing does not outsource responsibility. The responsible operator should understand why the test was commissioned, whether the method was appropriate and how the result affects the product. A laboratory certificate filed without critical review is not evidence of effective regulatory control. The producer must be able to explain the finding and demonstrate the decision that followed.

Analytical data are sometimes treated as a binary gateway: the product passes or fails. This is appropriate for certain clear specifications, but the wider regulatory function is more nuanced. Data identify trends, compare designs, support toxicological assessment, investigate failures and reveal uncertainty. A mature system uses measurements to reduce risk continuously rather than only to defend market entry.

The final decision should therefore answer several questions. Is the result scientifically reliable? Does it represent the marketed product? Is the exposure meaningful? Does it breach a legal or internal limit? Is the finding isolated or systematic? Can the source be identified and corrected? What populations are affected? What are the consequences of allowing, restricting or removing the product? What further evidence would materially change the conclusion?

Where those questions are answered openly, analytical evidence can support proportionate regulation. A clear and serious failure can trigger decisive action. A marginal or uncertain finding can lead to targeted investigation. A stable and consistently low-emitting product can remain on the market with appropriate monitoring. The decision becomes neither automatically permissive nor reflexively restrictive, but responsive to the strength and significance of the evidence.

The movement from laboratory result to regulatory action is therefore not an administrative final step appended to testing. It is the purpose for which the analytical system exists. Product definition, representative sampling, validation, accreditation, repeatability, batch control and uncertainty all converge at this point. If any part of that chain is weak, the decision may appear precise while resting on unstable evidence.

Analytical science cannot determine public policy by itself. It can show what was measured, under which conditions, with what confidence and at what likely exposure. Toxicology can evaluate the biological significance. Quality systems can determine whether the result represents a controlled product or a manufacturing failure. Regulators then decide what level of risk, uncertainty and corrective action is acceptable within the law and the wider public health context.

The strongest decisions preserve those distinctions. They do not convert detection into proof of harm, compliance into proof of safety or uncertainty into justification for inaction. They use analytical data to identify what is known, define what remains uncertain and select an intervention proportionate to both. That is the point at which laboratory testing becomes regulatory evidence rather than a collection of technically impressive numbers.

CHAPTER 5

Quality Systems and Manufacturing

A vaping product may be formulated correctly, tested competently and supported by a technically sound regulatory submission, yet still fail in the market if the manufacturing system cannot reproduce it consistently. Regulation often appears to focus most visibly on the product specification: nicotine concentration, ingredients, emissions, packaging, labelling and device characteristics. Those specifications matter, but they describe only what the product is intended to be. Manufacturing determines whether the product placed into each bottle, cartridge, pod or device actually corresponds to that intention. Quality systems provide the organisational structure through which the designed and assessed product is converted into repeatable commercial production, maintained through supply-chain change and corrected when performance departs from expectation. Without that structure, laboratory evidence remains connected to a development sample rather than to the thousands or millions of units eventually supplied to consumers.

The central problem of manufacturing is variation. No production process is perfectly identical from one batch to the next, and no component supplier produces materials without tolerances. Raw-material assay changes slightly, flavour concentrates vary within specification, electronic components are produced across different lots, filling equipment drifts, environmental conditions alter, operators change and production volumes increase. The purpose of a quality system is not to pretend that variation does not exist, but to identify which variation matters, define acceptable limits and ensure that deviations are detected before they become consumer exposure or regulatory failure. A product that performs well only when manufactured under unusually favourable conditions is not a controlled product. Control is demonstrated when the process continues to reproduce the required attributes during routine production, under normal operational pressures and through the ordinary changes that occur across a commercial lifecycle.

This distinction separates product development from manufacturing competence. During development, technical teams can select particular raw materials, prepare small batches carefully and test components under close supervision. Commercial manufacture introduces scale, repetition, multiple personnel, production schedules, supplier logistics, storage, transport and economic pressure. A formulation mixed successfully in a laboratory vessel may not behave identically in a large production tank. A component assembled correctly during engineering trials may vary when produced in large quantities across several subcontractors. A filling process that appears reliable during a short validation run may drift over a full production shift. Quality systems are therefore not an administrative layer applied after development. They are the means through which the assumptions made during development are tested against commercial reality.

The vaping sector has historically contained businesses with very different levels of manufacturing maturity. Some products are produced within highly structured facilities operating controlled processes, documented specifications and formal release systems. Others may pass through fragmented supply chains in which formulation, filling, component assembly, packaging and branding are performed by separate organisations with limited oversight of one another. A brand owner may possess no manufacturing facility and may rely entirely on external suppliers, yet remain responsible for the finished product placed on the market. Outsourcing changes where the work occurs; it does not remove the obligation to understand and control it. The more dispersed the supply chain becomes, the more important it is that responsibilities, specifications, records and change-notification requirements are defined clearly.

Quality management begins with the principle that the product must be designed and produced through controlled processes rather than inspected into compliance at the end. Finished-product testing is necessary, but it cannot detect every failure and should not be expected to compensate for a weak process. A laboratory may confirm nicotine concentration in selected bottles while missing a labelling mix-up affecting another part of the filling run. Device inspection may identify obvious defects while failing to reveal a component substitution that changes metal emissions after repeated use. A carbonyl test performed on a small number of units cannot prove that every coil has been assembled consistently. The stronger strategy is to build quality into the process through approved suppliers, defined materials, validated methods, trained personnel, calibrated equipment, controlled instructions and documented release decisions.

ISO 9001 provides one of the most widely recognised frameworks for organising such a system. It is not a vaping-specific manufacturing standard and does not prescribe the chemical composition, emissions limits or technical design of nicotine products. Its value lies in the principles it establishes around process control, customer and regulatory requirements, leadership, risk-based thinking, documented information, performance evaluation and continual improvement. Applied competently, these principles create a disciplined structure through which product and process requirements can be translated into routine operations. Applied superficially, they can produce a collection of procedures and certificates that appear impressive while daily production remains dependent on informal practice.

The difference lies in implementation. A quality manual stating that suppliers are approved has limited meaning unless approval criteria exist, evidence is retained and performance is reviewed. A procedure requiring equipment calibration is ineffective if instruments are used after calibration has expired or if calibration tolerances are unrelated to product requirements. A training record does not prove competence where operators cannot perform the process consistently. A corrective-action form does not establish improvement if root causes are not identified and repeated failures continue. The value of a quality system is shown by how it influences decisions, prevents recurrence and preserves product identity, not by the number of documents it generates.

Good Manufacturing Practice extends this discipline into the physical and procedural control of production. The term has its strongest and most developed meaning within pharmaceutical and regulated healthcare manufacturing, where detailed requirements govern premises, personnel, sanitation, materials, documentation, validation, production, quality control and release. Consumer vaping products do not always fall within pharmaceutical GMP systems, but the underlying principles remain highly relevant. Materials should be identified and protected against contamination. Production should follow approved instructions. Equipment should be suitable, maintained and cleaned. Labels and packaging should be reconciled. Batches should be traceable. Deviations should be investigated. Products should not be released until the required evidence has been reviewed.

The appropriate level of GMP-like control depends on the product, jurisdiction and regulatory pathway. A medicinal nicotine product requires a pharmaceutical standard of manufacture. A consumer vaping product may be regulated through a different legal framework, but the absence of a formal pharmaceutical requirement does not justify uncontrolled production. Nicotine is pharmacologically active, e-liquids are inhaled after heating and device components influence aerosol composition directly. These characteristics justify a higher level of manufacturing discipline than would be expected for an ordinary low-risk consumer good. The system should be proportionate, but proportionality should reflect product risk rather than commercial convenience.

Supplier control is one of the most important parts of this framework because a manufacturer can only produce consistently when incoming materials and components remain consistent. Nicotine, solvents, acids, flavour preparations, containers, seals, coils, batteries, plastics, electronics and printed packaging may each be sourced from different organisations. The finished-product manufacturer may control none of those original production processes directly. Supplier qualification and auditing therefore become extensions of the manufacturer's own quality system. The objective is not merely to obtain a certificate or questionnaire, but to understand whether the supplier can meet the defined requirements, whether its processes are stable and whether it will communicate changes before they affect the finished product.

A supplier audit should examine evidence rather than assurances. Specifications, production controls, traceability, calibration, non-conformance management, change control and previous performance all matter. For critical materials, the manufacturer should understand which process variables influence quality and whether the supplier has identified them. A flavour supplier may alter a carrier or constituent while retaining the same commercial name. A coil manufacturer may change alloy, wire diameter or wick source without changing the component code. A packaging supplier may substitute resin or closure design. Each change may affect stability, emissions, filling, leakage or regulatory status. Unless the supply agreement requires notification and the receiving organisation evaluates the change, the finished product can drift away from the version originally assessed without any deliberate decision by the brand owner.

Corrective and preventive action systems provide the formal mechanism for responding when such failures occur. Corrective action addresses an identified non-conformity and seeks to prevent its recurrence. Preventive thinking seeks to identify potential failure before it occurs, although modern quality systems increasingly incorporate prevention through risk management rather than through a separate administrative category. The distinction is less important than the discipline of moving beyond immediate correction. Replacing a failed bottle, repeating a laboratory test or retraining one operator may resolve the visible event while leaving the underlying cause untouched. Effective CAPA examines why the failure was possible, whether similar products or batches are affected and what change to the system will make recurrence less likely.

Root-cause analysis is central to that process. A nicotine result outside specification may arise from incorrect raw-material assay, calculation error, poor mixing, sampling bias, analytical failure or mislabelling. A leaking product may result from closure torque, container dimensions, seal material, filling temperature, transport damage or formulation interaction. A device complaint may reflect battery performance, coil assembly, software, liquid compatibility or user behaviour. Selecting the first plausible explanation and closing the investigation quickly produces administrative completion rather than quality improvement. The evidence should determine the cause, and where the evidence remains incomplete, the uncertainty should be recorded rather than hidden behind a convenient conclusion.

Change control performs the opposite function by assessing risk before a modification is introduced. Manufacturing systems must change because suppliers discontinue materials, equipment becomes obsolete, formulations are improved, sites move and regulations evolve. The problem is not change itself but uncontrolled change. A formal system requires the proposed modification to be described, its potential effects assessed and the necessary testing, validation, documentation and regulatory action identified before implementation. The assessment should consider the complete product, not only the component being altered. A change intended to improve one attribute may influence another. Increasing liquid viscosity may reduce leakage but impair wick supply. Replacing a coil alloy may reduce one metal while changing resistance and thermal behaviour. Moving production to a new facility may alter equipment, water, environment or operator practice even where the formulation remains unchanged.

Documentation connects all these activities into an auditable history. Specifications state what is required. Procedures describe how work is performed. Batch records show what occurred. Laboratory records support release. Deviation reports explain departures. CAPA records show how failures were addressed. Change controls record why modifications were accepted. Training records establish who was authorised. Supplier files show where materials originated. Complaint and recall records demonstrate what happened after market entry. The strength of the system lies in the connection between these records rather than in their individual existence.

Poor documentation creates both scientific and regulatory uncertainty. If a batch record cannot identify which nicotine lot was used, an impurity concern cannot be traced efficiently. If a device component code does not distinguish between two alloys, a metal-emissions finding cannot be connected to its source. If the current formulation is not linked to the submitted notification, it becomes difficult to determine whether the product remains the one originally described. If changes are communicated through informal emails or verbal instructions, later investigators may be unable to reconstruct why performance shifted. Documentation is therefore not bureaucratic memory; it is the evidence that product identity and decision-making were controlled.

Good documentation must also be usable. Excessively complicated procedures can be as damaging as missing ones because staff may work around them, create unofficial shortcuts or complete records retrospectively. Instructions should be clear, current and proportionate to the process. Records should be made at the time the work occurs, and corrections should remain visible. Electronic systems require access control, audit trails, version management and secure retention. Paper systems require legibility, controlled copies and protection against loss. In either format, data integrity depends on information being attributable, contemporaneous, accurate and complete.

Traceability converts documentation into practical control. Every finished unit should be connected, directly or through its batch, to the materials, components, process, testing and distribution history relevant to it. This connection enables targeted investigation and recall. Without it, a defect affecting one component lot may force action across an entire product range because the affected units cannot be distinguished. Strong traceability reduces consumer risk and unnecessary commercial disruption by allowing the response to match the actual scope of the failure.

Traceability must extend forward and backward. Backward traceability identifies which raw materials, suppliers and component lots entered a finished batch. Forward traceability identifies where the batch was distributed and, where practical, which customers or retailers received it. Internal traceability links the batch to production lines, personnel, equipment, test records and deviations. In global supply chains, importers, distributors and brand owners may each hold part of the record. Technical agreements should define how information will be shared when a concern arises, because delay during an incident can increase the scale of exposure and weaken the credibility of the response.

Complaint handling provides one of the most important post-market tests of the quality system. Complaints are not merely customer-service matters. They are signals about product performance, manufacturing variation, packaging, labelling, misuse and emerging risk. Reports of leaking, burnt taste, weak nicotine effect, unexpected harshness, battery failure, mislabelling or unusual colour may identify problems that were not visible during release testing. Each complaint should be recorded, assessed for seriousness, linked to the relevant product and batch and investigated to the level justified by the potential risk.

The value of complaint data lies in patterns as much as individual events. One report may be difficult to interpret, but repeated complaints involving the same batch, component, manufacturing date or failure mode may reveal a systematic problem. Trend analysis should therefore examine complaint rate, severity, product family, geography and recurrence. A low overall complaint rate can still conceal a concentrated serious defect. Conversely, an apparent increase may reflect higher sales volume rather than deterioration unless the data are normalised appropriately.

Complaint investigation should connect consumer information to retained samples, batch records, laboratory data and manufacturing history. Returned units may provide direct evidence, although they may have been used, damaged, stored poorly or altered. Retention samples show the condition of the batch under controlled storage. Comparing the two can help distinguish manufacturing failure from distribution, counterfeit supply or user-related effects. The investigation should not assume that the consumer is wrong because the product passed release, nor that the product is defective because a complaint was received. Evidence must link the event to a plausible cause.

Where a product presents a significant risk or fails materially to meet legal and quality requirements, recall may be necessary. Product recalls are among the most demanding tests of organisational readiness because they require rapid decision-making, accurate traceability, communication across the supply chain and evidence that affected products have been removed. A recall plan written only to satisfy an audit may fail when the organisation discovers that distribution records are incomplete, customers cannot be contacted or responsibilities are unclear.

Recall decisions should consider severity, likelihood, distribution, detectability and the availability of corrective action. Some issues may be managed through withdrawal before the product reaches consumers. Others require consumer-level recall, public communication or notification to authorities. The response should be proportionate but decisive. Delaying action while seeking perfect certainty can increase harm, while recalling excessively broad populations because traceability is poor creates avoidable disruption. Preparedness improves both speed and precision.

Mock recalls provide a practical means of testing readiness. The organisation selects a batch and attempts to trace its materials, production and distribution within a defined period. The exercise reveals gaps that procedures alone may not show. Distribution records may use inconsistent product identifiers. Retailers may retain incomplete contact information. Returned quantities may not reconcile with supplied quantities. A mock recall is valuable only when deficiencies lead to corrective action rather than being adjusted on paper to produce an acceptable result.

Continuous improvement brings these systems together. A quality system should not remain static after certification or initial regulatory submission. Data from deviations, complaints, supplier performance, analytical trends, audits, CAPA, recalls and process monitoring should be used to improve the product and the system. Improvement does not necessarily require constant alteration of the formulation or device. It may involve reducing process variation, strengthening supplier agreements, clarifying instructions, improving sampling, automating checks or simplifying documentation so that compliance becomes more reliable.

Continuous improvement requires measurement. Organisations cannot improve what they do not review. Suitable indicators may include batch rejection rate, deviation recurrence, complaint trends, supplier failures, CAPA completion time, calibration performance, audit findings and process capability. Metrics should support understanding rather than encourage superficial behaviour. A target of closing CAPA rapidly can lead to weak investigations if speed is valued more than effectiveness. A low deviation count may indicate excellent control or a culture in which problems are not reported. Quality indicators must therefore be interpreted within operational context.

Leadership influences whether the system functions honestly. Production pressure can encourage batches to be released despite unresolved questions. Commercial urgency can lead to undocumented supplier substitutions. Managers may discourage deviation reporting because failures reflect badly on performance. A mature quality culture treats the identification of problems as necessary information rather than disloyalty. Staff should be able to stop production, quarantine material and escalate concerns without fearing that doing so will be viewed as obstructive.

Quality culture is visible in routine decisions. It appears when a line is cleared properly despite time pressure, when an unfavourable laboratory result is investigated rather than retested repeatedly, when a supplier change is delayed until evidence is complete and when a recall is initiated because consumer protection requires it. Policies can state these expectations, but behaviour demonstrates whether they are real. The most detailed quality system will fail where incentives reward output while treating control as an administrative burden.

Regulators evaluate manufacturing systems because product compliance cannot be separated from the process that sustains it. A notification or technical dossier provides a snapshot. Quality systems determine whether the snapshot remains accurate. Ingredient specifications, emissions data and toxicological conclusions depend on the assumption that production continues to generate the same product. If the formulation changes without control, if component suppliers vary or if batch records are unreliable, the evidential foundation of the regulatory submission weakens.

The discussions that follow examines the machinery through which that continuity is maintained. It begins with ISO 9001 principles and the way process-based quality management can be applied to modern nicotine products. It then considers Good Manufacturing Practice as a practical standard of disciplined production, supplier auditing as the extension of quality control into the supply chain, CAPA as the system for investigating and preventing failure, and change control as the means of managing product evolution without losing regulatory identity. Documentation and traceability show how decisions, materials and batches remain connected. Complaint handling and product recalls extend quality responsibility beyond the factory and into the market. Continuous improvement then considers how evidence from the complete lifecycle can be used to strengthen both the product and the system that produces it.

Quality systems are sometimes dismissed as paperwork imposed after the real scientific work has been completed. In reality, they determine whether the chemistry, toxicology and analytical evidence generated during development survives contact with commercial manufacture. The formulation scientist defines the product, the toxicologist assesses it and the laboratory measures it, but the manufacturing system reproduces it. Where that system is weak, every later unit becomes an uncontrolled variation on the product originally assessed. Where it is strong, regulatory compliance becomes a continuing operational state rather than a document created once for market entry.

Figure 5.1 — Quality Systems and Manufacturing: QMS Operating Loop

The figure presents quality management as a continuous operating loop beginning with quality policy, leadership, customer requirements, regulatory obligations and risk-based thinking. ISO 9001 principles establish the organisational framework, while Good Manufacturing Practice translates those principles into controlled premises, trained personnel, approved materials, validated processes, in-process checks, documentation and product release. Non-conformities detected during manufacture, laboratory testing or post-market monitoring enter the corrective and preventive action system, where they are recorded, investigated and subjected to root-cause analysis. Corrective actions are then assessed for effectiveness, while required modifications are managed through formal change control to ensure that changes to formulations, components, suppliers, equipment or manufacturing processes do not alter the regulated product unintentionally.

Traceability connects raw materials, components, production batches, records and distribution channels, allowing complaints and emerging quality signals to be linked to the products and manufacturing conditions involved. Complaint handling feeds information back into CAPA and trend analysis, while serious or confirmed failures may require product withdrawal or recall. Recall outcomes, audit findings, performance indicators and accumulated quality data then support continuous improvement, returning knowledge to leadership and restarting the cycle. The diagram also identifies the principal outputs of the system—consistent product quality, regulatory compliance, consumer protection, business performance and stakeholder confidence—and the essential enablers of competent personnel, suitable infrastructure, controlled information, supplier management and legal and regulatory awareness.

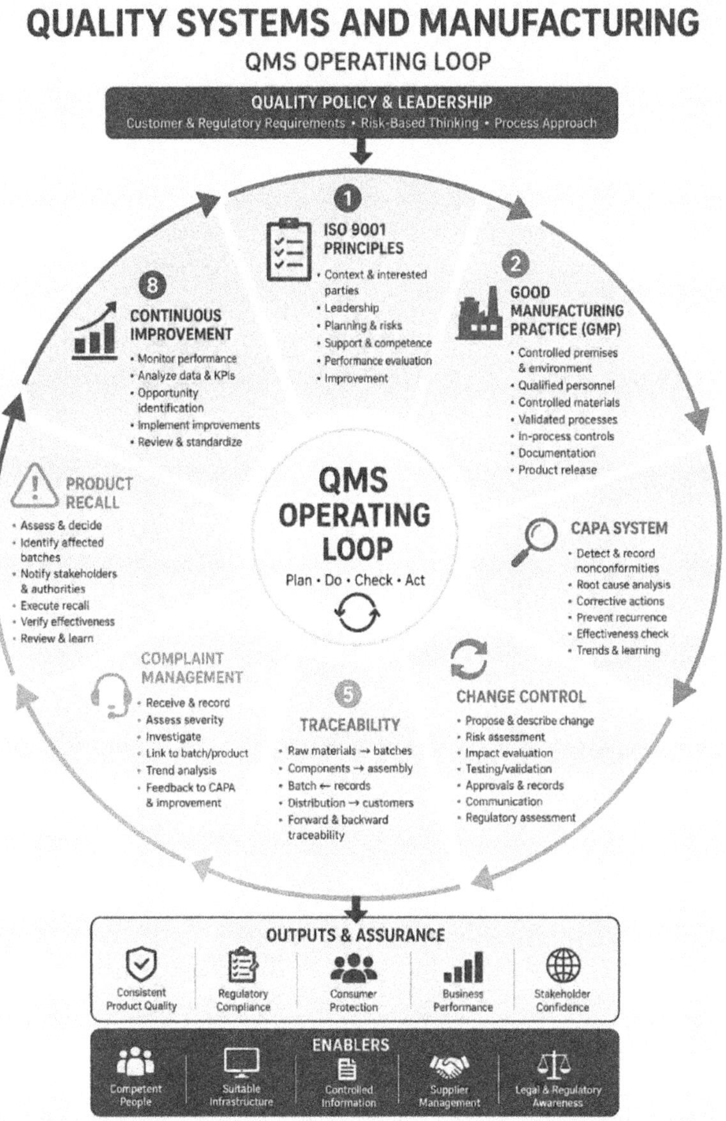

A risk-based, process-driven system that ensures products are designed, manufactured and maintained to meet quality, safety and regulatory requirements.

ISO 9001 Principles

ISO 9001 provides a general framework for establishing, operating and improving a quality management system, but its value in vaping manufacture depends entirely on how its principles are translated into product-specific controls. The standard does not define acceptable nicotine concentrations, emissions limits, coil materials or flavour requirements, and it does not replace the scientific, toxicological or regulatory assessment of the product. Its function is organisational rather than compositional. It requires a business to understand what it is trying to produce, identify the processes that affect that outcome, allocate responsibilities, control evidence, evaluate performance and respond when the system departs from expectation. For modern nicotine products, this framework is valuable because quality is rarely determined by one department or one manufacturing stage. Formulation, procurement, device engineering, filling, laboratory testing, packaging, distribution and post-market surveillance all contribute to whether the product supplied to consumers remains consistent with the product originally designed and assessed.

The starting point is the process approach. Rather than treating quality as the responsibility of a final inspection or quality-control laboratory, ISO 9001 requires the organisation to view its work as a connected system of inputs, activities and outputs. Raw materials, components, specifications and regulatory requirements enter the system; formulation, assembly, testing and release transform them; and finished products, records and market information emerge. Each process should have a defined purpose, responsible owner, required resources, operating criteria and method of evaluation. This is particularly important in vaping manufacture because the quality of the finished product depends on interactions between processes that may appear separate. A nicotine assay can be correct while the wrong label is applied. A liquid can meet formulation specification while an incompatible coil causes unstable emissions. A device can pass functional testing while a supplier substitution changes material composition. The process approach requires these relationships to be understood rather than allowing each department to optimise its own activity in isolation.

Process mapping is one practical means of achieving that understanding. A manufacturer should be able to describe how approved ingredients and components move from supplier qualification through receipt, quarantine, release, storage, production, filling, assembly, packaging, testing, batch release and distribution. The map should also show how deviations, complaints, changes and analytical findings feed back into the system. A process map is useful only where it reflects actual operations. A polished diagram that excludes informal workarounds, outsourced activities or unrecorded decisions provides little assurance. The purpose is to reveal where control is required, where information changes hands and where failure could occur without detection.

Customer focus is another central ISO 9001 principle, although in regulated nicotine products the meaning of "customer" must be interpreted carefully. The immediate customer may be a distributor, retailer or brand owner, but the ultimate recipient is the consumer using the product. Regulatory authorities and other interested parties also impose legitimate requirements that the organisation must satisfy. Customer focus therefore cannot be reduced to flavour preference, commercial demand or rapid delivery. It includes truthful labelling, predictable nicotine strength, reliable device performance, appropriate packaging, complaint response and avoidance of unnecessary exposure. A product that is commercially successful but manufactured outside its specification does not meet customer requirements in any meaningful quality sense.

The organisation should identify applicable needs and expectations before production begins. These include statutory requirements, technical dossier commitments, contractual specifications, product claims, retailer requirements and reasonable consumer expectations. Some are explicit, such as declared nicotine concentration or fill volume. Others are implicit, such as the expectation that nominally identical devices will operate consistently and that replacement pods will fit and perform as intended. The quality system should convert these expectations into measurable product and process requirements. Where expectations remain vague, the organisation cannot determine whether they have been achieved.

Leadership gives the quality system authority. ISO 9001 places responsibility on senior management because quality cannot be sustained where it is delegated entirely to a quality manager without the power to influence production, procurement or commercial decisions. Leaders must establish policy, assign responsibilities, provide resources and ensure that quality objectives align with business strategy. In practice, this means that production targets, launch deadlines and cost reductions should not override unresolved product concerns. A quality system loses credibility when senior management supports it formally but pressures staff informally to release batches, accept unsuitable suppliers or close investigations prematurely.

Leadership is also responsible for creating an environment in which problems can be reported honestly. Quality information is often inconvenient. A laboratory failure may delay release, a supplier audit may expose a critical weakness and a complaint trend may require costly investigation. Where staff believe that raising concerns will be treated as obstruction, the system becomes dependent on silence. Deviations are under-reported, records are adjusted and recurring problems remain hidden. A functioning ISO 9001 system therefore depends on quality culture as much as written procedure. Employees must understand that identifying a problem protects the product and the organisation, while concealing it increases both regulatory and commercial risk.

The organisation's context must be understood because quality systems do not operate in isolation. A small formulation and filling business has different risks from a multinational device manufacturer, but both must identify the external and internal factors that affect their ability to produce conforming products. External factors may include regulatory change, supplier concentration, import restrictions, technological development, market growth and enforcement activity. Internal factors may include staff competence, equipment age, site capacity, financial pressure, data systems and organisational structure. This review should not become an abstract corporate exercise. It should lead to practical conclusions about where the system is vulnerable and which controls require strengthening.

Interested parties should be considered in the same manner. Regulators require compliance and access to evidence. Consumers require product consistency and truthful information. Retailers require reliable supply and manageable returns. Laboratories require representative samples and clear test requests. Suppliers require defined specifications and feedback. Insurers, certification bodies and investors may require evidence of controlled risk. These expectations can conflict, and the quality system must resolve them without allowing commercial convenience to displace regulatory obligation.

Risk-based thinking is one of the most important ISO 9001 principles for nicotine-product manufacture. Not every material, process or failure carries the same consequence, and controls should reflect the level of risk. An error in decorative carton colour is not equivalent to an error in nicotine concentration, child-resistant closure or coil material. A supplier of outer packaging does not require the same technical scrutiny as a supplier of nicotine or heating elements. Risk assessment allows attention and resources to be concentrated on attributes that can affect product identity, exposure, legal status and consumer protection.

Risk-based thinking should begin during product and process design rather than being applied only after problems occur. The organisation should identify foreseeable failure modes, assess their consequences and determine how they will be prevented or detected. For a nicotine liquid, risks may include incorrect assay, inadequate mixing, oxidation, cross-contamination, mislabelling and packaging interaction. For a device, they may include battery failure, leakage, unstable power delivery, unsuitable materials, poor wick supply and component variation. The assessment should consider not only whether the failure can occur but whether existing controls would detect it before release.

The quality system should remain proportionate. Risk-based thinking does not require maximum control over every activity, nor should it become an excuse for minimal control wherever testing is expensive. The correct question is whether the selected control is sufficient for the consequence of failure. A critical raw material may require supplier audit, identity testing and periodic verification. A lower-risk consumable may require documented specification and incoming inspection only. The rationale should be recorded so that reduced testing or oversight remains an evidence-based decision rather than an undocumented economy.

Planning converts policy and risk assessment into objectives. Quality objectives should be specific enough to guide action and measurable enough to show whether improvement has occurred. General statements such as "maintain high quality" provide little operational value. More useful objectives might address batch-right-first-time performance, complaint recurrence, supplier non-conformance, traceability completion, CAPA effectiveness or analytical trend stability. The objective should have an owner, timeframe, method of measurement and response where performance falls short.

Targets require careful design because poorly chosen metrics can distort behaviour. A target to reduce deviations may encourage under-reporting rather than better control. A target to close corrective actions quickly may lead to superficial investigations. A target to reduce batch rejection may create pressure to widen specifications or repeat testing. Quality objectives should therefore measure meaningful system performance rather than rewarding the appearance of success. Their interpretation should consider context and unintended incentives.

Support processes provide the resources through which the system operates. Competent personnel, suitable infrastructure, controlled working environments, calibrated equipment, information systems and organisational knowledge all fall within this area. For vaping manufacture, competence must extend beyond general production training. Personnel handling nicotine require understanding of its hazards and concentration control. Analysts require method-specific competence. Device assemblers need clear acceptance criteria.

Staff reviewing suppliers, deviations or changes require sufficient technical knowledge to recognise their regulatory significance.

Training records alone do not establish competence. Employees should be assessed through supervised practice, observation, test results or other evidence relevant to the role. An operator may have attended a training session while remaining unable to perform the process consistently. Competence should also be maintained when procedures, equipment or responsibilities change. A revised filling line, new aerosol method or different electronic system can make previous training incomplete.

Infrastructure must be suitable for the product and process. This includes buildings, utilities, production equipment, storage, laboratory systems and digital records. The required controls should reflect actual risk. Nicotine handling may require segregation, controlled access and spill arrangements. Flavour storage may require temperature or light protection. Trace-metal testing may require low-contamination facilities. Device assembly may require electrostatic or cleanliness controls. The environment should be monitored where it can affect conformity rather than because monitoring is expected generally.

Organisational knowledge is often overlooked. Experienced personnel accumulate practical understanding of formulations, suppliers, equipment and failure modes, but this knowledge can be lost when staff leave or roles change. ISO 9001 requires organisations to identify and maintain the knowledge needed to operate their processes. In practical terms, important decisions should not depend entirely on one person's memory. Critical process parameters, known incompatibilities, supplier history and investigation outcomes should be incorporated into controlled procedures, technical files and training.

Communication is another support function with direct regulatory importance. Information must move accurately between formulation, procurement, production, quality, regulatory and commercial teams. A supplier change known to procurement may require emissions retesting, but only if regulatory staff are informed. A complaint trend identified by customer service may signal a manufacturing defect, but only if the data reach quality personnel. A revised specification is ineffective if production continues using an obsolete version. Communication should therefore be defined as part of the process rather than left to informal relationships.

Documented information creates evidence that the system is planned and operating. ISO 9001 is less prescriptive about specific documents than older quality frameworks, but this flexibility does not reduce the need for adequate records. The organisation must determine what documentation is necessary to control its processes and demonstrate conformity. For nicotine-product manufacture, this normally includes specifications, procedures, batch records, test methods, supplier approvals, calibration records, deviations, CAPA, change controls, training, complaints and release decisions.

Document control ensures that staff use the current approved version and that changes are authorised. Obsolete formulations, component drawings or test methods should not remain available for accidental use. Records should be protected, retrievable and retained for a period consistent with regulatory and business needs. Electronic systems should preserve audit trails and access controls, while manual records should remain legible and attributable. The quality system should make it possible to reconstruct what occurred without relying on retrospective explanation.

Operation is the point at which planning becomes manufacture. The organisation must control production and service provision according to defined criteria. This includes approved materials, instructions, equipment, monitoring, release and management of non-conforming output. Operational control should focus on critical parameters identified through product and process understanding. Mixing time, temperature, order of addition, filling accuracy, coil resistance, sealing conditions and software version may all require defined limits where they influence the finished product.

Validation is appropriate where the output cannot be verified fully through subsequent inspection or testing. A mixing process, cleaning procedure or automated assembly may need evidence that it performs consistently under defined conditions. End-product sampling cannot confirm every unit, so confidence must come from process capability. Validation should establish operating ranges, critical variables, acceptance criteria and response to failure. It should be repeated or reviewed when changes affect the basis on which the original conclusion was made.

Release controls should ensure that products remain quarantined until required evidence has been reviewed. The authorised reviewer should confirm not only that selected laboratory results pass but that the batch record is complete, materials were approved, deviations were resolved, yields reconciled and correct packaging used. Release is a quality decision involving the total batch history rather than a clerical action following a passing certificate.

Non-conforming outputs must be identified and controlled to prevent unintended use or distribution. This may involve segregation, status labelling, system blocking, rework, rejection or destruction. The organisation should determine whether similar batches or products are affected and whether the issue requires escalation. Rework must itself be controlled because it can alter composition, stability or traceability. A failed batch should not be adjusted informally until it passes without an approved and scientifically justified procedure.

Performance evaluation determines whether the system is achieving its intended results. Monitoring should include product data, process performance, supplier results, complaints, audits, quality objectives and customer feedback. The purpose is not to collect every available metric but to identify evidence capable of revealing loss of control. Trends are often more valuable than isolated outcomes because gradual drift may remain within specification until it becomes significant.

Internal audits test whether planned arrangements are followed and effective. They should examine actual practice, records and outcomes rather than merely confirm that procedures exist. Auditors require sufficient independence and competence to challenge the process. Repeatedly auditing only administrative details while avoiding critical manufacturing or supplier controls creates false assurance. Findings should be graded according to significance, corrected and reviewed for recurrence.

Management review brings system performance to leadership. It should consider audit results, complaints, supplier performance, process trends, non-conformities, CAPA, resource needs, risks, opportunities and changes. A management review that consists only of reading metrics without decisions provides little value. The outcome should include actions, priorities and allocation of resources. It is one of the principal mechanisms through which senior leadership demonstrates that quality is integrated into business governance.

Improvement completes the operating cycle. Non-conformities, audits, complaints and performance data should lead to correction, corrective action or wider system change. Continuous improvement does not require constant alteration of products or procedures. Stability is desirable where processes perform well. Improvement means reducing unnecessary variation, strengthening detection, simplifying controls, improving supplier performance and preventing recurrence. It should be evidence-led rather than driven by fashion or certification expectations.

The Plan–Do–Check–Act cycle provides a useful model for understanding this process. The organisation plans requirements, risks and controls; performs production through the defined system; checks results through monitoring, testing and review; and acts on findings through corrective action and improvement. The cycle then begins again with better information. Its value lies in repetition. Quality is not established permanently through one audit, validation or certification decision. It must be maintained as products, suppliers, staff and regulations change.

Certification to ISO 9001 can provide external assurance that the organisation has implemented a quality management system, but certification should not be confused with product approval. The certificate normally confirms conformity of the management system within a defined scope. It does not establish that a particular vaping product is safe, compliant or manufactured correctly. The scope, certification body and activities covered should be examined. A company certified for distribution or general administration may not have its formulation or manufacturing operations within scope.

Audits conducted for certification are also based on sampling. Assessors cannot observe every batch, record or employee. Certification therefore provides structured confidence rather than a guarantee of flawless operation. Its value is greatest where the organisation uses the framework to control genuine risks rather than treating the external audit as the principal objective. A business that prepares records only before audit and returns to informal practice afterwards may retain a certificate while failing to sustain the intended system.

For regulators and commercial partners, ISO 9001 certification should be treated as one element of supplier or manufacturer assessment. It can indicate that formal processes exist, but product-specific evidence remains necessary. Specifications, batch records, testing, change control, traceability and complaint performance must still be reviewed. A quality system should support regulatory evidence, not substitute for it.

The strongest application of ISO 9001 in vaping manufacture is therefore practical and integrated. Product requirements are translated into process controls, responsibilities are clear, risks determine priorities, competent staff use current information, evidence supports release and performance data drive improvement. Supplier, manufacturing, analytical and post-market processes remain connected, allowing the organisation to identify where a failure originated and what must change.

ISO 9001 does not make a product compliant through the existence of procedures. It creates the conditions under which compliance can be reproduced, demonstrated and improved. Its real contribution lies in turning isolated technical activities into one controlled operating system. Where these principles are embedded in daily decisions, the product described in the regulatory dossier is far more likely to remain the product manufactured and supplied. Where they exist only as certification language, the appearance of control can become more developed than control itself.

Good Manufacturing Practice

Good Manufacturing Practice provides the operational discipline through which a product specification is converted into controlled and repeatable manufacture. Whereas ISO 9001 establishes the broader management principles of process control, responsibility, risk, documentation and improvement, GMP focuses more directly on the conditions under which products are made, handled, tested, released and stored. Its central purpose is to reduce the possibility that quality, safety or identity depend on chance, operator memory or final inspection alone. In vaping manufacture, this is particularly important because the finished product combines chemical formulation, pharmacologically active nicotine, inhalation exposure, packaging integrity and device engineering. Failures can arise from contamination, incorrect concentration, unsuitable materials, component substitution, inadequate cleaning, poor environmental control, mixing error, filling variation or mislabelling, and many of these cannot be detected reliably by inspecting a small number of finished units.

GMP should therefore be understood as a system of prevention. The strongest manufacturing operation does not wait for the quality-control laboratory to discover whether a batch is acceptable; it designs the process so that unacceptable manufacture becomes less likely, more visible and easier to investigate. Materials are approved before use, equipment is qualified, instructions are controlled, operators are trained, critical parameters are monitored and batches remain quarantined until the evidence has been reviewed. Testing still has an important role, but it confirms the operation of a controlled process rather than replacing it. This distinction is fundamental because no practical sampling plan can prove the condition of every bottle, pod, coil or device in a large batch.

The term GMP is used most formally within pharmaceutical regulation, where it is supported by detailed legal and technical requirements governing premises, personnel, documentation, validation, production, quality control, release and distribution. Consumer vaping products do not always fall within pharmaceutical GMP regimes, and it would be misleading to suggest that every manufacturer operates under the same legal obligations as a medicinal-product facility. The underlying principles nevertheless remain highly relevant. Nicotine concentration must be accurate, raw materials must be suitable, containers must protect the contents, labels must be correct and the product must remain consistent with the version that was assessed and notified. The level of control should be proportionate to product risk and regulatory status, but proportionality should not be confused with informality.

A GMP-oriented operation begins with suitable premises. The facility should support orderly material flow, controlled storage, safe handling and prevention of mix-up or contamination. The required design depends on the activities conducted, but the basic principle is that the environment should not introduce avoidable risk to the product. Raw materials awaiting release should be segregated from approved materials, rejected stock should be prevented from re-entering production and finished goods should remain under controlled status until release. Different nicotine strengths, flavour systems and packaging materials should be organised in a way that reduces the likelihood of selection errors. The physical arrangement of the site should support the intended process rather than force staff to rely on memory or temporary labelling.

Material and personnel flow should be considered together. Ingredients, waste, returned products, cleaning equipment and finished goods should not move through the facility in ways that create unnecessary cross-contact or confusion. High-strength nicotine handling may require designated areas, restricted access and controls appropriate to occupational exposure and spill response. Device assembly may require clean, dry environments and protection of sensitive electronic components. Packaging areas require strong line-clearance and reconciliation controls because a correctly manufactured liquid placed into the wrong labelled container becomes a serious regulatory failure despite the chemistry being correct.

The condition of the premises also matters. Surfaces should be cleanable and maintained, lighting should allow errors and contamination to be seen, and ventilation should be suitable for the activities conducted. Pest control, waste handling, drainage and storage should be managed in a way that protects materials and products. These requirements may appear routine, but weak environmental control often produces recurring quality problems that are treated incorrectly as isolated incidents. Dust, condensation, uncontrolled temperature, poorly maintained seals or cluttered storage can affect product integrity without causing an immediate and obvious failure.

Environmental conditions should be controlled where they influence product quality. Temperature can affect nicotine stability, solvent viscosity, filling accuracy and packaging performance. Humidity may alter hygroscopic materials, electrical components, labels or analytical standards. Light exposure can contribute to degradation of nicotine and sensitive flavour constituents. The appropriate controls should follow the product and process rather than being adopted as generic facility requirements. A manufacturer should be able to explain why a particular range is acceptable and how excursions are assessed.

Personnel competence is another essential GMP element. Operators should understand not only how to perform a task but why the critical steps matter. A mixing instruction may specify order of addition, temperature and time because these parameters affect homogeneity, viscosity or chemical stability. A filling-line operator should understand the significance of line clearance, nozzle condition and correct label selection. Device assemblers should know which component variations are acceptable and which require escalation. Training that consists only of reading and signing a procedure is weak evidence of competence unless performance is also observed and assessed.

Responsibilities should be defined clearly. Production personnel operate the process, while quality personnel review evidence, approve or reject materials and batches, investigate deviations and control changes. The exact organisational structure may vary with company size, but the release decision should not be compromised by the same production pressures that created the batch. Independence does not necessarily require a large separate department, yet there must be sufficient authority for quality concerns to stop production, prevent release or require further investigation.

Personal hygiene and protective clothing should reflect the materials and risks involved. Nicotine solutions require controls that protect both personnel and product. Gloves, protective clothing and spill arrangements may be necessary, but protective equipment can itself create contamination or handling problems if selected poorly. Eating, drinking and storage of personal items should be controlled in production areas. Illness, wounds or other conditions capable of affecting product handling should be managed through clear procedures. The purpose is not ceremonial cleanliness but reduction of contamination and exposure pathways.

Raw-material control begins before the material reaches the site. Each ingredient and component should have an approved specification that defines the characteristics necessary for its intended use. For nicotine and formulation ingredients, this may include identity, assay, purity, water content, density, impurity limits and storage requirements. For device components, specifications may include dimensions, materials, resistance, surface condition, electrical performance and compatibility. For packaging, they may include fill volume, closure performance, material composition, print accuracy and child-resistant function where applicable.

Receipt procedures should confirm that materials correspond to the purchase order and approved supplier. Containers should be inspected for damage, contamination, tampering and correct labelling. Each lot should be assigned an internal status and traceable identifier. Materials should remain in quarantine until the required review or testing is complete. The term quarantine is important because it establishes that physical possession does not equal permission to use. A material can be present on site while remaining unavailable to production.

Sampling should be performed through controlled procedures. The sampling tool, location, quantity and container should be suitable for the material and analytical purpose. Sampling can itself introduce contamination, moisture or mix-up if conducted poorly. The number of containers sampled should reflect the criticality and expected uniformity of the shipment. Highly critical materials or suppliers with uncertain performance may require more extensive verification, while a well-controlled supplier with strong history may justify reduced testing under a documented programme.

Identity testing is particularly important where selection error could create a significant risk. Containers can be labelled incorrectly, documentation can be copied from an earlier lot and visually similar materials can be confused. Reliance on a certificate of analysis without any form of identity confirmation transfers too much confidence to paperwork. The level of verification should reflect the material, but the organisation should be able to demonstrate that the ingredient or component used was the one intended.

Certificates of analysis should be reviewed critically. The specification, method, result, unit, reporting limit and lot identity must align with the manufacturer's requirements. A supplier statement that a metal is "not detected" is incomplete without a method and detection capability. A nicotine assay must be understood on the correct chemical and concentration basis. A flavour certificate may not disclose every constituent relevant to inhalation assessment. Supplier documentation supports control, but it does not remove the receiving manufacturer's responsibility to determine whether the material is suitable.

Released materials should be stored under defined conditions and protected against deterioration, contamination and mix-up. Stock rotation should be controlled, usually according to expiry or retest date rather than convenience. Opened containers may require shorter use periods or additional protection because repeated exposure to air, moisture or handling can change the material.

Labels should remain legible, and partial containers should retain traceability to the original lot. Decanted materials require particular care because the new container can lose the identity and status information carried by the original.

Equipment used in production should be suitable for its intended purpose. Mixing vessels, pumps, balances, transfer lines, filling machines, torque devices, aerosol equipment and assembly tools should have the capacity, materials and precision required by the process. Equipment that is technically capable of operating does not necessarily mean it is suitable. A balance may function correctly while lacking the resolution needed for a concentrated nicotine addition. A pump may dispense reliably at one viscosity but not another. A mixing system may be adequate for a laboratory batch but fail to achieve homogeneity at commercial scale.

Equipment qualification provides evidence that the installed system is appropriate and performs as intended. Installation checks confirm that the equipment has been supplied and connected correctly. Operational checks establish that it functions across relevant settings. Performance qualification demonstrates that it can operate consistently within the actual manufacturing process. The terminology and formality may vary outside pharmaceutical manufacture, but the underlying sequence remains useful because it separates possession of equipment from demonstrated fitness for purpose.

Calibration and maintenance support continued control. Balances, thermometers, flow meters, pressure devices, timers and other measuring systems should be calibrated or verified against appropriate standards. Maintenance should be planned rather than limited to repair after failure. Worn seals, damaged impellers, blocked nozzles and degraded sensors can influence product quality before complete equipment breakdown occurs. Records should show when work was performed, what was found and whether any previous batches might have been affected.

Cleaning is another critical area. Equipment and contact surfaces should be cleaned sufficiently to prevent carryover, contamination and product degradation. Shared equipment used for multiple nicotine strengths or flavours presents an obvious cross-contact risk. The cleaning method should specify materials, concentrations, contact times, rinsing, inspection and release. The process should be practical enough to be followed consistently and effective enough to remove residues relevant to the next product.

Cleaning validation or verification should reflect the risk. A visually clean vessel may still contain nicotine or strongly active flavour residue. Where carryover could cause a material concentration error, analytical evidence may be required.

Worst-case products can be selected according to nicotine strength, solubility, flavour persistence, toxicity or difficulty of removal. The acceptable residue should be scientifically justified rather than based solely on whether contamination is visible or organoleptically obvious.

Line clearance prevents remnants from a previous operation entering the next. Packaging areas are especially vulnerable because labels, cartons, inserts and closures can be mixed easily. Before a new batch begins, obsolete materials should be removed, the area should be checked and the clearance documented. This simple control is one of the most effective methods of preventing mislabelling. Its reliability depends on disciplined execution, particularly when commercial pressure encourages rapid product changeover.

Production should follow an approved master manufacturing instruction. This document should define the formula, quantities, material identities, order of addition, equipment, process parameters, in-process checks, expected yields and packaging requirements. The instruction represents the approved method of manufacture and should be controlled through formal change procedures. Operators should not modify quantities, mixing time or process sequence informally, even where the adjustment appears sensible, because the change may affect composition, stability or the regulatory basis of the product.

The batch record documents what actually occurred. Material lot numbers, quantities, equipment, process conditions, dates, operators, yields, in-process results and deviations should be recorded contemporaneously. Preprinted or electronic templates can reduce omission, but they should allow the actual event to be captured rather than encouraging automatic confirmation of expected values. Entries made long after the activity weaken confidence because they depend on memory and may conceal abnormal events.

Weighing and dispensing require particular control where concentrated nicotine or acids are involved. Each material should be identified independently, the correct container selected and the amount verified. Critical additions may justify a second-person check or electronic verification. Corrections for raw-material assay should be calculated through approved methods. Units should remain consistent, and conversions between mass, volume and nicotine equivalent should be controlled. A small calculation error at this stage can affect the entire batch while remaining invisible visually.

Mixing parameters should be defined according to process understanding. Order of addition, speed, time, temperature and vessel fill level can affect homogeneity and product behaviour. A nominal instruction to "mix until uniform" is insufficient where uniformity cannot be judged visually. The process should be validated or demonstrated to produce a homogeneous batch under expected operating conditions. Samples from different vessel locations or stages of the filling run can confirm that the selected parameters are adequate.

Scale-up requires careful evaluation because mixing behaviour does not increase proportionally with batch size. Larger vessels can introduce dead zones, slower temperature equilibration and different shear conditions. Transfer lines and hold times may also change. A formulation manufactured successfully at small scale should not be assumed equivalent at commercial scale without supporting evidence. Scale-related differences can affect nicotine distribution, flavour concentration, dissolved gases, oxidation and filling consistency.

In-process controls provide information before manufacture is complete. Depending on the product, these may include appearance, density, pH, nicotine concentration, fill weight, closure torque, resistance, airflow or leak testing. The value of an in-process test lies in its connection to a controllable stage. A result that identifies a problem only after all material has been packaged may still be useful, but it does not provide the same opportunity for intervention as a check performed during mixing or filling.

Filling operations require control of volume or mass, container supply, line speed, temperature and nozzle performance. Product viscosity can influence pump accuracy, while temperature changes can alter both viscosity and density. Beginning, middle and end-of-run samples help identify drift. Containers should be inspected for damage, and closures should be applied consistently. Underfilling creates a consumer and compliance problem, while overfilling can affect headspace, leakage and economic control.

Packaging operations carry a high risk of identity error. The correct bottle, label, carton, insert and nicotine declaration must correspond with the batch. Barcode, vision or electronic systems can reduce error, but they require validation and control. Printed materials should be issued and reconciled, with unexplained discrepancies investigated. Excess labels and obsolete packaging should be destroyed or controlled securely. A chemically conforming product packaged under the wrong identity is not an acceptable batch.

Device manufacture requires additional controls around components and assembly. Coil resistance, wire type, wick material, battery specification, electronics and software should be defined. Assembly processes should prevent damage, loose connections, contamination and incorrect orientation. Functional testing may include activation, airflow, leakage, charging, protection circuits and output stability. The test should be capable of detecting the failure modes relevant to the design rather than providing only a general indication that the device powers on.

Firmware and software require version control where they influence power delivery, safety functions or user settings. A change in firmware can alter the thermal and emissions behaviour of the product without any external physical modification. The version installed should be traceable to the batch, changes should be assessed formally and programming systems should prevent unauthorised or incorrect software from being loaded.

Closed-system products require control of the liquid–device interaction because the two parts form one operating product. A pod that meets fill and nicotine specifications can still perform poorly if its wick, coil or airflow differs. Release testing and periodic verification should therefore include appropriate functional or aerosol measures where these attributes are critical. The exact extent should remain risk-based, but chemical and mechanical control should not be treated as unrelated.

Process validation provides evidence that the manufacturing operation can produce conforming output consistently. It is particularly important where final inspection cannot verify every unit or where the process influences hidden characteristics. Mixing, filling, sealing, cleaning, automated assembly and software loading may all require validation. A validation study should use approved protocols, defined acceptance criteria, representative operating conditions and sufficient repetition to show consistency.

Validation should challenge the realistic operating range rather than demonstrate success only at ideal settings. Minimum and maximum batch size, normal equipment variation, different operators and justified parameter limits may need to be considered. The purpose is to define a reliable operating window. If the process works only at one narrow and difficult-to-maintain setting, the manufacturer should recognise that vulnerability rather than declare the process generally validated.

Deviations are inevitable in real manufacturing, and GMP requires them to be recorded and assessed. A deviation may involve temperature, mixing time, equipment malfunction, incorrect material status, documentation error or failed in-process test. The immediate response should protect the product, often through quarantine or suspension of the operation. The subsequent investigation should determine what occurred, why it occurred and whether the batch or related products are affected.

The significance of a deviation depends on its relationship to product quality. A brief delay in a non-critical stage may have no material effect, while a small error in nicotine addition may be critical. The assessment should rely on process knowledge, data and risk rather than on a desire to avoid rejection. Repeated minor deviations may indicate a systemic problem even where each event is accepted individually. Trend review is therefore essential.

Non-conforming materials and products should be segregated and controlled. Rejected stock should not remain accessible for accidental use. Rework or reprocessing should occur only under approved instructions and after assessment of product quality, stability and regulatory implications. Informal adjustment of an out-of-specification batch is particularly dangerous because it can obscure the original failure and produce a product whose history no longer corresponds with the approved process.

Quality control laboratories support GMP by testing materials, in-process samples, finished products and stability samples. Laboratory methods should be validated or verified, equipment controlled and records reviewed. The laboratory should remain sufficiently independent to report unfavourable findings without commercial interference. Results should not be repeated selectively until a passing value is obtained. Out-of-specification and atypical results require investigation through controlled procedures.

Batch release is the point at which the organisation accepts responsibility for supplying the product. The decision should be made only after review of the complete batch history, including material status, manufacturing records, in-process controls, analytical results, deviations, yields, packaging and labelling. Release should be documented by an authorised person with sufficient competence and independence. The reviewer should be able to withhold release where evidence is incomplete, even if production schedules or customer commitments are affected.

Storage and distribution remain part of GMP control because a conforming product can deteriorate after manufacture. Finished goods should be stored under conditions consistent with their stability and packaging. Temperature, light, stacking, handling and transport can affect liquids, seals, batteries and devices. Distribution records should preserve batch traceability. Contractors and warehouses should be qualified where their activities can influence product condition.

Returned goods require controlled assessment. Products may have been exposed to unknown storage, opened, damaged or tampered with, and should not be returned automatically to saleable stock. The organisation should define when return to inventory is prohibited, when inspection is sufficient and when destruction is required. Returned products can also provide information about distribution failures, counterfeiting or market complaints and should be linked to the wider quality system.

Stability programmes confirm that the product remains within specification over its intended shelf life. Representative production batches should be stored in the marketed packaging under defined conditions and tested at planned intervals. Nicotine concentration, degradation, appearance, pH, leakage, device function and other critical attributes may be included according to product design. Stability should not be treated as a one-time development exercise if materials, packaging, process or manufacturing site change.

Retention samples provide evidence for later investigation. Sufficient finished units and, where appropriate, critical materials should be retained under controlled conditions for a justified period. These samples allow comparison with complaint, market or enforcement units. Their identity and storage history must remain traceable. A retained sample has limited value if it cannot be linked confidently to the batch or if its storage conditions were uncontrolled.

Self-inspection and internal audit test whether GMP controls operate as intended. Audits should examine actual practice, records, material status, line clearance, training, cleaning, maintenance and deviation handling. The purpose is not to produce a favourable checklist but to identify weaknesses before they contribute to failure. Findings should be assessed by risk, corrected and reviewed for effectiveness. Repeated findings indicate that the underlying system has not improved.

Contract manufacture requires explicit division of responsibility. The brand owner, manufacturer, testing laboratory and component suppliers should understand who controls specifications, approves changes, releases batches, investigates complaints and retains records. Technical agreements should be detailed enough to prevent responsibility gaps. A company cannot assume that the contractor will manage an issue that the contract does not define, nor can it rely on commercial ownership as proof that technical oversight exists.

Audits of contract manufacturers should examine product-specific controls rather than only general certification. Shared equipment, line clearance, segregation, supplier management, change control and data access all matter. The brand owner should retain enough technical information to understand the product and respond to regulatory questions. Outsourcing should not create a situation in which the responsible company cannot identify the materials, process or test methods used for its own product.

Data integrity supports every GMP activity. Records should reflect what actually occurred, not what was expected to occur. Entries must be attributable, legible, contemporaneous, original or appropriately controlled, accurate and complete. Electronic systems should preserve audit trails and prevent unauthorised alteration. Manual corrections should not obscure the original entry. Backdating, copied results, pre-completed forms and unrecorded changes undermine the evidential basis of the entire quality system.

A culture of compliance is therefore as important as technical procedure. Employees must be able to record mistakes, stop processes and escalate concerns without pressure to hide them. Management should not reward only output, speed or low deviation numbers. A facility can possess modern equipment and detailed procedures while remaining weak if staff are encouraged to meet targets at the expense of accurate records and proper investigation.

GMP is most effective when it remains connected to product science. Process controls should derive from formulation, engineering, analytical and toxicological understanding. A critical parameter should be controlled because its effect is known or plausibly significant, not merely because a generic template includes it. The quality system should be able to explain why the parameter matters, how it is measured and what happens when it moves outside the approved range.

This scientific connection is particularly important for vaping products because emissions can change even when conventional finished-product tests remain acceptable. A liquid may pass nicotine and density specifications while generating different carbonyls because of a formulation or device interaction. A device may pass electrical inspection while releasing more metal after a component change. GMP control should therefore extend beyond simple release attributes to the materials, processes and changes capable of influencing aerosol performance.

Periodic product review brings the evidence together. Batch results, deviations, complaints, supplier performance, stability, changes, returns and analytical trends should be examined collectively. The review can identify gradual deterioration or repeated weaknesses that individual batch decisions miss. It also provides an opportunity to confirm that the product remains aligned with its regulatory file and that the manufacturing process continues to operate within the validated or established state.

Good Manufacturing Practice ultimately provides confidence that conformity is not accidental. It establishes that materials were approved, processes were defined, equipment was suitable, personnel were competent, records were complete and release was based on evidence. It also ensures that failures remain visible and that changes are assessed before they alter the product. The value of GMP lies not in the ceremonial use of pharmaceutical language, but in its insistence that manufacturing should be controlled deliberately.

For vaping products, this discipline supports both consumer protection and harm-reduction credibility. A category intended to provide an alternative to combustible tobacco cannot depend on inconsistent nicotine strength, uncontrolled emissions, unsuitable materials or unreliable devices. Product quality is part of the risk profile. When GMP principles are applied competently, the finished product remains connected to its formulation, technical assessment and regulatory identity. When they are absent, the marketed product becomes progressively less predictable, and every later claim about its composition, performance or comparative risk rests on weaker ground.

Supplier Auditing

Supplier auditing extends the manufacturer's quality system beyond the walls of its own facility and into the organisations that provide the ingredients, components, packaging, services and technical evidence on which the finished product depends. A vaping manufacturer may control formulation, filling and release competently while remaining exposed to failures originating elsewhere in the supply chain. Nicotine can arrive with an incorrect assay or impurity profile, flavour concentrates can change composition without notice, bottles can vary in dimensions or permeability, coils can be produced from substituted alloys, batteries can differ in protection circuitry and printed labels can contain errors capable of converting a chemically correct product into a regulatory failure. The finished product is therefore only as reliable as the network of suppliers contributing to it, and auditing provides one of the principal means of determining whether those suppliers possess the systems, technical capability and organisational discipline required to meet defined expectations consistently.

The purpose of a supplier audit is not simply to confirm that a company appears professional, possesses certificates or maintains a clean facility. It is to evaluate whether the supplier can produce the specified material or service under controlled conditions, whether deviations and changes are likely to be detected, whether records can reconstruct what occurred and whether the manufacturer will be informed before a modification affects the regulated product. The audit should convert commercial confidence into evidence. A long-standing relationship, low price, rapid delivery or good personal contact may support business continuity, but none establishes that the material remains within specification or that the supplier's process has not changed. Auditing provides a structured challenge to assumptions that might otherwise remain untested.

Not every supplier requires the same level of scrutiny. A risk-based classification should determine the depth and frequency of qualification. Critical suppliers provide materials or services capable of affecting product composition, exposure, legal status or core performance. Nicotine suppliers, flavour houses, acid suppliers, coil manufacturers, battery and electronics suppliers, aerosol-testing laboratories and contract manufacturers will usually fall into this category because failure can alter the product materially or weaken the evidence supporting it. Suppliers of lower-risk items, such as secondary packaging or non-product-contact office materials, may justify simpler approval based on specification, questionnaire and performance history. The distinction should reflect the consequence of failure rather than the cost or commercial importance of the purchase.

Supplier criticality can be assessed through several factors. These include the material's direct contact with the liquid or aerosol, its pharmacological or toxicological significance, the possibility of substitution, the complexity of the supplier's process, the availability of independent verification, historical performance, geographic and regulatory environment, and the ease with which failure would be detected before market release. A highly critical material with limited incoming testing and a single-source supply arrangement creates a greater audit need than a low-risk item that can be inspected completely on receipt. The assessment should be documented so that audit frequency and scope remain connected to risk rather than to convenience or personal preference.

The supplier qualification process normally begins before the audit itself. The manufacturer should define the required specification, intended use, applicable regulatory expectations and information needed from the supplier. Initial due diligence may include questionnaires, certificates, technical data, safety information, declarations of composition, sample testing, references, financial stability and review of public enforcement history where relevant. These activities help determine whether the supplier appears suitable enough to justify further assessment. They should not be treated as substitutes for auditing where the material or service is critical, because questionnaires are self-reported and can describe intended systems more favourably than routine practice.

The quality or technical agreement should establish the relationship formally. It should define the approved specification, testing responsibilities, certificate requirements, batch traceability, record retention, complaint handling, deviation communication, audit rights and change-notification obligations. For critical materials, the agreement should state which changes require prior approval rather than retrospective notification. A flavour supplier should not alter a constituent, carrier, manufacturing site or raw-material source without informing the customer where the change could affect toxicology, emissions or regulatory notification. A coil supplier should not change alloy, wire diameter, wick material, weld process or resistance tolerance under the same part number without assessment. The strength of the agreement is measured by whether it prevents silent product drift rather than by how comprehensive it appears on paper.

Audit planning should begin with a clear objective and scope. A general corporate audit may review the supplier's overall quality system, while a product-specific audit examines the processes directly relevant to the material or component purchased. The strongest approach combines both. The auditor should understand what is being supplied, how it affects the finished product and which process stages are critical. An audit of a nicotine supplier should focus on raw-material identity, synthesis or extraction controls, purification, impurity management, assay, packaging, storage and contamination prevention. An audit of a coil manufacturer should examine wire sourcing, alloy verification, winding, welding, wick insertion, cleaning, resistance measurement and component traceability. A generic checklist applied identically to both would miss the risks that matter.

The audit team should possess sufficient technical competence to evaluate those risks. Quality-system knowledge is necessary, but it may not be sufficient where chemistry, electronics, aerosol performance or specialist testing are involved. A lead auditor may understand documentation and corrective action while requiring support from a formulation scientist, engineer or analytical chemist. The team should also remain independent enough to challenge the supplier objectively. Procurement personnel may provide valuable commercial context, but the final assessment should not be softened because the supplier is strategically important or difficult to replace.

Preparation should include review of previous audits, complaints, deviations, incoming-test results, changes, late deliveries and certificate discrepancies. Trends often reveal where the audit should concentrate. Repeated variation in nicotine assay may justify detailed review of standardisation and release testing. Inconsistent coil resistance may lead to examination of winding controls and measuring equipment. Packaging leakage may require review of resin grade, mould maintenance and dimensional inspection. Entering the audit without this history risks spending time on general presentation while missing known weaknesses.

The opening meeting should confirm the scope, schedule, confidentiality, communication routes and access required. It should also establish whether any significant organisational, process or site changes have occurred since qualification or the previous audit. A supplier may have transferred production, installed new equipment, outsourced part of the process or changed its own raw-material supplier. These modifications can affect the purchased material even where the product code and commercial description remain unchanged. The auditor should compare current practice with the assumptions under which the supplier was originally approved.

Quality management should be examined as an operating system rather than as a collection of documents. The audit should establish who is responsible for quality, whether quality personnel have authority to reject materials or stop release and whether management reviews performance meaningfully. Procedures should correspond with actual operations, and staff should be able to explain how they use them. An organisation that produces polished documentation but depends on informal decisions presents a significant risk because control may weaken when experienced individuals are absent or production pressure increases.

Document control is an early indicator of system maturity. Specifications, work instructions, drawings and test methods should be approved, current and available where used. Obsolete versions should be removed from routine access, and changes should be traceable. For device components, even a small drawing revision can alter dimensions, airflow or electrical contact. For formulations or flavours, a revised composition can affect toxicological review. The supplier should be able to show which version applied to a particular batch and when the change became effective.

Training and competence should be assessed through evidence of performance rather than signatures alone. Operators should understand critical process steps, acceptance criteria and escalation requirements. Analysts should be trained in the methods they perform. Personnel approving changes or deviations should possess sufficient technical knowledge to evaluate product impact. The auditor may observe staff carrying out tasks, ask them to explain the process or review results from competency checks. A training file that contains attendance records but no evidence of practical competence provides weak assurance.

Control of the supplier's own supply chain is equally important. A supplier may itself depend on subcontractors, raw-material manufacturers, laboratories or component vendors. The audit should determine how these upstream sources are qualified, monitored and changed. A flavour house that purchases complex ingredients without composition control cannot provide strong assurance to the vaping manufacturer. A coil assembler that sources wire from several mills without alloy verification may create variability that final resistance checks do not detect. The manufacturer should understand which parts of the supply chain are genuinely controlled and which rely mainly on commercial trust.

Incoming-material control should confirm identity, status and suitability before use. The supplier should have approved specifications, receiving inspection, quarantine and release arrangements proportionate to risk. Certificates should be checked rather than filed automatically. Sampling plans, test methods and acceptance criteria should be appropriate for the materials concerned. The auditor should examine how the supplier deals with damaged, expired, unlabelled or discrepant stock and whether rejected material is segregated effectively.

Traceability should allow the supplier to connect the delivered lot to the materials, equipment, personnel, process conditions and test records involved. For complex components, this may require traceability through several manufacturing stages. The system should also support forward tracing so that affected customers can be identified if a defect is discovered later. The auditor should test traceability practically by selecting a recent batch and following it backwards and forwards through the records. A traceability system that works only when explained by one experienced employee remains vulnerable.

Process control should be examined at the point of manufacture. The auditor should observe whether critical parameters are defined, monitored and recorded, whether equipment is suitable and whether operators follow the approved instructions. For chemical suppliers, this may include reaction conditions, purification, blending, storage and contamination controls. For component manufacturers, dimensions, material identity, assembly conditions, cleaning and functional testing may be central. The audit should focus on variables capable of affecting the customer's product rather than on every routine activity equally.

Equipment calibration and maintenance provide evidence that process measurements can be trusted. Balances, thermometers, resistance meters, flow devices, dimensional gauges and analytical instruments should be calibrated or verified at justified intervals. The acceptance tolerance should relate to process need. A measuring device can possess a valid calibration certificate yet still be unsuitable if its uncertainty is too large for the specification being controlled. Maintenance records should also reveal whether equipment failures could have affected previously released batches.

Cleaning and contamination control are particularly important for suppliers handling multiple chemicals, flavours or nicotine strengths. Shared equipment can create carryover that remains below visual detection but alters the delivered material. Cleaning procedures should define methods, responsibilities and verification. Where contamination could be critical, validation or analytical confirmation may be required. The audit should examine actual cleaning records and changeover practice rather than relying solely on the written procedure.

Laboratory controls deserve close review where the supplier issues certificates of analysis. Methods should be suitable, validated or verified, and capable of measuring the attribute at the required level. Standards, reagents, calibration, blanks, calculations and data review should be controlled. The auditor should compare reported certificate results with raw data and determine whether out-of-specification or atypical results are investigated. A certificate has little value where the underlying method is unsuitable or where failing data can be repeated until an acceptable result is obtained.

Data integrity is central to this assessment. Records should be attributable, contemporaneous, complete and protected from unauthorised alteration. Electronic systems should use individual access, audit trails and controlled changes. Manual records should preserve corrections and original entries. The auditor should look for pre-completed forms, unexplained overwriting, repeated identical values, missing raw data or inconsistent timestamps. These indicators do not automatically prove misconduct, but they justify deeper investigation because the reliability of every certificate and release decision depends on the integrity of the supporting data.

Non-conforming material should be identified, segregated and prevented from unintended use. The audit should examine recent examples to determine how failures were assessed and whether related lots or customers were considered. Rework or reprocessing should be controlled and scientifically justified. A supplier that routinely adjusts failed material until it meets specification may conceal an unstable process, particularly where the history is not disclosed to the customer.

Deviation and CAPA systems should demonstrate the supplier's ability to investigate failure rather than merely document it. Root causes should be supported by evidence, corrective actions should address the system and effectiveness should be checked. Repeated recurrence of the same issue indicates weak analysis or ineffective action. The auditor should examine whether commercial pressure influences closure and whether significant deviations are communicated to affected customers promptly.

Change control is one of the most important elements of supplier auditing because uncontrolled change can invalidate product evidence without producing an immediate failure. The supplier should have a system for assessing modifications to materials, equipment, methods, sites, subcontractors, specifications and software. The customer-notification process should be explicit. The auditor should compare recent changes with contractual obligations and determine whether relevant customers were informed. A mature supplier recognises that a change can remain within its own internal specification while still affecting the customer's regulatory assessment.

Silent change is especially problematic where proprietary materials are supplied. A flavour concentrate may retain the same sensory profile while its chemical composition changes. A battery may retain the same nominal capacity while its protection circuitry or cell source changes. A plastic may retain the same grade name while additives or manufacturing location differ. The supplier may consider such changes commercially minor, while the manufacturer considers them regulatory or toxicological changes. The audit should test whether these differing perspectives have been resolved through clear notification criteria.

Complaint handling should reveal how the supplier responds to customer feedback. Complaints should be recorded, investigated and trended by product, batch and failure type. Returned samples should be evaluated where available, and findings should feed into CAPA or change control. A supplier that treats complaints purely as commercial returns misses valuable quality information. The auditor should also determine whether complaints affecting multiple customers are recognised as systemic rather than handled separately.

Recall and incident preparedness should be proportionate to the supplier's role. The organisation should know how to identify affected lots, notify customers and support containment. Mock recalls or traceability exercises can demonstrate whether the system works. For critical suppliers, inability to trace distribution rapidly can force broader action by the vaping manufacturer because uncertainty replaces targeted control.

Business continuity should also be considered where supply interruption could encourage uncontrolled substitution. Single-source materials, specialist components and proprietary flavours create dependency. The supplier should have plans for equipment failure, utility loss, cyber incidents, fire, contamination or loss of key personnel. The manufacturer should understand whether alternative sites or materials would be introduced automatically during disruption and whether those alternatives have been approved. Continuity planning should preserve quality rather than prioritise supply at any cost.

Environmental and occupational controls may also matter where they affect product integrity or legal compliance. Nicotine handling requires appropriate protection, spill control and waste management. Chemical manufacture may involve solvents or reagents whose poor control can create contamination or regulatory risk. Device-component manufacture may involve metals, plating or cleaning processes. The audit should remain focused on product and supply-chain risk, but serious environmental or safety weaknesses can indicate broader management failure and potential instability.

Audit evidence should be recorded accurately and linked to the requirement or risk concerned. Findings should distinguish between critical, major and minor non-conformities according to potential impact. A critical finding may indicate a direct risk to product safety, data integrity or legal compliance. A major finding may reveal a significant system failure capable of affecting multiple batches. A minor finding may involve a limited departure that does not indicate systemic loss of control. Classification should reflect consequence and scope rather than the auditor's personal preference.

The closing meeting should present findings clearly, confirm factual accuracy and explain the next steps. The supplier should understand what evidence is required and by when. The auditor should avoid negotiating away valid findings merely to preserve the relationship, but should also remain open to evidence showing that an initial interpretation was incomplete. The purpose is to improve control and determine suitability, not to create confrontation.

Corrective-action responses should be reviewed critically. A promise to retrain staff or revise a procedure is not sufficient unless it addresses the identified root cause. The manufacturer should assess whether immediate containment was adequate, whether related products were considered and whether the action can be verified. Documentary closure may be acceptable for lower-risk findings, while critical issues may require follow-up audit, additional testing or suspension of approval.

Supplier approval should have defined outcomes. The supplier may be approved, conditionally approved, restricted to certain products or rejected. Conditional approval should include clear limitations and timescales rather than becoming indefinite acceptance of unresolved risk. Where no alternative supplier exists, the commercial difficulty should be acknowledged, but it should not be mistaken for quality assurance. Additional incoming testing, reduced order size, batch-specific approval or enhanced oversight may be required until the weakness is corrected.

Audit frequency should reflect ongoing performance. A critical supplier with strong systems, consistent materials and effective change communication may justify a longer interval between on-site audits, supported by periodic review. A supplier with repeated deviations, unexplained changes, poor responsiveness or inconsistent data should be audited more frequently or reconsidered. Remote audits and document reviews can support oversight, but they are less effective where direct observation of process, premises or data integrity is necessary.

Supplier monitoring between audits is essential because an audit provides only a snapshot. Incoming test results, certificate accuracy, complaints, delivery performance, deviations, change notifications and responsiveness should be reviewed over time. A supplier scorecard can help identify trends, but the indicators should be weighted by risk. One delayed shipment is not equivalent to a concealed formulation change. Numerical scores should support judgement rather than replace it.

Performance review should consider both quality and communication. A supplier may provide technically conforming material but fail to notify changes or investigate complaints adequately. Another may communicate openly and correct occasional failures effectively. Trust is strengthened not by the absence of every problem but by evidence that problems are detected, disclosed and resolved competently. A supplier that never reports deviations may be exceptionally controlled or may simply have a weak reporting culture.

Second-party auditing by the manufacturer does not remove the value of third-party certification. ISO 9001, ISO/IEC 17025, GMP or other recognised certifications can provide useful baseline assurance, depending on the supplier's activity. Their scope and credibility must be examined. A certificate may cover only part of the site, a different product family or general management activities. Certification audits are also based on sampling and may not address the specific material supplied. Product-specific auditing remains necessary where the consequence of failure is significant.

The manufacturer must also audit outsourced service providers where their work supports regulatory decisions. Contract laboratories, warehouses, transport providers, sterilisation or cleaning services and regulatory data processors can influence product quality or evidence. A laboratory audit should examine method scope, sample control, raw data, uncertainty, reporting and subcontracting. A warehouse audit should examine status control, temperature, security and traceability. The same principle applies: outsourced activity remains part of the manufacturer's controlled system.

Auditing should not become a checklist exercise detached from scientific understanding. The most valuable findings often arise from following one material or batch through the complete process and asking how each control proves what the supplier claims. Checklists help ensure coverage, but they can encourage superficial compliance where every box is answered without examining whether the system works. An auditor should compare procedures with practice, certificates with raw data, specifications with process capability and promises with historical evidence.

The audit process itself should be controlled. Auditors should be trained, conflicts of interest managed, reports reviewed and records retained. Consistency matters because suppliers should not receive fundamentally different evaluations depending on individual style. At the same time, standardisation should not prevent technical judgement. A supplier audit is not an inspection of identical facts across every business; it is an assessment of whether a particular organisation can control a particular material or service.

Supplier auditing ultimately protects the continuity of the regulated product. The analytical and toxicological evidence generated during development assumes that ingredients, components and services remain consistent with those originally assessed. Every uncommunicated supplier change weakens that assumption. Every uncontrolled process, incomplete record or unsuitable test introduces uncertainty into the finished product. Auditing reduces that uncertainty by examining the systems behind the certificate, component code and commercial assurance.

The strongest supplier relationship is therefore neither adversarial nor passive. It is based on clear expectations, technical transparency, timely communication and evidence that both parties understand how the supplied material affects the finished product. A competent supplier should be able to explain its process, disclose relevant changes, investigate failures and demonstrate control without treating customer oversight as hostility. A competent manufacturer should define its requirements clearly, review data critically and avoid imposing generic demands unrelated to risk.

Supplier auditing converts supply-chain dependence into managed responsibility. It does not guarantee that no supplier will fail, but it improves the likelihood that weakness will be identified before it becomes product failure, that changes will be assessed before implementation and that incidents can be traced and contained. In vaping manufacture, where a hidden change in flavour composition, coil material or nicotine quality can alter exposure without changing the brand or appearance of the product, that function is indispensable.

CAPA Systems

Corrective and preventive action systems provide the formal mechanism through which a manufacturing organisation identifies failure, determines why it occurred, controls its consequences and reduces the likelihood of recurrence. Within a vaping quality system, CAPA connects deviations, laboratory failures, supplier non-conformities, complaints, audit findings, stability concerns, equipment problems and post-market signals to a structured process of investigation and improvement. Its purpose is not merely to record that something went wrong. It is to distinguish the visible event from the underlying cause, identify whether other products or batches may be affected and implement actions that strengthen the system rather than simply restoring production. A CAPA programme becomes credible when repeated problems decline, process understanding improves and actions remain proportionate to the risk presented. It becomes ceremonial when investigations are closed quickly, explanations are selected for convenience and the same failure returns under a different reference number.

The distinction between correction, corrective action and preventive action is fundamental. A correction addresses the immediate non-conformity. A leaking pod may be removed from sale, an incorrect label may be replaced, a failed instrument may be recalibrated or a batch may be quarantined. These steps contain the immediate problem but do not explain why it became possible. Corrective action addresses the cause of an existing problem so that recurrence becomes less likely. Preventive action addresses a potential problem before failure occurs, although modern quality systems often integrate prevention into risk management, trend analysis, change control and process improvement rather than operating a completely separate preventive-action programme. The terminology matters less than the discipline of moving beyond the visible event. Replacing one defective device may satisfy the customer, but it does not correct a weak assembly process. Repeating a nicotine assay may produce a passing value, but it does not resolve an unstable formulation or unsuitable analytical method. Retraining an operator may appear decisive, but it does not repair an ambiguous procedure, poorly designed workstation or unrealistic production target.

A CAPA system should therefore begin with reliable detection. Problems can enter the system through many routes, and each source provides a different perspective on product and process performance. Internal deviations reveal departures during manufacture. Out-of-specification and out-of-trend results identify analytical or process concerns. Complaints and returns show how products behave after distribution. Supplier notifications and incoming inspection expose weaknesses in purchased materials. Internal audits identify gaps between procedure and practice. Regulatory inspections, market surveillance and enforcement testing may reveal failures not detected internally. Stability programmes show whether the product changes during storage, while equipment records can expose drift before a formal product failure occurs. The organisation should define which events require immediate CAPA, which require preliminary assessment and which can be managed through routine correction or local improvement.

Not every event warrants the same level of investigation. A minor administrative error with no product impact should not consume the same resources as a nicotine-strength failure, component substitution or battery-safety concern. Risk-based triage is therefore essential. The initial assessment should consider severity, likelihood, detectability, distribution, regulatory consequence and potential exposure. A one-off typographical error corrected before packaging may require simple documentation. A recurring label discrepancy, even if detected before release, may indicate a systemic control failure and justify formal CAPA. A single report of unusual metallic taste may not establish a product defect, but it may require escalation where the batch also shows elevated metal results or where similar complaints are increasing. The system should direct attention towards events with the greatest potential consequence without allowing recurrent lower-level failures to accumulate unnoticed.

Immediate containment protects consumers, prevents further manufacture and preserves evidence. Depending on the event, containment may include stopping the line, segregating materials, placing batches on hold, suspending a supplier, preserving laboratory samples, disabling electronic release or notifying distributors. The action should be broad enough to control the plausible scope of the problem while the investigation proceeds. Containment is not the final solution, and it should not be confused with corrective action. Repeatedly quarantining affected batches without addressing the underlying process may reduce immediate exposure while demonstrating that the system has failed to learn.

The initial scope assessment should determine what may be affected beyond the unit or batch in which the problem was discovered. A nicotine failure may involve one preparation, all batches made from the same raw-material lot or a wider period affected by a calculation error. A leaking closure may affect one mould cavity, one packaging lot or every product using the same container and formulation combination. A coil-alloy discrepancy may extend across several brands supplied by the same manufacturer. The investigation should not assume that the discovered event defines the full boundary. Traceability records, production history, supplier data and analytical trends should be used to identify related products, batches, sites and customers.

Problem definition is the next critical stage. Investigations often fail because the event is described too vaguely. Statements such as "high nicotine", "device failure" or "customer complaint" do not define the conditions under which the failure occurred. A useful problem statement identifies the product, batch, observed result, expected result, time, location, test method and scale. It should distinguish fact from interpretation. "Three of ten finished units from batch A measured above the approved nicotine specification using validated method B" is more useful than "mixing error suspected". The suspected cause should not be embedded in the problem definition before evidence has been collected.

A clear chronology helps reconstruct the event. Investigators should establish when the relevant materials were received, when manufacture occurred, which equipment and personnel were involved, when samples were taken, when the failure was detected and what actions followed. Time sequence can reveal relationships that are not obvious from isolated records. An equipment maintenance intervention may precede a sudden shift in fill weight. A supplier change may correspond with increasing leak complaints. A new analyst or revised method may coincide with apparent laboratory failures. Chronology does not prove causation, but it directs the investigation towards plausible mechanisms.

Evidence should be collected before memories fade or records are altered. Batch documentation, raw analytical data, instrument logs, calibration status, environmental records, supplier certificates, training records, retained samples, complaint products and electronic audit trails may all be relevant. Physical evidence should be preserved where possible. A returned device should not be disassembled immediately if later examination of its original condition may be important. A failed batch should not be adjusted before representative samples have been retained. The investigation should protect the evidence needed to distinguish between product, process, analytical and user-related causes.

Root-cause analysis is the central intellectual task within CAPA. The objective is not to identify someone who can be blamed, but to determine which conditions allowed the failure to occur and escape detection. Human error may be part of the event, but it is rarely a sufficient endpoint. An operator may have selected the wrong material, yet the deeper questions concern why the materials were stored together, why the labels were similar, why electronic verification was absent and why the error was not detected before use. A laboratory analyst may have prepared the wrong dilution, but the system may contain an unclear worksheet, poorly controlled units or inadequate independent review. Stopping at "operator error" removes the opportunity to strengthen the process.

Several root-cause tools can support investigation, although none replaces technical judgement. The five-whys approach encourages repeated examination of why each preceding condition existed. Cause-and-effect diagrams organise potential contributors under headings such as materials, methods, equipment, personnel, environment and measurement. Fault-tree analysis works backwards from the failure through possible combinations of events. Failure mode and effects analysis can help assess whether the discovered event reflects a broader process vulnerability. Trend analysis can show whether the failure is isolated or part of a developing pattern. These tools are useful when they structure evidence, but they can become formulaic if investigators complete them mechanically and then select the most convenient explanation.

The investigation should examine all plausible causal categories. Materials may be incorrect, contaminated, degraded or inconsistent. Equipment may be unsuitable, worn, miscalibrated or maintained improperly. Methods may be ambiguous, unvalidated or applied outside their intended range. Personnel may lack competence, supervision or realistic time to perform the work correctly. Environmental conditions may affect viscosity, stability, electronics or measurement. Management systems may encourage shortcuts, fail to communicate changes or prioritise output over control. Several contributing causes may operate together, and forcing every event into one primary cause can oversimplify complex failure.

Analytical failures require particular care because the laboratory can reveal a genuine product problem or generate an erroneous result. The first phase should assess instrument performance, standards, sample preparation, calculations, system suitability, blanks, quality controls and method execution. Retesting may be justified where an assignable analytical cause is suspected, but the original result should remain part of the record until invalidity is demonstrated. Repeating analysis until an acceptable value appears is not an investigation. The decision to retest, resample or invalidate data should follow a predefined procedure and documented scientific reasoning.

Out-of-trend results may require CAPA even where specification limits have not been exceeded. A progressive increase in carbonyl emissions, shift in nicotine concentration or widening variability in coil resistance can indicate deterioration before formal failure occurs. The significance lies in the pattern rather than one result. Trend-based CAPA is preventive in effect because it allows the organisation to intervene before non-compliant product is released. The quality system should therefore review data over time rather than treating each batch as an isolated pass or fail.

Supplier-related failures require collaboration but not transfer of responsibility. The supplier may perform its own investigation, yet the manufacturer should review the evidence critically and determine whether the response addresses the risk to the finished product. A supplier statement that staff were retrained or that the issue was isolated may be insufficient where the delivered material changed composition, failed identification or affected several customers. The manufacturer should consider incoming containment, additional testing, alternative sourcing, audit or suspension of approval while the issue remains unresolved.

Complaints can also initiate CAPA when seriousness or frequency indicates a possible systemic problem. The organisation should avoid dismissing complaints because retained samples passed or because the consumer cannot provide complete information. Some failures occur intermittently, after storage or only under specific use conditions. Complaint investigations may require analysis of returned units, batch history, device age, usage pattern and related market data. Where a credible mechanism connects the complaint to manufacturing or design, corrective action should address the source rather than only responding to the individual consumer.

Once root causes and contributing factors have been identified, the CAPA plan should define actions, responsibilities, timescales and required evidence. Actions should be specific enough to implement and evaluate. "Improve training" is weak unless it identifies which competence gap will be addressed, how the training will change and how effectiveness will be assessed. "Revise procedure" is incomplete unless the revision removes the ambiguity or control gap associated with the failure. "Monitor supplier" provides little assurance without defining which attributes, frequency and acceptance criteria will be used.

The strongest corrective actions alter the system so that recurrence becomes less likely or more readily detectable. Engineering and automated controls are generally stronger than repeated reminders. Barcode verification may reduce material-selection errors more effectively than another instruction to check labels. Interlocked software may prevent use of an obsolete formulation more reliably than email communication. A redesigned fixture may eliminate incorrect component orientation. Improved specification, supplier control or equipment capability may prevent variation at source. Training remains valuable where knowledge or skill genuinely contributed, but it should not be the default action for every failure.

Actions should also be proportionate to the root cause. A one-time transcription error in a well-controlled system may justify local correction and review. A recurring calculation problem may require software redesign, independent verification and retrospective batch assessment. A defective component may require supplier CAPA and enhanced incoming inspection. A fundamental product-design weakness may require reformulation or engineering change rather than procedural adjustment. The investigation should not choose the least disruptive action when the evidence supports a more substantial response.

Preventive actions can arise from the same analysis. An event affecting one product may reveal similar vulnerability elsewhere. If two nicotine strengths are easily confused, the organisation should examine whether other materials share similar labels or storage conditions. If one coil supplier changed alloy without notification, other critical suppliers may require stronger change-notification clauses. If one laboratory method lacked adequate matrix specificity, related methods may warrant review. CAPA should therefore consider horizontal application across products, sites, suppliers and processes rather than treating every event as isolated.

Change control should govern implementation where the CAPA alters formulation, equipment, materials, software, process parameters, test methods or documentation. Corrective urgency does not remove the need to assess wider consequences. A revised wick material may reduce dry-puff complaints but change aerosol yield and nicotine delivery. A new cleaning solvent may improve residue removal while affecting equipment seals or introducing new contamination. A tighter fill tolerance may require equipment qualification.

CAPA and change control should work together so that solving one problem does not create another unexamined risk.

Interim actions may be necessary where permanent correction requires time. Increased inspection, additional testing, reduced batch size, supplier restriction or temporary procedural checks can provide containment while engineering or process changes are developed. These controls should have clear duration and ownership. Temporary measures often become permanent through inertia, leaving the organisation dependent on labour-intensive checks rather than resolving the root cause. The CAPA record should identify when interim controls will be removed and what evidence is needed before that occurs.

Effectiveness verification distinguishes completed action from successful action. A revised procedure, training session or component change does not prove that recurrence has been prevented. The organisation should define in advance how effectiveness will be measured and over what period. Evidence may include absence of recurrence across a specified number of batches, improved process capability, acceptable audit results, reduced complaint rate, successful supplier performance or stable analytical trends. The metric should relate directly to the original failure and root cause.

The verification period should be long enough to capture realistic recurrence. Checking one batch may be insufficient where the failure occurred intermittently or depended on a particular supplier lot. A complaint-related CAPA may require market data over several months. A stability concern may require testing at future time points. Premature closure creates an appearance of completion while the outcome remains unknown. Where immediate closure is required administratively, the system should retain an open effectiveness review with a defined future date.

Failure of effectiveness should reopen the investigation or generate a new assessment rather than being explained away. Recurrence may indicate that the wrong root cause was selected, that the action was implemented inadequately or that several causes remain. Repeated CAPA for the same issue is a strong signal of system weakness. Management should review whether investigations are sufficiently rigorous and whether actions are constrained by cost, authority or culture.

CAPA records should remain complete and auditable. The file should include the source of the issue, risk assessment, containment, problem statement, investigation, evidence, root-cause conclusion, impact assessment, actions, approvals and effectiveness verification. Decisions not to take further action should also be justified. The record should allow an independent reviewer to understand what happened and why the chosen response was considered adequate. Excessive narrative without evidence is no stronger than a brief unsupported conclusion.

Timeliness matters because delayed investigations can allow affected product to remain in circulation and evidence to deteriorate. The system should establish target periods according to risk, with escalation where deadlines are missed. However, speed should not become the sole measure of CAPA performance. A complex technical investigation may require laboratory work, supplier data or stability evidence that cannot be produced immediately. The objective is timely risk control and competent analysis, not rapid administrative closure.

Extensions should therefore be controlled. The reason, remaining work, interim risk controls and new completion date should be documented. Repeated extensions may indicate inadequate resources or weak management attention. A large backlog can also reduce investigation quality because staff close older actions hurriedly to improve metrics. Management review should consider both timeliness and the substance of the work.

CAPA ownership should be assigned to someone with authority and technical understanding. The quality function normally coordinates the system and challenges weak investigations, but responsibility for action belongs to the process owner. Production, engineering, procurement, regulatory or laboratory personnel may each lead relevant actions. Cross-functional involvement is often necessary because failures do not respect departmental boundaries. A nicotine-strength issue can involve purchasing, formulation, production, analysis and labelling. A device complaint can involve supplier control, engineering, software and customer service.

Quality personnel should maintain sufficient independence to reject unsupported root causes, require wider impact assessment and prevent closure without effectiveness evidence. They should not become the sole authors of every CAPA because process owners may then view the system as a quality-department exercise rather than an operational responsibility. The most effective model combines process expertise with independent quality oversight.

Training in investigation methods should focus on reasoning, evidence and bias. Investigators may favour explanations that protect their department, avoid costly changes or align with previous assumptions. Confirmation bias can lead them to collect evidence supporting the preferred cause while ignoring alternatives. Familiarity with the process can create overconfidence, while unfamiliarity can produce superficial conclusions. Structured review, peer challenge and cross-functional investigation help reduce these weaknesses.

Management oversight is essential because some corrective actions require investment, supplier change, production interruption or product redesign. Senior leadership should review significant and overdue CAPA, recurrent failures and resource constraints. Management review should consider trends by source, root-cause category, product family and effectiveness outcome. A rising number of CAPA may indicate worsening control, improved reporting or broader product growth, so raw counts should be interpreted carefully.

Quality metrics should be designed to encourage meaningful improvement rather than gaming. Useful measures may include recurrence rate, overdue high-risk actions, effectiveness failures, repeated root-cause categories, investigation cycle time and CAPA originating from complaints or audits. A target of reducing the total number of CAPA can discourage reporting. A target of rapid closure can reward shallow investigation. The strongest metric is whether the system detects and resolves problems before they cause repeated consumer or regulatory impact.

Risk management should be updated when CAPA reveals new information. A failure may show that an assumed control was ineffective, that the probability of occurrence was underestimated or that the severity is greater than expected. Product and process risk assessments should therefore be living documents rather than static records created during development. Updating them ensures that lessons from one event influence future control strategies and preventive planning.

Regulatory implications should be considered throughout the process. A confirmed change in composition, emissions, materials or performance may affect the product's notification or technical file. Serious defects may require authority notification, withdrawal or recall. CAPA should not be confined to internal manufacturing correction where the marketed product or regulatory representation has changed. Regulatory personnel should participate early enough to assess reporting obligations and avoid delayed escalation.

Recall and field action may become part of the CAPA where affected products have already been distributed. The decision should consider severity, exposure, distribution and traceability. The CAPA investigation supports the scope of the recall by identifying affected batches and causes, while the recall provides additional evidence about the scale and effectiveness of containment. Post-recall review should determine whether the action reached the intended market and whether further corrective measures remain necessary.

CAPA also supports continuous improvement where the original event is not a formal failure. Audit observations, process capability data, near misses and employee suggestions may identify opportunities to strengthen control before non-conformity occurs. A near miss is particularly valuable because it reveals that the system almost failed but was protected by chance or one person's intervention. Treating near misses seriously allows prevention without waiting for consumer impact.

The strongest CAPA systems therefore operate as learning mechanisms. They preserve evidence, challenge assumptions, connect individual events to systemic risk and verify that actions change performance. They do not regard every failure as proof of individual carelessness, nor do they allow complexity to become an excuse for inconclusive investigations. They recognise that quality problems often arise from the interaction of design, process, materials, measurement and organisational pressure.

For vaping products, this discipline is critical because many failures are not visible to the consumer before use. Incorrect nicotine concentration, unstable thermal performance, metallic release, contamination or silent component substitution may remain hidden behind familiar packaging and branding. CAPA provides the pathway through which such evidence is converted into containment, technical understanding and durable improvement. When it functions properly, the same problem should not continue to reappear simply because each occurrence was treated as a separate incident. When it functions poorly, the records may show continual activity while the manufacturing system remains unchanged.

Change Control

Change control provides the formal mechanism through which modifications to a product, process, material, supplier, method, site, system or document are assessed before implementation. Manufacturing systems cannot remain static indefinitely. Raw materials become unavailable, suppliers alter their processes, equipment reaches the end of its service life, analytical methods improve, regulations develop and products are redesigned in response to complaints, performance data or commercial need. The objective of change control is therefore not to prevent change, but to prevent unexamined change. It ensures that modifications are introduced deliberately, that their consequences are considered across the complete product system and that the regulated product does not drift away from the version originally designed, tested and notified without a documented decision.

For vaping products, this discipline is particularly important because apparently minor modifications can affect several product attributes simultaneously. A change in propylene glycol and glycerol ratio can alter viscosity, wick replenishment, aerosol mass and carbonyl formation. A different acid can change nicotine protonation, pH, sensory character and chemical stability. A revised flavour concentrate may maintain a similar sensory profile while introducing different inhalation constituents. A change in coil alloy can alter resistance, heat distribution and metal emissions. A new plastic grade may appear physically equivalent while interacting differently with the formulation during storage. Firmware changes can modify power delivery without any visible alteration to the device. Change control provides the structure through which these connections are examined before the modified product reaches manufacture or the market.

The starting principle is that the regulatory product is defined by more than its commercial name and external appearance. It consists of a particular formulation, material set, device configuration, manufacturing process, packaging system, performance profile and body of supporting evidence. Analytical reports, toxicological assessments, stability studies and emissions data apply to that defined configuration. When a component or process changes, the organisation must determine whether the existing evidence remains applicable. The fact that the label, product code or consumer proposition remains unchanged does not establish technical equivalence. Change control protects the continuity between the product described in the technical file and the product actually supplied.

A robust system begins by defining what constitutes a change. Without a clear definition, modifications may be introduced informally because staff consider them too small to justify review. Changes can originate in product development, production, engineering, procurement, quality control, information technology, regulatory affairs, warehousing or external suppliers. They may involve ingredients, concentrations, raw-material specifications, manufacturing instructions, equipment, utilities, packaging, analytical procedures, software, cleaning, storage, distribution or documentation. The system should capture both planned improvements and changes imposed by circumstances, such as discontinuation of a component, emergency repair or regulatory intervention.

The scope should extend beyond physical modifications. A revised calculation formula, altered sampling plan, new reporting limit or change in software access can affect the reliability of product evidence. Moving a procedural step from one department to another may alter responsibility and oversight. Reducing test frequency changes the level of assurance applied to the process. Extending a shelf life changes the period for which the organisation claims product stability. These decisions may not alter the product immediately, but they change the system through which conformity is demonstrated and should therefore be controlled.

Change requests should describe the proposed modification clearly enough for an independent reviewer to understand what will be different. Vague statements such as "new supplier", "process improvement" or "update method" provide insufficient basis for assessment. The request should identify the current state, proposed state, reason for change, affected products and processes, implementation timetable and urgency. Supporting material may include supplier data, revised specifications, drawings, test results, risk assessments or regulatory correspondence. The description should distinguish the intended change from its expected benefit. A proposal to replace a wick may be intended to reduce leakage, but that expected benefit remains a hypothesis until demonstrated.

The reason for the change affects the assessment but does not determine its acceptability. Cost reduction, supply continuity, quality improvement, regulatory compliance, safety, capacity increase and process simplification can all be legitimate drivers. Commercial importance should not reduce the level of scrutiny. A change required to avoid production interruption may be urgent, but urgency does not make the technical consequences disappear. The system should allow rapid review where necessary while preserving risk assessment, authorisation and traceability.

Changes should be classified according to potential impact. The terminology may vary between organisations, but categories such as minor, moderate and major are useful where they are defined consistently. A minor change has little plausible effect on product identity, safety, performance or regulatory status and may require limited verification. A moderate change can influence controlled attributes and requires targeted evaluation. A major change alters a critical material, formulation, process, site, device function or regulatory commitment and may require extensive validation, toxicological review, emissions testing or notification. Classification should follow risk and scientific mechanism rather than the department proposing the modification.

A change to decorative secondary packaging may be minor if no mandatory information, barrier function or product identification is affected. A new bottle supplier may be moderate or major depending on material composition, dimensions, closure compatibility and stability evidence. A replacement coil described as technically equivalent may still be major where alloy, geometry or wick design differs. The same type of change can therefore receive different classifications according to the product and its potential consequences. The organisation should document the rationale rather than rely on a generic list alone.

Risk assessment is the central analytical stage. The reviewers should identify how the proposed modification could affect composition, manufacturing capability, emissions, nicotine delivery, stability, packaging, labelling, consumer use and legal status. The assessment should consider direct and indirect pathways. Replacing a solvent supplier may affect impurity profile directly, while a slight change in water content may influence viscosity and aerosol generation indirectly. Increasing production scale may not change the formula, but it may affect mixing homogeneity, oxygen exposure, transfer time and fill consistency. The strongest reviews follow the change through the complete product system rather than examining only the immediate process step.

Existing risk tools can support this work, but the reasoning must remain product-specific. Failure mode and effects analysis can identify possible failure modes and existing controls. Hazard analysis can focus attention on consumer exposure and product safety. Cause-and-effect mapping can show interactions between materials, equipment and measurement. The selected method should help the team identify what could change and what evidence is needed. Completing a standard scoring table without technical discussion creates the appearance of assessment while leaving important mechanisms unexplored.

Cross-functional review is essential because one department rarely sees every consequence. Procurement may understand supplier availability but not emissions implications. Engineering may understand the device but not the notification requirements. Regulatory personnel may understand legal commitments but not manufacturing capability. Toxicologists may identify exposure concerns that are not visible through conventional release testing. Quality personnel coordinate the process, but formulation scientists, engineers, analysts, production staff and commercial teams may all contribute depending on the change.

The review should also consider the consumer interface. A modified airflow, flavour description, fill volume or device setting may alter how the product is used even if the underlying chemistry remains acceptable. A new closure may affect accessibility, leakage or child resistance. A firmware update may change user behaviour by altering power limits or warning messages. Regulatory assessment should therefore consider not only what the product contains but how the change influences use and foreseeable exposure.

Supplier-originated changes require particular control because they can occur outside the manufacturer's immediate visibility. Technical agreements should require suppliers to notify relevant modifications before implementation. These may include raw-material source, composition, manufacturing site, process, specification, equipment, test method, packaging or subcontractor. The receiving organisation should decide whether the change is acceptable and what additional evidence is required. A supplier should not determine unilaterally that a modification is insignificant to the finished vaping product, because it may not understand the formulation, device interaction or regulatory commitments involved.

Silent supplier change is one of the greatest threats to product continuity. A flavour house may alter a carrier or replace one constituent with a sensory equivalent. A plastics supplier may change an additive package while retaining the same grade name. A coil supplier may move production to another factory using different tooling. A battery supplier may substitute an internal cell or protection board. The component may continue to meet the supplier's own specification while changing an attribute important to the finished product. Supplier auditing and incoming verification reduce this risk, but formal change notification remains necessary.

Raw-material changes should be assessed beyond headline specification. Two grades of glycerol may meet the same purity requirement while differing in water content, trace impurities or processing history. Nicotine from a new source may meet assay but have a different impurity profile. A new acid supplier may provide material with equivalent identity and concentration but different residual solvents or elemental contamination. Flavour ingredients are particularly complex because proprietary mixtures may change without full compositional disclosure. Comparability testing should therefore focus on attributes capable of influencing product quality and exposure.

Formulation changes require clear distinction between adjustment and redesign. A small change in flavour concentration may appear minor, yet it can affect total chemical load, aerosol composition and sensory use. Changing acid type, nicotine form, solvent ratio or water content can alter thermal and delivery characteristics. The assessment should identify whether previous toxicological and emissions data remain representative. Where the product family has been grouped for testing, the change may also alter the worst-case rationale on which read-across depended.

Device changes can be equally complex. Coil resistance, geometry, wire composition, wick material, airflow, reservoir design, power management and firmware interact to determine aerosol generation. Altering one component can change the thermal system even where measured output remains within a broad electrical specification. Comparability should therefore include functional and emissions endpoints where the mechanism supports them. Visual similarity and nominal resistance do not establish equivalent performance.

Equipment changes require consideration of both capability and product impact. Replacing a balance with an equivalent calibrated model may require straightforward qualification. Installing a new mixing vessel, filling line or automated assembly system may require process revalidation because scale, shear, hold time, transfer design or accuracy can differ. Equipment relocation can affect utilities, environment and workflow. Software upgrades may alter calculations, access, audit trails or data transfer. The assessment should determine whether the new equipment reproduces the established process or creates a materially different one.

Manufacturing-site transfer is usually a significant change because it can affect multiple variables simultaneously. Even where the formulation, equipment type and instructions remain nominally unchanged, the new site may differ in personnel, environmental conditions, utilities, water systems, material flow, storage, cleaning and quality culture. Technology transfer should include controlled documentation, training, comparative batches, analytical testing and confirmation that process capability has been maintained. The receiving site should not be treated as equivalent merely because it belongs to the same corporate group.

Analytical-method changes also require formal review. A new method may improve sensitivity, specificity or efficiency, but it can create apparent shifts in historical data. Changing the instrument, column, extraction, calibration model or reporting limit may alter results even when the product is unchanged. Bridging studies should demonstrate comparability or explain the expected difference. Trend records should identify the transition so that later reviewers do not interpret a methodological change as product drift.

Changing test frequency or removing an analytical parameter can be significant even where the method itself remains unchanged. Reduced testing may be justified through strong process capability and supplier history, but it changes the level of assurance. The decision should be supported by data and accompanied by conditions under which testing will increase again. Eliminating a test because failures have not occurred is different from demonstrating that another control detects the same risk more effectively.

Packaging changes should consider more than appearance. Product-contact materials can affect stability, permeability, adsorption, leaching and closure performance. Bottle dimensions influence filling, labelling and child-resistant function. Seal materials can interact with acids or flavours. Headspace and closure torque can affect oxidation and leakage. Secondary packaging changes may alter light protection, mandatory information or traceability. Shelf-life evidence generated in one container should not be transferred automatically to another without assessment.

Labelling changes require regulatory and quality review because they can alter consumer understanding, legal compliance and product identity. Changes to nicotine strength, warnings, flavour description, batch coding, instructions or claims may carry different consequences. Even a layout change can obscure mandatory text or create confusion between strengths. Artwork should remain controlled, approved and reconciled with the product specification. A printing correction should not be introduced informally where it changes regulated information.

Cleaning and sanitation changes can affect carryover and material compatibility. A new detergent, concentration, contact time or rinse procedure may improve cleaning but leave residues, damage seals or alter equipment surfaces. The change should be assessed against the substances and equipment involved, and cleaning verification should be updated where necessary. The same applies to environmental or hygiene controls where changes affect contamination risk.

Documentation changes range from purely editorial revisions to modifications that alter how the process is performed. Correcting spelling without changing meaning may require limited control, while revising a calculation, acceptance criterion or operating instruction requires technical review and training. The change-control system should avoid becoming overwhelmed by trivial corrections, but the distinction between editorial and substantive change should be defined. A small wording change can be significant if it affects operator interpretation.

Temporary changes need the same discipline as permanent ones. Equipment breakdown, material shortage or facility work may require temporary procedures, alternative equipment or substitute suppliers. The temporary nature of the change does not reduce its potential impact. The approval should define its scope, duration, affected batches, controls and expiry date. Temporary arrangements should not remain in place indefinitely because the organisation repeatedly extends them without completing a permanent assessment.

Emergency changes may be necessary to protect safety, maintain critical operations or respond to regulatory action. The system should permit expedited authorisation by designated personnel, but the rationale, risk controls and retrospective review must remain documented. An emergency pathway should not become a convenient route for bypassing normal scrutiny. Once the immediate situation is controlled, the organisation should complete the full impact assessment and determine whether the change should be retained, revised or reversed.

The evidence required before approval depends on the assessed risk. This may include supplier qualification, material certificates, laboratory comparison, engineering studies, process trials, stability work, emissions testing, toxicological assessment, packaging compatibility, software validation or user evaluation. The study design should target the mechanisms through which the change could affect the product. Repeating every historical test may be unnecessary, but performing only convenient tests can miss the relevant consequence.

Comparability studies are central where the organisation claims that the changed product remains equivalent to the previous version. Pre-change and post-change samples should be tested under the same conditions using suitable methods. The endpoints should reflect the change. A new nicotine supplier may require assay and impurity comparison. A coil change may require resistance, aerosol yield, nicotine delivery, carbonyl and metal analysis. A packaging change may require closure, leakage, extractables and stability assessment. Equivalence should be defined in advance rather than inferred after reviewing favourable results.

Statistical comparison can support the assessment but should not replace scientific judgement. A small sample may fail to detect meaningful differences, while a large sample may identify statistically significant changes with little regulatory importance. The reviewers should consider effect size, variability, measurement uncertainty and toxicological relevance. The objective is to determine whether the product remains materially the same for its intended regulatory and quality purposes, not merely whether a particular statistical test returns a preferred result.

Process validation or revalidation may be required where the change affects critical parameters or process capability. A larger mixing vessel, faster filling line, revised sealing temperature or new assembly machine may alter the operating window. Validation should demonstrate that the modified process produces consistent output under routine conditions. Where the change affects only one element, targeted requalification may be sufficient. The rationale should identify which aspects of the original validated state remain applicable and which require new evidence.

Stability assessment should consider whether the change can affect performance over time. New materials, suppliers, packaging, formulation composition or manufacturing conditions may change degradation, leakage, adsorption or device reliability. Full long-term stability may not always be available before implementation, particularly where supply continuity is threatened. Accelerated or comparative data may support an initial decision, but ongoing studies and defined review points should follow. The organisation should not make a long-term shelf-life claim based solely on short-term evidence without acknowledging the residual uncertainty.

Regulatory impact assessment must occur before implementation rather than after commercial production has begun. The reviewers should determine whether the change requires notification, updated technical documentation, authority approval, revised labelling or no external action. Requirements differ by jurisdiction and product classification, but the internal question remains consistent: does the modified product remain within the scope of the existing regulatory submission and supporting evidence? Regulatory staff should document the basis for the conclusion.

A change can be legally significant even where it appears to improve product quality. Reformulation to remove a concerning ingredient may require updated notification. Replacing a coil to reduce metals may alter other emissions and device specifications. Moving manufacture to another site may trigger changes in responsible economic operators or records. Regulatory compliance should not discourage improvement, but improvement must remain visible and controlled.

Approval authority should match change significance. Minor changes may be approved by the relevant process owner and quality representative. Major changes may require cross-functional or senior approval, including regulatory, toxicological and engineering review. The approval record should show that required evidence was considered and that outstanding actions are understood. Conditional approval may be appropriate where some evidence will follow, but the conditions, restrictions and deadlines should be explicit.

Implementation planning should define when and how the change enters use. The organisation should identify affected documents, training, materials, inventory, product codes, test methods, software and supplier agreements. The transition between old and new states must be controlled. Mixed use of obsolete and revised components can create batches that correspond to neither approved configuration. Effective dates, lot segregation and line-clearance arrangements should therefore be defined.

Inventory disposition is often overlooked. Existing raw materials, components, packaging and work in progress may remain after a change is approved. The organisation should decide whether they can be used, returned, reworked or destroyed. Using old and new materials concurrently may complicate traceability and comparability. Where phased implementation is necessary, each configuration should be identifiable and linked to the relevant batch.

Training should occur before revised procedures or equipment are used. The affected personnel should understand both the new method and the reason for the change, particularly where critical controls differ. Competence may require demonstration rather than attendance alone. Training records should identify the version and implementation date. Staff who were absent during the transition should not return later and use obsolete practice.

Documentation should be updated coherently. Specifications, master manufacturing instructions, drawings, analytical methods, risk assessments, technical agreements, labels and regulatory files may all require revision. Changing one document while leaving related records unchanged creates contradiction. The change-control record should include a document impact list and confirmation that obsolete versions have been withdrawn.

First-production or validation batches may require enhanced oversight. Additional sampling, testing or review can confirm that the change behaves as expected under routine conditions. The batch should remain clearly identified so that performance can be compared with pre-change data. Where the change is significant, commercial release may be delayed until predefined criteria are met. Where conditional release is justified, the residual risks and monitoring requirements should be documented.

Post-implementation review determines whether the change achieved its intended purpose without creating new problems. The review may examine batch results, process capability, complaints, deviations, supplier performance, stability and emissions. The timing should reflect the type of change. Equipment performance may be reviewed after several batches, while stability or complaint effects require longer observation. The review should compare actual outcomes with the assumptions made during approval.

A change should not be considered successful merely because implementation occurred without immediate failure. Some consequences develop gradually or intermittently. A new packaging seal may leak only after storage. A revised coil may accumulate deposits differently over time. A new flavour may alter stability after several months. The effectiveness criteria should therefore correspond to the expected mechanism and product lifecycle.

Unexpected results should trigger reassessment. The organisation may need additional testing, process adjustment, CAPA or reversal of the change. The change record should remain connected to any subsequent deviations or complaints so that the relationship can be identified. Treating post-change failures as unrelated events weakens organisational learning.

Closure should occur only after required actions have been completed or transferred into controlled follow-up. The record should show the final approved state, evidence reviewed, implementation date, affected batches and any ongoing commitments. Open stability studies or regulatory submissions may continue after operational implementation, but their ownership and deadlines should remain visible. Administrative closure should not cause outstanding technical obligations to disappear.

Cumulative change deserves particular attention. Several modifications that appear minor individually can alter the product substantially over time. A new flavour carrier, revised wick, alternative battery supplier and different filling site may each be approved separately, while the current product becomes materially different from the version originally assessed. Periodic product review should therefore examine the complete change history and determine whether cumulative reassessment is required.

This is especially important where read-across or product grouping supports the technical dossier. A series of changes can invalidate the basis on which one representative product was used for several others. The organisation should revisit worst-case assumptions, emissions evidence and stability claims rather than assuming that each separate approval preserves the original conclusion automatically.

Metrics can help evaluate the performance of the change-control system. Useful indicators include overdue changes, emergency changes, implementation errors, post-change deviations, failed effectiveness reviews and supplier changes received without notice. Raw numbers require interpretation. A low number of changes may indicate a stable operation or a culture in which modifications occur outside the system. A high number may reflect rapid innovation or excessive procedural fragmentation. The key measure is whether changes are identified early, assessed competently and implemented without unintended product impact.

Audits should test the system by comparing current operations with approved records and tracing recent modifications from proposal through implementation. The auditor should look for equipment, materials, software or practices that changed without formal review. Purchase records, supplier communications, engineering logs and production observations can reveal unrecorded changes. The existence of a detailed procedure offers little assurance if staff do not recognise when it applies.

Leadership influences the integrity of change control because commercial pressure often surrounds modifications. A cheaper supplier, faster line or accelerated launch may offer immediate benefit, while the required testing appears to create delay. Senior management should support the principle that implementation follows evidence rather than precedes it. Where leaders repeatedly approve retrospective changes, staff learn that documentation is a formality and that production urgency overrides control.

Quality culture is visible in whether employees raise changes before acting. An engineer who replaces a component with a near-equivalent part, an analyst who adjusts a method or a buyer who accepts a new supplier may not view the action as significant. Training should therefore explain the breadth of change control and the reasons for it. The system should be accessible enough that staff do not avoid it because initiation is unnecessarily burdensome. Control must be rigorous without becoming so bureaucratic that informal workarounds appear easier.

Change control and CAPA are closely related but serve different purposes. CAPA responds to existing or potential failure, while change control manages the modifications introduced as a consequence. A CAPA may identify the need for a new supplier, revised process or equipment redesign. The change-control system then assesses and implements that solution. Not every change arises from CAPA, and not every CAPA requires a material change, but the two systems should remain connected. An urgent corrective action should not bypass assessment simply because it responds to a real problem.

Change control also supports continuous improvement by allowing innovation without loss of regulatory discipline. A mature organisation should be capable of improving formulations, reducing emissions, modernising equipment and strengthening packaging while preserving traceability and scientific evidence. The objective is not to freeze the product at the point of initial notification. It is to ensure that evolution remains deliberate, documented and supported.

The strongest change-control systems therefore do more than approve forms. They preserve product identity across time. They connect supplier decisions, scientific evidence, manufacturing capability and regulatory obligations. They require the organisation to ask not only whether the proposed change appears reasonable, but what else it could affect, which evidence remains valid and what must be demonstrated before the modified product can be treated as equivalent.

For vaping products, that function is indispensable because performance arises from interaction between chemistry, materials and device operation. A small modification can alter exposure without changing the name or appearance presented to the consumer. Change control prevents commercial continuity from being mistaken for technical continuity. It ensures that the product placed on the market remains connected to the evidence used to justify it and that improvement occurs through controlled understanding rather than undocumented drift.

Documentation Systems

Documentation systems provide the evidential structure through which a quality management system becomes visible, repeatable and auditable. Manufacturing processes may be technically sound, personnel may be experienced and products may perform consistently, but without controlled documentation the organisation cannot demonstrate reliably what was intended, what was performed, which materials were used, why decisions were made or whether the finished product remained connected to its approved specification. In vaping manufacture, this is particularly important because the regulated product is defined through a combination of formulation records, component specifications, manufacturing instructions, analytical methods, batch data, supplier information, labels, technical assessments and post-market evidence. Documentation holds those elements together. It converts operational activity into a traceable history and allows the organisation, regulator, auditor or investigator to reconstruct the product and the decisions surrounding it.

The function of documentation is broader than record keeping. Documents establish requirements before work begins, while records provide evidence of what occurred. A specification defines the acceptable characteristics of nicotine, solvents, flavours, coils, plastics or finished products. A procedure describes how an activity should be carried out. A master manufacturing instruction defines the approved process. A batch record captures the actual quantities, materials, equipment, operators, timings and results for one production lot. A test method sets out the analytical procedure, while laboratory records show how that method was applied to a specific sample. These distinctions matter because a quality system fails when intended requirements and actual performance become confused. A completed procedure does not prove that the process was followed, and a result without an approved method cannot be interpreted with confidence.

A strong documentation system begins with document hierarchy. Policy documents express the organisation's overall commitments and responsibilities. Quality manuals or system descriptions explain how the management framework operates. Procedures define the controls used for activities such as supplier approval, production, testing, deviation management, complaints, recalls and change control. Work instructions describe detailed operational steps. Specifications establish acceptance criteria, while forms and templates provide a consistent means of recording evidence. Technical files, risk assessments and reports explain the scientific and regulatory basis for product decisions. The hierarchy should be logical enough that staff can understand which document governs an activity and where the evidence should be recorded.

Excessive hierarchy can become counterproductive. Some organisations create multiple layers of policy, procedure, instruction and guidance that overlap, contradict or repeat one another. Staff may then rely on unofficial summaries or personal memory because locating the current requirement becomes difficult. Documentation should be sufficiently detailed to control the process, but not so elaborate that the system encourages workarounds. The quality of documentation is measured by whether it supports correct and consistent action, not by the number of pages generated.

Every controlled document should have a clear identity. This normally includes a title, unique reference, version number, approval status and effective date. The document should identify its scope, purpose and responsibility where these are not obvious. Revision history should show what changed and why. The current version must be distinguishable from obsolete versions, and uncontrolled copies should be identified where they are used for reference only. These controls prevent a formulation, drawing, method or instruction from remaining in use after it has been superseded.

Version control is especially important in vaping manufacture because small changes can alter the regulated product. A revised nicotine concentration, solvent ratio, flavour code, coil resistance or warning statement may appear minor within one department while carrying wider analytical or regulatory consequences. The documentation system should allow the organisation to determine which version of a specification or manufacturing instruction applied to each batch. If a complaint arises, the investigator should be able to identify the exact formulation, component drawing, analytical method and label artwork in force at the time of manufacture.

Approval should be performed by individuals with appropriate authority and competence. A quality procedure may require approval by the quality function, while a formulation specification may also require scientific and regulatory review. Device drawings may require engineering approval, and labels may require quality, regulatory and commercial confirmation. The approval pathway should reflect the risk and content of the document rather than relying on one generic signatory for every record. Approval signifies that the reviewer accepts the requirement and its consequences, not merely that the document has been read.

Effective dates should be planned to allow associated changes to be implemented coherently. A revised manufacturing instruction may require new training, updated materials, changed software fields or different sampling. Introducing the document before those supporting controls are ready creates a gap between approved instruction and operational capability. Delaying its use after approval can leave staff following an obsolete process. The implementation plan should therefore coordinate documentation, training, inventory, equipment and regulatory actions.

Document distribution must ensure that the current version is available where work is performed. In paper systems, controlled copies should be issued, tracked and withdrawn when revised. In electronic systems, staff should access the approved version through a controlled platform rather than saving local copies that may become outdated. Production areas, laboratories and warehouses should not depend on printed documents whose status is uncertain. The system should make the correct document easier to use than an uncontrolled alternative.

Access should also be proportionate. Personnel need sufficient access to perform their roles, while sensitive formulations, proprietary data and personal information require protection. Electronic permissions should control who can view, edit, approve or archive documents. Shared accounts weaken accountability because later review cannot determine who performed an action. Physical records may require locked storage, controlled issue or restricted areas. Confidentiality should protect information without obstructing legitimate quality and regulatory review.

Document review should occur periodically and when change makes the existing content inaccurate. A procedure may remain valid for years if the process is stable, while a rapidly evolving device or regulatory process may require more frequent review. Periodic review should not become a ritual in which documents are reapproved without examination. The reviewer should confirm that the procedure reflects current practice, responsibilities, equipment, regulations and associated records. Where the document remains suitable, that decision should still be recorded.

Obsolete documents should be removed from routine use but retained where they provide historical evidence. Destruction of every superseded version would prevent later reconstruction of past manufacture. Retained copies should be marked clearly as obsolete and protected against accidental reissue. The retention period should reflect product shelf life, legal requirements, complaint and recall needs, contractual obligations and the potential delay between manufacture and later investigation.

The documentation system should distinguish between controlled documents and records. A controlled document directs future activity. A record captures completed activity and should not normally be rewritten to reflect what should have happened. Batch records, laboratory worksheets, calibration results, cleaning logs, training assessments and complaint files are records. Once completed, they should preserve the original evidence, including errors and corrections. Altering a record retrospectively to make it conform with expectation undermines data integrity even where the final product appears acceptable.

Good documentation practice requires entries to be attributable, legible, contemporaneous, original or appropriately controlled, accurate and complete. Each entry should identify who performed the activity and when. Records should be made at the time the work occurs rather than reconstructed later from memory. Data should be entered directly into the controlled record where practical, rather than transcribed repeatedly through notebooks, scraps of paper and spreadsheets. Corrections should preserve the original entry, explain the reason where necessary and identify the person and date responsible.

Blank spaces and unexplained omissions create uncertainty. A blank field may mean that the step was not performed, not applicable, forgotten or recorded elsewhere. The form should provide a defined means of indicating non-applicability. Pre-completed records are equally problematic because they create evidence before the activity occurs. Repeated identical values, improbable timing and retrospective signatures are indicators that documentation may be functioning as an administrative reconstruction rather than a real-time control.

The design of forms influences the quality of the resulting data. Forms should guide users through the required sequence, provide enough space for meaningful entries and avoid ambiguous fields. A poorly designed form can generate systematic omissions even among competent staff. Drop-down menus and predefined options can improve consistency in electronic systems, but they can also force complex events into unsuitable categories. Free-text fields may be necessary where investigation or explanation is required, though they should not substitute for structured data needed for trend analysis.

Batch documentation is one of the central elements of manufacturing control. The master manufacturing record defines the approved formulation and process, while the executed batch record demonstrates how a particular batch was produced. It should identify the product, batch number, intended size, raw-material lot numbers, quantities dispensed, equipment, process parameters, operators, timings, yields, in-process results, deviations and packaging details. The record should connect the batch to its analytical and release evidence.

Preprinted theoretical values should be distinguished from actual values. A form may state the target quantity or operating range, but the operator should record what was weighed, measured or observed. Where equipment captures data automatically, the electronic record should remain linked to the batch and protected from alteration. Copying expected values into the completed record defeats the purpose of documentation because the record no longer reflects the process.

Reconciliation is a significant part of batch documentation. The quantity of materials issued, used, returned, rejected and destroyed should be understood. Yield should be compared with expectation, and discrepancies should be investigated. Packaging materials require similar control, especially where labels or cartons identify nicotine strength, flavour or warning information. Unexplained label discrepancies can indicate mix-up, loss or unauthorised use and should not be dismissed as minor inventory variation.

Equipment records should establish suitability and status. Calibration, maintenance, cleaning, repair and qualification should be documented in a way that allows product impact to be assessed. If a balance is found outside tolerance, the organisation should be able to identify which batches were weighed since the last acceptable check. If a filling line develops a fault, its maintenance record should show when the condition began and whether previous batches require review. Equipment logs become valuable only when they connect the event to production history.

Cleaning records should identify the equipment, previous product, cleaning method, date, operator and verification. Shared equipment used for different nicotine strengths, flavours or formulations presents particular risk. The record should show that the required cleaning occurred before the next product entered the system. Where analytical verification is required, the result should be linked directly to the equipment release decision.

Laboratory documentation requires the same discipline. The test request should identify the sample, batch, purpose, method and required decision. Sample receipt records should describe condition, quantity, storage and chain of custody. Raw data should include instrument output, calibration, standard preparation, sample preparation, calculations, chromatograms or spectra, integration decisions, quality controls and deviations. The final report is a summary of this evidence, not a substitute for it.

Analytical calculations should be controlled. Spreadsheets, instrument templates and laboratory information systems can reduce transcription error, but they can also replicate hidden formula mistakes across many results. Calculation tools should be validated or verified according to their complexity and use. Formula changes should be authorised and traceable. Locked cells, version control and independent checks reduce the risk that results depend on an uncontrolled local file.

Manual transcription should be minimised because each transfer introduces the possibility of error. Where transcription is necessary, a second-person check or electronic verification may be appropriate. The original source should remain available so that the transferred value can be confirmed. A result copied from an instrument into a worksheet and then into a report should not lose its connection to the underlying data.

Audit trails are essential in electronic systems. They should record who created, modified, approved or deleted information and when the action occurred. The previous value should remain visible where relevant, together with the reason for change. An audit trail that exists technically but is never reviewed provides limited assurance. Review should focus particularly on critical changes, deleted data, repeated reprocessing and actions performed outside expected times.

Electronic records require control of system access, backup, recovery, cybersecurity and long-term readability. Data may be secure against accidental loss while remaining vulnerable to unauthorised alteration or ransomware.

Backup systems should be tested rather than assumed to work. Archived records should remain accessible after software upgrades or system replacement. The organisation should consider whether proprietary file formats will remain readable throughout the required retention period.

Cloud systems and outsourced platforms introduce additional responsibilities. The service provider may host data, manage backups or control software updates, but the regulated organisation remains responsible for record integrity and availability. Contracts should define ownership, access, retention, security, incident notification and data export. A platform should not be selected solely for convenience if the organisation cannot retrieve complete records or audit trails when required.

Hybrid systems combining paper and electronic records can create gaps. A batch may be documented partly on paper, partly in spreadsheets and partly within enterprise software. The organisation should define which source is the official record and how the parts remain linked. Duplicate systems can produce conflicting versions, while scanned documents may lose metadata or legibility. The system should support reconstruction without requiring staff to search through multiple uncontrolled locations.

Data integrity depends on culture as well as technology. Staff may enter data inaccurately because procedures are unclear, workloads are unrealistic or managers reward speed over accuracy. Systems should not force personnel to choose between meeting production targets and completing records properly. If documentation is consistently late or incomplete, management should examine process design and resources rather than assuming that every omission reflects individual carelessness.

Regulatory documentation should remain aligned with manufacturing records. The technical file may contain the approved formulation, ingredient information, device specification, emissions data and risk assessment. The quality system should ensure that these documents correspond with current production. A change-control record should trigger review of the technical dossier where materials, process or performance are affected. The regulatory file should not describe an earlier product while manufacturing records show a series of undocumented changes.

Supplier documentation is part of the same system. Approved supplier lists, quality agreements, certificates, audit reports, change notifications and performance reviews should remain linked to the materials received. A supplier certificate should correspond to the correct lot and specification. Where a supplier changes its own method or manufacturing site, the evidence should be retained with the approval decision. Commercial correspondence may contain important technical information and should not remain isolated in individual email accounts.

Specifications are among the most important controlled documents because they define acceptance. Raw-material, component, in-process and finished-product specifications should identify tests, methods, limits and any relevant sampling or storage requirements. Limits should be scientifically justified and consistent with legal and regulatory commitments. A specification copied from a supplier or historical template may not control the attributes that matter for the actual product.

The relationship between specifications and methods should remain explicit. A limit is meaningful only if the method can measure it adequately. Changing the method may alter sensitivity, bias or reporting basis and therefore require specification review. The document system should prevent a test method from being revised independently while the associated acceptance criteria remain unchanged without assessment.

Drawings and bills of materials control device identity. The bill of materials should specify the approved components, versions and suppliers where necessary. Drawings should define dimensions, materials, tolerances and critical features. Firmware or software versions should be identified where they affect operation. The batch record should show which component lots and versions were used. Without this connection, the manufacturer cannot demonstrate that the commercial device matches the tested and notified configuration.

Label and artwork control deserve the same rigour because mislabelling can create direct consumer and regulatory risk. Approved artwork should be version-controlled, reviewed for mandatory information and linked to the correct product code and nicotine strength. Printer proofs, issued quantities and reconciliation should be documented. Obsolete artwork should be removed from use. A formulation can be chemically correct and still be non-compliant or unsafe where the label is wrong.

Training documentation should show more than attendance. Records should identify the procedure or task, version, date, trainer and outcome. Competency assessment may include observation, practical demonstration, examination or review of completed work. Retraining should be triggered when procedures change, performance indicates weakness or personnel return after a long absence. The documentation system should prevent untrained staff from performing critical work independently.

Deviation and CAPA records should preserve the reasoning behind quality decisions. The file should contain the event, immediate containment, evidence, investigation, root cause, impact assessment, actions and effectiveness review. It should distinguish fact from assumption and show why batches or products were accepted, rejected or recalled. Weak documentation can make a sound technical decision appear arbitrary, while extensive paperwork cannot rescue an unsupported conclusion.

Change-control records should identify the current and proposed state, reason, affected documents, risk assessment, testing, regulatory impact, approvals and implementation evidence. The change should link to revised specifications, training, validation and post-implementation review. This prevents change control from becoming a standalone form disconnected from the documents and processes it modifies.

Complaint records should capture product identity, batch, consumer description, seriousness, investigation and outcome. Structured fields support trend analysis, while narrative allows unusual circumstances to be recorded. Returned-product analysis, retained samples and supplier findings should be linked. Privacy requirements should be observed, but consumer data should remain sufficient for legitimate investigation and follow-up.

Recall documentation should allow the organisation to show how the scope was defined, which batches were affected, who was notified, what quantities were recovered and whether the action was effective. Distribution records should support rapid identification of recipients. Mock recall results should also be retained and reviewed. A recall plan without evidence of tested traceability provides weak assurance.

Record retention should be based on product lifecycle and risk. Manufacturing and testing records should remain available long enough to support complaints, stability, regulatory review and potential legal action. The period may need to extend beyond shelf life because products can remain in distribution, storage or consumer possession. Different record categories may justify different retention periods, but the rationale should be documented and applied consistently.

Archiving should preserve integrity and accessibility. Paper records require protection from moisture, fire, pests and unauthorised removal. Electronic records require validated migration, backup and readable formats. Records should be indexed so that retrieval is efficient. An archive that technically contains the information but cannot produce it within a reasonable period is operationally weak.

Destruction should also be controlled. Once the retention period has expired and no legal hold, complaint or investigation requires continued preservation, records may be destroyed through approved methods. Confidential and personal information should not enter ordinary waste. Destruction should be documented where required so that the organisation can show that records were removed deliberately rather than lost.

Documented information should support trend analysis and management review. If deviations, complaints, supplier failures and laboratory results are recorded inconsistently, meaningful comparison becomes difficult. Standardised codes, product identifiers and failure categories improve analysis. Excessive coding, however, can oversimplify complex events. The system should balance structure with the ability to preserve context.

Quality metrics depend on reliable documentation. Batch-right-first-time rates, complaint frequency, CAPA recurrence, supplier performance and process capability can only be interpreted when the underlying records are complete and comparable. Poor documentation creates false metrics that may lead management towards the wrong conclusion. The quality of the decision cannot exceed the quality of the data collected.

Internal audits should examine documentation in use rather than reviewing only written procedures. Auditors should compare records with physical operations, interview staff and trace samples or batches through the system. They should look for missing data, inconsistent versions, unexplained corrections and gaps between written practice and actual behaviour. A document system may appear compliant at the level of templates while failing in routine execution.

External auditors and regulators often use documentation as the primary route into the manufacturing system. They cannot observe historical production directly, so records become the evidence of what occurred. Incomplete or contradictory documentation creates doubt that extends beyond the missing entry. If one batch record is unreliable, confidence in related release and traceability decisions may also weaken. Documentation failures therefore carry a broader reputational and regulatory consequence.

The doctrine that work not documented may be treated as work not done can appear harsh, particularly where staff are confident that the activity occurred. It reflects the practical reality that unrecorded actions cannot be verified later. Quality systems require evidence capable of surviving staff turnover, memory loss and dispute. Documentation preserves organisational knowledge beyond the individuals who performed the work.

This does not mean that every operational detail must be recorded. Over-documentation can obscure critical evidence and burden staff with low-value entries. The system should identify which information is necessary to control quality, reconstruct the batch and support decisions. Records should be proportionate to risk. The aim is disciplined evidence, not documentation for its own sake.

Continuous improvement should include the documentation system itself. Recurrent errors, late completion, duplicated data or unused fields indicate that documents may be poorly designed. Electronic automation may reduce transcription and improve retrieval, but only where it reflects the actual process. Simplification can strengthen compliance if it removes redundancy without losing critical control. Staff feedback is valuable because those using the documents daily can identify ambiguity and impractical requirements.

The strongest documentation systems create one coherent version of product history. Specifications, suppliers, materials, manufacturing, testing, release, distribution, complaints and changes remain linked through consistent identifiers and controlled records. A reviewer can begin with a finished unit and trace backwards to the raw materials and decisions that produced it, or begin with a supplier concern and trace forward to every affected batch and customer.

For vaping products, this coherence is essential because composition and performance can change without obvious visual evidence. A consumer cannot determine whether a coil alloy, nicotine source, flavour composition or firmware version has changed. Regulators cannot assess continuity if the manufacturer cannot reconstruct it. Documentation systems provide the chain that connects the physical product to its scientific and regulatory identity.

Documentation is therefore not a passive archive created after manufacture. It is an active control that directs work, prevents obsolete practice, supports release, exposes deviation and preserves accountability. Where it functions properly, the organisation can demonstrate not only that a product met specification, but how that conclusion was reached and whether the same product continued to be produced over time. Where documentation is fragmented, retrospective or unreliable, every other quality-system claim becomes harder to trust.

Traceability

Traceability is the ability to reconstruct the history, application, location and status of a product, material, component or batch through recorded identifiers and connected evidence. Within vaping manufacture, it provides the link between the finished unit placed on the market and the nicotine, solvents, flavours, acids, packaging, coils, batteries, electronic components, production conditions, analytical results and release decisions from which that unit arose. It also allows the manufacturer to determine where affected products were distributed when a problem is discovered. Traceability therefore operates in both directions: backwards from the finished product to its origins and forwards from a material, component or batch to every product and customer potentially affected.

A traceability system is not simply a batch number printed on a bottle or carton. The code has value only when it connects reliably to controlled records capable of reconstructing the product. A consumer-facing batch code should lead to the manufacturing date, site, formulation version, raw-material lots, component lots, filling or assembly line, analytical data, deviations, release decision and distribution history. If the code exists visually but the underlying records are incomplete, inconsistent or inaccessible, traceability is largely cosmetic. The objective is not merely to mark the product, but to preserve the chain of evidence required to understand what it was, how it was made and where it went.

This function is particularly important for vaping products because different commercial units may appear identical while containing materially different internal configurations. A pod can retain the same external shape and branding while its coil alloy, wick material, resistance, liquid composition or firmware changes. Two bottles can carry the same flavour name while being manufactured from different nicotine or flavour lots. Consumers, retailers and regulators cannot identify these differences from appearance alone. Traceability provides the hidden connection between the marketed product and the precise technical configuration represented by its records.

Three forms of traceability normally operate together. Backward traceability identifies the origin of materials and components used in a finished batch. Internal traceability follows those materials and components through manufacturing, testing, packaging and release. Forward traceability identifies the distributors, retailers, customers or markets to which the finished product was supplied. Weakness in any one direction limits the organisation's ability to investigate and contain failure. A manufacturer may know exactly which coil lot entered a batch but be unable to identify where the affected devices were sold. Alternatively, it may hold complete distribution records while being unable to determine which nicotine or flavour lot was used. Effective traceability requires the chain to remain intact from supplier to market.

Backward traceability begins with approved supplier and purchasing information. Each received material should be identified by supplier, supplier lot, internal receipt number, date, quantity and status. The organisation should be able to determine which purchase order and specification applied, whether the material passed incoming review and whether any supplier deviation or change notification affected it. A certificate of analysis should correspond to the precise lot received rather than to a generic product or earlier shipment. Where one delivery contains several supplier lots, each should remain distinguishable rather than being merged administratively into one internal code without preserving the original identities.

Internal relabelling must retain this connection. A drum of glycerol, nicotine solution or flavour concentrate may receive an internal warehouse label after receipt, but that new identifier should map back to the supplier lot and supporting documents. Decanting presents a common risk because material transferred into a smaller container can lose its original identity, expiry, storage requirement or release status. The receiving container should therefore carry sufficient information to preserve the chain, including the internal lot, material name, status, date and, where relevant, the person responsible for transfer.

Where raw materials are blended or repacked before use, traceability should show how the new lot was created. If several supplier lots are combined into one internal stock, the resulting code should connect to every contributing lot and the quantities involved. This allows later assessment of whether a defect associated with one source may have affected the full combined stock. Blending can improve uniformity operationally, but it can also broaden the scope of an investigation because one unsuitable lot becomes distributed through a larger quantity of material.

Nicotine requires particularly strong traceability because assay, impurity profile, form and storage history influence the finished product directly. Records should identify the nicotine supplier, lot, assay, chemical form, received concentration, expiry or retest date and any correction applied during formulation. Where nicotine is diluted into an intermediate stock, the preparation record should show the parent lot, quantities, solvent, final concentration, analytical verification and storage conditions. Every finished batch using that intermediate should then remain linked to it.

Flavour preparations can be more difficult because they are often proprietary mixtures supplied under commercial codes. Traceability should preserve the exact supplier code, lot and formulation version where available. If the flavour supplier changes the composition while retaining the same trade name, the manufacturer must be able to distinguish pre-change and post-change material. A generic internal description such as "mango flavour" is insufficient where several formulations or suppliers exist. The lot record should connect to the compositional and toxicological information used in the product assessment.

Device components require comparable control. Coil assemblies, wicks, reservoirs, seals, plastics, batteries, circuit boards, mouthpieces and housings should be identified at the level necessary to investigate performance. The appropriate level may differ by component. A decorative outer shell may require supplier and batch identification, while a heating element may require more detailed traceability to alloy, resistance specification, manufacturing lot and assembly date. The system should focus particularly on components capable of altering aerosol generation, electrical safety, leakage, metal release or product identity.

Bills of materials provide the formal structure linking component identity to the approved product design. The bill should specify the correct part numbers, versions and, where necessary, approved suppliers. Production records should show which actual component lots were consumed. If different supplier lots are used within one finished batch, that mixture should be recorded. A statement that the product used the approved coil is insufficient where several approved versions exist with different materials or performance characteristics.

Firmware and software must also be treated as traceable product elements where they influence device function. The installed version may control power delivery, temperature limitation, activation, charging and safety features. A device batch should therefore remain connected to the firmware version loaded during manufacture. Programming equipment, software release records and verification checks should demonstrate that the intended version was installed. If a field update is later issued, the manufacturer should be able to identify which products are eligible, which versions were replaced and whether the update was completed.

Internal traceability follows materials through each manufacturing stage. For e-liquid production, this includes dispensing, mixing, holding, transfer, filling, packaging and release. The batch record should identify the raw-material lots and quantities used, the equipment, operators, process parameters and any intermediate containers. If bulk liquid is divided across several filling runs or packaging formats, each finished lot should remain connected to the original bulk batch. Conversely, if one finished batch incorporates material from more than one bulk preparation, that relationship must be visible.

Intermediate products require clear identity and status. A mixed bulk liquid may await analytical release before filling, or it may be approved for immediate transfer under defined controls. The container should show product, batch, quantity, preparation date and status. Unlabelled or ambiguously labelled intermediate material creates a serious risk of mix-up. Temporary handwritten descriptions should not become the primary traceability mechanism where the process depends on accurate identity.

Transfer between vessels, rooms or sites can break the chain unless each movement is recorded. Bulk liquid sent from one manufacturing site to another for filling should carry documentation identifying the product, batch, quantity, release status, transport conditions and receiving confirmation. If the receiving site assigns a new internal lot, the mapping between the two identifiers should be retained. The commercial organisation should be able to trace across company or site boundaries without depending on personal knowledge.

Filling operations may create several layers of identity. The bulk batch may be filled into different bottle sizes, nicotine strengths or market-specific labels, each requiring a distinct finished-product code. The records should show which portion of the bulk entered each packaging configuration and during which period of the run. Beginning, middle and end-of-run samples should remain linked to the time or container sequence they represent. If a filling issue is detected, this information can help determine whether the problem affected the complete batch or a limited period.

Packaging traceability is critical because labels and cartons define product identity for the consumer. Issued packaging material should be linked to artwork version, product code, nicotine strength, flavour and market. Reconciliation records should show quantities issued, used, returned and destroyed. If an incorrect label is discovered, the organisation should be able to identify which batches and packaging periods may be affected. Treating packaging as a low-risk administrative item ignores the possibility that a chemically correct product can become unsafe or unlawful through wrong strength, warning or language.

Serialisation may provide unit-level traceability where justified, although many vaping products are controlled at batch level rather than by individual serial number. Unit-level identification can be valuable for high-value devices, firmware management, warranty, counterfeit control and targeted field action. Its usefulness depends on the code being unique, durable, readable and connected to reliable data. Printing a unique number without controlling duplicate generation, database integrity or scan history creates little real assurance.

Aggregation can link individual units to cartons, cases and pallets so that movement through distribution is captured efficiently. When a pallet is dispatched, the system can identify all included cases and units. This supports rapid location of affected stock and reduces the need for manual reconstruction. Aggregation is particularly useful in large or international supply chains, but it requires disciplined packing, scanning and exception handling. Repacked, split or damaged cases must be recorded so that the hierarchy does not become inaccurate after the initial shipment.

Batch coding should be designed for readability, uniqueness and durability. Codes that are too faint, easily rubbed away or confused with dates create problems during complaints and recalls. The format should not generate duplicate codes across products, sites or years unless another identifier resolves the ambiguity. A code visible only on discarded outer packaging may not support investigation where consumers retain the device or bottle but not the carton. The placement should reflect how the product is likely to be stored and used.

Date coding can support traceability but should not substitute for a batch identifier unless the manufacturing system ensures uniqueness. Production date, expiry date and batch number serve different functions. The expiry date relates to shelf life, while the batch code identifies manufacture. Where codes are compressed into one format, staff, distributors and regulators should be able to interpret them correctly. Undocumented or proprietary coding systems can delay an investigation if only one employee understands them.

Traceability should also connect the batch to analytical evidence. The sample tested by the laboratory must be identifiable as originating from the batch concerned. Sample labels, test requests and chain-of-custody records should preserve that connection. A laboratory report that names only a commercial product without batch or sample identification cannot support a specific release decision confidently. The batch record should show which sample was tested, which method was used, which result applied and who reviewed it.

Retained samples should carry the same level of identity. A retention sample labelled only with product name and approximate date provides limited value during a complaint investigation. It should identify batch, manufacturing date, storage condition and, where relevant, component or packaging configuration. The quantity retained should be sufficient for the intended future analysis.

Storage records should show that the sample remained under appropriate conditions and was not confused with development or market samples.

Chain of custody becomes especially important where evidence may support enforcement, litigation or serious safety investigation. The organisation should be able to show who collected the sample, how it was sealed, where it was stored, who accessed it and when it was transferred. Tamper-evident controls, photographs and controlled access may be appropriate. The purpose is to prevent later doubt about whether the tested item was the same item originally collected and whether its condition changed during handling.

Forward traceability begins at batch release and distribution. Dispatch records should identify the finished-product code, batch, quantity, destination and date. Where products move through distributors, wholesalers or fulfilment centres, contracts should require those organisations to maintain sufficient downstream records. The manufacturer may not know the identity of every final consumer, but it should be able to identify the next commercial recipient and require that recipient to continue the chain. In a recall, delay often arises because information is fragmented across organisations that did not plan in advance how records would be shared.

Distribution records should remain accurate when stock is transferred, returned, relabelled, repacked or re-exported. Products may move between warehouses, markets or legal entities after initial release. If the system records only the first destination, later containment may fail. Returns should preserve batch identity and reason for return. Reworked or relabelled products should be assigned controlled status so that the history remains visible rather than overwritten.

Online sales create additional opportunities and challenges. Direct-to-consumer systems may capture order and batch information more precisely than retail distribution, but only where the warehouse records which batch was supplied to each order. Many systems track product code and quantity without recording batch at pick-and-pack. That may be sufficient for stock management but not for targeted consumer notification. The appropriate level of traceability should reflect risk, volume and technical feasibility.

Retail channels may break the chain because individual units are sold without recording batch information. The manufacturer should nevertheless maintain batch-level records to the retailer or distributor. Where a serious recall occurs, public notices, retailer stock checks and consumer verification of batch codes may be required. Clear coding and communication then become essential. A traceability system should be designed with the practical recall route in mind rather than only with internal audit needs.

Complaint handling depends heavily on traceability. Customer-service staff should request product name, batch code, purchase location, date and relevant photographs where possible. The complaint system should use standard identifiers so that reports involving the same batch or component can be grouped. A free-text description may preserve detail but cannot support efficient trend analysis if the product code is missing or entered inconsistently.

Not every consumer can locate or read a batch code, and the system should allow partial identification through packaging, purchase records, serial number, device configuration or distribution date. Unidentified complaints should not be discarded, but their evidential limitations should be recognised. If repeated reports arise from one retailer or period, distribution records may narrow the likely batches even where individual consumers cannot provide the code.

Returned products should remain linked to the original complaint and consumer information. Once received, the unit should be assigned an investigation identifier while preserving the visible batch or serial number. Photographs should document its condition before disassembly or testing. Components removed during examination should remain labelled. Without this control, the investigation can lose the connection between observed defect, tested component and original product.

Traceability enables complaint trends to be examined across more than one level. Reports can be grouped by finished batch, raw-material lot, coil lot, manufacturing line, supplier, firmware version or distribution channel. A pattern that appears weak at product level may become clear when connected to one shared component. Several branded devices may show similar failures because they use the same coil supplier. Several flavours may show colour instability because they share one nicotine or bottle lot. This cross-product analysis depends on the underlying identifiers being structured consistently.

Recall effectiveness is one of the clearest tests of traceability. When a defect is confirmed, the organisation should identify the affected scope rapidly and with evidence. The recall may begin from a finished batch, raw-material lot, supplier component or date range. The traceability system should show every affected product, quantity and destination. It should also support reconciliation between quantity manufactured, distributed, held, returned, recovered and destroyed.

Poor traceability expands recall scope because uncertainty replaces targeted action. If the manufacturer cannot determine which batches used a defective coil lot, it may have to recall every product manufactured during a broad period. If distribution records do not show where batches went, all customers may need to be contacted. This increases cost and disruption while potentially reducing response speed. Strong traceability allows the intervention to remain proportionate to the evidence.

Mock recall exercises should test the system under realistic conditions. Selecting a finished batch and tracing it backwards and forwards reveals whether identifiers connect across records and organisations. A reverse exercise can begin with a raw-material or component lot and identify every affected finished product. The test should measure completeness and time, not merely whether an answer can eventually be constructed. Delays caused by archived spreadsheets, absent staff or inconsistent codes are operational weaknesses that should be corrected before a real incident.

The exercise should include reconciliation. Quantities received, consumed, manufactured, rejected, retained, distributed and remaining in stock should be compared. Perfect numerical equality may not always occur because of normal losses, sampling and destruction, but discrepancies should be understood. A traceability chain that identifies records without accounting for quantities may miss stock that entered or left the system outside authorised routes.

Contract manufacturing requires explicit traceability responsibilities. The contract manufacturer may hold production and component records, while the brand owner holds distribution and complaint data. The laboratory may hold raw test records, and the importer may hold customs and market information. Technical agreements should define which identifiers are shared, who retains each record and how quickly data must be supplied during investigation or recall. A fragmented system can function only when these interfaces are designed before an incident.

The brand owner should retain enough information to fulfil its own regulatory responsibilities. It should not depend entirely on the contractor's willingness or continued existence. At minimum, it should be able to identify the manufacturing site, batch, formulation or device version, release evidence and distribution route. Where commercially sensitive details remain with the contractor, contractual access should be guaranteed for regulatory and safety purposes.

Supplier traceability should extend upstream where necessary. A coil assembler may purchase wire, wick and solder from separate sources. A flavour house may blend ingredients from several manufacturers. The immediate supplier should be able to identify the relevant upstream lots when a concern arises. The vaping manufacturer may not need direct routine access to every sub-supplier, but it should verify through qualification and audit that the chain exists and can be activated.

Complex proprietary supply chains create additional risk. A supplier may refuse to disclose detailed composition or source information for commercial reasons. Confidentiality arrangements can protect legitimate intellectual property, but they should not prevent investigation of safety or regulatory concerns. The responsible manufacturer must have a route to obtain enough information to assess affected products, even if some data are shared directly with a regulator, toxicologist or authorised third party rather than through normal commercial channels.

Counterfeit and diverted products create another traceability challenge. Genuine packaging, codes and identifiers can be copied, reused or fabricated. A valid-looking batch number does not prove authenticity. Serialisation, secure code generation, tamper evidence and verification databases can strengthen authentication, but no single feature is sufficient. The organisation should compare physical construction, distribution route, packaging details and analytical profile when counterfeit supply is suspected.

Duplicate or impossible codes may indicate falsification, but they can also result from weak internal coding. The manufacturer should ensure that its own system does not create avoidable ambiguity. Codes should not be reused across sites or years without a clear differentiator. Market surveillance should monitor reports of codes that do not correspond to production records or that appear in implausible quantities.

Traceability data are increasingly held electronically, and system design influences reliability. Enterprise resource planning systems, warehouse platforms, laboratory systems and complaint databases may each contain part of the chain. Integration reduces manual transcription, but mismatched product codes and data fields can create hidden breaks. The organisation should define master identifiers and ensure that each system uses them consistently or maps them through controlled tables.

Barcode and scanning systems can improve accuracy by reducing manual entry. Materials can be scanned during dispensing, components during assembly and finished products during packing and dispatch. Automated checks can prevent use of an unapproved or expired lot. These controls are powerful when validated and maintained, but they can create false assurance if labels are duplicated, scanners bypassed or software mappings incorrect. Physical verification and exception review remain necessary.

System validation should establish that traceability records are captured, stored, retrieved and protected correctly. Changes to software, code formats or integrations should be controlled. User access should prevent unauthorised alteration. Audit trails should record critical changes. Backup and recovery should be tested because traceability data become especially important during incidents, when system failure would have the greatest consequence.

Manual systems can also be effective where operations are smaller, provided they are disciplined and coherent. Controlled batch logs, warehouse records and distribution files may support full reconstruction without sophisticated software. Their weakness often lies in duplication, handwriting, local spreadsheets and dependence on one individual's knowledge. The system should remain retrievable and understandable by others, including after staff turnover.

Data quality is more important than technological complexity. An advanced platform populated with incomplete or inaccurate information provides weaker traceability than a simple system used consistently. Required fields, validation rules, reconciliation and routine review help maintain accuracy. Staff should understand that scanning or recording a lot is a quality activity, not an administrative inconvenience.

The level of granularity should be risk-based. Recording the supplier and batch of every critical component may be essential, while tracing every low-risk consumable individually may add little value. Excessive detail can burden operations and reduce compliance if staff regard the system as impractical. Insufficient detail prevents meaningful investigation. The correct level is the one that allows the organisation to identify and contain plausible failures without collecting information that has no realistic use.

Batch size influences the consequence of traceability granularity. A very large finished batch may incorporate several component or raw-material lots, broadening the potential recall if one becomes suspect. Smaller or segmented batches improve containment but increase record complexity and cost. The organisation should balance operational efficiency with the need to isolate failure. Where large batches are unavoidable, sub-lot or time-based identification can help narrow the affected portion.

Process segregation can improve traceability by preventing uncontrolled mixing of materials and configurations. Dedicated lines, defined campaign periods or staged component issue can reduce ambiguity. Where multiple lots are used during one run, the changeover point should be recorded. If the exact point cannot be determined, the affected scope should be widened conservatively. Accurate time stamps and consumption records can support more precise assessment.

Rework and reprocessing create special challenges because material leaves the ordinary sequence and re-enters later. The traceability record should show the original batch, reason for rework, method, quantity, destination and final status. Reworked material should not disappear into a new batch without preserving its history. The decision should also assess whether combining batches complicates stability, regulatory identity or future recall.

Waste and destruction records contribute to reconciliation. Materials rejected or destroyed should remain accounted for so that the organisation can show they did not enter unauthorised production or distribution. High-strength nicotine, labels and branded packaging deserve particular control because diversion could create safety or counterfeit risks. Destruction should be documented by quantity, identity, date and authorised personnel.

Samples consumed during testing should also be recorded where they affect quantity reconciliation. Laboratory, stability and retention samples may explain differences between manufactured and distributed totals. Without these records, normal quality activities can appear as unexplained stock loss. The system should avoid excessive precision where quantities are small, but the overall material balance should remain credible.

Traceability supports stability and shelf-life assessment by connecting stored samples to representative production batches. If a stability result changes unexpectedly, investigators should be able to review raw-material lots, packaging, process and related market batches. Where several products share packaging or ingredients, traceability may reveal whether the trend is product-specific or associated with a common material.

It also supports analytical trend interpretation. A rise in metal emissions may correspond with one coil lot, while a shift in nicotine assay may correspond with a raw-material or equipment change. Without traceability, the result appears as unexplained variation. With it, the organisation can identify plausible causes and design targeted investigation.

Regulatory submissions and notifications depend on the assumption that marketed products correspond to the assessed configuration. Traceability provides evidence that this continuity has been maintained. During inspection or technical review, the manufacturer may be asked to show that a tested or notified formulation matches current production. The organisation should be able to select a market batch and reconstruct the approved version, ingredients, components and release evidence without relying on retrospective assertion.

Where substantial changes occur, traceability should distinguish the pre-change and post-change populations. Effective dates, first affected batch and distribution should be clear. If a later concern is associated only with the revised version, the earlier product should not be included unnecessarily. Conversely, if the change point cannot be established, both populations may need to be treated as affected.

Traceability also supports legal accountability and commercial dispute resolution. Where a supplier denies that its material entered a failed product, lot records can establish the connection. Where a retailer reports receiving defective stock, dispatch records can confirm quantities and batches. Where a counterfeit product is alleged to be genuine, the code and distribution history can be examined. The system provides factual evidence where memory and commercial interest may differ.

Record retention must be long enough for traceability to remain useful throughout the product lifecycle. Records should remain available beyond manufacture and initial distribution because complaints, stability concerns and enforcement action may arise later. The period should consider shelf life, expected consumer possession, legal requirements and potential latency of product concerns. Destroying upstream or distribution records too early can make later investigation impossible even where the finished product remains in circulation.

Archived records should remain readable and retrievable. A batch code is useless if its supporting data are stored in obsolete software or inaccessible contractor systems. Migration, backup and contractual retention should therefore be planned. The organisation should periodically test retrieval from older records rather than assuming that archive status guarantees accessibility.

Internal audits should challenge traceability practically. Auditors can select a finished product and trace backwards to materials and forwards to customers, or select a critical raw-material lot and identify every affected finished batch. They should compare electronic and physical records, examine quantity reconciliation and identify manual breaks. The exercise should be performed without advance preparation where possible because an emergency will not allow weeks to reconstruct missing data.

Audit findings often reveal that traceability appears complete within departments but fails at interfaces. Procurement may use supplier lot numbers, production internal codes, the laboratory sample identifiers and distribution commercial stock codes. Unless those systems are mapped, the chain becomes difficult to follow. Cross-functional traceability tests expose these gaps more effectively than reviewing each department separately.

Management should review traceability performance through mock-recall times, reconciliation accuracy, coding errors, missing batch data and delayed supplier responses. Metrics should focus on operational capability rather than record volume. A system that captures extensive data but requires several days to identify affected customers may not meet the organisation's risk needs.

Training should explain why accurate traceability matters. Operators, warehouse staff and customer-service teams may see lot recording as routine administration until a complaint or recall occurs. Understanding the consequence of missed scans, unclear handwriting or discarded labels improves compliance. Staff should also know how to escalate mismatched, damaged or unreadable codes rather than correcting them informally.

Leadership determines whether traceability remains intact under pressure. Production urgency can encourage use of material before system receipt, manual substitution of components or delayed record completion. Commercial teams may distribute samples or promotional stock outside ordinary channels. Engineering may introduce trial components without clear segregation. Each shortcut creates a population of products whose history is less certain. Management should ensure that exceptions are controlled rather than accepted because the quantities are small or the deadline is urgent.

Traceability should not be treated as a system used only after failure. It supports daily control by preventing use of unapproved materials, identifying stock status, linking tests to batches and preserving product identity through change. It also creates the data needed for trend analysis, supplier review, stability assessment and continuous improvement. Its value increases when records are used actively rather than stored for hypothetical future investigation.

The strongest traceability system allows the organisation to begin with any important point in the product lifecycle and move confidently in either direction. From a consumer complaint, it can identify the finished batch, manufacturing conditions, component lots and suppliers. From a supplier concern, it can identify every affected batch, market and customer. From an analytical result, it can locate related products sharing the same material or process. From a regulatory change, it can distinguish which products and batches correspond to each technical configuration.

For vaping products, this capability is indispensable because many of the characteristics that determine exposure are not visible after manufacture. The consumer cannot identify the nicotine lot, coil alloy, flavour version or firmware from ordinary use. The regulator cannot verify continuity without records, and the manufacturer cannot contain failure without knowing where materials and products travelled. Traceability preserves that hidden history and converts product identity from a commercial label into an evidential chain capable of supporting investigation, recall and regulatory accountability.

Complaint Handling

Complaint handling is the process through which information from consumers, retailers, distributors, healthcare professionals and other external parties is converted into evidence about product quality, performance and potential risk. Within a vaping quality system, complaints are not merely customer-service interactions or reputational problems to be resolved through replacement, refund or apology. They are post-market signals that may reveal failures not identified during development, batch release or routine surveillance. Leakage, mislabelling, inconsistent nicotine delivery, burnt taste, metallic taste, battery malfunction, charging failure, colour change, unexpected harshness, contamination, packaging damage and device incompatibility may all first become visible through user reports. A competent complaint system preserves those reports, assesses their significance, connects them to the relevant product and batch, investigates plausible causes and determines whether corrective action, market withdrawal, recall or regulatory notification is required.

The importance of complaints arises from the limitations of pre-market and release testing. Development programmes examine selected samples under defined conditions. Batch release testing confirms that specified attributes were acceptable in the units tested. Neither process can reproduce every storage condition, distribution route, device age, consumer behaviour or intermittent manufacturing defect. A component may fail only after repeated charging, a seal may begin leaking after temperature cycling, a coil may behave differently after prolonged use and a flavour system may change after months of storage. Consumers therefore encounter product states that laboratories and production teams may not have observed directly. Complaint handling provides the route through which those real-world observations return to the quality system.

The system should begin with a broad and practical definition of a complaint. Any communication alleging a deficiency in the identity, quality, durability, reliability, safety, performance, packaging, labelling or regulatory status of a distributed product should be considered for complaint assessment, regardless of the language used by the reporter. Consumers may not describe the issue technically. A statement that a product "tastes wrong", "hits too hard", "does nothing", "gets hot", "spits", "leaks everywhere" or "does not last" may correspond to a formulation, device, packaging or use-related problem. Staff receiving the report should capture the observation without forcing it prematurely into a technical conclusion.

Not every negative comment is necessarily a quality complaint. Dislike of a flavour that conforms to specification may be a preference issue, while dissatisfaction with price or delivery may be commercial rather than technical. The organisation should define classification criteria so that genuine quality signals are not lost within general customer-service data and routine service matters do not overwhelm the investigation system. Where classification remains uncertain, the report should enter preliminary quality review rather than being excluded automatically.

All relevant routes of receipt should feed into one controlled system. Complaints may arrive through email, telephone, social media, retailer reports, distributor returns, online reviews, regulatory enquiries, sales representatives or informal messages to employees. A fragmented system creates the risk that each channel holds partial information and no one sees the complete pattern. Customer-service staff, commercial teams and social-media managers should understand which reports require escalation and how quickly they must be transferred to quality personnel.

The initial record should preserve the reporter's own description alongside any standard coding. Product name, nicotine strength, flavour, batch or serial number, purchase location, purchase date, date of first use, date of the event, storage conditions, device configuration and photographs may all be relevant. Where the complaint concerns a reusable or adjustable device, the power setting, coil type, liquid used, charging equipment and duration of use may be important. Where the complaint concerns a disposable or closed system, remaining liquid level, visible damage, leakage and activation behaviour may help define the failure.

The quality of the investigation depends heavily on the quality of this initial information. Staff should ask structured questions without leading the reporter towards a preferred explanation. A consumer who reports a burnt taste should be asked when it began, whether the product was new, whether the liquid level was low, whether the device had been used continuously and whether any visible damage occurred. They should not be told immediately that the product was probably used incorrectly. Leading questions can distort the account and create confirmation bias before technical review begins.

Consumer identity and contact information should be collected only to the extent needed for legitimate follow-up, privacy and regulatory purposes. The complaint record should remain linked to the individual where further information, medical follow-up or return of the product may be necessary. Personal data should be protected through controlled access and retention. Privacy requirements should not prevent adequate investigation, but unnecessary personal information should not be collected simply because the system allows it.

Product identification is one of the most important elements. Batch number, serial number, barcode, packaging code and photographs should be obtained where possible. Consumers often discard outer packaging, and codes may be small, faint or damaged. The organisation should design product coding so that the unit retained by the consumer remains identifiable. Where exact batch information is unavailable, purchase date, retailer, product appearance and distribution records may help narrow the likely manufacturing period.

Complaints without complete traceability should not be dismissed automatically. A report may still contribute to a wider signal, particularly where similar issues arise from the same market, product or period. The evidential weight is lower because the affected batch cannot be confirmed, but the observation remains relevant. The complaint system should distinguish between confirmed product identity, probable identity and unverified identity rather than treating all reports as either complete or useless.

Initial triage should assess seriousness, urgency and potential scope. The reviewer should consider whether the event may involve injury, fire, overheating, toxic exposure, incorrect nicotine strength, child access, contamination, mislabelling, counterfeit supply or another condition requiring immediate escalation. A report of minor cosmetic damage does not require the same response as a battery venting event or a product labelled at one nicotine strength but suspected of containing another. Triage should determine containment and investigation priority, not the final cause.

Serious events may require immediate action before the full investigation is complete. The organisation may place related stock on hold, suspend distribution, notify senior management, contact the reporter for urgent information or request return of the product. Where an event involves fire, injury or suspected poisoning, preservation of physical evidence becomes critical. The unit, charger, packaging, photographs, medical information and circumstances should be documented before the item is altered or discarded.

The complaint should be assessed for possible adverse-event reporting or regulatory notification obligations. Quality complaints and adverse events overlap but are not identical. A leaking product can be a quality complaint without reported injury. Dizziness or nausea may be an adverse event with or without confirmed product defect. The organisation should have a process for identifying reports that require clinical, toxicological or regulatory review and for escalating them within applicable timescales.

The complaint should also be assessed for possible counterfeit, tampered or diverted product. Packaging discrepancies, invalid codes, unusual construction, unexpected formulation or purchase outside authorised channels may indicate that the item did not originate from the approved supply chain. Counterfeit suspicion should not be used as a convenient explanation for every unexpected product, but it should be investigated where the evidence supports it. Authentication may require comparison of packaging, batch records, internal construction, chemical profile and distribution history.

Returned products provide valuable evidence but must be handled carefully. The organisation should issue clear instructions for safe return, particularly where the product has leaked, overheated or contains a damaged battery. The returned item should receive a unique investigation identifier while preserving the original batch or serial information. Its condition should be photographed and recorded on receipt before cleaning, disassembly or testing begins.

Chain of custody may be necessary where the complaint could lead to legal action, regulatory enforcement or significant recall. Records should show who received, stored, transferred, opened and tested the item. Tamper-evident packaging and controlled access may be appropriate. Even for routine complaints, clear sample control prevents units and components from being confused during investigation.

A returned product should not be assumed to remain in the same condition as when the event occurred. It may have been used further, exposed to temperature, cleaned, damaged in transit or stored for days before return. The investigator should compare the consumer's original account, photographs and receipt condition. Differences do not invalidate the complaint, but they affect which conclusions can be drawn from later testing.

Retained samples provide a controlled comparator. A retention sample from the same batch can be examined for appearance, nicotine concentration, leakage, device performance, emissions or other relevant attributes. If both returned and retained units show the same defect, a batch-related issue becomes more plausible. If only the returned unit is abnormal, the cause may be intermittent manufacturing variation, distribution damage, use conditions, tampering or isolated component failure.

Passing retained samples do not prove that the complaint is invalid. A batch may contain intermittent defects, and the returned item may represent one of them. Sampling and release testing cannot establish uniformity of every unit. The investigation should therefore consider the frequency and mechanism of the failure rather than using one conforming retained unit to dismiss the report.

The investigation plan should follow the failure mode. A complaint about nicotine effect may require verification of liquid concentration, fill volume, device output and aerosol delivery. A burnt taste may justify inspection of wick saturation, coil condition, airflow, power delivery and carbonyl emissions. Metallic taste may lead to examination of device components and elemental analysis. Leakage may require container dimensions, seal material, torque, transport and formulation-viscosity review. Applying the same standard laboratory panel to every complaint wastes resources and may fail to answer the actual question.

Batch and manufacturing records should be reviewed for deviations, equipment issues, process trends and component changes. The investigator should determine whether the affected unit was manufactured during an abnormal period, whether the same material lots were used in other products and whether complaints correspond with a known supplier or process change. The complaint may be the first external sign of a deviation already visible internally, or it may expose a condition that production records did not identify.

Supplier involvement may be necessary where the suspected cause lies in a component or raw material. The supplier should receive enough information and evidence to conduct its own investigation, but the manufacturer should retain oversight. Supplier conclusions should be reviewed critically, particularly where they attribute the failure to misuse without supporting evidence. The responsible product company remains accountable for the final assessment and action.

Complaint coding supports trend analysis. Each report should be assigned product, batch, market, failure mode, seriousness, cause status and outcome. Codes should be defined consistently so that similar events are grouped. "Leakage", "wet packaging", "liquid around mouthpiece" and "pod seepage" may represent one underlying category and should not be separated arbitrarily.

Conversely, broad categories such as "device issue" provide too little resolution to identify mechanisms.

Coding should not replace narrative. Complex or unusual events require detail that predefined categories cannot capture. The record should preserve the reporter's description, investigator observations and evidence. Structured data support statistical review, while narrative preserves context. Both are necessary.

Trend analysis should consider complaint rate rather than absolute count alone. Ten complaints from ten thousand units represent a different signal from ten complaints from one million units. Sales volume, distribution period and market exposure should therefore be incorporated where reliable. The rate may be expressed per thousand or million units, but the denominator should match the product and time period accurately.

Severity should remain visible within trend analysis. A low number of serious battery incidents may be more important than a high number of minor cosmetic complaints. Weighted systems can help, but they should not hide individual critical events within an overall score. Serious complaints should be reviewed separately even where the total complaint rate appears low.

Time trends can reveal process drift or delayed-life failures. Complaints may cluster shortly after manufacture, after several months of storage or near the end of device life. Plotting event date, manufacture date and purchase date can help distinguish immediate defects from ageing or distribution effects. A packaging seal that fails only after temperature exposure may not produce complaints until later, while mislabelling may appear immediately.

Geographic trends may indicate distribution, climate, retailer or counterfeit issues. Leakage concentrated in hot markets may suggest temperature-sensitive packaging performance. Failures associated with one distributor may indicate handling or storage problems. A cluster in a market with known counterfeit activity may require authentication review. Geographic concentration should guide investigation without becoming a substitute for product evidence.

Cross-product analysis can reveal common causes. Several brands or flavours may share the same coil, battery, bottle or nicotine supplier. Complaints recorded only under the commercial product name may appear unrelated until component traceability is examined. A strong complaint system allows data to be analysed by shared material, component, site and supplier as well as by finished product.

Complaint thresholds and escalation criteria should be defined, but they should not be applied mechanically. A threshold may trigger investigation when the complaint rate exceeds historical expectation, yet a single serious event may require action regardless of frequency. Conversely, a minor increase may reflect improved reporting or product growth rather than deterioration. Statistical signals require technical and contextual review.

Absence of complaints should not be interpreted as proof of product quality. Consumers may not report issues, retailers may replace products without informing the manufacturer and chronic exposures may not produce obvious immediate symptoms. Complaints are one source of post-market evidence and should be considered alongside market surveillance, analytical testing, returns, warranty data and regulatory information.

Root-cause analysis should distinguish confirmed cause, probable cause, possible cause and unresolved outcome. Some complaints cannot be reproduced or explained definitively. The system should not force certainty where evidence is incomplete. An unresolved complaint can still contribute to trend analysis and may become meaningful when similar reports accumulate. Recording it as "no fault found" should not imply that no defect occurred, only that the investigation did not establish one.

"No fault found" outcomes require caution because they can conceal inadequate test conditions. A returned device may pass basic functional checks while failing only intermittently, under heat, after repeated use or with a particular charging sequence. The investigation should attempt to reproduce the reported conditions where reasonable. Testing a product under ideal laboratory conditions may not address a complaint arising under foreseeable real-world use.

User behaviour should be considered without becoming the default explanation. Misuse, incompatible charging equipment, incorrect filling, operation outside recommended settings and poor storage can contribute to failure. The organisation should determine whether the behaviour was clearly contrary to instructions, reasonably foreseeable or encouraged by product design. A failure arising from common foreseeable use may still indicate that the product or instructions require improvement.

Where the complaint results from misunderstanding, labelling and instructions should be reviewed. Repeated reports of the same "misuse" may indicate that the product is not intuitive, warnings are unclear or design allows easy error. Quality systems should not place unlimited responsibility on the consumer where the manufacturer can reduce foreseeable failure through better design or communication.

Complaint disposition should identify both the individual response and the quality-system outcome. The consumer may receive a refund or replacement, but that commercial resolution does not close the technical issue. The quality record should show whether the complaint was confirmed, whether other units were affected, whether CAPA was opened and whether regulatory action was considered. Customer-service closure and quality closure are separate decisions.

Serious or recurring complaints should enter the CAPA system. The CAPA should address the underlying cause, affected scope, corrective action and effectiveness. Complaint data may provide the baseline against which improvement is measured. If a new seal is introduced to reduce leakage, subsequent complaint rates should be reviewed to confirm that the action worked. A fall in complaints may support effectiveness, but changes in sales volume or reporting route should also be considered.

Change control should govern modifications arising from complaints. Reformulating a liquid, changing a coil, revising firmware or replacing packaging may solve the reported issue while affecting emissions, nicotine delivery or stability. The urgency of complaint correction does not remove the need to assess wider consequences. The modified product should be supported by appropriate comparability and validation evidence.

A complaint can trigger market action before root cause is fully established where the potential consequence is serious. Batch quarantine, distribution suspension, targeted withdrawal or recall may be justified while investigation continues. The decision should consider severity, plausibility, distribution and uncertainty. Waiting for complete proof can expose more consumers, while disproportionate action can create unnecessary disruption. The complaint system should feed rapidly into the organisation's risk and recall decision pathways.

Communication with the complainant should be accurate and respectful. The organisation should acknowledge receipt, explain what information or product return is required and avoid promising a conclusion before investigation. Technical uncertainty should be communicated honestly. Statements that the product is safe because no fault has yet been found, or that the consumer caused the issue before evidence is reviewed, undermine trust and may create legal or regulatory difficulty.

Where an investigation is completed, the consumer should receive an appropriate outcome, although confidential technical or supplier information may not be disclosed in full. The response should distinguish what was confirmed from what remained uncertain. Where a safety issue is identified, clear instructions should be provided regarding product use, return or disposal.

Retailers and distributors should have defined routes for reporting complaints and returns. They may resolve minor customer issues directly, but quality-related information should still reach the manufacturer. Commercial agreements should require timely forwarding of serious or repeated reports. Retail staff should know how to preserve batch details and returned products rather than discarding them after refund.

The manufacturer should review whether intermediaries are filtering complaint information unintentionally. A distributor may report only issues that generate returns, while social-media teams may delete or respond to comments without quality escalation. Periodic reconciliation between customer-service, returns and warranty systems can identify missing signals.

Complaint records should be retained for a period consistent with product lifecycle, legal requirements and potential delayed investigation. The record should remain linked to returned units, photographs, laboratory data, correspondence, CAPA and regulatory submissions. Fragmented storage weakens later trend review and makes it difficult to reconstruct why a decision was made.

Electronic complaint systems should support consistent identifiers, audit trails, access control and reporting. Required fields can improve completeness, but rigid forms should not prevent capture of unusual events. The system should avoid duplicate records where the same issue is reported by consumer, retailer and distributor. Duplicate detection should preserve the separate sources while linking them to one event.

Data integrity applies to complaint handling as strongly as to manufacturing and laboratory records. Dates, product identity, seriousness and outcome should not be altered to improve metrics. Closing complaints without investigation, downgrading severity or splitting related reports can conceal emerging problems. Quality oversight should review coding consistency and significant closures.

Internal audits should examine complaint handling from receipt to outcome. Auditors should sample complaints across seriousness levels, compare source communications with system records, review timeliness, trace returned products and assess whether CAPA or recall decisions were justified. They should also test whether all complaint channels feed into the controlled system.

Management review should consider complaint trends, serious events, recurrence, investigation quality, overdue cases and effectiveness of actions. Raw complaint counts should be interpreted alongside sales and market exposure. Management should ask whether complaint data identify product, supplier or process weaknesses requiring investment. A review that treats complaints only as a customer-satisfaction measure misses their quality and regulatory value.

Timeliness should be monitored, but rapid closure should not become the dominant metric. Complex investigations may require supplier examination, laboratory testing or long-term observation. The priority is timely containment and competent conclusion. Overdue complaints should be escalated, and extensions should explain remaining work and interim risk controls.

Complaint-handling personnel require training in product knowledge, questioning, seriousness assessment, data protection and escalation. Customer-service staff do not need to become analytical scientists, but they should recognise which details matter and avoid speculative technical advice. Quality investigators require competence in failure analysis, manufacturing records, device operation and relevant regulation.

Leadership determines whether complaint information is welcomed or suppressed. Complaints can be commercially uncomfortable, particularly when they threaten a successful product or important supplier. A mature organisation treats them as evidence rather than as attacks. Staff should not be rewarded for minimising complaint numbers through restrictive classification or discouraged from escalating serious reports.

The strongest complaint systems create a closed information loop between the market and the manufacturer. Reports are captured consistently, serious events are contained, product identity is traced, evidence is investigated, trends are reviewed and actions are verified. The result is not merely better customer service but improved understanding of how the product behaves outside controlled development and laboratory conditions.

For vaping products, this function is essential because quality and exposure depend on interactions between formulation, device, storage and use. A complaint may be the first indication that a seal degrades, a coil varies, a liquid ages unexpectedly or a label has been applied incorrectly. When complaint handling is integrated with traceability, CAPA, change control and recall systems, these observations become actionable evidence. When it is treated only as a commercial nuisance, the organisation loses one of its most direct sources of information about the product actually experienced by consumers.

Product Recalls

Product recalls represent the most visible and operationally demanding response available within a quality system because they require an organisation to move from internal assessment to external intervention, often under conditions of uncertainty, commercial pressure and public scrutiny. A recall may be initiated because a product presents a potential safety risk, fails to comply with a legal requirement, does not correspond with its approved specification or has been manufactured under conditions that undermine confidence in its quality. In vaping manufacture, the initiating issue may involve incorrect nicotine concentration, mislabelling, contamination, battery malfunction, leakage, unsuitable materials, excessive emissions, defective child-resistant packaging, counterfeit substitution or an undocumented component change. The recall process must determine which products are affected, where they have been distributed, how consumers and commercial partners will be notified, what action they should take and how the organisation will verify that the intervention has been effective. These decisions must be made rapidly enough to protect consumers, but not so hastily that the scope becomes arbitrary or the communication creates unnecessary confusion.

A recall should not be understood as a single event or announcement. It is a controlled sequence of detection, risk assessment, containment, decision, notification, recovery, reconciliation, investigation and effectiveness review. The quality system should define this sequence before any incident occurs because the organisation will have limited time to design it while affected products remain in distribution. Responsibilities, communication routes, authority contacts, decision criteria, distribution records and record-retention arrangements should therefore be established in advance. A written procedure alone is insufficient if key personnel do not understand their roles, customer information is incomplete or batch records cannot be linked quickly to dispatch data. Recall readiness depends on whether the organisation can convert its documented system into action under pressure.

The distinction between withdrawal and recall should remain clear, even though terminology varies between jurisdictions and organisations. A withdrawal generally removes product from distribution before it has reached the consumer or where the concern does not require direct consumer action. A recall normally involves product already supplied to retailers, distributors or consumers and may require public communication. Some situations can be contained through quarantine of warehouse stock, suspension of shipment or return from trade channels without wider notification. Others require consumers to stop using the product immediately and return or dispose of it according to defined instructions. The classification should reflect distribution status and risk rather than the organisation's preference for less visible terminology.

The first stage is immediate containment. Once a credible concern is identified, the organisation should prevent additional affected stock from leaving its control. Relevant batches may be placed on hold, production suspended, supplier deliveries blocked and electronic release status changed. Warehouses and contract manufacturers should be informed rapidly, with clear instructions that prevent further dispatch, repacking or transfer. Containment should also preserve evidence. Retained samples, returned units, raw materials, component lots, analytical records and production documentation may be needed to determine the cause and scope. Adjusting, destroying or redistributing material before the investigation is complete can make the recall less precise and weaken later regulatory defence.

The scope of containment should be based on the plausible extent of the problem, not merely the first batch in which it was detected. A nicotine-concentration failure may affect one vessel, several filling runs, all products manufactured from the same raw-material lot or a longer period involving an incorrect calculation. A leaking package may affect one bottle mould, one closure lot or every formulation using the same container system. A defective heating element may be present across several branded products assembled from the same component lot. The initial action may need to be broader than the final recall while the organisation determines where the failure begins and ends. It is generally easier to release unaffected stock later than to recover product that continued to move while the scope remained uncertain.

Risk assessment should consider both the hazard and the circumstances of exposure. A product containing the wrong nicotine concentration may create different consequences depending on the magnitude of the error, declared strength, user population and likelihood of repeated use. A battery defect may have low occurrence but severe potential consequence. A labelling error may create immediate risk where a high-strength product is presented as a lower strength, while a minor formatting defect may be primarily a compliance issue. A metal or carbonyl finding may require assessment of measured level, frequency, product variability and realistic exposure. The recall decision should therefore consider severity, probability, detectability, duration on the market, number of units distributed and whether consumers can identify or avoid the hazard.

Scientific uncertainty does not remove the need for action. In serious cases, the organisation may need to act before the root cause has been confirmed. A credible indication of fire, poisoning, contamination or substantial mislabelling can justify precautionary suspension or recall while investigation continues. The decision should document what is known, what remains uncertain and why the selected action is proportionate. Waiting for complete certainty can increase exposure, while treating every unconfirmed report as proof of widespread danger can produce disproportionate disruption. The quality system should support decisions that are conservative where the possible consequence is severe without abandoning scientific discipline.

The recall classification system should reflect urgency and required consumer response. Higher-risk recalls generally require immediate communication, rapid market removal and direct involvement of regulatory authorities. Lower-risk recalls may allow more controlled recovery through distribution channels. The organisation should not rely solely on internal categories because regulatory bodies may apply their own terminology or reporting expectations. The internal system should nevertheless define practical escalation levels so that staff understand whether the issue requires senior management, legal, regulatory, medical, toxicological or public-relations involvement.

A recall committee or crisis team should be established with clear authority. Its membership may include quality, regulatory affairs, manufacturing, supply chain, legal, communications, customer service, technical specialists and senior leadership. The composition should reflect the nature of the issue. A battery event may require engineering expertise, while a nicotine error requires formulation and toxicological input. One person should coordinate the process, maintain the decision log and ensure that actions do not become fragmented between departments. The committee should be able to make rapid decisions without waiting for normal approval cycles, while still recording the rationale and evidence considered.

Regulatory notification should occur according to applicable legal requirements and agreed timescales. Authorities may require information about the product, hazard, batches, distribution, risk assessment, proposed action and public communication. The organisation should provide accurate information without delaying notification until every detail is known. Preliminary reports can be updated as the investigation develops. Delayed, incomplete or inconsistent communication weakens confidence and may lead authorities to impose broader or more restrictive action than would otherwise have been necessary.

The manufacturer or responsible economic operator should not assume that distributors, retailers or contract manufacturers will notify authorities on its behalf unless responsibility is defined explicitly. In complex supply chains, several legal entities may hold obligations, and their communications should be coordinated to avoid contradictory statements. The technical agreement should identify who leads notification, who supplies distribution data and who communicates with consumers. During an incident, uncertainty about ownership can waste critical time.

Product identification must be unambiguous. The recall notice should state the product name, nicotine strength, flavour, format, pack size, batch code, serial number, production date or other identifiers needed to distinguish affected units. Photographs can assist where packaging is similar across variants. The notice should explain where the code is located and how consumers or retailers can determine whether their product is included. Vague statements referring only to a brand or product family can cause unaffected consumers to stop using products unnecessarily while failing to identify the actual affected population.

Where traceability is weak, the recall scope may need to expand. If the organisation cannot identify which batches used a suspect component, all products manufactured during the possible period may require inclusion. If the batch code is unreadable or absent on units already in use, the recall may need to rely on purchase date, retailer or physical characteristics. Poor traceability therefore converts uncertainty into commercial and regulatory consequence. It increases the number of units affected, delays communication and makes effectiveness harder to measure.

Forward traceability should identify the quantity and destination of affected stock. The organisation should know how many units were manufactured, how many remained in its control, how many were supplied to distributors, retailers, online customers or export markets and how many were already returned or destroyed. Where intermediaries hold downstream records, they should provide them promptly. The recall team should not depend on one spreadsheet maintained by an absent employee or on commercial systems that record only total product code without batch information.

Distribution mapping should include stock transferred between warehouses, markets and legal entities. Product may have been repacked, relabelled or redistributed after initial sale. Parallel trade and informal resale can complicate recovery, particularly for popular vaping products. The organisation should identify authorised channels first, while monitoring whether affected units appear elsewhere. Online marketplaces and social media may provide evidence of continuing availability after formal distributors have stopped supply.

Consumer communication should be clear, specific and proportionate. The message should explain the affected product, the reason for the recall, the risk, what the consumer should do and how refunds, replacement, return or disposal will be handled. Technical language should be translated into instructions that can be followed safely. A battery-related recall may require consumers not to charge, puncture or post the device without specialist packaging. A leaking nicotine product may require protective handling and advice about skin contact. A mislabelled product may require immediate cessation of use.

The communication should avoid both minimisation and alarmism. Statements such as "out of an abundance of caution" can be appropriate but should not obscure the actual reason for action. Equally, describing detection of a substance without context may create disproportionate fear. The organisation should distinguish between legal non-compliance, quality defect and confirmed health hazard. Consumers need to know what action to take more than they need technical detail, but the underlying explanation should remain truthful.

Consistency across communication channels is essential. Authority notices, press statements, website information, retailer instructions, social-media posts and customer-service scripts should all describe the same scope and action. Inconsistent wording can create doubt about whether different products are affected. A controlled communication document should be approved and updated centrally, with obsolete versions withdrawn when new information becomes available.

Retailers and distributors should receive practical instructions covering quarantine, stock count, consumer enquiries, returns and record submission. They should stop sale immediately where required and identify stock in warehouses, stores and transit. Products should be physically segregated and labelled to prevent accidental resale. Retailers should not dispose of units before quantities, batch codes and evidence have been recorded unless the organisation or authority directs otherwise.

Direct-to-consumer sales can support targeted notification where order records include batch information. Where they do not, all purchasers of the product during the relevant period may need to be contacted. Email, text, account notification and postal communication may be used depending on available data and seriousness. The message should be repeated where necessary, particularly if response rates are low. Consumers may overlook one notification or assume that the notice does not apply to them.

Product return arrangements should be designed around the nature of the hazard. Ordinary postal return may be inappropriate for damaged lithium-ion batteries, leaking nicotine or contaminated products. Collection, retailer return or specialist disposal may be required. The organisation should provide clear packaging and handling instructions where return is safe. A recall that asks consumers to take impractical or hazardous steps is less likely to succeed.

Where physical return is not necessary, disposal instructions should comply with environmental and safety requirements. Vaping devices contain batteries, electronics and residual liquid and should not be directed routinely into ordinary household waste. The recall plan should consider local disposal routes and provide realistic guidance. Consumers should not be left with a product they have been told not to use but no safe means of removing it.

Recovered products should be controlled on receipt. They should be identified, counted, segregated and stored according to the risk. Returned units may provide valuable evidence and should not all be destroyed immediately. Representative samples should be preserved for technical investigation, regulatory review or legal purposes. The remainder should be destroyed or reworked only through an approved process after the organisation has determined that further examination is unnecessary.

Rework after recall requires exceptional caution. A product recalled for a packaging or labelling defect may sometimes be corrected, but the process must preserve identity, quality and traceability. Products recalled because of uncertain composition, contamination, device failure or storage history are less likely to be suitable for rework. The decision should consider whether the product has remained under controlled conditions and whether the correction can be verified. Commercial value should not override uncertainty about quality.

Quantity reconciliation is central to recall control. The organisation should account for units manufactured, held, distributed, returned, destroyed, reworked and unaccounted for. The figures should be reviewed by batch and destination. Differences may arise through samples, damage, theft, data error or stock movement, but unexplained discrepancies should be investigated. A recall cannot be considered effective simply because many units were returned; the organisation must understand the proportion of the affected population recovered or otherwise controlled.

Effectiveness checks determine whether recall communication reached the intended recipients and whether they acted. The organisation may contact a sample or all distributors, retailers or consumers to confirm receipt of the notice, identification of stock and completion of required action. The depth of checking should reflect risk. A serious recall may require direct confirmation from every distributor and targeted consumer follow-up, while a lower-risk withdrawal may justify sample verification.

Response rate alone does not measure effectiveness. A distributor may acknowledge the notice without removing stock, or a consumer may read the message but continue using the product. Follow-up questions should confirm that affected inventory was identified and controlled. Retail surveillance, mystery purchasing or online monitoring may be appropriate where there is concern that units remain available. Authorities may conduct their own checks, and the organisation should cooperate fully.

Low recovery does not automatically mean that the recall failed because some products may already have been consumed, discarded or sold beyond traceable channels. The organisation should estimate the likely status of unrecovered units and consider whether additional communication is needed. The effectiveness conclusion should be evidence-based and should not present incomplete recovery as success merely because further action would be difficult.

Mock recalls are one of the strongest tests of readiness. A simulated exercise can begin with a finished batch and trace backwards to materials and forwards to customers, or it can begin with a suspect component lot and identify every affected product. The exercise should include realistic time limits, quantity reconciliation, contact verification and escalation. It should not be announced so far in advance that records are prepared specially for inspection, because a real incident will not provide that opportunity.

The value of a mock recall lies in exposing weakness. Missing distribution data, inconsistent product codes, delayed supplier response and unclear authority should generate corrective action. A mock recall that is adjusted until it appears successful teaches the organisation nothing. The exercise should be reviewed by management and repeated after major system changes, site transfers or significant supply-chain expansion.

Recall plans should be tested across organisational boundaries. Contract manufacturers, warehouses, distributors, retailers and laboratories may each hold essential information. An internal exercise that stops at the first distributor does not demonstrate consumer-level capability. Technical agreements should require participation and define expected response times. The organisation should understand whether partners operate in different time zones, languages or regulatory systems that could delay action.

The investigation into root cause should continue alongside recovery activity. Recall removes affected product but does not correct the system that produced it. The investigation should review materials, suppliers, manufacturing records, laboratory data, equipment, changes, complaints and distribution conditions. The organisation should determine whether the defect arose from design, manufacture, storage, counterfeit supply or misuse. Where several causes contributed, corrective action should address each one.

CAPA should capture the findings and assign permanent actions. These may include supplier replacement, process redesign, revised specifications, additional testing, training, equipment modification, packaging change or stronger traceability. The actions should be verified for effectiveness. A recall is not complete when products have been recovered if the same defect can recur in the next batch.

Change control should govern any modification introduced as a corrective response. Replacing a coil, seal, flavour ingredient or software version can affect other product attributes. Urgency does not remove the need for validation, comparability and regulatory assessment. The organisation should avoid solving the immediate recall cause while creating a new unexamined risk.

The scope of retrospective review should extend beyond recalled batches. The investigation may reveal that earlier products used the same material or process. Complaint and analytical records should be examined to determine whether the issue existed previously. Future batches should also remain under enhanced monitoring until the corrective action is proven. A narrow review limited to the first failed batch may miss the true duration of the problem.

The recall decision and investigation should consider whether other brands or customers are affected. Contract manufacturers and component suppliers may provide the same product or part to several companies. A defect identified under one brand may therefore have wider market implications. Confidentiality should not prevent necessary safety communication. Suppliers should notify all affected customers, and regulators may coordinate broader action where common sources are involved.

International recalls require coordination across different legal systems, languages and distribution structures. A product may be lawful or packaged differently in one market while sharing the same defect. The responsible organisation should determine which countries received affected batches and which authorities require notification. Consumer instructions should be translated accurately, and local disposal or return arrangements should be practical. A global statement may need local adaptation without changing the underlying scope or risk message.

Timing is critical throughout the process. The organisation should record when the issue was detected, when containment began, when management decided, when authorities and customers were notified and when recovery started. Delays should be explainable. A recall initiated days after a serious concern was confirmed will attract scrutiny, particularly if commercial discussions or additional testing postponed action without adequate containment.

At the same time, the organisation should avoid issuing repeated inaccurate notices because initial information was not reviewed carefully. Rapid preliminary communication can be followed by updates, but basic product identity and consumer instructions should be verified before release. The recall team should distinguish information that must be confirmed immediately from details that can be refined later.

Decision records are essential. The file should show the evidence considered, participants, risk assessment, alternatives and rationale. It should also document why particular batches, markets or products were included or excluded. This record allows later review by auditors, regulators, courts or senior management and protects against retrospective reconstruction. Important decisions made by telephone or informal meeting should be captured promptly.

Legal and insurance considerations may influence the process but should not control technical judgement. Legal advisers can assist with notification, wording and liability, while insurers may impose reporting requirements. Neither function should suppress accurate safety communication or delay necessary action. The quality and regulatory assessment should remain grounded in evidence and consumer protection.

Public communication may attract media attention, particularly where the defect involves fire, children, poisoning or contamination. The organisation should designate trained spokespeople and avoid speculative statements. The message should remain consistent with regulatory notifications and technical evidence. Overly defensive communication can damage credibility, while premature admission of unconfirmed causes can complicate the investigation. Transparency about known facts and uncertainty is generally stronger than categorical reassurance.

Social media can spread both recall information and misinformation rapidly. The organisation should monitor public discussion, correct false claims where necessary and respond to consumers seeking identification help. Deleted posts or hostile responses can create the appearance of concealment. Social-media teams should use approved information and escalate reports of additional incidents into the complaint system.

Counterfeit products can complicate recall communication. A notice concerning genuine products may be used by counterfeiters to redirect consumers or may reveal invalid codes that were never issued. The organisation should explain how to verify authenticity where possible. If counterfeit units present the same or a different hazard, a separate warning may be needed. The investigation should not assume that every invalid code proves counterfeiting because coding or distribution records may themselves be weak.

Recall records should be retained according to legal and product-lifecycle requirements. The file should include the initiating evidence, risk assessment, authority correspondence, notices, distribution lists, recovery data, effectiveness checks, investigation, CAPA and final review. Returned-product examination, photographs and destruction certificates should remain linked. The record should permit full reconstruction years later if further claims or regulatory questions arise.

Final closure should occur only when the organisation has completed the required recovery, assessed effectiveness, reconciled quantities, concluded the investigation and initiated or completed corrective actions. Some CAPA or stability work may continue after formal recall closure, but ownership and deadlines should remain visible. Closure should not be driven solely by administrative age or commercial desire to move on from the incident.

A post-recall review should examine how the process itself performed. The organisation should ask whether the concern was detected early, whether decisions were timely, whether traceability worked, whether communications were clear and whether partners responded as expected. Weaknesses in the recall system should generate their own corrective actions. A technically correct recall can still reveal poor preparedness if information was assembled manually, responsibilities were unclear or consumer contact was incomplete.

Management review should consider recall trends and lessons across the organisation. Even one recall may expose broader weaknesses in supplier control, change management, complaint handling or leadership. Repeated recalls involving different products may share a common organisational cause, such as poor document control or inadequate validation. The event should therefore inform quality objectives, audit plans, supplier strategy and resource allocation.

Product recall is sometimes viewed as evidence that the quality system has failed completely. The defect leading to the recall may indeed reveal a failure, but the willingness and ability to act decisively are also measures of system maturity. An organisation that identifies a problem, communicates transparently, recovers affected stock and corrects the cause demonstrates stronger control than one that conceals, delays or narrows action without evidence. The objective of quality management is not to claim that failure can never occur, but to ensure that it is detected, contained and prevented from recurring.

For vaping products, recall capability is particularly important because consumers cannot see many of the attributes that determine exposure and safety. Incorrect nicotine concentration, substituted coil materials, unstable batteries or contaminated formulations can remain hidden within familiar branding. Once such a problem is identified, traceability, complaint data, batch records and supplier information must be converted rapidly into protective action. A recall system that functions only on paper leaves the organisation dependent on improvisation at the moment when precision matters most.

The strongest recall programmes are therefore built long before the first affected product is discovered. They combine accurate coding, complete distribution records, tested communication routes, clear authority, risk-based decision criteria and a culture willing to place consumer protection ahead of short-term commercial discomfort. When those elements are present, a recall can be targeted, timely and scientifically defensible. When they are absent, the same defect becomes harder to contain, more expensive to correct and more damaging to public confidence than the original manufacturing failure alone.

Continuous Improvement

Continuous improvement is the process through which a quality system learns from experience, reduces unnecessary variation and strengthens the controls that preserve product quality over time. It is not a final activity performed after manufacturing, auditing, complaint handling and corrective action have been completed, but the mechanism that connects those activities into an evolving system. Every batch result, deviation, complaint, supplier failure, audit finding, recall, process trend and analytical investigation provides information about how the product and organisation are performing. Continuous improvement ensures that this information is used deliberately rather than stored as isolated evidence. Its purpose is to move the organisation from repeated reaction towards greater process understanding, earlier detection and more reliable prevention.

The concept is sometimes misunderstood as a requirement for constant visible change. A stable and capable manufacturing process does not need to be altered merely to demonstrate improvement. Unnecessary modification can introduce new risk, weaken validation and create confusion in documentation and training. Improvement may instead consist of reducing variability, clarifying instructions, strengthening supplier oversight, improving data quality, simplifying a process, increasing traceability or eliminating recurring causes of deviation. The objective is not perpetual reinvention, but progressive control. A mature quality system changes when evidence supports change and preserves stability where the process is already performing effectively.

For vaping products, continuous improvement is particularly important because formulation, device design, materials, software and regulation continue to evolve. The commercial product may remain on the market for several years while its suppliers, manufacturing equipment, laboratory methods and consumer use patterns change. The technical file and initial validation provide a starting point, but they cannot anticipate every later operating condition. Quality data generated across the lifecycle show whether the original assumptions remain valid and whether the product continues to correspond with the evidence used to support it.

Improvement begins with reliable information. An organisation cannot identify meaningful trends when records are incomplete, complaint categories are inconsistent, batch data are stored in disconnected systems or deviations are closed without clear causes. Data quality therefore becomes a prerequisite for improvement. Product identifiers, batch numbers, supplier lots, component versions, test methods and failure categories should remain consistent enough to support comparison across time. Narrative context should also be preserved because numerical summaries can obscure unusual circumstances or changes in operating conditions.

The quality system should identify the data sources that reveal performance most effectively. These may include raw-material results, finished-product assays, process yields, in-process checks, device resistance, aerosol output, carbonyl and metal trends, stability results, supplier non-conformities, complaint rates, product returns, audit findings, CAPA effectiveness, recall performance and training outcomes. The selected indicators should reflect the product and process rather than follow a generic template. A refill-liquid manufacturer and a device-assembly operation require different measures, although both depend on consistent materials, controlled processes and reliable release decisions.

The value lies not in collecting the largest possible quantity of data, but in identifying which data reveal loss of control, emerging risk or opportunity for improvement. Excessive reporting can obscure the few indicators that matter. A dashboard containing dozens of metrics may appear sophisticated while management attention remains dispersed. The organisation should understand why each measure is collected, what normal performance looks like and what action follows when the result changes. Indicators without decision criteria become descriptive rather than operational.

Trend analysis is one of the principal tools. Individual batches may pass specification while the process moves gradually towards a limit. Nicotine concentration may rise slowly because of a raw-material or weighing shift. Fill weight may become more variable as equipment wears. Carbonyl emissions may increase after a coil or wick change. Complaint rates may rise after packaging is sourced from a new supplier. These changes can remain invisible when each result is reviewed only as an isolated pass or fail. Plotting performance over time reveals direction, stability and variation.

Control charts can distinguish common-cause variation from signals suggesting a specific change in the process. Common-cause variation reflects the ordinary behaviour of a stable system, while special-cause variation may arise from equipment failure, supplier change, operator error or environmental disturbance. The distinction is important because the response differs. Common-cause variation generally requires improvement of the process itself, whereas special-cause variation requires identification and removal of the specific source. Treating every fluctuation as a local operator problem creates repeated intervention without improving the underlying system.

Statistical process control should not become a mathematical exercise detached from product science. A result may be statistically unusual without being toxicologically or operationally important, while a small but consistent shift may matter because it approaches a legal or safety boundary. The interpretation should consider the product specification, analytical uncertainty, process capability and potential effect on exposure. Statistical tools reveal patterns, but technical judgement determines their significance.

Process capability analysis provides another perspective by examining whether a stable process can operate comfortably within its specification. A process whose mean lies close to one limit may produce repeated failures even where its short-term variability appears modest. A process with wide variation may depend on end-product testing to separate acceptable from unacceptable batches. Improvement should aim to centre critical processes around the intended target and reduce the spread relative to the permitted range. This creates margin for ordinary variation and reduces reliance on retrospective sorting or repeated testing.

The distinction between specification limits and control limits should remain clear. Specification limits define acceptable product performance or regulatory boundaries. Control limits describe the observed behaviour of the process. A result can remain within specification while falling outside the expected process pattern, indicating that something changed. Conversely, a process can be statistically stable while centred incorrectly and therefore produce consistently non-conforming output. Improvement requires attention to both stability and capability.

Quality objectives should be linked to these findings. Broad statements such as improving customer satisfaction or reducing defects provide little direction without measurable outcomes and defined ownership. Objectives may include reducing repeat leakage complaints, improving right-first-time batch performance, lowering supplier deviation rates, shortening traceability response time or reducing variation in nicotine assay. The objective should identify a baseline, target, timeframe and method of review. It should also avoid creating incentives that distort reporting.

Metrics can be gamed when their purpose is misunderstood. A target to reduce the number of deviations may lead staff to stop recording them. A target to close CAPA quickly may encourage weak root-cause analysis. A target to lower complaint numbers may lead customer-service teams to reclassify reports. Improvement metrics should therefore focus on system effectiveness rather than favourable appearance. Recurrence, severity, effectiveness and process performance are often more informative than raw counts.

The Plan–Do–Check–Act cycle provides a practical model. The organisation plans the intended improvement, defines evidence and assesses risk; implements the action under controlled conditions; checks the resulting performance; and acts on the findings by standardising success, revising the approach or abandoning an ineffective change. The cycle is valuable because it prevents improvement from ending at implementation. A revised procedure, component or process is not successful simply because it was introduced. Its effect must be measured.

Small-scale trials can support this approach. Before a major process change is applied across all production, it may be tested on a limited batch, one line or a controlled period. The trial should have predefined acceptance criteria and should remain traceable through change control. This allows the organisation to learn while limiting exposure to unintended consequences. Informal experimentation outside the approved system should be avoided because it can introduce untraceable product variation.

Continuous improvement depends heavily on CAPA. Corrective action identifies why failure occurred and introduces changes intended to prevent recurrence. The effectiveness stage determines whether improvement was achieved. Repeated CAPA involving the same failure indicates that the system has not learned sufficiently. Management should examine whether root causes are being selected weakly, whether actions are too superficial or whether resource constraints prevent durable correction.

Horizontal review strengthens the process by asking whether the lesson from one failure applies elsewhere. A mislabelling event may reveal similar risk across other strengths or products. A supplier change made without notification may indicate weakness in other technical agreements. A calculation error may exist in several spreadsheets built from the same template. Improvement becomes more powerful when it addresses the systemic vulnerability rather than the single event in which it was first discovered.

Near misses provide particularly valuable information because they reveal that the system almost failed but was protected by chance, one alert employee or an unrelated control. A material selected incorrectly but noticed before use, a label mix-up detected before packing or a supplier substitution discovered before manufacture all show where control is weak. Treating near misses seriously allows the organisation to improve without waiting for consumer exposure or batch loss.

Audit findings should also feed improvement. Internal and external audits identify gaps between planned and actual practice, but the value of the finding depends on what follows. Correcting one missing signature or obsolete document may close the immediate finding while leaving the process design unchanged. The organisation should ask why the issue occurred, whether similar gaps exist and whether the audit programme itself focuses on meaningful risks. Repeated minor findings in one area may reveal a larger weakness in training, supervision or document usability.

The audit programme should evolve with the organisation. Processes with strong performance and few changes may require less frequent or more focused review, while new sites, suppliers, methods or technologies require greater attention. Complaint trends and CAPA data should influence audit priorities. An audit schedule based solely on fixed annual repetition can miss emerging risks and spend excessive time reviewing areas already well controlled.

Supplier performance forms a major part of improvement because many product characteristics originate outside the manufacturer's direct control. Supplier scorecards may include material conformity, change notification, complaint response, delivery, documentation and audit findings. The assessment should distinguish between commercial performance and quality risk. A supplier that delivers on time but changes composition without notice is not performing acceptably.

Supplier improvement can involve joint investigations, clearer specifications, better communication, process capability work or increased verification. In some cases, the correct improvement is supplier replacement. Long-standing relationships should not protect persistent weakness. At the same time, suppliers should receive clear feedback and realistic requirements. A manufacturer cannot expect improvement where specifications are ambiguous or where it communicates problems only through rejection.

Periodic supplier review should consider trends rather than individual incidents. One isolated deviation may be managed effectively, while repeated smaller issues can indicate declining control. Changes in ownership, site, key personnel or subcontracting may also alter risk even before material performance changes. Improvement depends on recognising such signals early.

Manufacturing process improvement should focus on removing dependence on memory, judgement and manual intervention where stronger controls are feasible. Automated material verification, barcode scanning, electronic recipes, interlocks and real-time process monitoring can reduce selection and transcription errors. Engineering changes can improve mixing, filling, sealing and assembly consistency. Automation should not be introduced solely because it appears modern. The system must be validated, maintained and designed around the actual process.

Manual systems can remain effective where scale is smaller and controls are disciplined. Improvement may involve redesigning forms, simplifying workflows, improving segregation or making status more visible. The correct solution is the one that reduces risk reliably. A complex electronic system can create new failure modes through software mapping, access, data migration and user workarounds.

Standard work provides a basis for improvement because performance cannot be compared when each operator uses a different method. Procedures should define critical steps and acceptable operating ranges while allowing justified professional judgement where necessary. Once a better method is demonstrated, it should be incorporated into controlled documentation, training and validation. Improvement should become the new standard rather than remaining dependent on the individuals who developed it.

Employee participation is essential because the people performing the process often recognise inefficiency and risk before management does. Operators see repeated minor equipment issues, difficult instructions, awkward material flows and points where errors are likely. Analysts see method weaknesses, manual calculations and recurring interference. Customer-service staff recognise complaint patterns before they appear in formal trend reports. The quality system should provide routes for these observations to be raised and assessed.

Suggestion schemes are useful only where feedback is reviewed and acted upon transparently. Repeatedly requesting ideas without response discourages participation. Staff should understand whether the proposal was accepted, rejected or requires more evidence. Rejection should not be interpreted as resistance to improvement where the change introduces greater risk than benefit.

A culture that punishes error also suppresses improvement because staff conceal the information needed to strengthen the system. Accountability remains necessary where procedures are deliberately ignored, but most process failures arise from combinations of human, organisational and technical factors. Management should distinguish honest reporting from negligence. The objective is not to remove responsibility, but to ensure that the system learns rather than driving evidence underground.

Training should itself improve continuously. Competence data, audit findings, deviations and observed performance should show whether training is effective. Repeating the same presentation annually does not demonstrate that staff understand critical controls. Practical assessment, targeted retraining and updated materials may be required. Where errors persist despite repeated training, the process or instruction should be examined rather than assuming that every operator failed independently.

Documentation systems also require improvement. Forms may contain redundant fields, procedures may contradict actual workflow and electronic systems may require duplicate entry. These weaknesses increase administrative burden and encourage inaccurate completion. Simplification can improve compliance where it preserves critical evidence. The objective is not to reduce documentation indiscriminately, but to make correct recording more direct and useful.

Data should be collected once where possible and reused through controlled integration rather than transcribed repeatedly. Batch, laboratory, warehouse and complaint systems should share consistent identifiers. This supports trend analysis and reduces error. Integration should be validated so that automated transfer does not create incorrect mappings or silent loss of information.

Laboratory methods evolve as equipment, standards and scientific understanding improve. Continuous improvement may involve lower detection limits, better specificity, reduced uncertainty, increased automation or more representative aerosol collection. Method changes should remain controlled because improved sensitivity can create apparent shifts in product performance. Bridging studies and clear trend annotation are needed so that data before and after the change remain interpretable.

Improvement should focus on fitness for purpose rather than sensitivity alone. Detecting more compounds at lower concentrations may provide useful information, but it can also generate findings of uncertain regulatory significance. Analytical development should address the questions relevant to product control, exposure and decision-making. A method that is more complex but less reproducible may not represent an improvement.

Product design can also be improved through manufacturing evidence. Repeated leakage may indicate that the tolerance stack between bottle, seal and closure is too narrow. Variable carbonyl emissions may show that the device operates too close to liquid-starvation conditions. Metal findings may reveal unsuitable materials or manufacturing debris. Complaint and batch data can identify designs that require excessive process control to remain acceptable. Redesign may be more effective than continually strengthening inspection around an inherently fragile product.

Design for manufacture seeks to create products that can be produced consistently within realistic tolerances. A formulation that requires an exceptionally narrow viscosity range, a coil that depends on precise manual wick placement or a closure that leaks after small dimensional change creates long-term quality risk. Improvement should therefore consider whether the product can be made robustly, not only whether one ideal batch performs well.

Design for quality also considers how failure is detected. Features may be introduced that prevent incorrect assembly, verify component presence or make product status visible. A component that can be installed only in the correct orientation is stronger than an instruction warning the operator to check it. A connector coded by size or shape can reduce mix-up. Such changes remove opportunities for error rather than relying entirely on human vigilance.

Complaint data should feed product and process improvement systematically. Repeated reports of weak delivery, burnt taste, leaking or difficult activation may reveal issues that remain within formal specification but reduce consumer confidence and product performance. The organisation should examine whether the complaint rate differs by batch, supplier, age or market. Improvements should address the observed mechanism and should be verified through later complaint and testing data.

Returns and warranty information can provide additional insight, particularly for reusable devices. The reason for return, age at failure, component version and repair findings should be recorded. Parts replaced during service may reveal common failure modes. A high return rate attributed generally to user dissatisfaction may conceal a specific design or manufacturing weakness.

Recall experience should produce substantial learning. The organisation should review not only the defect but how effectively the recall system operated. Delays in identifying distribution, inconsistent communication, poor recovery or weak quantity reconciliation all require improvement. Mock recalls should then verify that the revised controls work. A recall closed without improving the underlying product and recall system leaves the organisation vulnerable to repetition.

Traceability performance should also be measured. The time required to identify affected batches, components, suppliers and customers provides a practical indicator. Missing codes, inconsistent systems and unreconciled quantities should be corrected. Improved traceability allows later interventions to remain narrower and faster, reducing both consumer risk and unnecessary disruption.

Management review is the formal point at which these data and improvement opportunities are considered together. Senior leadership should examine performance against objectives, trends, audits, complaints, supplier results, CAPA, changes, recalls and resource needs. The discussion should lead to decisions rather than simply acknowledge reports. Actions should identify ownership, priority, funding and timeframe.

Management review should also consider whether the quality system remains appropriate to the scale and complexity of the business. A system designed for small-batch filling may become inadequate after rapid growth, international expansion or introduction of device assembly. Additional automation, staff, technical expertise or governance may be required. Growth without quality-system development creates hidden fragility because informal controls that worked at small scale fail under increased volume.

Resource allocation is therefore part of improvement. Persistent backlogs, delayed investigations, overdue calibration or incomplete supplier oversight may indicate insufficient staffing or capability rather than poor individual performance. Management should recognise when the system asks personnel to perform more than available time and tools allow. Improvement requires investment where structural constraints are the cause.

Quality cost analysis can support decisions. Prevention and appraisal costs should be compared with failure costs such as rejected batches, complaints, returns, recalls, legal action and reputational damage. Reducing quality control indiscriminately may create short-term savings while increasing total cost. Conversely, excessive low-value inspection can consume resources without improving outcomes. The objective is an economically sustainable system that prevents significant failure and uses evidence efficiently.

Continuous improvement should not be driven solely by cost. Some changes are justified by consumer protection, regulatory obligation or scientific development even where financial return is indirect. Reducing emissions, strengthening child resistance or improving battery safety may increase production cost while supporting the legitimacy and long-term sustainability of the category.

Benchmarking can help organisations understand whether their performance and controls are reasonable compared with peers, recognised standards or other regulated sectors. Direct comparison must remain cautious because products, scales and risk profiles differ. Pharmaceutical practices may provide useful principles without every control being necessary for consumer vaping manufacture. Benchmarking should stimulate questioning and adaptation rather than copying procedures without understanding their purpose.

External scientific and regulatory developments should also feed improvement. New evidence may identify compounds, materials or use conditions requiring additional control. Standards may be revised, analytical methods improved and enforcement expectations clarified. The organisation should monitor relevant developments and assess their applicability to current products. Continuous improvement includes updating earlier assumptions when better evidence becomes available.

Change control remains essential because improvement actions can create unintended consequences. A new material, process, method or software system should be assessed, validated and implemented through the approved system. Improvement does not justify uncontrolled experimentation. The organisation should preserve traceability between the problem, proposed solution, evidence and final implementation.

The cumulative effect of small improvements should also be reviewed. Multiple process, supplier and product changes may gradually transform the operating system. Periodic product review should confirm that the current product remains aligned with its regulatory and scientific basis. Improvement should strengthen continuity rather than produce undocumented divergence.

Effectiveness verification should be designed before the action begins. The organisation should define what evidence would show that performance improved, over how many batches or months and against which baseline. Without this definition, teams may declare success based on one favourable result. The verification period should reflect the recurrence pattern. An intermittent defect may require a longer observation period than a simple procedural error.

Unexpected negative effects should be treated as new evidence rather than concealed to protect the improvement project. A packaging change may reduce leakage but increase closure difficulty. A tighter wick may improve stability while reducing aerosol output. A revised cleaning process may remove residues but damage equipment. The improvement cycle should allow revision or reversal where the total outcome is unfavourable.

Successful improvements should be standardised. Procedures, specifications, training, validation and technical files should be updated, and obsolete practices removed. The learning should be communicated to other sites, products or suppliers where relevant. Local improvements that remain undocumented are vulnerable to loss when personnel change.

Knowledge management is therefore part of continuous improvement. Investigation reports, validation studies, supplier history and technical decisions should remain accessible. Lessons should not depend on memory or individual experience. Repeatedly rediscovering the same information wastes resources and allows previous failures to return.

The organisation should distinguish continuous improvement from innovation, although the two can overlap. Continuous improvement generally strengthens an existing product or process through incremental learning. Innovation may introduce a substantially new formulation, device or technology requiring broader development and regulatory assessment. Both should use quality principles, but innovation should not be presented as a minor improvement where the product has changed materially.

Improvement should remain connected to consumer and public health outcomes. A process can become more efficient while product quality deteriorates, or manufacturing costs can fall through supplier substitution while emissions increase. The organisation should consider whether the change improves consistency, exposure, reliability and truthful presentation as well as operational productivity. Quality improvement is not synonymous with faster or cheaper manufacture.

For harm-reduction products, this connection is especially important. A vaping product must be sufficiently reliable and acceptable to support switching away from smoking, while avoiding preventable exposure and failure. Inconsistent nicotine delivery, leakage, burnt taste or device malfunction can undermine confidence and contribute to relapse or abandonment. Manufacturing improvement therefore supports both product quality and the wider public health function the product is intended to serve.

The strongest continuous-improvement systems combine scientific understanding, operational evidence and organisational honesty. They recognise that failures and near misses are sources of information, that stable processes still require review and that improvement must be demonstrated through results rather than declared through activity. They do not change products merely to satisfy management targets, nor do they preserve weak processes because they have not yet caused a formal failure.

Continuous improvement completes the quality-system operating loop because it returns knowledge from manufacture and the market to the point where new decisions are made. ISO 9001 principles provide the framework, GMP controls production, supplier auditing extends oversight, CAPA investigates failure, change control manages modification, documentation preserves evidence, traceability connects the product history, complaints reveal real-world performance and recalls contain serious failure. Continuous improvement ensures that these systems do not operate as separate administrative functions. It uses their combined evidence to strengthen the product and the organisation that produces it.

A quality system reaches maturity when it no longer depends primarily on inspection, emergency correction or individual experience. Processes become more capable, variation becomes more visible, suppliers become more reliable and failures are identified earlier. The objective is not a claim of perfection, but a demonstrable reduction in uncertainty and repeated error. In that form, continuous improvement converts quality management from a static body of procedures into an active system of learning, one capable of preserving product integrity as science, manufacturing and regulation continue to develop.

CHAPTER 6

Product Notifications and Compliance

Regulation rarely encounters a product in the form experienced by the consumer. The regulator does not ordinarily begin with the sealed bottle, the filled pod, the assembled device, the vapour produced during use or the manufacturing line from which the finished unit emerged. It begins with information. The product first enters the regulatory system as a name, an identifier, a formulation table, a sequence of chemical descriptions, a collection of analytical results, a technical specification, a toxicological argument and a declaration made by a responsible economic operator. Before the authority sees the physical object, it sees a representation of that object, and much of modern product regulation depends upon whether that representation is complete, accurate and capable of remaining connected to the product sold in the market.

This creates a second product alongside the physical one. The first is manufactured, packaged, distributed and used. The second exists within regulatory databases, submission portals, technical files and controlled records. It is made from data rather than liquid, metal, polymer and electronic components, but it is no less important to legal market access. The physical product may be well designed and manufactured consistently, yet still fail if its regulatory representation is incomplete, contradictory or incorrectly submitted. Conversely, a polished dossier may describe a product convincingly while the goods reaching consumers have drifted away from the formulation, components or processes originally declared. Compliance exists only where these two versions remain equivalent.

That equivalence is more difficult to maintain than it first appears. A vaping product is not static. Ingredients are sourced through supply chains that change, flavour preparations may be reformulated, analytical methods may be revised, component manufacturers may substitute materials, packaging may be redesigned and production may move between facilities. Commercial teams may alter names, descriptions or market presentation without recognising that the underlying regulatory identity is being affected. Engineers may improve a coil or airflow system while assuming that the change is too small to matter outside device performance. Procurement teams may accept a replacement material because its specification appears similar, even though its impurity profile, thermal behaviour or chemical identifier differs. The product can therefore change in numerous small increments without anyone making one dramatic decision to create a new product.

The regulatory record, by contrast, tends to preserve a defined moment. It captures what the producer stated the product was at the time of submission. The formulation has specified quantities, the device has defined components, the laboratory reports refer to tested samples and the technical description reflects an approved configuration. That record provides the authority with a fixed point against which later questions can be asked. If a complaint arises, if surveillance testing identifies an unexpected substance, if a retailer supplies a product with altered packaging or if a regulator suspects that a product has changed, the original notification becomes part of the evidential baseline. The central compliance question is not merely whether a product was notified once, but whether the product now present in the market is still the product described within that notification.

This distinction exposes a common misunderstanding. Notification is often treated commercially as a gateway event: the dossier is prepared, the submission is made, the product appears on a register and the compliance project is considered complete. That interpretation reflects the needs of launch planning but not the nature of regulatory responsibility. A notification is not the ceremonial end of development. It is the beginning of an accountable relationship between the producer, the product and the competent authority. The information supplied may later be relied upon during inspection, investigation, enforcement, corrective action or policy review. Every submitted statement therefore carries forward into the product's commercial life.

Nor does successful submission transform uncertainty into approval. A portal can accept files, validate mandatory fields and generate reference numbers without independently confirming every scientific proposition made by the producer. A product may appear within a published database without the competent authority having reproduced its analytical work, audited each supplier, verified every ingredient identity or endorsed the broader commercial proposition. Regulatory visibility and regulatory approval are different conditions, although market language frequently blurs them. Retailers may describe products as approved because they appear on an official list. Consumers may assume that every listed product has undergone an individual safety determination. Manufacturers may use acceptance of a submission as evidence that their scientific reasoning was correct. These assumptions assign the regulator a level of prior assessment that notification systems were not necessarily designed or resourced to provide.

The distinction matters because responsibility remains with the economic operator placing the product on the market. The producer is not merely delivering information for government storage. It is making a series of representations: that the product has been identified correctly, that the composition is known, that relevant evidence has been considered, that the physical product corresponds to the information submitted and that continuing systems exist to manage what happens after sale. A weak notification culture sees the authority as the final checker. A mature compliance culture recognises that the authority is receiving information generated under the producer's responsibility and may later test the reliability of that information against events in the market.

This information-based model creates a profound asymmetry between responsible and irresponsible operators. A compliant business must know what it is selling. It must obtain supplier information, define specifications, commission testing, control product identity, retain records and place its name behind the submission. An unlawful supplier may operate through rapidly changing brands, opaque import channels, disposable companies and products whose declared characteristics bear little relationship to their actual construction. The responsible operator therefore carries the cost of producing regulatory visibility, while the non-compliant operator may benefit commercially from remaining difficult to see.

The effectiveness of notification regulation depends on whether the state can convert information into control. A database containing thousands of product records creates potential intelligence, but only if authorities can search it, compare entries, identify anomalies and connect the records to physical goods, importers, manufacturers, retailers and test results. Large volumes of poorly structured or inconsistent information can create administrative density without regulatory understanding. The system may know that many products exist while remaining unable to determine which formulations are effectively identical, which ingredients recur across the market, which products have changed, which declarations conflict and which records correspond to goods actually being sold.

Modern regulatory systems are therefore not simply repositories. They are information architectures. Their design influences what authorities are capable of seeing. A field that requires a single ingredient name may hide complexity that matters toxicologically. A structure built around one product identifier may struggle with modular devices or families of related variants. A portal that distinguishes formulation data from emissions data may support meaningful analysis; one that treats all chemical information as equivalent may blur the difference between substances intentionally added and substances formed during heating. The categories chosen by the system become part of the regulatory reality because information that cannot be entered clearly is difficult to compare, monitor or enforce.

This creates tension between standardisation and scientific accuracy. Regulators require consistent fields, units, identifiers and formats so that submissions can be processed at scale. Science does not always fit neatly within those fields. Commercial mixtures may contain numerous substances. Natural materials may vary. Chemical identities may be uncertain, proprietary or dependent on form. Device performance may change with operating conditions. Toxicological evidence may support a qualified interpretation rather than a simple declaration of safety or risk. The submission system nevertheless demands that this complexity be translated into discrete entries and structured attachments.

Translation inevitably involves judgement. Someone must decide which name best represents the ingredient, which identifier applies, which test result belongs to which configuration and how uncertainty should be expressed within a system designed for administrative consistency. These decisions may appear minor, but they shape how the product is understood later. An incorrect chemical identifier can connect a substance to the wrong hazard record. A generic ingredient description can prevent meaningful comparison. A device entered under an unsuitable category can create confusion over the evidence expected. A result reported without sufficient operating context can appear more definitive than the underlying experiment justifies.

The quality of the notification therefore depends on more than the presence of documents. It depends on whether the organisation has converted product knowledge into regulatory knowledge without losing meaning. The chemist understands the formulation, the engineer understands the device, the laboratory understands the method, the toxicologist understands the weight of evidence, the manufacturer understands the process and the commercial team understands the product presented to the consumer. The dossier must bring those perspectives together into one controlled account. Where functions operate separately, each may hold accurate information that becomes inconsistent when assembled. One department may use the supplier's trade name, another the chemical name and another an internal material code. One may refer to the prototype, another to the production version and another to the retail pack. Every statement can be locally correct while the combined submission remains unreliable.

This is why notification work often reveals organisational weaknesses that were previously hidden. The process forces a company to answer apparently simple questions with precision. What exactly is the product? Which formulation is current? Which supplier specification applies? Which device was tested? Which report supports the marketed version? Who owns the master record? Which change created the present configuration? Where uncertainty or contradiction exists, the notification does not create the problem; it exposes the absence of an authoritative answer.

For smaller companies, this exposure can be severe. Early vaping markets often developed through rapid iteration, informal supplier relationships and product families that multiplied more quickly than technical records. Product knowledge might reside with founders, formulators or external suppliers rather than within controlled systems. The arrival of formal notification requirements therefore demanded more than the completion of government forms. It required businesses to transform practical knowledge into reproducible organisational knowledge. What had previously been understood through experience now had to be documented in a form capable of surviving personnel changes, supplier disputes, regulatory challenge and the passage of time.

Larger organisations may possess stronger data infrastructure, but scale introduces different risks. Multiple departments, global suppliers, contract manufacturers and national affiliates can generate parallel records. The same product may be assigned several codes, adapted for different markets or supported by different versions of analytical evidence. A central regulatory system can improve control, yet it can also create distance between the official record and local manufacturing reality. Sophisticated software does not guarantee integrity when the source information is wrong, ownership is unclear or changes are not communicated.

The legal status of the information adds further weight. Regulatory records are not ordinary working notes. They may become evidence. A submission can be examined years after it was prepared, often by people who were not involved in the original decisions. Assumptions that seemed obvious at the time may no longer be understood. Informal justifications may have disappeared with staff turnover. Supplier emails may be inaccessible. The dossier must therefore contain enough context to show not merely what was decided, but why the decision was defensible on the evidence available.

This temporal dimension is easily overlooked. Compliance systems operate across product lifecycles, while commercial attention tends to move towards the next launch. The regulatory record must remain intelligible after the development team has dispersed, the supplier has changed and the original submission software has been updated or replaced. Data retention is not simply an archival obligation. It preserves the chain of reasoning that connects past decisions to present responsibility.

Notification also shapes the market at a structural level. Every evidential demand, data field, fee and waiting period creates a cost of lawful entry. Some cost is necessary because products containing nicotine and intended for inhalation should not circulate without accountable producers and defined technical information. The difficulty lies in ensuring that the burden corresponds to regulatory value. A system can become so administratively complex that substantial resources are spent transforming the same underlying information into slightly different national formats without improving consumer protection. The result may be market consolidation, delayed innovation and commercial advantage for firms large enough to maintain extensive regulatory departments.

At the same time, an excessively permissive system can permit weakly characterised products to enter with minimal scrutiny. The regulatory problem is not solved by choosing between documentation and innovation. It is solved by designing information requirements that reveal what authorities genuinely need to know and by removing requirements that generate volume without insight. The purpose of notification should be to make the market legible: to identify products, locate responsibility, expose relevant risks, support surveillance and enable intervention when the product no longer corresponds to the lawful record.

The market becomes illegible when names change rapidly, formulations remain proprietary, importers disappear, identifiers are reused and products are redesigned around regulatory boundaries. In such conditions, the notification system may retain a formal list of lawful products while physical trade moves beyond it. A register can then become a historical map of what producers once declared rather than an accurate picture of what consumers can buy. Restoring the connection requires more than stricter submission rules. It requires integration with customs, retail inspection, analytical surveillance, complaints, enforcement intelligence and supply-chain traceability.

The central problem of product notification is therefore one of correspondence. The data must correspond to the product, the product must correspond to the market presentation, the marketed units must correspond to controlled manufacture and the regulatory record must continue to correspond as the product evolves. Once any of those relationships breaks, compliance becomes unstable. The product may still appear lawful because an identifier exists, yet the evidence attached to that identifier no longer describes what is being sold.

Product notification is the point at which all earlier regulatory work becomes visible and testable. It exposes whether the formulation has been defined, the toxicology understood, the analytical evidence connected to the correct product and the quality system capable of preserving it. A strong notification does not manufacture compliance through paperwork. It demonstrates that compliance has already been designed, assessed and controlled, and that the organisation possesses the information systems needed to maintain that position as the product, evidence and regulatory environment continue to change.

I will now discuss regulation at the point of translation between the material and informational product, they're concerned with how product knowledge becomes a regulatory record, how that record acquires authority and how easily authority can be weakened when data are incomplete, inconsistent or detached from manufacturing reality. Notification is often presented as paperwork because paperwork is its visible form. In substance, it is a test of whether an organisation knows its own product well enough to describe it precisely, defend it scientifically and keep that description true over time.

Figure 6.1. Product notifications and compliance: the notification operating loop.

This diagram presents product notification as a continuous regulatory process rather than a single administrative submission. It begins with the foundation inputs required to support a defensible dossier, including formulation data, analytical results, toxicological assessments, manufacturing information, quality-system records and applicable regulatory requirements. These inputs feed into an operating loop covering dossier construction, chemical-identifier control, ingredient databases, toxicological summaries, submission platforms, regulatory timelines, common submission failures, data management, cross-border compliance and the continuing maintenance of notified products. The circular structure emphasises that notification remains dependent on accurate data, controlled change and ongoing review after market entry. The outputs include compliant submissions, regulatory acceptance, market access, reduced regulatory risk, continuing compliance and product sustainability, supported by competent personnel, robust systems, controlled processes, reliable suppliers, regulatory awareness and organisational integrity.

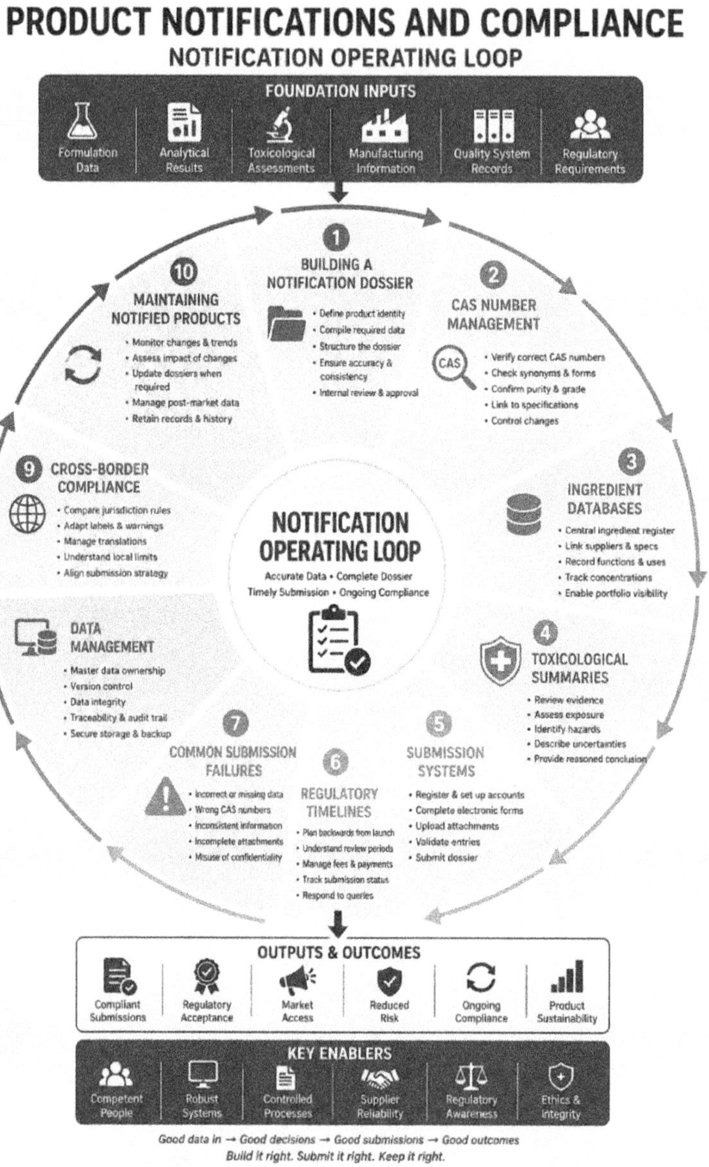
PRODUCT NOTIFICATIONS AND COMPLIANCE
NOTIFICATION OPERATING LOOP
FOUNDATION INPUTS
Formulation Data
Analytical Results
Toxicological Assessments
Manufacturing Information
Quality System Records
Regulatory Requirements
1
BUILDING A NOTIFICATION DOSSIER
• Define product identity
• Compile required data
• Structure the dossier
• Ensure accuracy & consistency
• Internal review & approval
2
CAS NUMBER MANAGEMENT
CAS
• Verify correct CAS numbers
• Check synonyms & forms
• Confirm purity & grade
• Link to specifications
• Control changes
3
INGREDIENT DATABASES
• Central ingredient register
• Link suppliers & specs
• Record functions & uses
• Track concentrations
• Enable portfolio visibility
4
TOXICOLOGICAL SUMMARIES
• Review evidence
• Assess exposure
• Identify hazards
• Describe uncertainties
• Provide reasoned conclusion
5
SUBMISSION SYSTEMS
• Register & set up accounts
• Complete electronic forms
• Upload attachments
• Validate entries
• Submit dossier
6
REGULATORY TIMELINES
• Plan backwards from launch
• Understand review periods
• Manage fees & payments
• Track submission status
• Respond to queries
7
COMMON SUBMISSION FAILURES
• Incorrect or missing data
• Wrong CAS numbers
• Inconsistent information
• Incomplete attachments
• Misuse of confidentiality
DATA MANAGEMENT
• Master data ownership
• Version control
• Data integrity
• Traceability & audit trail
• Secure storage & backup
9
CROSS-BORDER COMPLIANCE
• Compare jurisdiction rules
• Adapt labels & warnings
• Manage translations
• Understand local limits
• Align submission strategy
10
MAINTAINING NOTIFIED PRODUCTS
• Monitor changes & trends
• Assess impact of changes
• Update dossiers when required
• Manage post-market data
• Retain records & history
NOTIFICATION OPERATING LOOP
Accurate Data • Complete Dossier
Timely Submission • Ongoing Compliance
OUTPUTS & OUTCOMES
Compliant Submissions
Regulatory Acceptance
Market Access
Reduced Risk
Ongoing Compliance
Product Sustainability
KEY ENABLERS
Competent People
Robust Systems
Controlled Processes
Supplier Reliability
Regulatory Awareness
Ethics & Integrity
Good data in → Good decisions → Good submissions → Good outcomes
Build it right. Submit it right. Keep it right.

Building a Notification Dossier

A notification dossier is the controlled regulatory representation of a product at a defined point in its lifecycle. It brings together the information needed to identify the product, explain its composition and construction, demonstrate that relevant scientific and technical questions have been considered, and show that the manufacturer or importer accepts responsibility for placing it on the market. Although the visible output may be a set of electronic forms and supporting attachments, the dossier itself should exist before any portal is opened. It is not created by the submission system. It is created through the disciplined organisation of product knowledge, and the portal merely receives a jurisdiction-specific version of that knowledge. Where businesses begin with the submission fields and attempt to gather information as each question appears, the resulting record is usually fragmented, inconsistent and dependent on last-minute interpretation. A defensible dossier is built from a controlled master source and then translated into the format required by the competent authority.

The first task is to define the exact regulatory object being notified. This is more demanding than naming the brand, flavour or device. The dossier must establish which specific formulation, nicotine strength, container format, device configuration, component set and commercial presentation are covered. A product family may contain many closely related variants, but each variant must be understood well enough to determine whether shared evidence is scientifically and legally appropriate. Two liquids may use the same base formulation but differ in flavour composition. Two devices may share the same housing but use different coils, power limits or reservoir systems. A refill container may be sold independently and also supplied as part of a kit. These relationships need to be described clearly because the authority must be able to distinguish products without being forced to infer their identity from inconsistent names or marketing descriptions.

The product identity should be anchored by internal codes that remain stable even if commercial naming changes. Brand names are useful for market recognition but are vulnerable to redesign, translation, retailer abbreviations and regional adaptation. An internal product code, formulation code, device code and packaging code provide a more reliable framework. These identifiers should appear consistently across specifications, laboratory reports, toxicological assessments, artwork approvals, manufacturing records and notification forms. Where the tested sample is identified only by a generic flavour name while the dossier refers to a later commercial name, the connection between evidence and product may become uncertain. Every major supporting document should therefore contain enough identifying information to demonstrate that it applies to the notified product rather than to an earlier prototype, a similar variant or an unspecified member of a wider range.

Once the product identity has been fixed, the dossier architecture can be established. The exact modules will vary between jurisdictions, but the underlying logic remains consistent. The record should identify the responsible economic operator, describe the product and its intended market, define its composition and components, present relevant analytical and toxicological evidence, explain manufacturing responsibility, include required declarations and preserve the records needed to support continuing compliance. The strongest structure mirrors the way the product itself is understood. Product identity sits at the centre, with formulation, device, packaging, manufacturing and scientific evidence connected to it through controlled references. The dossier should not be a loose collection of files held in separate folders with no clear hierarchy. It should be possible to open the master index and determine immediately which documents describe the current product, which versions are approved and how the evidence fits together.

A formal dossier index is therefore essential. This document should list every controlled record, its title, unique reference, revision number, approval status and relationship to the product. It should also distinguish between mandatory submission documents, internal supporting records and external source documents. A regulator may not require every supplier certificate, method-validation report or quality procedure to be uploaded at the point of notification, but the producer should still retain them within the supporting technical file. The absence of a portal field does not remove the underlying responsibility. If a question later arises concerning an ingredient, analytical result or manufacturing change, the organisation must be able to produce the evidence on which its original declaration relied.

The formulation section should describe the product quantitatively and unambiguously. Each deliberately added substance should be identified by a controlled name, chemical identifier where appropriate, function, supplier or material code, specification and concentration. Units must be consistent, and the total formulation should reconcile mathematically. Apparent minor differences, such as reporting a component as a percentage by mass in one document and as a mass concentration in another, can create discrepancies if density assumptions are not stated. The dossier should therefore use one approved formulation basis and explain any necessary conversion. Where a flavouring material is itself a mixture, the relationship between the commercial flavour and its constituent substances must be controlled. The manufacturer cannot treat a flavour name as a complete chemical identity merely because the mixture was purchased from a reputable supplier.

Confidential formulations require particular care. A flavour house may be willing to disclose constituent information only under a confidentiality agreement or directly to an appointed toxicologist or competent authority. Such arrangements can protect legitimate intellectual property, but they must not leave the producer unable to manage the product. The legal entity placing the product on the market must know enough to assess whether the mixture contains restricted substances, whether supplier changes are material, whether the toxicological assessment remains valid and whether the notified composition is accurate. A dossier built around unidentified proprietary mixtures is structurally weak because the organisation cannot demonstrate control over substances it cannot see.

Nicotine data should be treated with the same precision. The dossier should distinguish the declared finished-product concentration from the assay and purity of the nicotine raw material used during manufacture. It should identify whether the formulation contains freebase nicotine or a salt, the acid used where relevant, the target concentration and the evidence showing that production batches meet that target within an appropriate tolerance. If the product is described commercially by one strength but laboratory testing or formulation calculations use another basis, the difference must be resolved rather than hidden through rounding. The submitted concentration, packaging declaration, batch specification and analytical verification should tell the same story.

For devices and prefilled systems, the dossier must define the component configuration that influences performance and exposure. This can include the heating element, coil resistance, power range, control circuitry, reservoir capacity, airflow, wick material, battery characteristics, materials in contact with liquid or aerosol and any user-adjustable settings. The purpose is not to describe every cosmetic feature, but to preserve the technical identity of the system that was assessed. A change in colour may be commercially important but scientifically negligible. A change in coil alloy, resistance, power delivery or reservoir material may alter emissions, thermal behaviour or compatibility. The dossier should therefore distinguish critical technical attributes from non-critical presentation features and explain how those attributes are controlled in production.

Product photographs and drawings can support identity, but they should not replace specifications. Images show visible form, while compliance often depends on characteristics that are not visible. A device may look identical after a component substitution that materially changes performance. Technical drawings, bills of materials, approved component specifications and configuration records provide the more reliable basis. These need not all be submitted routinely, but they should be available within the supporting file and linked to the notification record.

The analytical section should demonstrate that the data belong to the notified product and that the conditions under which they were generated are understood. Reports should identify the exact sample, batch or prototype tested, the method used, the laboratory, the date, the operating conditions and the results. Where the test item differs from the final production version, the organisation must justify why the evidence remains applicable. This is particularly important in rapidly developing product programmes, where testing may begin before every commercial detail has been frozen. A dossier should not quietly attach reports from an earlier configuration because they are convenient or expensive to repeat. The relevance of each report must be established through a documented comparison.

Method descriptions should be sufficiently detailed to explain what the result means. Emissions data produced under one puffing regime cannot be interpreted as universal product performance. Nicotine verification from a liquid sample does not necessarily demonstrate delivered nicotine consistency from the device. Stability results from one packaging material may not apply after a container change. The dossier should preserve these boundaries rather than presenting every analytical result as a broad certificate of quality. Evidence is strongest when its scope is stated precisely.

Toxicological documentation should then interpret the formulation and emissions evidence rather than merely duplicate it. The dossier needs a coherent scientific rationale explaining why identified substances and measured exposures are considered acceptable within the regulatory framework being applied. This may involve substance-specific summaries, mixture assessment, exposure estimation, read-across, weight-of-evidence reasoning and consideration of thermal degradation products. The toxicological narrative should be connected directly to the final formulation and device. A general assessment prepared for an ingredient database may provide the foundation, but the product-specific dossier must still consider concentration, intended use and measured or estimated exposure.

The scientific evidence should also be internally consistent. If the toxicological assessment states that a substance is present below a particular concentration, the formulation record and submission data must confirm the same value. If the emissions report identifies a compound of concern, the dossier should show how the result was interpreted and whether any corrective action was taken. Unexplained results create a gap between data generation and regulatory judgement. A regulator does not need to agree automatically with the producer's conclusion, but it should be possible to follow the reasoning from the evidence to the decision.

Manufacturing information provides the link between the assessed product and the batches placed on the market. The dossier should identify the manufacturer or manufacturers, relevant sites, outsourced activities and the controls used to ensure that production follows the approved specification. A notification is weakened if it describes a precise formulation and device but says little about how that configuration is maintained. The supporting file should therefore contain or reference approved manufacturing instructions, raw-material controls, in-process checks, finished-product acceptance criteria, release procedures and change-control arrangements. The authority may require only a description or declaration at submission, but the producer should be able to substantiate that statement through controlled records.

Where more than one manufacturing site is used, the dossier should explain whether all sites follow the same specification, methods and quality requirements. Site transfer should not be treated as a purely logistical change. Differences in equipment, mixing scale, filling processes, environmental control or component sourcing can affect the product. The organisation must determine whether additional verification, stability work or regulatory action is required. The original dossier should be structured so that these relationships can be updated without losing the history of the notified version.

Packaging and labelling form another controlled part of the dossier because they define how the product is presented and what information accompanies it. The approved artwork should be linked to the same product identity used throughout the technical file. Mandatory warnings, ingredient information, nicotine declaration, volume, instructions, batch coding and responsible-operator details must be accurate and legible. The dossier should preserve both the final approved artwork and evidence that the printed packaging reflects it. A regulatory submission may contain correct information while the commercial pack uses an outdated version. This disconnect is particularly common where artwork proceeds through separate marketing and production workflows.

The claims made on packaging and promotional materials should also be reviewed against the product's regulatory status. Statements implying therapeutic benefit, absolute safety, purity or official approval can create legal risk even where the technical dossier is otherwise competent. Notification does not authorise claims that belong to a medicinal, clinical or formal risk-modification pathway. The dossier should therefore contain a record of claim review and the basis on which any performance or comparative statements are permitted.

The responsible economic operator section should identify who is legally accountable for the product in the target market. This may be the manufacturer, importer, authorised representative or another defined entity depending on the jurisdiction. The relationship between the brand owner, contract manufacturer, importer and distributor should be clear enough to avoid uncertainty over responsibility. A dossier that identifies one company as submitter while packaging, invoices and supply records point to others can make enforcement and corrective action difficult. The legal and operational chain should therefore be mapped before submission.

Regulatory declarations must be treated as substantive commitments rather than routine signatures. A declaration that the information is accurate, that manufacturing processes ensure conformity or that the product complies with applicable requirements should be approved only after the supporting evidence has been reviewed. The person signing should have access to the relevant information and authority within the organisation. Declarations made merely to complete a portal create personal and corporate risk because they may later be examined against internal records showing unresolved concerns or missing data.

Document control determines whether the dossier remains reliable during preparation. Every file should have a unique reference, revision status, author, reviewer and approval record. Drafts should be distinguishable from approved versions, and superseded documents should be retained without remaining available for accidental use. File names alone are insufficient because informal naming conventions become unreliable when several people are working on the submission. A controlled register allows the organisation to see which evidence is current and prevents obsolete formulations, reports or labels from entering the final package.

The master dossier should also include a data-reconciliation review. Before submission, the organisation should compare every repeated value across the file. Product names, codes, nicotine concentrations, ingredient quantities, capacities, materials, manufacturer details and dates should match wherever they appear. This review is different from ordinary proofreading. It tests whether the dossier describes one coherent product. A spelling correction may improve presentation, but a reconciliation review can reveal that the laboratory tested a different strength, that the label uses an old capacity or that the toxicological assessment refers to a superseded ingredient list.

A formal gap assessment should follow. Each regulatory requirement should be mapped against available evidence, and any missing or weak area should be classified according to significance. Some gaps may be resolved through clarification or document correction. Others may require supplier information, analytical testing, reformulation, additional toxicological work or changes to manufacturing control. The assessment should not be manipulated to preserve the planned launch date. Where the evidence is inadequate, the product is not submission-ready regardless of commercial pressure.

Internal review benefits from separating scientific, regulatory and quality perspectives. The toxicologist should verify the scientific reasoning, the regulatory specialist the jurisdictional requirements, the quality function the controlled status of documents and manufacturing links, while the product owner confirms that the dossier reflects the item intended for market. No single reviewer is likely to identify every problem. Cross-functional review is particularly valuable because submission failures often occur at the boundaries between disciplines rather than within one technical document.

The dossier should then be frozen formally for submission. This creates a baseline defining the product and evidence package at that date. Any change made after the freeze must be assessed against the baseline, even if manufacturing or commercial launch has not yet begun. Without this control, minor late changes can enter production after the evidence review has closed, leaving the submitted record already obsolete at the moment of market entry.

A well-built notification dossier does not attempt to overwhelm the authority with volume. It provides the information required, supported by a deeper technical file that can be produced when needed. Excessive attachments can obscure the regulatory argument just as easily as missing data can weaken it. The aim is coherence, traceability and scientific relevance. Each document should serve a defined purpose, and the relationship between the product, the evidence and the declarations should remain visible throughout.

The final dossier therefore functions as more than an application package. It is the baseline against which later product changes, complaints, investigations and regulatory questions will be assessed. Its quality depends on whether the organisation has defined the product precisely, reconciled the data, controlled the evidence and preserved the reasoning behind its decisions. Where those conditions are met, the submission process becomes the formal expression of an already mature compliance system. Where they are absent, the portal becomes the place where the organisation first discovers that it cannot describe its own product with certainty.

CAS Number Management

Chemical Abstracts Service Registry Numbers are among the most widely used identifiers in scientific and regulatory documentation because they provide a concise means of linking a substance to a defined chemical identity. In product notification systems, a CAS number may appear to be a minor data field beside the ingredient name, concentration and function, yet its importance extends well beyond administrative completeness. It connects formulation records to supplier specifications, toxicological literature, analytical methods, hazard classifications, regulatory databases and market submissions. When the number is correct and applied to the correct chemical form, it improves consistency across the entire dossier. When it is copied inaccurately, assigned too broadly or used without understanding the substance it represents, it can direct every subsequent assessment towards the wrong material. CAS number management is therefore not a matter of filling gaps in a spreadsheet. It is a controlled process for preserving chemical identity throughout development, notification, manufacture and post-market maintenance.

The apparent simplicity of the system can create overconfidence. Each CAS Registry Number follows a standard numerical format and is intended to identify a unique substance recorded within the Chemical Abstracts Service registry. This allows scientists and regulators to distinguish chemicals that may possess several names, regional spellings, trade names, abbreviations or historical synonyms. A compound known by a common flavour name may also have an International Union of Pure and Applied Chemistry name, an alternative systematic name and several supplier descriptions. Using the correct CAS number provides a common point of reference across these naming conventions. It does not, however, eliminate the need to understand the chemistry. The registry number identifies the substance associated with that number; it does not confirm automatically that the substance in the formulation is the same material, purity, stereochemical form, salt, hydrate or commercial mixture that the assessor assumes.

This distinction is particularly important in vaping products because formulations often combine simple solvents, nicotine, acids and numerous flavour compounds supplied through complex commercial chains. Propylene glycol, glycerol and water are generally straightforward to identify, although even these materials require control over grade, purity and specification. Flavour substances are more difficult. A supplier may sell a material under a familiar sensory name that describes its odour or taste rather than its precise chemical identity. Another supplier may use a trade name containing several substances, solvents and processing aids. A natural extract may contain many constituents and vary between batches. A proprietary flavour concentrate may be represented by one mixture identifier even though the toxicological assessment depends on its individual components. Assigning a single CAS number to such materials can create an appearance of precision without providing an accurate description of what is actually present.

The first requirement of sound CAS management is therefore to determine whether the ingredient is a single defined substance or a mixture. Single substances can usually be linked to a specific registry number once their chemical form has been confirmed. Mixtures require a different approach. Some mixtures have their own CAS identifiers, but that does not mean that the identifier provides enough information for inhalation assessment or regulatory notification. A mixture number may describe a broad commercial or natural material with variable composition. It may be useful for supply-chain recognition while remaining inadequate for toxicological evaluation. The dossier may still need the identity and concentration of individual constituents, particularly where those constituents contribute materially to exposure or hazard. A regulatory team should never assume that the existence of a CAS number removes the need for compositional disclosure.

Chemical form creates another recurring source of error. A free base, salt, acid, ester, hydrate and stereoisomer may each possess a different CAS number even where their names appear closely related. Nicotine provides a clear example. The freebase compound, particular salts and different stereochemical forms are not interchangeable identifiers. A formulation described only as containing nicotine may conceal whether the material is freebase nicotine, a protonated form generated in situ or a premanufactured nicotine salt. The acid used, stoichiometry and resulting composition affect the product's chemistry and may influence analytical interpretation, sensory characteristics and regulatory reporting. Copying the CAS number for freebase nicotine into every nicotine-containing formulation is not necessarily correct merely because nicotine remains the pharmacologically active component.

The same issue applies to acids and flavour compounds. Citric acid, for example, may be supplied in anhydrous or hydrated form. Optical isomers may differ in biological or sensory behaviour. A flavouring material may be described by a common name that covers more than one structural form.

Toxicological literature may relate to one form while the supplier provides another. If the regulatory database treats these materials as identical because their names appear similar, the wrong evidence may be attached to the product. Verification must therefore begin with the actual supplier specification and not with a generic internet search or a previously used ingredient list.

Supplier documents are an important source of CAS information, but they should not be accepted without review. Safety data sheets frequently provide registry numbers, yet those documents are prepared primarily for workplace hazard communication and transport requirements rather than for detailed formulation disclosure. They may omit non-hazardous constituents, list only components above disclosure thresholds or use broad identifiers for proprietary mixtures. A certificate of analysis may confirm assay and purity without stating a CAS number at all. A technical data sheet may use an internal material description inconsistent with the safety data sheet. Where several documents disagree, the organisation must resolve the discrepancy before the ingredient enters the approved database.

Resolution may require direct contact with the supplier. The regulatory team should ask whether the material is a single substance or mixture, which chemical form is supplied, whether the stated CAS number applies to the complete product or only to one constituent, and whether composition has changed since the previous specification. Where confidentiality is involved, disclosure may be made under a non-disclosure agreement or directly to an appointed toxicologist. Commercial sensitivity does not justify maintaining a regulatory record known to be incomplete. The producer must have enough information to identify restricted substances, evaluate inhalation hazards, control formulation changes and confirm that the notified data represent the material being purchased.

A central ingredient database is the most reliable mechanism for controlling this information. Each approved substance should have one master record containing its preferred chemical name, recognised synonyms, CAS Registry Number, molecular formula where relevant, chemical form, supplier, trade name, grade, purity, specification reference, functional role, concentration limits and toxicological status. The record should also state whether the number has been verified, by whom and against which source. This prevents the same substance from being entered repeatedly under different names and reduces the risk that one department uses the trade name while another uses the systematic name and a third assigns an unrelated identifier.

Synonym control is essential because chemical names are rarely used consistently across suppliers, laboratories and regulatory portals. A single compound may appear under an abbreviated name in a formulation, a systematic name in the analytical method and a common flavour name in the toxicological literature. The master record should preserve these synonyms while establishing one preferred name for regulatory use. Searches of scientific literature should include relevant alternatives, but the final dossier should use a consistent description. Without this control, duplicate assessments can be created for the same substance, or separate substances can be merged because their commercial names are similar.

The master database should not be editable by every user with access to the formulation system. CAS changes should follow a controlled approval process because an alteration can affect multiple products and submissions simultaneously. A user correcting what appears to be a typographical error may unintentionally replace a valid number with one representing a different isomer or salt. Changes should therefore require supporting evidence, scientific review and documentation of the reason for amendment. The original value should be retained within the audit trail, together with the date, approver and list of affected products.

This audit trail becomes important during regulatory inspection or when historical submissions are reviewed. An authority may identify that a product was notified under one CAS number and later records show another. The organisation must be able to explain whether the ingredient changed, the earlier entry was corrected or the supplier documentation was revised. An unexplained discrepancy can appear to indicate an undeclared formulation change even where the physical material remained the same. Good CAS governance preserves the distinction between changes to the product and corrections to the information describing it.

Verification should normally involve more than one source. The supplier specification establishes what the purchased material is intended to be. An authoritative chemical registry or recognised scientific database can confirm that the stated number corresponds to the named substance. Analytical evidence may provide additional confirmation where identity is critical or uncertainty remains. The objective is not to reproduce the work of the registry but to ensure that the organisation has connected the correct number to the correct material. Informal websites, retailer listings and unverified online compilations should not be treated as primary evidence because errors can be copied across multiple sources and gain false credibility through repetition.

The CAS number must also agree with the substance used in toxicological assessment. Literature searching often begins with the registry number because it can improve specificity, particularly where names are ambiguous. If the number is wrong, the literature review may retrieve evidence for another compound and exclude evidence relevant to the actual ingredient. The resulting toxicological summary can then appear methodical while being scientifically misdirected. The assessor should cross-check the registry number, chemical name, structure and molecular formula before relying on retrieved data. This is especially important for closely related compounds where one substitution, stereochemical difference or oxidation state may alter biological activity.

Read-across assessments depend even more heavily on accurate identity. Where direct inhalation evidence is unavailable, an assessor may use structurally related substances to inform hazard evaluation. The scientific justification rests on understanding molecular similarity, functional groups, metabolism and expected biological behaviour. A mistaken CAS number can distort this process by assigning the substance to the wrong chemical category. Correct identification does not guarantee that read-across is valid, but incorrect identification makes a valid assessment impossible.

Analytical laboratories also rely on registry numbers when selecting standards, developing methods and reporting results. A test request that lists the wrong CAS number may lead the laboratory to purchase the wrong reference material or search for an inappropriate analyte. Where compounds share names or exist as related forms, the risk is not theoretical. The laboratory report may then contain a result that appears connected to the formulation but actually concerns another substance. Test requests should therefore be generated directly from the approved ingredient record rather than manually retyped from uncontrolled spreadsheets or emails.

Emissions testing creates an additional challenge because substances detected in aerosol may not have been deliberately added to the formulation. Thermal degradation products, impurities, metals, contaminants and reaction products must be entered into the scientific database with their own identities and evidence. They should not be confused with formulation ingredients simply because both appear under CAS-numbered lists. The system should distinguish the source and status of each substance: intentionally added ingredient, known impurity, material-derived constituent, process contaminant or aerosol-generated product. This distinction affects how the substance is interpreted and which control measures are appropriate.

The concentration basis must also remain separate from identity. A correct CAS number does not validate the quantity entered beside it. Regulatory submissions often require ingredient concentrations, but the number assigned to the substance says nothing about its amount, purity or exposure. A flavour concentrate may contain a constituent at a low percentage, while the dossier mistakenly reports the percentage of the complete concentrate as though it were the concentration of the constituent. This can overstate exposure substantially. The database should preserve the relationship between raw-material composition, formulation inclusion rate and final-product concentration so that toxicological calculations are based on the actual substance level.

Confidential flavour compositions are especially vulnerable to this error. A supplier may provide a constituent list with concentration ranges rather than exact percentages. The producer then has to determine how these ranges are translated into the finished formulation and reported within the applicable regulatory system. Conservative assumptions may be appropriate, but they must be documented. Assigning CAS numbers without preserving concentration context produces a chemical inventory that looks complete but cannot support meaningful exposure assessment.

Cross-border submissions increase the need for disciplined control because national portals may use different naming conventions, validation rules and expectations. One authority may accept a mixture identifier, while another expects constituent-level disclosure. Translation can introduce further inconsistency where chemical names are converted into national languages but registry numbers remain constant. The CAS number can provide continuity across jurisdictions, yet only if the same substance is being described. The master ingredient record should therefore remain the authoritative source, with market-specific fields mapped from it rather than recreated independently for each country.

Regulatory portals may reject a valid submission when the CAS format is incorrect, spaces or punctuation are misplaced, or the number fails an automated checksum. Such failures are administrative rather than scientific, but they can delay market entry. Data validation should therefore include format checks before upload. The final digit of a CAS Registry Number functions as a check digit derived from the preceding digits, allowing many transcription errors to be detected automatically. Software can apply this validation, but it cannot determine whether a technically valid number belongs to the intended substance. Both format and identity must be checked.

Common data failures include transposed digits, missing hyphens, use of a European Community number in the CAS field, insertion of an internal supplier code and assignment of the parent substance number to a salt or derivative. Another frequent problem is the use of "not available" without evidence that the ingredient genuinely lacks a suitable identifier. Some substances and mixtures will not have a single appropriate CAS number, but this should be a scientific conclusion rather than the result of incomplete searching. The record should explain why no number is assigned and how the material is otherwise controlled.

Duplicate records require regular review. The same ingredient may enter the database through different suppliers under different trade names, leading to several records with the same CAS number. This is not always an error because supplier specifications, grades and impurity profiles may differ. The database should distinguish the chemical identity from the purchased material identity. One chemical master record can link to several approved supplier materials, each with its own specification and qualification status. This structure avoids confusing chemical sameness with material equivalence.

The reverse situation also occurs: one supplier material may contain several CAS-numbered constituents. Treating the commercial material as one ingredient for procurement purposes while controlling its components for toxicology and notification requires linked records rather than forced simplification. The database should reflect both realities. Procurement needs to know which material to order, manufacturing needs the approved formulation code, and regulatory teams need the chemical composition. A good system connects these perspectives without allowing one to replace the others.

Periodic review is necessary because chemical information changes. Suppliers revise specifications, regulatory classifications are updated, new toxicological evidence emerges and restricted-substance lists develop. The CAS number itself may remain constant while the interpretation of the substance changes. A review programme should therefore examine both identity and regulatory relevance. It should confirm that the material remains sourced from the approved supplier, that the specification is current, that no change in chemical form has occurred and that the toxicological assessment still reflects available evidence.

Change control should be triggered when a supplier alters composition, carrier, purity, manufacturing route or source. Even where the same CAS number remains on the safety data sheet, the material may no longer be equivalent for product purposes. A revised impurity profile can affect emissions or toxicology.

A change from synthetic to natural origin may introduce compositional variability. A new carrier in a flavour concentrate may alter formulation percentages or aerosol behaviour. CAS identity is one element of sameness, not proof that every relevant property is unchanged.

The organisation should also review the impact of correcting historical errors. If a wrong CAS number has appeared in a notified product, simply updating the internal database is insufficient. The regulatory team must determine whether the authority requires an amendment, correction or new submission. Toxicological assessments and analytical requests based on the incorrect identity may need to be repeated or justified. A documented impact assessment should identify every affected product, jurisdiction, report and label. The seriousness of the response should reflect whether the error was purely clerical or whether it undermined the scientific evaluation.

Responsibility for CAS governance should be defined clearly. Regulatory affairs may own the submission fields, but chemical identity requires input from formulation scientists, suppliers, toxicologists, analytical laboratories and quality personnel. One function should maintain the master record, while changes are reviewed by those with the expertise to assess their consequences. Fragmented ownership encourages parallel spreadsheets and conflicting values. Central ownership with cross-functional approval provides a more reliable model.

Training should explain why these numbers matter rather than teaching staff merely where to enter them. Procurement teams need to recognise that a supplier change may alter identity or composition. Formulators must understand the difference between trade materials and chemical substances. Toxicologists should confirm structure and form before searching the literature. Regulatory personnel should know that portal acceptance does not validate the scientific correctness of the entry. Quality auditors should be able to trace a notified identifier back to the purchased raw material and forward into the products in which it is used.

An effective audit can begin with one CAS number selected from a notification and follow it through the entire system. The auditor should be able to locate the corresponding substance name, supplier material, specification, certificate of analysis, formulation concentration, toxicological review, analytical relevance, affected products and change history. The same exercise can be performed in reverse by selecting a raw material from the warehouse and tracing it to every regulatory submission in which its constituents appear.

Where the chain breaks, the organisation has identified a weakness in data integrity rather than merely a missing document.

CAS number management ultimately provides the chemical backbone of the notification dossier. It allows evidence generated by different departments and external organisations to remain connected to the correct substance over time. Its value lies not in the number itself but in the discipline surrounding it: verification, synonym control, material linkage, version control, impact assessment and continuing review. A correct identifier cannot make an unsuitable ingredient safe, and it cannot replace toxicological judgement, exposure assessment or analytical evidence. It does, however, ensure that those activities are directed towards the substance actually present in the product.

Where CAS numbers are treated as decorative metadata, errors spread quietly across formulations, submissions and scientific assessments. Where they are governed as controlled chemical identities, they support consistency, traceability and rapid regulatory response. The difference is not visible in the appearance of the final dossier, because both systems may contain complete-looking tables. It becomes visible when a regulator asks what a substance is, where it came from, which products contain it and whether the evidence attached to it genuinely applies.

Ingredient Databases

An ingredient database is not simply a catalogue of substances used in formulation. It is the controlled scientific record through which a manufacturer understands what enters its products, why each material is present, where it comes from, which specifications define it, how it is assessed and which products may be affected when knowledge or regulation changes. In a weak system, ingredients are stored as names in spreadsheets assembled for individual submissions, often copied from supplier documents and duplicated across product files. In a mature system, the database operates as a central source of truth connecting chemical identity, supplier qualification, formulation control, toxicology, analytical testing, manufacturing, regulatory notification and lifecycle management. Its value lies not in the number of fields it contains, but in whether those fields preserve the relationships needed to explain a material from receipt through to use, exposure and eventual regulatory review.

The first challenge is deciding what the database is actually intended to represent. A purchased raw material, a chemical substance and a regulatory ingredient are not always the same thing. A flavour concentrate may be procured as one commercial material, manufactured under one trade name and assigned one internal stock code, yet contain numerous constituent substances requiring separate toxicological consideration and regulatory disclosure. Conversely, the same chemical may be purchased from several suppliers under different trade names and grades. Treating every supplier material as a unique ingredient creates duplication, while treating every material sharing the same chemical name as equivalent can conceal differences in purity, carrier, impurity profile and manufacturing route. The database therefore needs linked levels of identity: the chemical entity, the commercial raw material, the approved supplier source and the products in which the material is used.

The chemical entity record should contain the preferred name, recognised synonyms, relevant identifiers, molecular form, structural information where appropriate, functional category and regulatory status. The supplier-material record should identify the trade name, manufacturer, specification, grade, composition, carrier system, purity, certificate requirements, storage conditions and qualification status. These records must be linked without being collapsed into one another. Propylene glycol from two qualified suppliers may represent the same chemical substance but remain separate materials for quality purposes because the approved specifications, impurity limits and documentation differ. A proprietary flavour mixture may remain one procurement item while linking to multiple disclosed constituents for toxicology and notification. This layered structure reflects the reality of how materials move through commercial, scientific and regulatory systems.

Naming control is fundamental because ingredient names are rarely consistent across the supply chain. Suppliers may use common names, flavour descriptions, abbreviations, systematic chemical names or internal codes. Laboratories may report analytes using different terminology from that used in formulations. Toxicological literature may rely on historical synonyms. Regulatory portals may expect controlled names that differ from the language used in manufacturing. Without a defined naming convention, the same substance can appear several times within the database, creating duplicate assessments and conflicting concentration records. The database should therefore maintain one preferred name for internal and regulatory use while preserving synonyms for searching, cross-referencing and historical traceability. Synonym management is not cosmetic. It ensures that a literature search, supplier document, analytical result and product submission can be recognised as referring to the same substance.

The ingredient record must also preserve function. A substance may act as a solvent, flavouring agent, acid, sweetener, coolant, colourant, stabiliser, processing aid or impurity. Function provides important context because it explains why the material is present and whether its concentration is consistent with its intended role. A compound recorded as a flavouring constituent may deserve different scrutiny if it is present at a concentration more typical of a carrier or active modifier. Function can also affect regulatory interpretation, particularly where certain classes of additive are prohibited or restricted. Recording function allows the organisation to identify unnecessary complexity, challenge ingredients with no clear technical purpose and distinguish deliberately added substances from constituents introduced through carriers or raw-material impurities.

Concentration data must be managed with equal care. Ingredient databases frequently contain nominal values copied from master formulations, but these values can be misleading unless the basis of calculation is defined. Concentrations may be expressed as percentage by mass, percentage by volume, milligrams per millilitre, parts per million or ranges supplied under confidentiality. A flavour concentrate may contain a constituent at one concentration, while the concentrate itself is added to the finished formulation at another. The final-product concentration must therefore be calculated through the complete compositional hierarchy. If the database records only the inclusion rate of the commercial mixture, the toxicological assessor may overestimate or underestimate the level of an individual constituent. Each concentration field should state its unit, basis, source, calculation method and degree of certainty.

Ranges require particular discipline. Suppliers may disclose constituent levels as broad bands to protect intellectual property, and the manufacturer may need to use the upper bound for conservative exposure assessment. That assumption should be visible rather than hidden within a calculated value. Where exact composition is unavailable, the database should distinguish measured concentration, formulation target, supplier-declared range and conservative assessment value. Combining them into one number produces false precision and makes later review difficult. A regulator or internal assessor should be able to determine whether a value is exact, estimated or deliberately conservative.

The database should also preserve the relationship between intended ingredients and unintended substances. A product may contain deliberately added compounds, known raw-material impurities, contaminants, extract constituents, leachables from packaging, metals from device components and thermal degradation products generated during use. These categories should not be merged merely because every substance can be assigned a chemical name. Their origin determines how they should be controlled. An intentionally added flavour compound may be assessed through formulation concentration and inhalation exposure. A contaminant may require specification tightening or supplier corrective action. A thermal degradation product may require device or formulation redesign. The database should therefore classify substances by source as well as identity.

Toxicological information belongs within the ingredient system, but the database should not become a repository for uncontrolled literature. Each chemical record should link to an approved assessment status showing whether the substance has been reviewed, which evidence was considered, what concerns were identified and whether restrictions or concentration limits apply. The underlying references may be stored in a separate document-management system, while the database preserves the current regulatory conclusion. This separation is important because scientific evidence changes. A substance assessed several years earlier may require review when new inhalation data, classification decisions or regulatory restrictions emerge. The database should show the date of assessment, reviewer, version, conclusion and next review trigger.

A simple status model can provide practical control. Substances may be classified as approved, approved with restrictions, under review, not approved, prohibited or obsolete. The meaning of each status should be defined clearly. "Approved" should not imply that the substance is universally safe or acceptable at any concentration. It should mean that its use is permitted within specified conditions, product types and concentration limits on the evidence available. "Approved with restrictions" may indicate a maximum level, market limitation, supplier requirement or need for product-specific review. "Under review" should prevent uncontrolled use until the assessment is complete. These statuses allow formulators and regulatory teams to make consistent decisions without repeatedly interpreting the entire evidence base.

Product linkage transforms the database from a reference library into a regulatory control system. Every approved ingredient should be connected to the formulations and products in which it is used. This enables rapid impact assessment. If a supplier changes a material, a classification is revised or a competent authority restricts a substance, the organisation can identify the affected portfolio immediately. Without this linkage, the response depends on manual searching through individual formulations, increasing the risk that products are missed. The ability to move from substance to supplier, formulation, market and batch is one of the most valuable functions of a well-designed system.

The same linkage supports portfolio rationalisation. Large product ranges often contain ingredients used in only one formulation, duplicate flavour systems performing similar functions and legacy substances retained because no one has reviewed whether they remain necessary. Database analysis can reveal these patterns. A substance used in one low-volume product but requiring extensive toxicological control may create disproportionate compliance burden. A supplier material used across many products may represent a concentration of risk if its specification changes. The database allows these decisions to be made with visibility rather than through intuition.

Supplier integration is essential because ingredient data are only as reliable as the information received. Approved materials should link to current safety data sheets, specifications, certificates, compositional disclosures and change-notification agreements. The system should record the date and revision of each document so that outdated evidence can be identified. A safety data sheet revised for transport classification may not indicate a formulation change, while a new technical specification may alter impurity limits without changing the product name. Document revision alone should therefore trigger review rather than automatic rejection or acceptance.

Supplier notifications must be assessed against the ingredient record. Changes in manufacturing route, source material, carrier, concentration, purity, natural origin or processing aid may affect toxicology, stability or emissions even where the trade name and primary chemical identifier remain unchanged. The database should allow the previous and current material versions to be compared and should preserve the decision on whether the change is acceptable. If the material is used in multiple products, the assessment must extend across the complete portfolio rather than only the formulation that first drew attention to the change.

Confidential information creates a structural challenge. Flavour suppliers may resist full disclosure of proprietary compositions, while producers require sufficient knowledge to satisfy notification and toxicological obligations. The database must accommodate different levels of access without fragmenting the scientific record. Sensitive fields may be restricted to authorised personnel, but the existence of the information, its review status and its relevance to affected products should remain visible to those responsible for compliance. Access control should protect commercial information without preventing the quality system from knowing that an assessment exists or that a change requires action.

A database that stores confidential composition without robust security creates commercial and legal risk. User permissions, audit trails, encrypted storage, backup, retention and access review are therefore part of scientific governance. Every change to a critical ingredient field should be attributable to an identified user and accompanied by an approval record. Deleting a historical value should normally be prohibited; the system should supersede rather than erase. Regulatory investigations often require reconstruction of what was known at a particular time, and an audit trail allows the organisation to distinguish between the product as originally assessed and later corrections or updates.

Version control must operate at both record and relationship level. An ingredient identity may remain unchanged while its assessment status, supplier specification or permitted concentration changes. A formulation may continue to use the same ingredient but under a new supplier-material revision. The database should preserve these distinctions. If only the current value is visible, historical submissions may become impossible to reconstruct. The organisation should be able to show which ingredient version supported a product notification, which specification applied to a manufactured batch and when a later change became effective.

Integration with formulation software reduces transcription errors, but system connectivity introduces its own risks. Automatic transfer is reliable only when field definitions are aligned. A concentration field in one system may represent the raw-material inclusion rate, while the receiving system assumes the concentration of the chemical constituent. An ingredient name may be shortened during export, or a mixture may be flattened into one record. Interface mapping should therefore be validated, with reconciliation checks confirming that identities, quantities and units remain correct after transfer. Automation can reproduce errors at greater speed if the underlying data model is poorly designed.

Regulatory submissions should draw from the approved ingredient database rather than from locally prepared spreadsheets. This ensures that the same controlled identity, concentration and assessment status are used across markets. Jurisdiction-specific rules may require different reporting formats, but the scientific source should remain common. A market requiring constituent-level disclosure may extract more detail than one accepting mixture-level data, yet both should derive from the same underlying record. Recreating data independently for each portal encourages divergence and makes later change management unnecessarily complex.

Cross-border regulation also requires market-specific status fields. A substance may be acceptable in one jurisdiction, restricted in another and subject to additional reporting elsewhere. The database should distinguish global scientific assessment from local legal permission. An ingredient can be toxicologically supportable but commercially unusable in a market because legislation prohibits its function or classification. Conversely, the absence of a local prohibition does not establish scientific acceptability. Maintaining both dimensions prevents legal status from being mistaken for safety assessment.

Data quality should be measured rather than assumed. Useful indicators include the proportion of active ingredients with verified identities, current specifications, completed toxicological reviews, confirmed supplier documents and mapped product relationships. Duplicate records, missing units, expired assessments and unresolved supplier discrepancies should be reported as quality issues. These metrics allow management to see whether the database is functioning as a control system or gradually becoming an archive of incomplete information.

Periodic audit should test the database vertically and horizontally. A vertical audit follows one substance from supplier documentation through chemical identity, assessment, formulation, notification and batch use. A horizontal audit examines one field, such as supplier status or assessment date, across the whole database. Both methods reveal different weaknesses. Vertical review tests traceability, while horizontal review identifies systemic inconsistency. Sampling should include simple materials, complex mixtures, high-use ingredients and substances with restricted status.

Human judgement remains essential because no database design can resolve every ambiguity automatically. Chemical mixtures, natural extracts, incomplete supplier disclosure and emerging evidence require scientific interpretation. The system should support that judgement by making uncertainty visible rather than forcing premature certainty. Fields such as "identity unconfirmed", "composition range", "assessment pending" and "supplier clarification required" can be valuable where they trigger controlled action. Hiding uncertainty behind completed fields weakens the database while creating the appearance of order.

An ingredient database becomes strategically valuable when it is used before formulation rather than only after development. Formulators can screen proposed materials against approved status, concentration limits, existing toxicological evidence and market restrictions before investing in prototypes. Procurement can identify approved suppliers. Regulatory teams can anticipate submission complexity. Toxicologists can focus on novel or higher-risk substances rather than reassessing familiar materials. This turns the database into a product-development control rather than a retrospective compliance exercise.

The strongest systems preserve both precision and context. They identify the chemical, the material purchased, the supplier, the concentration, the function, the evidence, the products affected and the decisions made. They allow information to be updated without destroying history and permit changes to be assessed across the whole portfolio. A weak database can still contain thousands of entries, yet fail when the organisation needs to answer a simple regulatory question about where a substance is used and why it was considered acceptable. A mature ingredient database provides that answer directly, with the evidence and traceability necessary to defend it.

Toxicological Summaries

Toxicological summaries sit at the point where ingredient data, analytical results and product design are converted into a regulatory judgement about whether a vaping product can be placed on the market responsibly. They are not generic chemical profiles or abbreviated safety data sheets. They are product-specific assessments explaining what each ingredient is, why it is present, how much is used, what happens when it is heated, what the consumer is likely to inhale and whether the available evidence supports that exposure. They allow reviewers to understand the reasoning without reconstructing it from scattered supplier documents, literature, laboratory reports and formulation spreadsheets. A strong summary combines chemical identity, hazard information, exposure context, thermal behaviour and uncertainty into one controlled narrative. It should show that the manufacturer has assessed an inhaled aerosol system rather than assumed that substances acceptable in food, cosmetics or oral products are suitable for vaping.

The starting point is the approved formulation. Toxicological summaries should not be built from an early development recipe, a marketing flavour name or a supplier's headline description. Each substance must be linked to the concentration used in the finished liquid, its function and the products in which it appears. Formulations containing propylene glycol, vegetable glycerol, nicotine and few flavour compounds may be straightforward. Complex flavour systems can contain dozens of chemicals, carriers, sweeteners, cooling agents, acids and processing aids. The summary must distinguish between the commercial flavour concentrate and the individual constituents creating the inhalation exposure. A statement that a product contains "strawberry flavour" has no toxicological meaning. The assessor needs their identities and concentrations, with enough information to identify respiratory hazards, sensitisation concerns, genotoxic alerts or problematic thermal degradation.

This creates a persistent industry difficulty: flavour houses protecting formulations as confidential intellectual property. Confidentiality is commercially understandable, but it cannot remove the producer's responsibility to know what is being inhaled. Where suppliers withhold full composition, the manufacturer should establish confidential disclosure to a qualified toxicologist, regulatory consultant or competent authority. The summary should record that the composition has been reviewed, identify limitations in disclosure and make clear whether the assessment covers every constituent or only those above a supplier reporting threshold. A complete-looking summary is misleading if undisclosed components remain outside review. Supplier reformulations must also trigger reassessment because a flavour sold under the same trade name may change composition without any obvious alteration to the finished product's branding or sensory character.

Ingredient-by-ingredient hazard review forms the core of the summary, but hazard identification alone is insufficient. Many substances cause adverse effects at some dose or route. The relevant question is whether the substance, at the concentration used and under intended operating conditions, creates an unacceptable inhalation risk. The assessor should consider respiratory irritation, sensitisation, systemic toxicity, genotoxicity, reproductive toxicity, carcinogenicity and organ-specific effects relevant to the evidence. Nicotine requires separate treatment because it is pharmacologically active, dependence-forming and capable of acute toxicity at sufficient exposure. The summary should address finished-product concentration, chemical form and expected delivery rather than treat nicotine as another flavour ingredient. Acids used in nicotine-salt formulations require consideration of identity, concentration, pH contribution and aerosol exposure. Cooling agents, sweeteners and sensory modifiers require review for inhalation evidence, thermal instability, concentration and necessity.

The route of exposure must remain central. Much of the available toxicological information for flavour chemicals comes from oral use, occupational handling or dermal exposure. These data can inform weight of evidence but cannot transfer directly to the respiratory tract. The lungs lack several protective and metabolic processes associated with ingestion, while aerosol deposition exposes epithelial surfaces directly. A substance with a long history of safe food use may still have little evidence supporting repeated inhalation. The summary should identify other-route evidence, justify extrapolation and state remaining uncertainty. "Food grade" should never be the principal justification for inclusion. Food-use history may inform toxicology; it does not establish respiratory suitability.

Thermal behaviour makes vaping toxicology distinct from conventional ingredient assessment. Consumers do not inhale the original unheated liquid. Liquid is drawn into a wick, exposed to a heated coil and converted into an aerosol under conditions affected by power, coil resistance, airflow, viscosity, puff duration, ageing and user behaviour. Some ingredients remain unchanged; others degrade, react or form new compounds. The summary should connect formulation data with emissions testing and known thermal decomposition pathways. Substances associated with carbonyl formation, reactive intermediates or unstable structures deserve closer scrutiny. Absence from the ingredient list does not prevent consumer exposure. Formaldehyde, acetaldehyde, acrolein and other emissions can arise during heating and must be interpreted as product-generated exposures rather than deliberately added ingredients.

Device conditions are equally important because the same liquid can produce different emissions in different hardware. A formulation used in a low-power pod may behave differently in a higher-power open device. Coil material, resistance, temperature control, wick saturation and aerosol mass influence exposure. Summaries for prefilled pods, cartridges or disposable devices should therefore be tied to the specific device configuration in which the liquid will be sold. For refill liquids, the assessment should define tested conditions and limits of extrapolation. A result generated under severe dry-puff conditions may identify a failure mode but should not be presented as normal consumer exposure. Unrealistically mild testing can underestimate foreseeable use. The summary should explain why the selected regime is relevant and how stress conditions were interpreted.

Exposure estimation converts hazard information into regulatory meaning. The assessor should use the concentration of each ingredient in the liquid, the amount transferred into aerosol, measured emissions where available and a justified assumption about daily consumption or puffing behaviour. A conservative screening calculation may suffice; measured aerosol concentration is needed where transfer efficiency is uncertain or thermal transformation likely. The summary should state whether the estimate represents ingredient content, aerosol yield, inhaled dose or deposited dose, because these are not interchangeable. Assumptions for body weight, consumption and frequency should be explicit. Conservative inputs are appropriate where uncertainty is material, but they should remain realistic enough to support decisions rather than creating implausible exposures that obscure the principal risks.

A margin of exposure may be useful where a suitable toxicological reference point exists, but it should not be applied mechanically. Many vaping ingredients lack inhalation-specific reference values, and oral limits may be inappropriate. Where a point of departure comes from another route or species, the summary should explain uncertainty factors and limitations. A large margin reassures only when the reference point suits the endpoint and route. The absence of a formal threshold does not automatically require rejection. Structural alerts, analogue data, exposure, analytical evidence and product function may require weight-of-evidence reasoning. The argument should be transparent enough that another toxicologist can understand how the conclusion was reached.

Read-across is particularly important because direct inhalation studies are unavailable for many flavour compounds. It can reduce unnecessary animal testing and make use of existing knowledge, but it depends on accurate identity and a defensible analogue. Similar odour, flavour or use does not establish toxicological similarity. The assessor should compare structure, functional groups, physicochemical properties, metabolism and known biological activity. The summary should identify the source substance, explain why it is relevant and describe differences weakening the comparison. Conflicting analogue evidence should be stated, not resolved selectively in favour of inclusion. Read-across is a scientific argument, not a convenient substitute for missing data.

Mixture assessment adds another difficulty because e-liquids expose consumers to combinations rather than isolated chemicals. Summaries often assess ingredients separately and accept the product because none exceeds a concern threshold. This can miss additive irritation, shared metabolic pathways or combined exposure to compounds with similar effects. Full mixture toxicology is rarely possible, but the summary should identify ingredients with common endpoints, including respiratory irritation, sensitisation or carbonyl formation potential. Numerous weak irritants may warrant reformulation even where each appears acceptable alone. The assessment should also consider whether unnecessary complexity can be reduced, because every additional constituent introduces uncertainty, variation and thermal chemistry.

Certain ingredient classes require explicit treatment because of recurring vaping concerns. Diacetyl and structurally related diketones should be identified and controlled through supplier specifications and appropriate testing. Cinnamaldehyde and other reactive aldehydes may require scrutiny for irritation and cytotoxicity. Menthol and synthetic coolants can affect sensory exposure and use patterns despite differing toxicology. Sweeteners may degrade during heating or contribute to coil fouling and altered emissions. Oils, lipids, vitamins, pharmacologically active substances and materials with established respiratory hazards should trigger strong justification or exclusion. The summary should show how absence of prohibited substances was verified and maintained through supplier control and analysis.

Analytical results must be incorporated into the toxicological conclusion rather than attached as an unrelated appendix. If testing identifies elevated carbonyls, metals or unexpected volatiles, the summary should assess significance, sources and corrective action. A finding cannot be dismissed because it was not predicted from the formulation. The assessor should compare concentrations with relevant benchmarks where available, consider method uncertainty and determine whether the result reflects normal use, product variability or abnormal operation. Repeated detection carries different weight from an isolated result near the reporting limit. The summary should distinguish detection, quantification and toxicological relevance.

Quality and manufacturing information affect toxicological confidence. An acceptable formulation can become unacceptable if identity, purity or concentration are uncontrolled. The summary should reference raw-material specifications, impurity limits, supplier qualification and nicotine verification where these influence the assessment. Metals and contaminants may arise from device components, production equipment or poor-quality materials. Flavour composition may drift between supplier batches. The conclusion applies only to the assessed material and configuration, so preserving controls must be identified. This is particularly important where acceptability depends on low concentrations or the verified absence of a substance of concern.

Uncertainty should be presented directly. Vaping products lack decades of inhalation evidence for every ingredient and configuration. The assessor should distinguish minor gaps from those materially affecting the conclusion. Uncertainty may be managed through conservative assumptions, concentration limits, supplier controls, additional emissions testing, targeted literature review or ingredient exclusion. A summary noting missing data without explaining gap management is incomplete. A summary that converts every absence of evidence into a declaration of safety is indefensible. The purpose is to show how uncertainty was recognised and reduced to a level considered acceptable for the intended product.

For regulatory notification, the summary should be written in a format that survives separation from the dossier. It should identify the product, formulation revision, device configuration, evidence sources, assessment date and reviewer, so that its conclusion cannot be applied to another variant. Generic wording copied across flavour ranges is dangerous because superficially similar products may differ in aldehydes, cooling agents, acids or supplier mixtures. Product-specific authorship and version control prevent one assessment from being stretched across a portfolio it was never designed to cover.

The conclusion should be product-specific, conditional and capable of supporting a regulatory decision. It should state whether the formulation is toxicologically acceptable for the defined device, nicotine strength and use conditions, identify restrictions and specify triggers for reassessment. Acceptability may depend on a maximum concentration, approved supplier, particular coil specification or emissions remaining within an established range. The conclusion should not use absolute language such as "safe" or "non-toxic". Vaping is not risk-free, and the summary is not intended to prove the absence of all harm. Its function is to determine whether avoidable hazards are controlled and evidence supports market placement.

Toxicological summaries must remain living records after notification. New literature, supplier changes, complaints, surveillance and restrictions can alter the assessment. If a flavour house changes composition, a regulator raises concern about a cooling agent or market testing detects an undeclared compound, the affected summaries and notifications must be reviewed together. Historical versions should show which evidence supported the product at each stage. Summary quality reveals whether compliance rests on science or paperwork assembled for submission. A weak summary repeats hazard phrases, relies on food-use history and ignores the device. A strong summary follows the formulation through heating, aerosol generation, exposure, uncertainty and lifecycle control, producing a defensible judgement tied to the product used.

Submission Systems

Submission systems are the administrative machinery through which vaping products become visible to regulators. Portal design determines how a product is described, validated, searched, compared and maintained. For competent authorities, it provides an architecture for receiving product records consistently. Vaping products are chemically, technically and commercially complex, while electronic submission systems depend on standardisation. A portal must process that complexity at scale without simplifying it so far that essential scientific and regulatory meaning is ultimately lost.

European vaping regulation made this problem particularly visible through the EU Common Entry Gate. EU-CEG was designed to provide a common electronic route for manufacturers and importers submitting information on tobacco products, electronic cigarettes and refill containers to national authorities. Economic operators could use a shared structure and direct submissions to intended markets. This created consistency across product identity, ingredients, emissions, toxicology, components and commercial presentation. It did not create complete regulatory uniformity, because fees, publication practices, national interpretation and enforcement remained partly domestic, but it established a common language for product notification.

The United Kingdom inherited much of this logic through the MHRA notification framework. Nicotine vaping products are submitted through structured systems requiring product definition, ingredient and emissions information, and compliance declarations. It gives the authority an auditable record and supports publication. Electronic acceptance must still be distinguished from scientific approval. A portal can confirm completed fields, attached files and generated identifiers. It cannot determine automatically whether a toxicological argument is sound, whether a flavour mixture has been fully disclosed, whether the tested device matches the marketed product or whether the manufacturing process will maintain the notified specification.

This distinction shapes how submissions should be prepared. The portal should be the final destination of approved data, not the place where product information is first assembled. Entering information directly from supplier emails, uncontrolled spreadsheets or draft laboratory reports creates inconsistency and weakens traceability. A manufacturer should maintain a master dossier containing the authoritative product identity, formulation, component specification, analytical evidence, toxicological assessments, packaging information and responsible-operator details. The submission system should then receive a mapped version of that approved record. This allows the organisation to reconcile data before upload, retain the context that may not fit within portal fields and reproduce the submission later if the system changes or a regulator requests clarification.

Product hierarchy is one of the most difficult features to manage. Vaping portfolios often contain families of related liquids, nicotine strengths, pod formats, devices and kits. Some elements are shared; others are product-specific. A submission system may require each variant to be entered separately while allowing certain components or evidence to be reused. The regulatory team must determine when shared data are justified and when a difference creates a distinct product. A flavour change can alter toxicology and emissions. A nicotine-strength change affects formulation and exposure. A coil change can alter thermal behaviour. A packaging change may be administratively minor unless it affects mandatory information or product presentation. The system should not dictate the scientific conclusion, but its structure forces the manufacturer to classify the relationship between variants.

Identifiers are central to this architecture. Submitter identifiers, product identifiers, formulation references, component codes and national publication numbers help regulators distinguish one record from another. They also create the basis for later amendments, market checks and enforcement. These identifiers must be controlled internally and connected to manufacturing and commercial records. A product code used only within the portal has limited value if the same code does not appear in the dossier, artwork, laboratory reports or change-control system. Likewise, a marketing team should not rename a product or introduce a regional variant without confirming how the change affects the regulatory record. Stable identifiers allow the physical product, electronic submission and internal quality system to remain aligned.

Structured ingredient fields create both value and risk. Standardised names, CAS numbers, functions and concentrations make it possible for authorities to search across thousands of formulations and identify recurring substances. They also expose weaknesses where suppliers use trade names, proprietary mixtures or incomplete disclosures. A portal may require one chemical identifier for a material that is actually a complex flavour concentrate. It may permit a mixture-level entry while toxicological evaluation requires constituent-level information. The organisation must therefore understand what the field is asking and preserve any scientific detail that the electronic structure cannot capture. Completing a field in the only technically permitted way does not absolve the producer from maintaining a more accurate supporting record.

Units and concentration bases require equally careful control. Submission systems may specify percentage by mass, milligrams per millilitre or another format. Internal formulation systems may use different units or calculate concentrations from supplier mixtures. Converting values during manual data entry creates obvious opportunities for error. A flavour constituent present at five per cent within a concentrate added at two per cent to the finished liquid is not present at five per cent in the product. Density assumptions, rounding rules and concentration ranges should be defined centrally. Automated validation can identify totals that do not reconcile or values outside permitted formats, but it cannot detect every scientifically incorrect conversion.

Attachments provide the space for evidence that cannot be reduced to data fields, yet they create their own management problems. Laboratory reports, toxicological summaries, product descriptions, manufacturing statements and declarations must be uploaded under the correct categories and linked to the correct product version. File names should identify the product, document type and revision without exposing uncontrolled internal language. A technically valid attachment may still be wrong if it relates to an earlier formulation or a different device. Submission teams should use an approved attachment schedule showing which document supports each field and confirming that all files are final, signed where required and readable after upload.

Portal validation messages are often treated as technical obstacles rather than regulatory signals. Some errors are simple, such as an invalid identifier format, missing mandatory field or unsupported file type. Others reveal deeper contradictions, including mismatched quantities, duplicated product records or absent component relationships. The team should investigate the cause rather than merely find wording that allows the system to accept the entry. Repeated attempts to bypass validation can produce a formally complete submission that no longer reflects the underlying dossier. The purpose of validation is not always scientifically sophisticated, but it provides a useful final check on consistency.

Submission status terminology also requires careful interpretation. Draft, validated, submitted, accepted, published, withdrawn and rejected can mean different things between systems. Commercial teams may assume that "accepted" means the product is legally cleared for immediate sale, while the authority may use it only to indicate successful receipt. Publication may occur after a waiting period or further administrative processing. Some markets operate notification, others registration or formal premarket authorisation. The legal significance of a status must therefore be confirmed against the applicable framework rather than inferred from ordinary language. Launch decisions should be based on the statutory condition for market entry, not on an optimistic reading of a portal message.

User access and account governance are important because submission systems contain commercially sensitive and legally significant information. Access should be limited according to role, with named users rather than shared credentials. Departing employees and external consultants should lose access promptly. Multi-factor authentication, password control and recovery procedures should be managed as part of regulatory continuity. A business that cannot access its account may be unable to amend a product, respond to authority questions or retrieve evidence of submission. Reliance on one consultant or one employee creates an avoidable operational risk.

External consultants can add expertise and capacity, particularly for smaller vaping businesses, but outsourcing data entry does not transfer legal responsibility. The manufacturer or importer must approve the information submitted in its name and retain copies of the final records, identifiers, correspondence and attachments. Consultants should work from controlled source data, document assumptions and return a complete submission archive. Where the consultant maintains the only working files, the business becomes dependent on a third party for its own regulatory history. Contracts should define data ownership, confidentiality, access, correction of errors and support during authority enquiries.

Submission systems also produce correspondence that must be controlled. Regulators may request clarification, additional evidence, correction of fields or explanation of an apparent inconsistency. These exchanges form part of the product's regulatory history and should be retained with the dossier. Responses should be scientifically reviewed and approved rather than treated as informal customer-service messages. A clarification can effectively modify the authority's understanding of the product, and an unsupported answer may create a contradiction with the original submission. The organisation should record what was asked, how it responded and whether any internal or market action followed.

Amendments require particular discipline because portals differ in how they handle product changes. Some allow selected fields to be updated, while others require a new submission for substantial modifications. The manufacturer must assess the change scientifically and legally before deciding which function to use. An editable field does not necessarily mean that every change is permitted without a new notification. Conversely, creating a new product record for a minor correction can generate duplicates and confuse publication lists. The amendment decision should be documented through change control, with a clear explanation of whether the physical product changed or only the information describing it was corrected.

Cross-border use adds complexity because a common system does not eliminate national requirements. One EU-CEG submission may be directed to several Member States, but fees, language expectations, national identifiers, publication rules and market restrictions may differ. A product can be technically submitted to a country yet remain commercially unsuitable because local flavour, retail, labelling or distance-sales rules prohibit its intended presentation. Northern Ireland and Great Britain may also require different regulatory planning. Submission management must therefore be integrated with market-access assessment rather than treated as proof of universal legality.

Data extraction and reconciliation should follow every completed submission. The final electronic record, acknowledgement, payment evidence, identifiers and uploaded files should be archived in a format that can be reviewed independently of the live portal. Staff should compare the submitted output against the approved master dossier to ensure that no field was altered, truncated or misapplied during entry. Screenshots alone are insufficient where structured export files or formal submission reports are available. The archive should allow the organisation to reconstruct exactly what the authority received on the submission date.

System outages, software changes and platform migrations create further risks. Regulatory portals may be unavailable close to deadlines, validation rules may change and older records may become difficult to retrieve. Businesses should not leave submission until the final permissible day, and they should retain evidence of failed attempts where technical problems occur. Internal data should be maintained in formats independent of the portal so that it can be remapped if the authority introduces a new system. A submission process dependent entirely on one external interface lacks resilience.

The regulatory value of these systems depends ultimately on data quality and regulatory use. A portal can collect enormous volumes of ingredient and emissions information, but the public-health benefit arises only when authorities can analyse the data, identify patterns, target products for review and connect records to enforcement. Poorly standardised entries, duplicate products and inconsistent terminology reduce that value. Manufacturers contribute to the effectiveness of the system by submitting accurate, structured and current information rather than treating the portal as a hurdle to be cleared with the minimum possible detail.

For the vaping industry, submission systems are therefore both gateways and continuing control mechanisms. They determine how products enter the legal market, how they are identified by regulators and how later changes are managed. Their limitations should not be confused with irrelevance. Electronic acceptance does not certify safety, but the record creates accountability. Standardised fields cannot capture every scientific nuance, but they make market-wide comparison possible. The strongest compliance approach uses the portal as one layer of a broader regulatory system: a controlled interface fed by an authoritative dossier, supported by quality management and maintained throughout the product lifecycle over time.

Regulatory Timelines

Regulatory timelines determine whether a vaping product reaches the market lawfully, reaches it late, or fails because scientific and technical work were never aligned. In nicotine product regulation, timing is not an administrative detail added after development. It is part of product strategy from the moment a formulation, device or product family is proposed. A manufacturer must understand how long ingredient disclosure, toxicological review, emissions testing, stability work, packaging approval, submission preparation, authority processing and any mandatory waiting period will take. Where these stages are treated separately, businesses commit to launch dates that the evidence cannot support, creating rushed testing, obsolete packaging and stranded stock.

The European requirement is the six-month period between notification and intended market placement for nicotine-containing electronic cigarettes and refill containers under the Tobacco Products Directive framework. That interval gives competent authorities visibility before products enter national markets, but it also reshaped the commercial rhythm of vaping. Businesses accustomed to rapid product turnover could no longer assume that a new flavour, nicotine strength, pod or device modification could move directly from development into retail. The notification date must precede launch by the required period, and a substantial modification may restart the clock. Regulatory time therefore became part of the product specification itself.

The waiting period is only the visible part of the timeline. A submission filed six months before launch may require several months of preparation. Ingredient composition must be complete, supplier documentation current, chemical identifiers verified and toxicological summaries approved. The final formulation must be frozen early enough for laboratory testing to represent the product that will actually be sold. Device testing may depend on production-equivalent coils, reservoirs, batteries and firmware. Packaging cannot be approved confidently until nicotine declaration, warnings, responsible operator and market language are settled. A company beginning dossier preparation six months before launch has normally started too late.

Backward planning is therefore essential. The intended launch date should be converted into milestones, each with an owner, dependency and contingency. The submission deadline sits before the statutory waiting period. Before submission come final review, data reconciliation and approval. Before those come laboratory reports, toxicological conclusions, ingredient verification and product specification. Before testing come product freeze and representative sample manufacture. Before sample manufacture come supplier qualification, component confirmation and formulation development. The plan must expose the true critical path rather than assume every activity can proceed in parallel. One unresolved flavour disclosure can delay toxicology, submission, production and distribution together.

Vaping businesses face timing pressure because product cycles are short and consumer preferences move quickly. Flavours, device formats and nicotine-delivery systems can change within months, while regulatory preparation takes longer. This mismatch creates a temptation to launch first and regularise later, especially when competitors introduce similar products rapidly. That approach transfers commercial urgency into legal risk. A product sold before completion of the applicable notification or authorisation process may be unlawful regardless of technical quality. Retailers may hold stock they cannot supply, distributors may demand reimbursement and enforcement authorities may require withdrawal. Speed gained before launch can therefore produce greater delay and cost afterwards.

Product freeze is one of the most important timing decisions. The product cannot remain fluid while testing and submission continue. At a defined point, the formulation, device configuration, container, nicotine strength and materials must be locked sufficiently for the evidence to apply. Cosmetic matters may continue under control, but scientific and regulatory attributes should not change casually after freeze. If a flavour house modifies a concentrate, a coil supplier changes resistance tolerance or a reservoir material is replaced, the organisation must decide whether existing tests remain valid. Late changes can invalidate months of work and restart the regulatory timetable completely.

Laboratory capacity must be reserved early because emissions testing is not an instantaneous service. Experienced laboratories may have long lead times, particularly when many manufacturers face the same regulatory deadline. Sample shipping, conditioning, method agreement, test failure, repeat analysis and report review all add time. A completed report may still require correction if product identifiers, units or device conditions are unclear. Manufacturers should not assume that testing begins close to the date an approved report becomes available. Planning should include quotation, protocol approval, sample production, analysis, quality review, toxicological interpretation and the possibility of repeating work after unexpected results.

Toxicological assessment has similar dependencies. The assessor cannot complete a summary where ingredient composition is partial or the finished concentration remains unsettled. Proprietary flavour information may take weeks to obtain, especially where confidentiality agreements or several suppliers are involved. Literature review and read-across require time, and concerns may lead to reformulation or additional testing. Toxicology should influence development early rather than appear as a final signature before submission. A substance rejected near the filing date can force a new formulation, new samples, revised analytical work, altered artwork and a complete reset of the planned notification date.

Stability timelines are difficult to reconcile with fast-moving vape markets. Real-time evidence requires time by definition, yet businesses may wish to launch before the full claimed shelf life has elapsed. A justified programme may combine real-time data, accelerated studies, packaging compatibility and continuing monitoring, depending on the product and regulatory expectation. Shelf-life claims should be planned rather than invented to suit commercial stock cycles. If the dossier relies on continuing studies, review and escalation dates must remain active after submission. Early evidence of nicotine loss, colour change, leakage, flavour deterioration or packaging interaction may require corrective action before distribution begins.

Packaging development has its own critical path. Statutory warnings, leaflet content, ingredient information, nicotine strength, container volume, responsible-operator details and identifiers must be finalised for each market. Translation and legal review take time, while printers require approved artwork, lead times and minimum order quantities. If artwork is released before the notification data are frozen, later corrections can create large volumes of unusable packaging. If printing waits until every regulatory step is finished, launch may miss its commercial window. Staged approval is therefore preferable, with provisional design work followed by final release only after all regulatory data have been reconciled.

Fees and administrative prerequisites also affect the timetable. Companies may require submitter registration, portal access, payment arrangements, local responsible operators or national accounts before product data can be filed. Account creation and identity verification should be completed long before submission. A finished dossier is of little value if the organisation cannot access the system or direct the product to the intended jurisdiction. National fees may need payment before review or publication, and failure to match payment with the correct product identifier can delay progress. These procedural matters belong within the project plan rather than being left to the final week.

The meaning of the regulatory clock differs between notification and authorisation systems. In a notification model, the producer supplies prescribed information and may enter the market after the required period, subject to national rules and unresolved authority concerns. In an authorisation model, submission begins an assessment whose duration may be uncertain and whose outcome is not guaranteed. The United States premarket pathway illustrates this distinction because filing an application does not itself permit lawful marketing of a new tobacco product. Companies must distinguish a predictable waiting period from an open-ended review. Commercial forecasts based on the wrong model can become catastrophically inaccurate.

Requests for clarification can extend either type of process. A competent authority may identify inconsistent formulation totals, missing toxicological support, unclear product relationships or incomplete manufacturing information. Response periods may be short even where the dossier took months to prepare. Organisations should therefore preserve expert availability after submission. Consultants, laboratories and suppliers may be needed to explain or correct data quickly. A submission is not finished when the upload succeeds. The regulatory project remains active until the product reaches the appropriate status, every question is resolved and evidence of that status is archived within the controlled dossier.

Cross-border launches multiply the timetable because one technical dossier may enter several systems with different requirements. Language, fees, local contacts, publication practices and national restrictions may prevent simultaneous filing. One market may accept the planned flavour while another prohibits it. One may publish products quickly, while another requires additional processing. The business must choose between a coordinated regional launch and a phased sequence. Phasing can reduce risk and allow lessons from the first market to improve later submissions, but it complicates packaging, inventory and distributor expectations. Simultaneous launch creates commercial impact while concentrating regulatory risk around one deadline.

Northern Ireland and Great Britain require careful separation because post-European arrangements can create different procedural routes even where products appear commercially identical. A company should not assume that a notification valid for one territory automatically covers the other. Market destination must be defined before stock is produced. Product codes, packaging and supply records should show which version is intended for which jurisdiction. Where one version supports several markets, the dossier should demonstrate that the applicable requirements have been met in each. Regulatory timelines become unreliable when geographical scope remains ambiguous or is decided only after manufacturing has begun.

Substantial modification is another point where timing and scientific judgement interact. A change may appear commercially minor but be significant regulatorily. Altering flavour composition, nicotine concentration, coil design, power output, reservoir materials or aerosol performance can affect the notified evidence. The organisation must decide whether the change can be managed as an amendment or requires a new notification and waiting period. That decision should occur before procurement or production commitments. Treating every change as minor preserves speed but risks supplying an unnotified product; treating every correction as a new product creates unnecessary delay. A documented change-classification procedure is therefore indispensable.

Seasonal and promotional launches expose poor timeline control quickly. A flavour intended for a summer campaign or limited retail window may lose commercial value if development begins too late for notification. Regulatory requirements do not shorten because the opportunity is temporary. The company must begin earlier, reuse defensible platform evidence or abandon the launch. Pressure to compress science to fit a promotional calendar shows that commercial planning has overtaken compliance. Limited editions are not exempt from ingredient assessment, emissions testing, submission or lifecycle responsibility merely because fewer units will be sold or the product will appear briefly.

Inventory timing should follow regulatory certainty. Manufacturing too early creates stock at risk if the submission is delayed, rejected or affected by a rule change. Manufacturing too late may leave the business unable to supply retailers when lawful launch arrives. A staged approach can separate validation batches, submission samples, packaging procurement and commercial-scale manufacture. Contracts with suppliers and distributors should recognise that regulatory dates can move. Forecasts should include retesting, authority questions, artwork correction and market-specific delay. Compliance planning is strongest when commercial agreements reflect uncertainty rather than pretending that every regulatory milestone will occur exactly as predicted.

Regulatory intelligence must remain active throughout development because rules can change before launch. New flavour restrictions, packaging controls, duties, device prohibitions or submission guidance may affect a product already in preparation. A dossier built to yesterday's rules may be complete but commercially obsolete. The organisation should monitor legislation, competent-authority guidance, consultations and enforcement trends continuously. Major policy changes may require a pause, redesign or accelerated filing before a transitional deadline. Transition provisions must also be interpreted carefully because manufacture, importation, placement on the market and final retail sale may have different cut-off dates. Inventory decisions depend on understanding which event controls.

Post-market obligations continue after the apparent end of the launch timetable. Stability review, complaint monitoring, adverse-event reporting, annual reporting where applicable, renewal fees, data updates and change assessment can all carry future deadlines. A lifecycle calendar should therefore replace the one-off launch chart once the product reaches the market. The responsible team must know when evidence expires, supplier documents require renewal and regulatory payments or reports are due. A mature vaping business starts with the legal market date and works backwards through product control, evidence and submission, then continues forwards through maintenance. Disciplined timing is what prevents a successful launch from becoming an unlawful one.

Common Submission Failures

Vape product submissions often fail for mundane reasons rather than scientific inadequacy. A manufacturer may commission emissions testing, obtain supplier declarations, review ingredient toxicology and invest heavily in packaging, yet the submission can still fail because the information does not describe one coherent product. Most failures arise where formulation, device, laboratory, quality and regulatory records develop separately and meet only at filing. The system exposes those disconnections. It forces the business to define the marketed product, its supporting evidence and whether every declaration, attachment and field refers to the same controlled version.

The most common failure is unstable product identity. Brand names, flavour descriptions, nicotine strengths and internal codes may differ between the submission form, laboratory report, toxicological summary and packaging artwork. A liquid tested under a development code may later receive a commercial name, while the portal entry uses a shortened description and the label adds a regional variation. Each document may appear understandable, yet the authority cannot be certain they concern the same product. The risk increases across large flavour ranges, where similar names and repeated nicotine strengths encourage copying. A robust submission requires one stable internal identifier linked to every record, with commercial names treated as secondary descriptors.

Formulation inconsistency is another persistent cause of failure. Ingredient tables may not total correctly, concentrations may be expressed on different bases, or one document may report a flavour concentrate while another lists its individual constituents. A formulation written as percentage by mass cannot be compared directly with a portal field expecting milligrams per millilitre unless density and conversion assumptions are documented. Nicotine may be declared as the strength of the finished liquid in one place and as the assay of the raw material in another. Small rounding differences can become significant when dozens of constituents are involved. Authorities may interpret these discrepancies as poor control or undeclared reformulation, where the manufacturer cannot identify which record is authoritative.

Incorrect chemical identifiers create failures that are both administrative and scientific. CAS numbers are frequently copied from safety data sheets without confirming whether they refer to the complete material, one hazardous constituent, a salt, an isomer or a carrier. A valid number entered against the wrong substance can pass format validation while directing the toxicological review towards the wrong chemistry. Mixtures present a particular problem because suppliers may provide one trade name and one broad identifier for a preparation containing many components. A complete ingredient table may conceal insufficient disclosure. Where identifiers, names and supplier documents do not align, the submission may be queried or considered unreliable even if the underlying material itself has not changed.

Proprietary flavour compositions often produce the largest data gaps. Flavour houses may provide only partial constituent lists, concentration bands or declarations that omit substances below internal reporting thresholds. The producer may submit the flavour name as a single ingredient or rely on supplier assurance of suitability. This is not enough for a product-specific inhalation assessment. The responsible operator must understand what is present, at what level and whether any constituent raises respiratory, thermal or regulatory concern. Confidentiality can be managed through non-disclosure agreements or direct disclosure to an assessor, but it cannot be used to explain why the submission lacks the composition needed to support toxicology.

Toxicological summaries fail when they are generic, route-insensitive or detached from the final formulation. Common weaknesses include reliance on food-use status, copied safety data sheet phrases and statements that no adverse effects are expected without exposure reasoning. A summary may list hazards but never calculate the concentration likely to reach aerosol. It may discuss the unheated ingredient while ignoring decomposition during vaping. It may be written for one flavour and reused across a product family whose constituents differ materially. Authorities are likely to question assessments that do not address inhalation, device conditions, measured emissions and uncertainty. The summary must show how evidence applies to the specific liquid and hardware.

Analytical reports commonly fail through poor sample traceability. The laboratory may identify the test item by a generic name, handwritten label or code that does not match the notified product. The tested sample may be a prototype, an earlier nicotine strength or a device fitted with a different coil from the commercial version. Where development continues after dispatch, the final product can drift from the evidence unnoticed. Teams sometimes attach the available report because repeating the work would delay launch. Unless equivalence is documented scientifically, this creates a weak dossier. The report must show that the tested sample represents the marketed configuration.

Test-method descriptions can also be inadequate. Emissions results without puff duration, interval, airflow, power setting, coil condition or sample preparation provide little basis for interpretation. A laboratory may use an unsuitable standard regime or operate adjustable hardware at one setting without explaining why it reflects foreseeable use. Severe dry-puff conditions can exaggerate carbonyl formation, while mild conditions can understate normal exposure. If the method is not reproducible or relevant, numerical results may satisfy an attachment requirement without supporting a regulatory conclusion. Failures occur when the business treats laboratory completion as scientific adequacy and does not review data generation.

Nicotine data are another recurring problem. The declared concentration may not match laboratory verification, packaging or formulation calculations. Differences can arise from raw-material assay, salt conversion, density assumptions, degradation or simple transcription error. Some businesses report the nicotine salt mass rather than nicotine equivalent, producing an apparent discrepancy against the labelled strength. Others rely on a single result from one batch without defining an acceptable manufacturing tolerance. Near a legal concentration limit, even a modest analytical or production difference may become significant. A submission should reconcile target, measured result, specification and label before filing, with a clear explanation of the basis used.

Device specifications fail when they describe appearance rather than critical performance attributes. Photographs may show the correct housing while internal components differ from those assessed. Coil resistance, alloy, wick material, firmware, power limits, airflow and reservoir capacity can influence emissions and nicotine delivery. A supplier may change one of these features while retaining the same model name and external design. If the submission contains only marketing specifications, the producer may be unable to demonstrate that the commercial units match the tested device. The failure reflects insufficient control over the system generating the inhaled aerosol.

Capacity and refillability declarations create specific compliance problems. Manufacturers may rely on nominal reservoir volume, while enforcement testing finds that usable capacity exceeds the declared value. Devices described as refillable may not function meaningfully as reusable products, or may depend on components that consumers cannot replace. Kits can also combine pods, reservoirs and devices in ways that make the notified configuration unclear. A submission may pass validation yet fail surveillance because the physical product does not satisfy the declared technical requirement. Measurements should be based on defined methods, production-equivalent units and the exact assembly sold to consumers.

Manufacturing information is often too vague to support the declarations made. Statements that a product is manufactured under good practice or within a quality system are weak if the dossier does not identify the site, process, release controls or relationship between the brand owner and contract manufacturer. Submissions can fail when several factories produce nominally identical goods without evidence of equivalent specifications and controls. A site may change after testing, or a second source may be introduced to meet demand. Unless manufacturing responsibility and change control are documented, the notified product can become detached from the batches entering the market.

Packaging and submission data frequently diverge because artwork follows a separate commercial workflow. The portal may contain one nicotine strength, responsible operator or ingredient description while printed packs show another. Mandatory warnings may be incomplete, obscured or translated inaccurately. Product names may be changed for retail appeal after notification without assessing whether the regulatory identity is affected. Old packaging can remain in stock after a data correction, producing two versions in the market. A pre-submission artwork reconciliation should compare every regulated statement against the approved dossier and ensure that the production file, not merely the visual proof, is controlled.

Administrative failures remain common. Incorrect portal accounts, expired credentials, unpaid fees, invalid file formats, missing signatures and attachments uploaded under the wrong product can delay otherwise competent dossiers. Shared logins make it difficult to identify who changed data. External consultants may retain the only access to the account or the only copy of the submission archive. A company can therefore lose control over its regulatory record. Submission readiness should include account governance, authorised users, payment arrangements, naming conventions and a complete export of what was filed, rather than focusing only on scientific content.

Duplicate and copied submissions create further risk. Product families encourage teams to duplicate earlier records and edit the apparent differences, but hidden fields, attachments and identifiers may remain linked to the original product. One flavour can inherit another flavour's constituent list or toxicological summary. A nicotine-free template may be adapted for a nicotine product without every relevant field being updated. Duplicate records may also be created accidentally when a correction is submitted as a new product rather than an amendment. These errors can confuse publication lists, national authorities and internal lifecycle management. Templates are useful only when every copied element receives independent review.

Timing failures often convert minor problems into submission crises. Testing may be commissioned before formulation freeze, supplier data may arrive after toxicology has begun, and packaging may be printed before the dossier is approved. When the filing deadline approaches, unresolved discrepancies are rationalised rather than corrected. Commercial pressure encourages teams to describe gaps as minor, assume authority acceptance or plan to amend data after launch. The statutory waiting period then magnifies the consequence of delay. A product that misses submission may lose an entire retail season. Strong governance makes the launch date follow evidence readiness.

Cross-border submissions fail when businesses assume that one notification creates universal compliance. A product record may be technically accepted through a common portal while national fees, language requirements, local responsible-person rules or product restrictions remain outstanding. Packaging lawful in one country may be defective in another. A flavour permitted in one jurisdiction may be prohibited elsewhere. Great Britain, Northern Ireland and European Union markets can require distinct procedural planning even where the formulation is identical. Market access should therefore be confirmed country by country, with each submitted version linked to the specific product, artwork and distribution route intended for that territory.

Post-submission maintenance is another failure point. Businesses may treat publication or portal acceptance as the end of responsibility and make later changes without reassessing the dossier. Flavour suppliers reformulate, coil manufacturers substitute materials, nicotine sources change and packaging is redesigned. Each modification may affect composition, emissions, stability or legal identity. If the notification is not updated appropriately, the listed record becomes a description of an obsolete product. Authorities may discover the discrepancy through complaints, testing or inspection. The failure then concerns not only the change itself but the absence of a system capable of recognising and controlling it.

The most serious submissions fail through false confidence. Every mandatory field may be complete, every attachment present and every status marked as accepted, yet the information can remain scientifically inconsistent or disconnected from production. Electronic validation confirms structure, not truth. Publication confirms regulatory visibility, not universal approval. The responsible operator must therefore conduct a final cross-functional review asking whether the dossier, physical product, packaging and manufacturing system still describe the same article. Common vape submission failures are rarely isolated clerical mistakes. They are symptoms of weak product definition, fragmented data ownership and poor lifecycle control. Preventing them requires the submission to be treated as the controlled expression of the product, not as paperwork assembled around a launch date.

Data Management

Data management is the infrastructure that allows a vaping business to demonstrate that the product described to a regulator is the same product designed, manufactured, tested, notified, distributed and monitored throughout its life. Regulatory compliance depends on accurate data moving between formulation, procurement, toxicology, testing, manufacturing, packaging, submission and surveillance. Where those functions maintain separate spreadsheets and informal naming conventions, the organisation may hold extensive information without possessing a reliable product record. Effective vape data management is not simply an information-technology function. It is a regulatory control system governing product identity, scientific evidence, market status and legal responsibility.

Each product should have one authoritative master record. That record should define the formulation, nicotine strength, device configuration, component specifications, packaging version, manufacturing site, responsible economic operator and jurisdictions in which the product is notified or otherwise authorised. Commercial names are insufficient because branding changes across markets and retailers. Stable internal identifiers should link the product to every supporting record, including supplier documents, laboratory reports, toxicological summaries, artwork approvals, batch records and submission references. If several departments use different names for the same product, the data system must preserve those synonyms while ensuring that all activity points back to one controlled identity.

Product and formulation relationships must be explicit. A single formulation may support several nicotine strengths or package formats, while one commercial product may be revised through successive formulation versions. The database should show which formulation version applied to each notified product and its effective date. Historical versions must remain accessible because a complaint, laboratory investigation or regulatory enquiry may concern stock manufactured under an earlier specification. Replacing the current formulation in a shared spreadsheet without preserving the previous version destroys the ability to reconstruct what consumers actually received and which evidence supported the original submission.

Ingredient data require a layered structure. The system should distinguish the chemical substance, the purchased raw material, the approved supplier and the finished-product concentration. A proprietary flavour concentrate may be one stock item but contain numerous constituents requiring separate toxicological and regulatory treatment. The same chemical may come from suppliers with different specifications and impurity limits. Collapsing these levels creates ambiguity over what was purchased, what was assessed and what was reported. Linked records allow procurement, manufacturing, toxicology and regulatory affairs to work from the same information without forcing each function to interpret the material through its own uncontrolled terminology.

Data ownership must be assigned clearly. Regulatory affairs may own submission records, formulation science the master recipe, quality the approved specifications, toxicology the assessment status and laboratories the analytical data. Shared responsibility still requires defined ownership. Each critical field should have an identified owner authorised to approve changes and accountable for accuracy. Other users may propose amendments, but changes to nicotine concentration, CAS numbers, supplier materials, device components or market status should not occur without controlled review. A central system with unrestricted editing can become less reliable than a controlled spreadsheet because errors spread instantly.

Access control is therefore a regulatory safeguard. Users should receive permissions according to role, with sensitive flavour composition, personal information and commercial data restricted appropriately. Shared accounts should be avoided because they remove accountability. Every addition, correction and approval should be attributable to an individual and recorded within an audit trail. Departing staff and consultants should lose access promptly, while the business retains every regulatory record. Dependence on one employee or external consultant for portal credentials, submission files or ingredient data creates a serious continuity risk if that relationship ends unexpectedly.

Version control should apply to data fields as well as documents. Document systems identify revisions of reports and specifications, but regulatory datasets change at field level. A supplier address may be corrected without altering product science, while a coil alloy change may affect emissions, toxicology and notification status. The system should record what changed, why, who approved it, when it became effective and which products or submissions were affected. Historical values should be superseded rather than deleted. This distinguishes clerical corrections from product modifications and explains discrepancies between current records and earlier notifications.

Source traceability determines whether data can be defended. Every significant regulatory value should connect to evidence. An ingredient concentration should trace to the approved formulation; a CAS number to verified supplier or chemical identity records; a nicotine result to a signed laboratory report; a tank capacity to an engineering specification or validated measurement; and a market status to an official submission acknowledgement or publication record. Repeated manual copying gradually separates values from their source and introduces transcription errors. The data system should preserve provenance so that reviewers can identify where each value originated and whether it remains current.

Manual data entry remains one of the main sources of failure in vaping submissions. Ingredient lists are copied from supplier files into formulation spreadsheets, from spreadsheets into toxicological templates and then into regulatory portals. At each stage names may be abbreviated, decimal places altered, units changed or mixture concentrations confused with constituent concentrations. Automation can reduce these errors, but only where field definitions are aligned. A percentage by mass in one system may be interpreted as percentage by volume in another. Interfaces should therefore be validated, and transferred data should be reconciled against the approved source before use.

Units require especially strict governance. Vaping data may be expressed as percentage by mass, percentage by volume, milligrams per millilitre, micrograms per puff, milligrams per device, milligrams per gram or concentration in collected aerosol. These values are not interchangeable. The database should store the unit with the number, define the calculation basis and prevent values from being exported without context. Density assumptions, dilution factors and conversion equations should be documented. A nicotine strength reported incorrectly because the system separated the number from its unit can create labelling, legal-limit and consumer-safety consequences.

Laboratory data should enter the system with full sample context. A numerical emissions result has limited meaning unless linked to the tested product, batch, device configuration, puffing regime, laboratory method, reporting limit and report revision. The same formulation tested in another coil or at another power may produce different results. Data management should therefore preserve the test conditions rather than extracting only the final numbers for submission. Where results are reanalysed, corrected or repeated, the relationship between reports must remain visible. Selecting the most favourable result without documenting the complete analytical history would undermine integrity.

Toxicological conclusions also require structured control. The database should show whether each ingredient is approved, restricted, under review, rejected or obsolete, together with applicable concentration limits, supplier conditions and product restrictions. The conclusion should link to the approved assessment version and review date. Formulators should be prevented from selecting a substance whose status is unresolved or whose permitted concentration would be exceeded. This allows toxicology to influence product design before notification rather than acting as a retrospective check after commercial decisions have been made.

Submission data should be generated from approved master records wherever possible. Rebuilding a product separately within each national portal encourages divergence. One market may receive an outdated ingredient list, another an incorrect nicotine strength and another a laboratory report belonging to an earlier device. Jurisdiction-specific requirements still need separate fields, languages, warnings and identifiers, but the underlying scientific information should originate from one controlled source. The system should record what was submitted, when, by whom, to which authority and under which product version.

Regulatory status must be represented precisely. Terms such as draft, submitted, validated, accepted, published, authorised, withdrawn and discontinued have different legal implications. A commercial dashboard that reduces them to "approved" can mislead sales and distribution teams. The database should distinguish portal status from lawful market status and should record any waiting period, fee requirement, market restriction or unresolved authority query. Distribution controls can then prevent stock from being released into a country before the appropriate condition has been satisfied.

Packaging data must remain connected to the regulatory record. Each market version should link to approved artwork, nicotine declaration, warning text, ingredient information, responsible-operator details, batch coding and language. Commercial teams should not be able to release revised artwork without confirming whether the change affects the notification or legal presentation. The system should show which packaging revision was used for each production batch. This becomes critical where old and new packs coexist during a transition or where an authority investigates a product found with inconsistent labelling.

Manufacturing integration provides the physical confirmation that the regulatory data are being applied. Batch records should identify the formulation version, raw-material lots, component versions, manufacturing site, production date and release decision. Where contract manufacturers use their own enterprise systems, data exchange must be defined and audited. The brand owner should not depend on summary certificates that omit the records needed to investigate variation. If a supplier changes a coil, flavour or nicotine source, the change should enter the regulatory data system before the modified product is released.

Change control is where data management becomes lifecycle compliance. A proposed change should identify every affected record, assessment, test, label, market and submission. The system should support impact assessment rather than simply replacing old data with new. A flavour supplier change may affect constituent disclosure, toxicology, emissions and several notified products. A device colour change may affect only artwork. By mapping relationships in advance, the organisation can distinguish changes requiring a new submission from those requiring an internal update and preserve evidence supporting the decision.

Complaint and vigilance data should connect back to the same product and batch structure. Reports of leakage, irritation, abnormal taste, battery failure or inconsistent nicotine delivery are difficult to interpret if the consumer product cannot be identified precisely. Brand name alone may be insufficient where counterfeit goods or multiple variants exist. The data system should capture photographs, batch codes, retailer, market, device type and relevant use information where available. Repeated signals can then be analysed across formulations, suppliers, components and production periods.

Data retention should reflect the product lifecycle and legal risk rather than ordinary office housekeeping. Discontinued products may still generate complaints, enforcement questions or liability claims years later. Submission records, supporting evidence, change histories and batch traceability should remain accessible for defined periods after final supply. Migration to new software must preserve metadata, relationships and audit trails, not merely transfer current files. An archive that cannot be searched or reconstructed does not provide meaningful regulatory continuity.

Cybersecurity and backup are also compliance issues. Ingredient compositions, nicotine-product submissions and supplier records are commercially sensitive, while loss or corruption could prevent the business from demonstrating compliance. Systems should use secure backups, recovery testing, access monitoring and controlled export. Cloud storage does not remove the need to understand where data are held, who can access them and how they would be recovered. A ransomware incident or account failure should not erase the regulatory history of an entire product portfolio.

Data quality should be measured through routine review. Useful indicators include missing supplier specifications, expired toxicological assessments, unresolved duplicate ingredients, submissions lacking final archives, products without current artwork links and batches manufactured against obsolete records. Vertical audits can trace one marketed vape from pack and batch back through submission, formulation, ingredients and testing. Horizontal audits can examine one field, such as CAS verification or market status, across the portfolio. These exercises test whether the system supports regulatory decisions rather than simply storing information.

The strongest vape data systems do not attempt to replace scientific judgement. They make relationships, uncertainty and responsibility visible. They show which product was assessed, which evidence applies, what changed and whether the regulatory record remains current. Poor systems produce polished dossiers by copying data at the last moment, while mature systems generate submissions from information already controlled through development and manufacture. In vaping regulation, data management is ultimately the mechanism that keeps the digital product aligned with the physical one. When that alignment is maintained, notification, surveillance and corrective action become credible. When it breaks, the organisation may no longer know whether the product being sold is the product the regulator was told existed.

Cross-Border Compliance

Cross-border vape compliance begins with a simple problem: a product does not carry its lawful status automatically when it moves from one market to another. The same e-liquid, prefilled pod, device or kit may be lawful in one jurisdiction, restricted in a neighbouring country and prohibited elsewhere. Differences can arise from nicotine limits, tank capacity, flavour rules, notification procedures, labelling, excise duty, product classification, age restrictions, advertising controls and responsible-person requirements. A manufacturer that treats international expansion as a matter of shipping identical stock into several territories misunderstands the structure of modern vape regulation. Cross-border compliance requires each destination to be assessed as a separate legal and regulatory environment.

The European Union created a degree of harmonisation through the Tobacco Products Directive and the EU Common Entry Gate, but harmonisation is not uniformity. Article 20 established common requirements for nicotine-containing electronic cigarettes and refill containers, including notification, ingredient and emissions data, nicotine concentration limits, refill-container and reservoir limits, warnings and technical protections. Manufacturers could prepare a common technical foundation and submit products to several Member States through one electronic gateway. National authorities nevertheless retained powers over fees, publication, domestic advertising, age-of-sale rules, distance sales, flavour restrictions, taxation and enforcement. A product notified through EU-CEG may therefore possess a common European dossier while still requiring separate national market-access decisions.

The first cross-border task is to define the regulatory category in every intended market. A nicotine-containing refill liquid, a nicotine-free e-liquid, a disposable device, a prefilled pod, a nicotine pouch and a medicinally presented inhaled nicotine product may follow entirely different pathways. Classification is affected by composition, presentation, claims and intended use. A product treated as a consumer vaping product under tobacco-related legislation in one country may be regarded as a medicine, prohibited nicotine product or unregulated consumer article in another. The business should confirm classification before adapting packaging or appointing distributors because every later obligation depends on that decision.

Product identity must remain stable across markets while allowing lawful national variation. Commercial teams often change flavour names, nicotine descriptions, artwork, language and pack sizes to suit local consumers. These changes can create regulatory divergence if they are not controlled. The organisation should maintain one global product identity linked to market-specific versions. Each version should show its formulation, device configuration, packaging, responsible operator, submission status and countries of supply. Where the formulation changes to meet a national flavour restriction or nicotine limit, it should receive a distinct controlled identity rather than being treated as the same product merely because the brand name remains unchanged.

Great Britain, Northern Ireland and the European Union illustrate why geographical precision matters. The United Kingdom's departure from the European Union created different procedural and legal relationships across these territories. Businesses must determine which submission route applies, which competent authority receives the information and whether one notification can support more than one destination. A product listed for Great Britain should not be assumed to be compliant automatically in Northern Ireland or an EU Member State. Packaging, responsible-person details and market records should reflect the actual territory of supply. Warehousing and distribution systems must prevent stock prepared for one regime from being diverted casually into another.

Nicotine concentration is one of the most visible cross-border variables. European-style systems commonly apply a maximum concentration of 20 milligrams per millilitre for consumer vaping products, while other markets permit higher strengths, impose lower limits, restrict nicotine to prescription pathways or prohibit commercial nicotine liquids entirely. Nicotine salts complicate interpretation because the label may refer to nicotine equivalent, salt mass or percentage strength. The regulatory team must confirm the legal basis used in each jurisdiction and ensure that formulation calculations, analytical results and labels use the same basis. Relabelling a stronger product without reformulation does not create compliance.

Volume and device-capacity restrictions require similar control. A refill container, pod or reservoir lawful in one market may exceed legal limits elsewhere. Manufacturers sometimes attempt to create one hardware platform and alter only the labelled capacity. This is unacceptable if the physical capacity remains greater than declared. The device specification, tooling, filling volume and production controls must correspond to the permitted configuration. Where separate versions are produced, component codes and packaging must prevent mixing. Cross-border compliance depends on the physical product matching the national requirement, not on the wording printed on the pack.

Flavour regulation is becoming one of the most fragmented areas. Some countries permit broad flavour ranges, others restrict descriptors, prohibit selected ingredients or limit products to tobacco, menthol or narrowly defined categories. A flavour accepted toxicologically may still be unlawful because of national policy. Conversely, a flavour permitted legally may remain unsuitable if its constituents present inhalation or thermal concerns. The organisation should therefore maintain separate scientific and legal status fields within the ingredient database. Market permission should never be interpreted as evidence of safety, and scientific acceptability should never be mistaken for legal permission.

Labelling requires more than translation. Mandatory warnings, leaflet content, ingredient disclosures, nicotine statements, batch information, responsible-operator details and recycling marks differ between jurisdictions. Direct translation can introduce technical errors where legal phrases have prescribed wording. Font size, placement, contrast and pack coverage may also be specified. Local language review should involve regulatory competence rather than ordinary commercial translation. The final artwork should be reconciled against the market-specific dossier and approved before printing. A centrally correct English label can become non-compliant through poor translation, omitted wording or the use of a contact address unacceptable in the destination country.

Responsible economic operators must be identified clearly. Some markets require a locally established manufacturer, importer, authorised representative or responsible person. Distributors may assume that they fulfil this role without understanding the legal obligations attached to it. Contracts should define who submits notifications, pays fees, maintains records, reports adverse events, manages recalls and responds to authorities. The brand owner should not assume that appointing an importer transfers every responsibility. Likewise, a local partner should not be named on packaging unless it has accepted the required duties and possesses access to the technical information needed to perform them.

Cross-border distance sales create another layer of regulation. A website accessible internationally does not mean that lawful supply is permitted everywhere. Countries may prohibit cross-border distance sales, require registration, impose age-verification standards or restrict online advertising and payment methods. The seller must control where orders are accepted, how age is verified, which stock is offered and whether tax and reporting obligations are triggered. Generic website disclaimers are inadequate. Geographical blocking, market-specific catalogues and shipping controls may be necessary to prevent consumers purchasing products that are not lawful in their location.

Customs classification and import documentation must align with the regulatory identity of the product. Incorrect commodity codes, vague descriptions or inconsistent declared values can delay shipments and attract scrutiny. Customs authorities may examine nicotine content, product type, origin, excise status and compliance documentation. A shipment described simply as "electronic accessories" may contain regulated nicotine devices and create suspicion of concealment. Commercial invoices, packing lists, certificates and product identifiers should use language consistent with the notified product. Importers should retain evidence that the goods correspond to lawful market versions rather than assuming that supplier documents are sufficient.

Excise duties and tax stamps increasingly influence cross-border vape supply. A product may be technically compliant yet unlawful for sale because duty has not been paid, the importer is unregistered or the pack lacks a required fiscal mark. Duty can apply by liquid volume, nicotine content or product category, and implementation dates may differ from product-notification timelines. Businesses must integrate fiscal compliance with regulatory planning, warehousing and inventory control. Stock produced before a duty change may require transitional treatment. Untaxed goods entering through another jurisdiction can create both customs and product-law offences.

Advertising and commercial communication rules vary considerably. Claims permitted in one market may be prohibited in another, particularly statements concerning cessation, health, reduced risk or official approval. The same social-media campaign can reach consumers across borders and trigger national restrictions even where the business has no local shop. Product names, influencer content, retailer materials and comparative statements should be reviewed for destination-specific compliance. A notification does not authorise promotional claims. Companies should separate the technical right to place a product on the market from the legal right to advertise it in a particular manner.

Enforcement intensity also varies. One country may conduct frequent retail inspections and laboratory testing, while another relies mainly on documentary checks. This does not justify applying weaker controls in less active markets. Products can move between countries, authorities share intelligence and non-compliance discovered in one jurisdiction may expose the entire portfolio. A failed sample may lead regulators elsewhere to review related products. Cross-border compliance should therefore be built to the applicable legal standard in every market and supported by one internal quality system capable of responding consistently to investigations.

Market surveillance data should be consolidated internationally. Complaints, adverse events, leakage, battery failures, labelling problems and counterfeit reports may appear first in one country. If local distributors retain these data independently, the manufacturer may miss a wider pattern. Contracts should require prompt transfer of safety and quality information using common product identifiers. The central system should compare signals across markets, batches, components and formulations. A problem that appears isolated nationally may become significant when combined with reports from several territories. Regulatory reporting obligations should then be assessed separately for each authority.

Counterfeit and grey-market products complicate cross-border responsibility. Genuine products intended for one country may be diverted into another where the packaging, nicotine strength or flavour is non-compliant. Counterfeits may copy notification numbers, branding and warnings while differing chemically or technically. Authentication features, controlled distribution and batch traceability help distinguish lawful stock from diverted or false goods. Manufacturers should monitor marketplaces and work with importers, retailers and authorities where misuse of their identity is detected. A product appearing under a familiar brand cannot be assumed to have originated from the notified supply chain.

Change control must consider every market in which the product is supplied. A supplier substitution, flavour adjustment, coil revision or artwork change may be acceptable in one jurisdiction but require amendment, renotification or withdrawal in another. The impact assessment should identify affected submissions, labels, duties, stock and transition dates country by country. Global changes should not be released until each market has been classified. Local changes should remain isolated so that one national version does not drift into another supply chain. Effective enterprise data systems make these relationships visible before procurement and manufacturing begin.

Cross-border expansion should therefore proceed through a formal market-entry gate. The business should confirm classification, composition limits, device requirements, notification status, fees, responsible operator, labelling, taxation, sales-channel rules and enforcement expectations before approving supply. The gate should include legal, regulatory, scientific, quality, logistics and commercial review. Distributor enthusiasm or retailer demand should not substitute for this assessment. A market that appears commercially attractive may require reformulation, new testing, local representation or a timetable incompatible with the planned launch.

Regulatory intelligence must continue after entry because requirements change independently. A product compliant at launch may become restricted through new flavour rules, duty arrangements, packaging standards or online-sales controls. Local partners should report legislation and authority guidance, but the manufacturer should verify developments centrally. Transition periods require careful interpretation because manufacture, import, placement on the market and final retail sale may have different deadlines. Advance monitoring allows stock, artwork, submissions and contracts to be adjusted before lawful supply is interrupted.

The strongest cross-border compliance model uses one controlled scientific dossier supported by market-specific legal modules. The common core contains product identity, formulation, toxicology, analytical evidence, manufacturing and quality controls. Each national module defines the lawful version, submission route, warnings, taxes, claims, sales restrictions and responsible parties. This avoids duplicating science while recognising that market access is never automatic. For the vaping industry, international compliance is not the movement of one product through many borders. It is the controlled placement of correctly defined product versions into distinct regulatory systems, with evidence, accountability and lifecycle oversight preserved in every destination.

Maintaining Notified Products

Maintaining a notified vaping product is the discipline of keeping the marketed article aligned with the product originally described to the competent authority. Notification captures a defined formulation, device configuration, manufacturing arrangement, packaging presentation and responsible economic operator at a particular moment. Commercial life begins afterwards, when suppliers change, components become unavailable, artwork is revised, new batches are produced and evidence develops. The principal compliance risk is therefore not that the original dossier was incomplete, but that the physical product gradually moves away from the submitted record while the notification remains unchanged. Lifecycle maintenance exists to prevent that separation.

The first control is a clearly defined regulatory baseline. The organisation should preserve the exact formulation revision, nicotine concentration, flavour composition, device specification, reservoir capacity, coil configuration, packaging version, manufacturing sites and analytical reports supporting the notified product. This baseline should be frozen at submission and linked to the official product identifier. Every later decision should be assessed against it. Without a baseline, teams compare proposed changes against current practice rather than against what was actually notified, allowing several individually small modifications to accumulate into a materially different product.

Change control is therefore central. Any proposed alteration to an ingredient, supplier, manufacturing process, component, device setting, label, pack format or market name should enter a formal assessment before implementation. The assessment should consider whether the change affects product identity, toxicological conclusions, emissions, nicotine delivery, stability, labelling or the legal status of the existing notification. Commercial pressure frequently encourages teams to classify changes as minor, particularly when the outward appearance remains unchanged. Vaping products, however, can be altered materially by changes that consumers cannot see, including coil alloy, wick density, firmware limits or flavour-carrier composition.

Supplier changes deserve particular scrutiny because they are a common source of unnoticed product drift. Two raw materials with the same chemical name or CAS number may differ in purity, impurity profile, carrier, manufacturing route or specification. A replacement flavour concentrate sold under the same sensory description may contain a different balance of constituents. A new nicotine source may meet headline assay requirements while introducing different degradation products or storage behaviour. The notified product remains defensible only when equivalent materials are demonstrated rather than assumed. Supplier change notifications, comparative specifications and targeted analytical confirmation should support the decision.

Flavour houses present a distinctive lifecycle challenge. Proprietary formulations may be adjusted for ingredient availability, cost, regulatory pressure or sensory consistency, sometimes without a change in trade name. The producer should require contractual notification of compositional changes and maintain access to updated constituent information. If a flavour is reformulated, the toxicological assessment, ingredient database, finished-product concentration calculations and relevant submissions must be reviewed together. Accepting a supplier assurance that the flavour remains "equivalent" is insufficient when the regulatory record depends on individual chemical identities and inhalation exposure.

Device component obsolescence creates similar pressure. Coils, batteries, seals, plastics and electronic controls may be substituted during a product's commercial life because original parts are discontinued or manufacturing moves to a new source. A replacement component can alter heating behaviour, aerosol mass, leakage, metal emissions or nicotine delivery even where dimensions and appearance are unchanged. Engineering equivalence should therefore be demonstrated through controlled comparison. Critical attributes such as resistance, alloy, power output, airflow and materials in contact with liquid should be defined within specifications and verified before the revised device enters production.

Manufacturing-site changes also require more than administrative update. Moving production between facilities can affect mixing scale, filling accuracy, environmental control, cleaning, component handling and batch release. The receiving site should be qualified against the notified specification, with transfer protocols, validation batches and comparable analytical results where appropriate. Contract manufacturers should not introduce local process changes without approval from the responsible economic operator. The brand owner remains accountable for the product placed on the market, even where the physical manufacturing activity is performed elsewhere.

Routine batch control keeps the notified product stable between formal changes. Raw-material release, in-process checks, nicotine verification, fill-volume control, device inspection and finished-product release should confirm that each batch remains within approved limits. Trend analysis is more valuable than isolated pass-or-fail decisions. Gradual movement in nicotine concentration, pH, colour, viscosity or emissions can reveal supplier drift, equipment wear or formulation instability before specification failure occurs. A notified product should therefore be monitored as a continuing process rather than treated as a static recipe reproduced indefinitely.

Stability programmes should remain active after launch. Real-time data may reveal changes not predicted by accelerated studies, including nicotine loss, oxidation, flavour degradation, darkening, seal failure, leakage or interaction with pod materials. These findings should be assessed against shelf-life claims and consumer exposure. Where stability trends approach limits, corrective action may include shorter shelf life, revised storage instructions, packaging changes or reformulation. Any action affecting the notified specification must then be evaluated regulatorily. The original shelf-life claim should not be defended simply because it was accepted at submission.

Post-market complaints provide another source of evidence about whether the product remains under control. Reports of harshness, unusual flavour, leakage, overheating, inconsistent vapour, battery failure or unexpected nicotine effect should be coded and linked to product version, batch, device and market. Individual complaints may reflect misuse or unrelated factors, but repeated patterns can reveal manufacturing or design failures. Complaint investigation should compare the marketed unit with the notified baseline and determine whether the issue is confined to one batch, one component source or a broader product change.

Adverse-event and vigilance systems require similar precision. The organisation should be able to identify which product was used, whether it was genuine, which batch was involved and whether the consumer combined it with other substances or devices. Reports should be assessed scientifically and escalated according to legal requirements. A suspected association does not prove causation, but recurring signals may justify targeted testing, label revision, market communication or withdrawal. Maintaining notification compliance includes demonstrating that new safety information is collected and acted upon rather than merely filed.

Market surveillance should not be left entirely to authorities. Manufacturers and importers should sample products from normal distribution channels and compare them with approved specifications. Warehouse samples alone may not reveal transport damage, retail substitution or counterfeit activity. Periodic checks can confirm nicotine concentration, capacity, packaging, authenticity and component configuration. Surveillance is particularly important for widely copied disposable or pod brands, where counterfeit products may use similar packaging while containing different liquids or oversized reservoirs. The existence of a valid notification does not protect the brand from unlawful imitation.

Packaging changes must remain connected to the regulatory record. Marketing teams may revise colour, typography, descriptors or pack format without intending to alter compliance. Yet warning placement, nicotine statements, ingredient information, responsible-operator details and product identity can be affected. Artwork revision should therefore pass through regulatory and quality review before printing. Old and new packaging should be controlled during transition, and batches should be traceable to the exact artwork version used. A notified product sold in packaging inconsistent with the submission can create enforcement concern even where the formulation remains unchanged.

Product naming also needs control. Retailers and distributors may abbreviate names, create bundle descriptions or translate flavours in ways that obscure the official identifier. The business should maintain a controlled list of permitted commercial names and aliases linked to the notified product. Where a name change affects flavour description, youth appeal or market-specific restrictions, the regulatory impact should be assessed. Rebranding should not be used to preserve an old notification for a product whose composition or presentation has changed materially.

Regulatory portals and publication lists must be monitored throughout the product's life. Fees may require renewal, authority correspondence may remain outstanding, and product status can change following review or enforcement action. The company should retain evidence of current status and reconcile public listings with its internal portfolio. Products discontinued commercially should be marked appropriately without destroying historical records. Products still sold should not rely on outdated listings that no longer correspond to the current formulation or responsible operator.

Cross-border maintenance complicates every change because one product may be notified in several markets under different rules. A modification acceptable as an amendment in one jurisdiction may require a new notification or be prohibited elsewhere. The impact assessment should identify every affected country, submission, pack and distributor before implementation. Market-specific stock must remain segregated where versions differ. A globally approved supplier change cannot be released automatically until each national regulatory consequence has been resolved.

Regulatory intelligence is therefore part of maintenance. Ingredient restrictions, flavour rules, packaging controls, taxes, environmental measures and device definitions evolve while products remain on sale. The organisation should monitor competent-authority guidance, legislation, enforcement trends and scientific developments. New evidence may affect an ingredient that was acceptable when notified. A regulatory change may impose a transition period requiring reformulation, relabelling or withdrawal. Lifecycle compliance depends on recognising these developments early enough to act deliberately rather than responding after stock becomes unlawful.

Internal audits should test whether notified products remain aligned with reality. An auditor can select a product from the market and trace it back through the current submission, formulation, supplier records, laboratory evidence, manufacturing batches and artwork. The reverse exercise can begin with a notified record and confirm that the corresponding product is still manufactured and sold as described. Differences should be investigated rather than explained away informally. The audit objective is to identify drift before an authority, retailer or consumer does.

Management review should consider portfolio risk, not only individual product status. Large flavour ranges and frequent device variants can create more notifications than the organisation can maintain competently. Products with low sales but complex supplier or toxicological requirements may no longer justify continuation. Portfolio rationalisation can reduce regulatory burden and improve control by concentrating resources on products that remain commercially and scientifically defensible. Discontinuation should be planned, with stock, submissions, complaints and record retention managed through a controlled process.

An annual product review can consolidate this evidence into one decision on continuing suitability. It should examine batch trends, complaints, adverse events, stability, supplier performance, analytical surveillance, regulatory changes and outstanding corrective actions. The review should confirm whether the notified dossier remains current, whether further testing is needed and whether continued supply is justified. This prevents lifecycle maintenance from becoming a collection of disconnected reactions and gives management a documented basis for retaining, modifying or discontinuing each vaping product within portfolio.

Where a product no longer meets requirements, corrective action must be proportionate and timely. Options include stopping manufacture, quarantining stock, correcting labels, amending the notification, reformulating, withdrawing affected batches or recalling products from consumers. The decision should consider the nature of the defect, exposure, distribution and legal obligations. Delaying action to protect sales can transform a manageable compliance issue into a wider enforcement and reputational failure. Authorities should be informed where required, with clear records of the investigation and measures taken.

Discontinued products remain part of the regulatory history. Complaints, adverse events or authority questions may arise after final sale, and retained stock may remain within distribution. Technical dossiers, submission records, batch data, change histories and correspondence should be preserved for defined periods. The organisation should know when final units entered the market and when responsibilities can reasonably close. Deleting records because a product has disappeared from the catalogue destroys evidence needed to understand past manufacture and exposure.

Maintaining notified vaping products is ultimately the practice of preserving correspondence between the regulatory record and the evolving commercial product. It requires disciplined change control, supplier oversight, batch monitoring, surveillance, regulatory intelligence and decisive corrective action. Notification provides lawful visibility at one moment; maintenance determines whether that visibility remains truthful. A product that was compliant at launch can become non-compliant through accumulation of unmanaged changes, while a well-controlled product can remain defensible for years because every alteration is recognised, assessed and documented. The strength of the system is measured not by how many products appear on a register, but by whether each listed product still exists in the market exactly as the regulator has been led to understand it.

CHAPTER 7

Global Regulatory Models

A vaping product does not change chemically when it crosses a national border, yet its legal identity can change completely. The same liquid may be treated as a lawful consumer product in one country, a therapeutic good in another, a tobacco product elsewhere and a prohibited import in the next. Its nicotine concentration, aerosol composition, battery chemistry and toxicological profile remain unchanged, but the regulatory meaning assigned to those characteristics depends on the jurisdiction in which the product is manufactured, imported, advertised, sold or used. Geography therefore becomes an invisible component of the product. It determines not only whether the product may enter the market, but which evidence must be generated, which claims may be made, which consumers can obtain it and which institutions assume responsibility for controlling it.

This fragmentation is not unique to vaping, but vaping exposes it with unusual clarity. Medicines, foods, cosmetics, chemicals and electrical goods are also regulated differently across the world, yet their established categories provide a degree of shared legal understanding. Vaping entered international markets without such stability. It combined a nicotine formulation, an electrical device, an inhaled aerosol, a smoking-like behaviour and a consumer proposition that could not be contained comfortably within any existing category. Governments were required to classify the technology before they could regulate it, and that first classification decision shaped almost everything that followed.

Where the product was placed within tobacco law, policy tended to emphasise nicotine dependence, youth initiation, advertising restrictions and the historical conduct of cigarette companies. Where it entered medicines law, the focus shifted towards quality, safety, efficacy, controlled manufacturing and therapeutic purpose. Where it remained primarily within consumer-product legislation, electrical safety, chemical disclosure and general obligations not to supply unsafe goods became more prominent. Some governments treated vaping principally as an alternative to smoking. Others treated it as a new route into nicotine use. Each interpretation produced a different regulatory architecture from the same underlying technology.

These differences demonstrate that regulation is not simply the scientific assessment of a product followed by the application of neutral controls. It is the institutional interpretation of what the product represents. A vaping device may be viewed as a smoking substitute, a recreational nicotine product, a cessation aid, an environmental burden, a youth-attractive commodity or an extension of the tobacco market. None of these descriptions captures the whole product, yet each can become the organising principle of national policy. Once selected, it influences which evidence receives greatest weight and which outcomes are regarded as regulatory success.

A system centred on smoking substitution is likely to ask whether adult smokers can obtain products capable of competing with cigarettes. It may value nicotine delivery, sensory acceptability, product variety and retail accessibility because these characteristics influence whether consumers switch completely. A system centred on prevention is more likely to ask whether flavours, packaging, price and availability encourage nicotine initiation among people who would otherwise remain abstinent. A medicalised system may ask whether a defined product can demonstrate therapeutic benefit under controlled conditions, while a prohibitionist system may conclude that uncertainty itself provides sufficient reason to prevent legal supply.

The scientific evidence does not change merely because these questions differ, but its interpretation does. A study showing that a vaping product exposes users to fewer combustion-related toxicants than cigarettes may support regulated market access in one jurisdiction. Another authority may regard the same evidence as insufficient because it does not establish long-term safety or population benefit. Evidence of smoking cessation may be treated as proof of harm-reduction potential, or discounted because the product has not received medicinal authorisation. Evidence of youth use may justify targeted age enforcement in one system and broad product prohibition in another. The regulatory outcome depends not only on what the research demonstrates, but on the comparator, population and public objective selected by the state.

This makes international comparison scientifically valuable. Different legal systems operate as large-scale policy experiments. They alter product availability, price, nicotine concentration, flavour choice, retail access, advertising, consumer perception and the structure of the lawful market. These differences influence who uses vaping products, what they use, how they obtain them and what they might otherwise have consumed. Regulation therefore becomes an exposure variable in its own right. It changes the products present in the population and the behaviours through which health outcomes emerge.

The results are rarely simple. A permissive market may encourage rapid switching away from smoking while also allowing aggressive promotion, product proliferation and youth access. A restrictive market may reduce lawful product visibility but stimulate informal supply, personal importation or illicit trade. A prescription model may provide clinical oversight while limiting access for smokers who do not engage with healthcare services. A demanding premarket authorisation system may improve the quality of evidence required from lawful manufacturers while concentrating the market among companies capable of financing extensive submissions. Prohibition may reduce recorded legal sales without eliminating consumer demand.

Observed outcomes must therefore be interpreted carefully. Low lawful sales do not necessarily demonstrate low use if products are entering through informal channels. High notification numbers do not prove that regulators have assessed every product in depth. A decline in vaping prevalence may appear beneficial while smoking, illicit nicotine use or cross-border purchasing increases. Conversely, growth in vaping can indicate successful substitution among smokers, new uptake among non-smokers or both. Regulatory evaluation must look beyond the indicator most favourable to the chosen policy.

The global market also reveals the limits of regulating products through national borders. Formulations may be developed in one country, manufactured in another, branded in a third and sold online to consumers across several jurisdictions. Components travel through international supply chains before final assembly. Flavour houses, nicotine suppliers, device factories, laboratories, importers and distributors may each operate under different legal systems. A national authority can control domestic sale, but it cannot assume that the product's entire history has occurred within its own regulatory environment.

Digital commerce makes this problem more acute. Online marketplaces can present consumers with products that are absent from domestic registers, exceed local nicotine or capacity limits, or carry packaging intended for another country. Social-media promotion crosses borders more easily than regulated advertising. Small parcels can enter through postal and courier networks that were not designed to inspect every nicotine product individually. A system may impose detailed obligations on domestic manufacturers while consumers purchase non-compliant goods directly from overseas suppliers that remain beyond effective enforcement.

This creates an asymmetry between the regulated and unregulated market. Lawful businesses must interpret national requirements, prepare dossiers, pay fees, adapt packaging, observe waiting periods and maintain responsible operators. Suppliers outside the jurisdiction may avoid those costs and reach consumers through channels that are difficult to police. The stricter the lawful pathway becomes, the greater the potential economic advantage available to those willing to bypass it. Regulatory strength must therefore be judged partly by the state's ability to control the market beyond the businesses already inclined to comply.

International divergence also affects product design. Manufacturers do not develop products in a legal vacuum. They design around nicotine ceilings, container limits, prohibited ingredients, refillability definitions, flavour restrictions and evidential requirements. A device developed for a market permitting higher nicotine concentrations may be unsuitable for a jurisdiction with a lower limit unless aerosol performance is altered. A product designed around one legal definition of reusability may be prohibited under another. Packaging may need to accommodate different warnings, languages, tax stamps and responsible-person details. Regulation becomes embedded within the engineering and formulation of the product.

The resulting product may no longer be genuinely global. The brand appears international, but the physical and regulatory versions differ. One market receives a lower nicotine strength, another a restricted flavour range, another a prescription product and another no lawful product at all. These differences complicate manufacturing, data management and post-market surveillance. Complaints associated with the same brand may concern materially different formulations or devices. Laboratory findings generated in one jurisdiction may not apply directly to the version sold elsewhere. Global brand recognition can therefore conceal significant technical variation.

The distinction between notification and authorisation is especially important in international comparison. A notification system places responsibility primarily on the manufacturer or importer to submit prescribed information and comply with legal requirements. The authority receives visibility and may intervene where concerns arise, but it does not necessarily make an affirmative premarket judgement on every product. An authorisation system requires the regulator to determine that the evidence satisfies a defined statutory threshold before lawful marketing. These approaches differ in cost, speed, evidential depth and market effect.

Neither model guarantees control. Notification can permit a wide variety of products while leaving authorities with more data than they can analyse effectively. Authorisation can demand extensive evidence while unauthorised products continue to circulate. A register can be mistaken for approval, and an authorisation can be misunderstood as a declaration that the product is safe. Both systems depend on accurate manufacturer data, competent scientific review, market surveillance and enforcement. The legal gateway is only one part of the regulatory model.

Regulatory capacity varies enormously between countries. Some authorities maintain specialist teams in toxicology, aerosol science, engineering, data analysis and market surveillance. Others must regulate vaping within departments already responsible for medicines, tobacco, chemicals, food or consumer products. A technically sophisticated law may therefore exceed the resources available to implement it. Authorities may receive extensive ingredient and emissions data without possessing the laboratory capacity or analytical systems needed to evaluate them. Enforcement officers may be expected to distinguish lawful from unlawful devices without reliable access to product records or testing.

International organisations and larger regulatory jurisdictions consequently exert influence beyond their formal legal boundaries. Countries with limited domestic capacity may adopt definitions, warnings, prohibitions or technical limits developed elsewhere. This can accelerate the introduction of basic protections and prevent markets from operating without oversight. It can also transfer assumptions from one social, economic and epidemiological context into another. A policy designed for a wealthy country with declining smoking prevalence, extensive enforcement and accessible cessation services may not produce the same outcome where smoking remains high, healthcare access is limited and illicit trade is widespread.

Economic conditions matter because regulation changes the relative attractiveness of lawful products. Notification fees, laboratory requirements, taxation and import controls raise the cost of compliant supply. In high-income markets, consumers may absorb some of that cost. In lower-income markets, modest price increases can shift demand towards cigarettes, informal refills or unregulated imports. A product standard that appears proportionate in one economy may remove lawful products from another entirely. Global regulation cannot be assessed separately from affordability, commercial scale and enforcement capacity.

Cultural and political attitudes towards nicotine also shape national models. Some societies accept continuing nicotine use where it occurs through substantially less hazardous delivery systems. Others define success as movement towards complete nicotine abstinence. Some governments trust regulated consumer markets; others prefer medical, state-controlled or highly restricted access. The influence of tobacco companies, independent vaping businesses, public health organisations and consumer groups varies between jurisdictions. Historical experience with cigarette industry conduct can lead authorities to distrust all commercial nicotine innovation, while experience of consumer-led switching can produce greater tolerance of regulated access.

These differences make claims of a single correct global model difficult to sustain. Scientific principles can be shared: accurate ingredient disclosure, controlled manufacture, reliable testing, protection of children, truthful communication, traceability and effective corrective action are relevant everywhere. The policy balance surrounding those principles is more contested. Governments assign different weight to adult autonomy, youth prevention, smoking displacement, precaution, environmental harm and commercial freedom. International comparison can reveal which systems perform better against specified outcomes, but it cannot remove the need to state which outcomes matter.

The danger lies in mistaking regulatory uniformity for scientific coherence. Applying identical restrictions to all products and countries may appear consistent, yet ignore differences in toxicological risk, smoking prevalence, healthcare access and market behaviour. At the same time, uncontrolled national divergence creates duplication, trade barriers, inconsistent consumer protection and opportunities for regulatory arbitrage. The challenge is to identify which elements require international consistency and which should remain adaptable to local conditions.

Modern nicotine regulation therefore operates between two competing realities. Products and supply chains are global, while legal authority remains national. Scientific evidence crosses borders, but policy objectives do not always travel with it. A laboratory method can be standardised internationally; the judgement made from its result may still differ. A chemical identifier can mean the same thing in every country; the substance it represents may be permitted, restricted or prohibited according to local law. A common technical dossier can support several markets, but no dossier can erase differences in classification, claims, taxation, retail control or political purpose.

Global regulatory models reveal more than variations in legal drafting. They reveal how societies understand nicotine, risk and responsibility. They determine whether harm reduction is treated as a consumer transition, a medical intervention, a tightly controlled exception or an unacceptable compromise. They show how regulation can create lawful markets, suppress them, concentrate them or drive them beyond official visibility. Most importantly, they demonstrate that regulatory outcomes cannot be judged from the severity of the rules alone. The meaningful question is whether the system produces a safer, more accountable and more intelligible nicotine market than the one that would exist without it.

Figure 7.1. Global Regulatory Models for Vaping: Jurisdiction Comparison Matrix.

This matrix compares the principal regulatory approaches applied to vaping products across major jurisdictions and developing markets. It organises each jurisdiction according to four connected elements: the primary regulatory model, the route through which products gain lawful market access, the principal technical and legal controls applied, and the overall regulatory posture created by those controls. The colour key at the top distinguishes notification-based systems, authorisation-heavy systems, medicalised models, mixed or fragmented regimes and developing frameworks, making the differences in regulatory philosophy immediately visible.

The European Union is presented as a harmonised notification-based model operating through the Tobacco Products Directive. Its framework combines pre-market notification with defined nicotine and volume limits, ingredient and emissions reporting and technical product requirements, while still allowing national variation in taxation, retail controls, flavours and enforcement. The United Kingdom is shown as retaining a closely related consumer-product model administered through the MHRA, with structured notification, publication, vigilance and due-diligence expectations adapted to the post-Brexit regulatory environment.

The United States is positioned as an authorisation-heavy system because lawful market access depends on the Premarket Tobacco Product Application pathway and the granting of a written marketing order. This contrasts sharply with notification systems, since the applicant must provide product-specific scientific evidence capable of satisfying a demanding population-level statutory standard before the product can remain lawfully marketed. Australia is shown as a medicalised and restrictive model, in which access has been shaped through therapeutic, pharmacy and prescription-led controls rather than an ordinary consumer market.

New Zealand is presented as a regulated consumer harm-reduction model. Its system allows comparatively accessible adult market access while applying product notification, specialist retail controls, marketing restrictions, product standards and youth-protection measures. Canada occupies a more layered position, combining federal consumer-product requirements with nicotine, packaging, promotion and reporting controls, alongside provincial rules that can alter retail access and product presentation.

Asia is represented as highly fragmented because there is no single regional model. Countries within the region range from notification and standards-based systems to prescription control, import restriction and outright prohibition. The Middle East is similarly shown as mixed and rapidly evolving, with some jurisdictions moving towards formal standards, product registration and import oversight while others retain restrictive or inconsistent approaches. Emerging markets are presented as transitional systems in which limited regulatory capacity, borrowed legal models, taxation pressures and illicit-trade risks often influence the pace and direction of formalisation.

The lower section identifies the common regulatory levers used across these otherwise different systems: product classification, notification, authorisation, technical standards, labelling, marketing controls, taxation and enforcement. These levers show that jurisdictions often regulate the same scientific and commercial issues through different legal mechanisms. A country may use notification where another requires authorisation, or taxation where another relies on prescription control, yet all are attempting to manage product identity, nicotine exposure, consumer protection, youth access and market accountability.

The figure should be read as a comparison of regulatory structure rather than a ranking of which jurisdiction is most protective or effective. A demanding model does not necessarily produce stronger market control if unauthorised products remain widely available, while a notification-based model does not necessarily imply weak oversight where data quality, surveillance and enforcement are robust. The matrix therefore establishes the central analytical question for the chapter: not simply how strict each regime appears, but how effectively each model translates scientific evidence, legal authority and enforcement capacity into a controlled vaping market.

CHAPTER 7 – GLOBAL REGULATORY MODELS

JURISDICTION COMPARISON MATRIX

Notification-based | Authorisation-heavy | Medicalised | Mixed / fragmented | Developing frameworks

	PRIMARY MODEL	MARKET ACCESS ROUTE	KEY REGULATORY FEATURES	OVERALL POSTURE
EUROPEAN UNION	TPD consumer product framework	Pre-market notification	20 mg/mL nicotine cap; 2 mL tank and 10 mL refill limits; ingredient and emissions reporting	Harmonised baseline with national variation
UNITED KINGDOM	MHRA-administered consumer framework	Pre-market notification	Notification list; ingredient and emissions data; vigilance and due-diligence expectations	Structured and transparent post-Brexit continuity
UNITED STATES (PMTA)	Tobacco product authorisation	PMTA marketing order	Product-specific scientific review; high evidential burden; FDA enforcement focus	Highly demanding authorisation model
AUSTRALIA	Therapeutic / prescription-led model	Medical or controlled supply pathways	Prescription focus; tight retail controls; therapeutic standards	Medicalised and restrictive
NEW ZEALAND	Regulated consumer harm-reduction model	Notification and retail compliance	Specialist vape retail; product standards; youth and marketing controls	Accessible but actively regulated
CANADA	Federal consumer framework	Product compliance plus reporting	Promotion restrictions; nicotine and packaging controls; federal and provincial layers	Balanced but tightening
ASIA	Mixed regional approaches	Country-specific approvals or restrictions	Wide diversity: notification, restriction or prohibition depending on market	Highly fragmented
MIDDLE EAST	Mixed and often restrictive	Country-specific registration or import control	Standards-based control; import oversight; variable national rules	Rapidly evolving, unevenly regulated
EMERGING MARKETS	Developing frameworks	Interim rules or borrowed models	Capacity constraints; tax pressure; illicit-trade risk; gradual formalisation	Transitional and diverse

COMMON REGULATORY LEVERS

Classification | Notification | Authorisation | Product standards | Labelling | Marketing controls | Taxation | Enforcement

European Union

The European Union created the first harmonised regulatory framework designed specifically for consumer vaping products. Its importance extends beyond the twenty-seven Member States because the model established a route between unrestricted consumer sale and pharmaceutical authorisation. Instead of requiring every nicotine-containing electronic cigarette to become a medicine, the Union placed these products within tobacco-related legislation and imposed notification, composition, packaging, technical and post-market obligations. The result was not a declaration that vaping was equivalent to smoking, but a legal compromise through which a non-combustible nicotine product could remain available while becoming visible to public authorities. Directive 2014/40/EU entered into force in May 2014 and became applicable across the Union in May 2016.

The framework rests on the dual legal objectives of improving the functioning of the internal market and securing a high level of human health protection. Those objectives explain both its strengths and its tensions. Harmonisation was necessary because electronic cigarettes had previously been classified and controlled differently between countries, creating barriers to trade and inconsistent consumer protection. Public health protection required controls over nicotine, ingredients, emissions, packaging and product performance. Yet the Directive also left significant authority with Member States, so the European market became harmonised at its technical core while remaining fragmented in taxation, flavour policy, retail rules, enforcement and aspects of product presentation.

Article 20 supplies the regulatory centre of the model. It applies to electronic cigarettes and refill containers that are not authorised as medicinal products. Manufacturers and importers must notify the competent authorities of the Member States in which products are intended to be placed on the market, generally six months before market entry. The information includes product identity, ingredients, emissions, toxicological data, nicotine dose and uptake, components, manufacturing processes and declarations of responsibility. Notification is therefore a pre-market information duty rather than a conventional authorisation. The authority receives a structured representation of the product, but inclusion within a national record does not mean that every scientific statement has been independently verified or that the product has received an affirmative safety approval.

This distinction enabled a diverse consumer market to survive. Full pharmaceutical assessment for every flavour, nicotine strength and device variant would have imposed costs and development times incompatible with much of the early independent vaping sector. Notification lowered the evidential gateway while retaining producer accountability. It also transferred responsibility to manufacturers and importers. They must ensure that submitted data are accurate, that ingredients meet the required standards, that products remain compliant after notification and that corrective action is taken when safety or quality concerns arise. The European model therefore depends heavily on the competence and integrity of the economic operator.

The Directive established numerical limits that reshaped product design. Nicotine-containing liquid may not exceed 20 milligrams per millilitre; refill containers are limited to 10 millilitres; and tanks or cartridges are generally limited to 2 millilitres. Products must be child-resistant and tamper-evident, protected against breakage and leakage, and capable of refilling without leakage where applicable. Ingredients other than nicotine must meet high purity expectations, while nicotine delivery should remain consistent under comparable conditions of use. These requirements created measurable boundaries that enforcement authorities could inspect and laboratories could test.

Their scientific meaning is more limited than their legal precision suggests. Nicotine exposure is not determined by concentration alone. Device power, coil design, aerosol mass, nicotine chemistry, puff duration and consumer behaviour all influence delivered dose. A 2-millilitre reservoir does not limit daily consumption when it can be refilled repeatedly, and a 10-millilitre bottle does not control cumulative purchasing. The limits nevertheless forced manufacturers to design products capable of satisfying smokers within fixed constraints. Improvements in aerosol efficiency, pod design and acidified nicotine formulations partly emerged within this regulatory environment. The law did not stop innovation; it redirected it towards performance within prescribed boundaries.

Ingredient regulation is similarly principle-based rather than exhaustive. Producers must avoid prohibited additives and ensure that ingredients do not pose a risk to human health in heated or unheated form. This creates a demanding scientific obligation because many flavour substances possess extensive oral-use histories but limited inhalation evidence. The Directive does not provide a complete positive list of permitted e-liquid ingredients or a universal toxicological threshold for every compound. Manufacturers must therefore combine supplier disclosure, literature review, exposure assessment, emissions testing and professional judgement. The quality of compliance varies according to the data available and the sophistication of the producer's scientific systems.

EU-CEG, the European Union Common Entry Gate, provides the information architecture supporting these obligations. It allows manufacturers and importers to submit structured information on tobacco products, electronic cigarettes and refill containers to the relevant Member States through one technical gateway. The system was intended to reduce administrative burden and improve comparability by standardising fields for ingredients, emissions, toxicological information, product characteristics and submitter identity.

EU-CEG is one of the model's most significant achievements, but also reveals the difference between data collection and regulatory intelligence. A common format can require the same categories of information without guaranteeing that chemical names, CAS numbers, toxicological summaries or emissions methods are scientifically comparable. Proprietary flavour mixtures may be reported inconsistently. Similar products can generate separate records, while product families may be difficult to group. National authorities vary in their ability to analyse large datasets. The portal can confirm technical completion, yet it cannot determine automatically whether an ingredient assessment is adequate or whether the tested product matches commercial manufacture.

Packaging and consumer information complete the core product framework. Nicotine-containing products must carry prescribed warnings and provide instructions concerning use, storage, contraindications, possible adverse effects, addictiveness and toxicity. The pack must not present the product as beneficial to health, environmentally preferable or otherwise misleading. These requirements acknowledge that the vape is both a chemical exposure system and a consumer article used without professional supervision. Their value depends on clarity. Dense leaflets and repetitive warnings may satisfy formal requirements while contributing little to safe use, whereas simplified communication can omit information necessary for vulnerable consumers, accidental exposure prevention or correct device operation.

Post-market responsibility extends beyond passive complaint collection. Manufacturers and importers must maintain systems for recording suspected adverse effects, investigate products believed to be unsafe or non-compliant and notify authorities of corrective measures. This creates a lifecycle obligation connecting the original dossier with batches sold years later. In practice, vigilance quality depends on traceable product identifiers, distributor cooperation and the ability to distinguish genuine products from counterfeits.

Weak reports may identify only a brand or flavour, leaving the responsible operator unable to determine the formulation, device, batch or market version involved. The European model is strongest where notification, manufacturing traceability, complaint investigation and authority reporting function as one continuous evidence system rather than separate administrative duties. That continuity determines whether early regulatory visibility becomes sustained consumer protection throughout commercial life.

The European system therefore operates through shared legislation but decentralised implementation. Each Member State designates competent authorities, receives submissions, sets or collects fees where applicable, publishes information according to national arrangements and enforces domestic law. This division respects national responsibility while permitting different levels of scrutiny and market control. A manufacturer can use a common dossier foundation, but still encounters different administrative practices, languages, charges and enforcement expectations. Harmonisation reduces duplication; it does not remove the need for country-specific regulatory intelligence.

National discretion has expanded as Member States respond to youth use, environmental waste and political pressure. Some have adopted flavour restrictions, retail controls or prohibitions affecting disposable electronic cigarettes. By mid-2026, the Commission had issued decisions concerning national measures notified by France, Bulgaria, Ireland and Austria, illustrating how Article 24 mechanisms can permit stronger national action within the wider European framework. This produces a market in which the core product rules remain European while the commercial conditions of access become increasingly national.

Advertising regulation reinforces that fragmentation. The Directive restricts cross-border commercial communications and sponsorship, but domestic controls can differ. Manufacturers cannot assume that a product notified lawfully may be promoted uniformly across the Union. Claims concerning cessation, health or reduced risk are especially sensitive because they may trigger medicines law, consumer-protection rules or tobacco-advertising prohibitions. This creates an information problem: companies must not imply that vaping is harmless or officially approved, yet overly broad restrictions can also make truthful communication about the absence of combustion and relative exposure difficult.

Market surveillance is the test of whether the model controls real products rather than compliant paperwork. Notification databases help authorities identify responsible operators and compare declared characteristics, but they do not prevent oversized, unnotified or counterfeit products from entering shops and online markets. Legal manufacturers observe waiting periods, pay fees, commission testing and limit capacities, while unlawful suppliers can move rapidly through changing brands and import channels. The public-health value of Article 20 therefore depends on inspection, sampling, laboratory capability, customs cooperation and effective penalties. A sophisticated submission system cannot compensate for weak enforcement at the point of sale.

The model also generates market-structure effects. Regulatory costs improved documentation and removed some poorly characterised products, but they favoured businesses able to finance testing, toxicology and regulatory staff. Smaller independent companies could remain within a notification system more readily than under pharmaceutical authorisation, yet still faced substantial costs across multiple variants and Member States. Larger tobacco and consumer-goods companies possessed greater capacity to absorb these burdens. Regulation consequently improved formal control while contributing to consolidation and a market increasingly divided between well-resourced lawful operators and rapidly moving illicit suppliers.

The European approach remains closely connected to the precautionary principle. Legislators acted before long-term epidemiological evidence was available, reasoning that nicotine-containing inhalation products should not develop without controls. The Court of Justice upheld Article 20 in the Pillbox 38 litigation, recognising the legislature's discretion in a technically complex field characterised by uncertainty and divergent national rules. Legal validity, however, does not establish that every limit is scientifically optimal. It confirms that the Union was entitled to adopt proportionate controls within a broad public-health mandate.

A decade of implementation has revealed where the architecture has aged. The Directive was developed around refill liquids, early tank systems and first-generation electronic cigarettes. The later market introduced nicotine salts, compact pods, disposable products, rechargeable hybrids and devices marketed through claimed puff counts rather than transparent liquid volume. Fixed definitions and capacity limits have been tested by products designed around their boundaries. Regulatory interpretation has had to evolve without equivalent speed in the primary legislation.

The Commission's 2021 application report recognised the Directive's achievements while identifying problems involving data quality, enforcement, emerging products and national divergence. The wider evaluation of the tobacco-control legislative framework, published in April 2026, assessed effectiveness, efficiency, relevance, coherence and European added value within the objective of a tobacco-free generation by 2040. It concluded that the framework required development to respond to market and public-health change, and the Commission began preparing further legislative action.

Future reform will have to decide whether harmonisation should deepen or permit further national experimentation. EU-wide flavour rules, environmental requirements, taxation and broader nicotine-product definitions could reduce fragmentation and regulatory arbitrage. They could also impose one policy balance across countries with different smoking rates, consumer behaviours and enforcement capabilities. A centralised approach may improve consistency, but scientific proportionality depends on preserving distinctions between combustible products, vaping products and other nicotine systems rather than regulating every category through inherited tobacco assumptions.

The European Union model remains influential because it made vaping governable without forcing it wholly into medicines law or leaving it under general consumer safety rules. It established a common product identity, a structured notification pathway and minimum protections across a large market. Its enduring weakness is the gap between harmonised data obligations and uneven real-world control. The next stage must make the information already collected more usable, strengthen connections between notifications and enforcement, and ensure that restrictions aimed at youth or environmental protection do not erase the toxicological distinction between combustion and non-combustion. European regulation will succeed only where legal consistency, scientific competence and enforceable market control remain aligned.

United Kingdom

The United Kingdom occupies a distinctive position in global vaping regulation because it combines a permissive harm-reduction policy with a structured consumer-product framework. Nicotine-containing vapes are not ordinary consumer goods, yet most do not require medicinal authorisation before sale. The principal route remains notification under the Tobacco and Related Products Regulations 2016, administered by the Medicines and Healthcare products Regulatory Agency. This arrangement preserved much of the European Tobacco Products Directive architecture while allowing domestic priorities after withdrawal from the European Union. The model accepts vaping as materially different from smoking but surrounds that acceptance with stronger controls over product design, retailing, advertising, taxation and environmental impact.

The regulatory foundation is Part 6 of the Tobacco and Related Products Regulations 2016. These Regulations define requirements for nicotine-containing electronic cigarettes and refill containers supplied as consumer products. They limit nicotine concentration to 20 milligrams per millilitre, refill-container volume to 10 millilitres and tank or cartridge capacity to 2 millilitres. Products must be child-resistant and tamper-evident, protected against breakage and leakage, and designed to deliver nicotine consistently under normal conditions. Packaging must carry prescribed warnings and information, while manufacturers and importers must notify products before lawful supply. These requirements created a measurable market baseline and remain central to compliance in Great Britain.

The Medicines and Healthcare products Regulatory Agency is the competent authority for the notification scheme. Producers submit product identity, formulation, ingredient, emissions, toxicological, component and manufacturing information through the system. Products completing the process are published on a list, allowing retailers, consumers and enforcement officers to check whether a nicotine-containing vape has been notified. Publication does not amount to medicinal approval, independent safety certification or confirmation that every scientific statement has been verified. It records that required information has been provided and the product has entered the regulatory system under the manufacturer's or importer's responsibility.

This distinction between notification and authorisation is fundamental to the British model. The producer remains responsible for product quality, safety, conformity and continuing accuracy of the submitted information. The MHRA can review data, request clarification, investigate concerns and support corrective action, but it does not reproduce every emissions study, audit every manufacturing site or approve every formulation in the pharmaceutical sense. The framework therefore depends heavily on the quality systems and scientific competence of economic operators. A complete portal entry cannot compensate for an unidentified flavour constituent, an inappropriate aerosol method, an unqualified supplier or a device that no longer matches the configuration originally tested.

The United Kingdom also preserves a separate medicinal pathway. A vaping product intended to treat nicotine dependence, support smoking cessation through authorised therapeutic claims or enter formal healthcare supply may seek a medicines marketing authorisation. This route demands substantially greater evidence of quality, safety, efficacy, manufacturing consistency and benefit-risk. It offers the possibility of approved therapeutic claims and integration into clinical pathways, but the development cost, stable product specification and regulatory timescale differ sharply from those of the consumer market. The coexistence of the two routes reflects an unresolved but pragmatic distinction: vapes may be used by consumers to stop smoking without every product being regulated as a medicine.

Post-market vigilance forms an important part of the system. Producers must maintain arrangements for collecting information about suspected adverse effects and must investigate products that may be unsafe, poor quality or non-compliant. The MHRA's Yellow Card arrangements provide a route for reporting suspected safety problems associated with nicotine-containing vapes and e-liquids. Reports do not prove causation, but repeated patterns can identify issues involving leakage, overheating, unexpected reactions, defective batteries or inconsistent product performance. Effective vigilance requires accurate product names, batch codes and supply-chain information, because a complaint linked only to a brand may concern a counterfeit, an outdated version or a product manufactured outside the notified specification.

Enforcement is distributed rather than concentrated within the MHRA. Trading Standards services lead retail inspection, age-of-sale compliance, sampling and action against non-compliant products. Border and customs authorities address imports, while environmental regulators, advertising bodies and local authorities control other parts of the market. This division reflects the vape's simultaneous status as a nicotine product, electrical device, chemical mixture, packaged article and excisable good. It also creates coordination challenges. A sophisticated notification database has limited effect if local services cannot inspect shops, test capacity, confirm nicotine strength or trace imported products to responsible operators.

The United Kingdom's public-health stance has historically distinguished vaping from smoking more clearly than many other jurisdictions. National policy has recognised that complete substitution away from combustible cigarettes can reduce exposure to combustion-related toxicants, while maintaining that vaping is not risk-free and should not be promoted to children or people who do not smoke. This dual position supported broad adult consumer access, specialist retailing and the use of vaping within smoking-cessation practice. It also created communication difficulties. Regulators must prevent unsupported claims of safety or medicinal benefit while ensuring that smokers understand why non-combustible nicotine products are not equivalent to cigarettes.

Youth uptake has altered the political balance. Rapid growth in colourful, low-cost and highly convenient products produced concern that the market was extending beyond adult smokers. The response has moved British regulation beyond the original technical controls of the 2016 Regulations. Product presentation, flavour descriptions, retail display, advertising, age verification and enforcement have become central policy issues. This shift does not remove the harm-reduction rationale, but it places greater emphasis on separating adult access from youth appeal. The scientific difficulty is that characteristics supporting successful substitution for smokers, including flavour, simplicity and effective nicotine delivery, can also increase attractiveness to inexperienced users.

The prohibition on the sale and supply of single-use vapes from 1 June 2025 demonstrated how environmental law can reshape nicotine regulation. Disposable devices combine plastics, electronic components and lithium batteries in products designed for brief use. The ban also responded indirectly to enforcement and youth concerns associated with rapid brand turnover and highly visible formats. It did not prohibit vaping; it redirected the lawful market towards reusable products. Its effectiveness depends on whether replacements are genuinely refillable and rechargeable rather than merely redesigned to satisfy the minimum legal definition.

The Tobacco and Vapes Act 2026 marks a broader transition from inherited European-style product rules towards a more comprehensive domestic nicotine-control regime. Receiving Royal Assent on 29 April 2026, the Act created powers and offences extending across tobacco, vaping and other nicotine products. For vaping, its significance lies in the ability to regulate packaging, product standards, flavours, displays, retail licensing, advertising and sponsorship more extensively than under the earlier framework. The Act establishes the legal machinery, but many practical effects depend on commencement provisions and secondary regulations. Regulatory impact will therefore be determined by the detailed rules, transition periods and enforcement arrangements made under it.

A comprehensive ban on advertising and sponsorship of vaping and nicotine products is intended to come into force across the United Kingdom from 1 June 2027. This represents a substantial change from a system in which certain domestic promotional channels remained available despite restrictions on cross-border advertising. The policy seeks to reduce commercial exposure and youth appeal, while preserving a defence for qualifying public-health communications. Its success will depend on the treatment of factual product information, retailer communication and harm-reduction messaging. A ban that prevents lifestyle promotion can protect young people; one that also obstructs accurate information for adult smokers may weaken informed substitution.

The Act also broadens the regulatory treatment of nicotine products beyond traditional nicotine-containing e-cigarettes. Earlier controls did not always apply consistently to nicotine-free vapes or newer oral nicotine products. Extending age restrictions, licensing and product powers across categories reduces opportunities for suppliers to move products outside narrow definitions. It also requires technical precision. Nicotine-free liquids, reusable devices and products with no tobacco content do not present identical hazards, and a common legal framework should not become a claim of toxicological equivalence. Proportionate implementation requires controls to follow product function, exposure and likely users rather than terminology alone.

Fiscal regulation now forms another major layer. Vaping Products Duty applies from 1 October 2026 to qualifying vaping liquids produced in or imported into the United Kingdom, whether or not they contain nicotine. The duty is set at a flat rate, accompanied by a duty-stamp scheme for retail packaging. Manufacturers and importers must operate within HM Revenue and Customs approval, record-keeping and payment arrangements. The system converts vaping from a notified consumer category into an excisable product with additional controls over production, importation, warehousing and release. This changes compliance profoundly because technical legality, MHRA notification and tax status must all align before lawful supply.

The duty may improve traceability and provide enforcement tools against undeclared products, but it also affects the economics of harm reduction. A flat charge based on liquid volume is administratively clear, yet it does not correspond directly to nicotine delivery, toxicological risk or smoking-substitution value. The Government has paired the new duty with an additional increase in tobacco duty to preserve a price differential between vaping and smoking. Whether that differential remains sufficient will depend on retail pricing, compliance costs, illicit trade and consumer behaviour. If lawful vaping becomes substantially more expensive while cigarettes and untaxed imports remain accessible, fiscal policy could weaken the incentive to switch.

Duty stamps may become a practical market-authentication tool, although they cannot prove that a product meets every technical requirement. A stamped pack can indicate participation in the fiscal system while still containing an incorrectly notified, mislabelled or defective product. Conversely, pre-existing retail stock may remain lawfully saleable during transitional arrangements even when unstamped. Retailers and enforcement officers will therefore need to distinguish fiscal status, notification status and product conformity rather than treating one visible mark as universal approval. Integration between HMRC records, MHRA identifiers, customs information and Trading Standards intelligence would make the system substantially more effective.

The distinction between Great Britain and Northern Ireland remains important. Products may follow different procedural arrangements because Northern Ireland retains particular relationships with European rules, while Great Britain operates a domestic notification and publication system. Manufacturers must identify the intended territory before submission, packaging and distribution. A product listed in Great Britain should not be assumed to satisfy every requirement applicable in Northern Ireland. Supply-chain controls must prevent national versions from being mixed, especially where identifiers, responsible persons, submissions or future secondary regulations diverge.

The British model is therefore becoming more layered rather than replacing one regime with another. The 2016 product framework continues to govern nicotine concentration, capacity, composition, notification and vigilance. Environmental regulation has removed single-use products from lawful supply. The 2026 Act introduces wider powers over presentation, retailing and promotion. Excise duty adds fiscal registration, stamps and manufacturing controls. These systems involve different authorities and legal purposes, yet they converge on the same physical product. Manufacturers must understand their interaction rather than treat each requirement as an isolated compliance project.

This layered structure has strengths. It retains a lawful consumer route for adults seeking alternatives to smoking, requires formal product identification and creates mechanisms for surveillance, enforcement and correction. It also allows the state to address youth appeal, environmental waste and illicit trade without forcing every vape into medicines law. Its weakness is cumulative complexity. Notification, testing, packaging, retail licensing, advertising restrictions, environmental rules, duty and local enforcement can burden smaller responsible businesses. Complexity may improve control, but it can also favour large operators and create space for illicit suppliers ignoring every layer.

The future effectiveness of United Kingdom regulation will depend less on the number of powers available than on the precision with which they are used. Product standards should address demonstrable risks, flavour and packaging controls should target youth appeal without eliminating products important to adult switching, and taxation should preserve a meaningful advantage over smoking. Enforcement must focus on oversized, unnotified, counterfeit and untaxed products rather than burdening only businesses already inclined to comply. The British model remains internationally significant because it attempts to hold two positions simultaneously: vaping should be controlled rigorously, and combustible smoking should remain the dominant comparator. Its credibility will depend on maintaining both.

United States PMTA

The United States Premarket Tobacco Product Application system represents a demanding market-access pathway. Unlike the European and British notification models, it does not allow a manufacturer to enter the market after disclosing prescribed information. A new electronic nicotine delivery system must receive a written marketing order from the Food and Drug Administration before lawful marketing. The decision is not based on whether the product is safe, because no tobacco product is assessed through the pharmaceutical standard of safety and efficacy. It depends on whether permitting that product to be marketed would be appropriate for the protection of the public health, a population test that considers both users and non-users.

The statutory foundation lies in section 910 of the Federal Food, Drug, and Cosmetic Act. A "new tobacco product" is generally one not commercially marketed in the United States on or before 15 February 2007, or a product modified after that date. Because the modern vaping market barely existed, almost every e-cigarette, pod, e-liquid and disposable device falls within the new-product category. The FDA's 2016 Deeming Rule extended federal tobacco-product authority to electronic nicotine delivery systems and nicotine-containing e-liquids, bringing manufacture, importation, labelling and marketing within the agency's jurisdiction.

The public-health standard distinguishes PMTA review from ordinary product-safety regulation. FDA must consider the risks and benefits to the population as a whole, including users and non-users. It examines whether existing tobacco users would be more or less likely to stop using tobacco products if the new product were available and whether people who do not use tobacco would be more or less likely to begin. For vaping, this creates a balance between adult smoking substitution and youth or non-user initiation. The same product characteristic can support both sides: effective nicotine delivery may help smokers move away from cigarettes while increasing dependence potential among inexperienced users.

A PMTA must therefore describe more than composition. The applicant is expected to define the product precisely, including its design, components, ingredients, additives, properties and principles of operation. It must provide information concerning manufacturing, product specifications, harmful and potentially harmful constituents, stability, laboratory methods, health-risk investigations, consumer perception, patterns of use and environmental effects. The final PMTA rule, effective from November 2021, established content, format and recordkeeping requirements. The application must include information known to, or reasonably expected to be known to, the applicant, including unfavourable evidence rather than favourable studies alone.

Product identity is important because authorisation is product-specific. A marketing order applies to the product described in the application, not automatically to an entire brand or technology platform. Differences in nicotine concentration, flavour, device configuration, coil, reservoir, formulation or package size can create separate products requiring individually specified evidence. FDA permits grouped submissions, but each product within the group remains a separate application and requires its own identifying information and environmental assessment. This structure discourages the assumption that evidence generated for one tobacco-flavoured pod can be transferred to numerous flavoured variants without explaining relevant differences in exposure, behaviour and population effects.

The review process begins with intake and acceptance, followed by filing and scientific review. Acceptance examines whether the submission contains the basic elements needed to enter the process. Filing determines whether the application is sufficiently complete for substantive assessment. Scientific review then evaluates chemistry, engineering, toxicology, manufacturing, behavioural evidence and the population-level public-health case. FDA may issue deficiency letters requesting clarification or additional information. The possible outcomes include a marketing granted order, a marketing denial order, refusal to accept or refusal to file. Submission alone creates no legal entitlement to sell, and the pendency of an application is not a safe harbour from enforcement.

Chemistry and manufacturing evidence matter because FDA must understand what consumers will receive consistently, not merely what was tested once. Applicants should characterise nicotine, solvents, flavour chemicals, impurities, aerosol constituents and materials that may transfer from the device.

Manufacturing descriptions must explain how specifications are maintained, how suppliers and processes are controlled and how deviations are investigated. Stability data should support the proposed shelf life and show whether nicotine, flavour constituents, leachables or emissions change over time. A sophisticated prototype cannot support authorisation if commercial production is insufficiently controlled to reproduce it. The PMTA is both a product assessment and examination of the system that will manufacture the product.

For electronic nicotine delivery systems, aerosol generation connects formulation chemistry with device engineering. FDA review can consider power output, coil resistance, heating-element materials, airflow, wick performance, reservoir design, firmware and foreseeable operating conditions. Emissions testing must be tied to the product and method used, with suitable sensitivity and an explanation of variability. Carbonyls, volatile organic compounds, metals, nicotine and other constituents may require characterisation. A result obtained from one device setting or fresh coil cannot automatically describe performance across the product's life. The application must explain why the test regime represents intended and reasonably foreseeable use and how abnormal conditions were distinguished from normal operation.

Toxicological evidence must interpret these measurements in relation to exposure. Reduced emissions compared with cigarettes can support the proposition that complete switching may lower individual harm, but comparative chemistry alone does not establish that marketing the product benefits the population. FDA may consider nonclinical studies, human evidence, abuse liability, nicotine pharmacokinetics and uncertainties concerning repeated inhalation. The applicant must connect the formulation and aerosol to the expected users and use. A product capable of reducing toxicant exposure for smokers may still fail the statutory standard if its likely uptake among young people or non-users is judged to outweigh that benefit.

Behavioural evidence is central rather than supplementary. Applicants may need to examine whether adult smokers understand the product, whether they are likely to switch completely, whether dual use persists and how labelling or marketing affects perception. Complete switching is more relevant to risk reduction than adding vaping while maintaining substantial cigarette consumption. FDA considers initiation, experimentation and progression among non-users. Product appeal, flavour, nicotine delivery, design and marketing plans become regulatory evidence. The PMTA pathway evaluates not only what the aerosol contains, but what the availability of the product is expected to cause people to do.

Flavoured products have become the most contested part of this standard. FDA has required evidence that the added benefit to adult smokers is sufficient to outweigh the increased risk of youth initiation and use. Many applications for non-tobacco flavours received marketing denial orders because the submitted evidence did not demonstrate that balance. In March 2026, FDA issued draft guidance describing its current thinking on assessing youth risk and the additional adult benefit needed for flavoured electronic nicotine delivery systems compared with tobacco-flavoured products. The non-binding draft makes explicit that flavour is evaluated as a population-behaviour variable rather than merely an ingredient choice.

The history of PMTA implementation has been shaped by enforcement policy. Products already on the market when the Deeming Rule took effect in August 2016 were temporarily allowed to remain while applications were prepared. Following federal litigation, manufacturers of eligible deemed products were required to submit applications by 9 September 2020. FDA received submissions covering millions of products, many consisting of e-liquid variants generated through combinations of flavour, nicotine strength and container size. The scale demonstrated both the diversity of the American vape market and difficulties of applying product-by-product authorisation to a category built around rapid variation.

The burden of the pathway has altered market structure. Preparing a credible PMTA can require analytical chemistry, toxicology, behavioural research, manufacturing documentation, environmental assessment, legal review and long-term regulatory support. Large tobacco companies and well-capitalised manufacturers are better able to finance this work than small independent businesses. Grouping can improve efficiency, and platform evidence may be shared where justified, but it does not remove the need to characterise each product. The system can therefore eliminate weakly documented products while also excluding competent smaller manufacturers whose failure is insufficient capital rather than an identified scientific defect.

Marketing granted orders must be interpreted. FDA authorisation means that the agency concluded the statutory public-health standard was met for the product under specified conditions. It does not mean that the product is safe, approved as a medicine or endorsed for non-users. Orders may impose post-market reporting, recordkeeping, marketing and surveillance requirements, and FDA can withdraw authorisation if the statutory standard is no longer met. The authorised product must remain aligned with the application; material changes may require further regulatory action. Authorisation begins a controlled lifecycle rather than ending scrutiny.

The pattern of authorisations has evolved. Early electronic-cigarette marketing orders concentrated heavily on tobacco-flavoured products, reflecting FDA's concern about youth appeal. Subsequent decisions included menthol products, and in May 2026 the agency authorised four Glas nicotine pod products, including its first non-tobacco and non-menthol ENDS authorisations. FDA stated that each pod contained 50 milligrams per millilitre of tobacco-derived nicotine. These decisions demonstrate that the pathway is capable of authorising products beyond tobacco flavour where the agency concludes that the evidence satisfies the population standard, although the evidential threshold remains demanding.

The weakness of the American model is the gap between the statutory gateway and the physical market. Numerous unauthorised disposable and flavoured products have remained available through domestic retail, online sales and imports despite the legal requirement for marketing orders. FDA has issued warning letters, civil money penalties, import alerts and other actions, but product turnover and complex supply chains make enforcement difficult. As of 2026, the agency stated that it had issued hundreds of warning letters to firms and more than a thousand to retailers concerning unauthorised tobacco products. A rigorous authorisation system cannot deliver its intended public-health effect if unlawful products remain easier to launch and replace than authorised products.

This enforcement asymmetry imposes the greatest costs on businesses attempting to comply. An authorised manufacturer must maintain specifications, reporting, marketing restrictions and post-market records, while an unauthorised supplier can introduce new flavours or devices without waiting for scientific review. Retailers may struggle to distinguish lawful products from brands claiming pending applications or relying on outdated enforcement assumptions. FDA has emphasised that a pending application does not ordinarily create a safe harbour and that products lacking required authorisation are marketed unlawfully, subject to limited case-specific stays or enforcement policies. Searchable product databases and import controls help, but they must be matched by rapid action against suppliers and distributors.

The PMTA model nevertheless makes an important scientific contribution by forcing explicit population reasoning. It does not assume that lower toxicant emissions alone establish public-health benefit, nor that any youth uptake automatically defeats adult harm reduction. It requires the regulator to weigh both pathways, although the evidence needed to quantify them remains uncertain. Population effects depend on future behaviour, competitor products, smoking prevalence, enforcement and communication. Applications therefore combine measured product data with predictions about real-world use. The apparent precision of the legal standard should not obscure the judgement involved in deciding how much adult switching benefit is sufficient to offset initiation risk.

FDA has attempted to improve the process through guidance, electronic submission systems, application grouping and engagement with smaller manufacturers. In 2026 the agency reported efforts to accelerate acceptance review and held a roundtable focused on PMTA submissions from small electronic nicotine delivery system manufacturers. Such measures may reduce avoidable administrative delay, but they cannot remove the statutory requirement for persuasive scientific evidence. Greater predictability would nevertheless benefit both applicants and public health by clarifying study expectations, reducing repeated deficiencies and allowing resources to be directed towards questions that genuinely determine risk and behaviour.

The United States therefore offers the clearest example of authorisation-heavy vaping regulation. Its strength lies in requiring product-specific evidence and an affirmative public-health determination before lawful marketing. Its weakness lies in cost, delay, market concentration and the presence of unauthorised products. The model can distinguish assessed products from speculative claims only when enforcement preserves that distinction in commerce. PMTA regulation will ultimately be judged not by the volume of applications processed or denied, but by whether the authorised market provides adult smokers with credible non-combustible alternatives while preventing the uncontrolled expansion of products that have never met the statutory test.

Australia

Australia has constructed one of the most medicalised and restrictive regulatory models for vaping in the world. Rather than treating vaping products principally as consumer alternatives to cigarettes, the federal framework places lawful products within therapeutic-goods legislation and confines consumer supply to pharmacies for smoking cessation or the management of nicotine dependence. The model does not prohibit every vape, but it prohibits the ordinary retail market that exists in the European Union, the United Kingdom, New Zealand and parts of North America. Tobacconists, specialist vape shops, convenience stores and general online retailers cannot lawfully sell vaping goods. Since July 2024, the importation, domestic manufacture, commercial possession, supply and advertising of non-therapeutic vapes and disposable products have been prohibited, regardless of whether nicotine is present.

Lawful access is consequently defined by therapeutic purpose, compliant product standards and a controlled pharmacy pathway rather than by ordinary adult consumer choice.

This architecture developed from Australia's earlier decision to regulate nicotine for vaping through medicines and poisons controls. Before the 2024 reforms, nicotine vaping products generally required a prescription and access operated through unapproved-therapeutic-goods pathways. The later reforms tightened control over all vaping goods, including nicotine-free products, because enforcement had been complicated by products declared as nicotine-free while containing nicotine and by retailers operating around narrow chemical definitions. From 1 July 2024, the Therapeutic Goods and Other Legislation Amendment (Vaping Reforms) Act 2024 became the centrepiece of the system. It shifted the legal question from whether a product contained nicotine towards whether the vaping good formed part of a lawful therapeutic supply chain. This broader definition allowed authorities to act without first proving nicotine content through laboratory analysis and brought devices, liquids, pods and accessories within a more coherent enforcement structure.

The consumer pathway changed again on 1 October 2024. Adults aged eighteen or over may obtain therapeutic vapes containing no more than 20 milligrams per millilitre of nicotine from a participating pharmacy without a prescription, where supply is clinically appropriate and permitted under state or territory law. The pharmacist must verify identity and age, explain that the product is not included in the Australian Register of Therapeutic Goods, obtain informed consent, discuss approved cessation options, advise on dose and medicine interactions, and limit supply to one month's quantity during one month. Products above 20 milligrams per millilitre remain prescription only, as do products supplied to people under eighteen where local law permits access. Pharmacists are not obliged to stock or supply vapes, even where a patient presents a prescription. The model therefore creates legal availability without guaranteeing practical availability in every community.

This pharmacy-only route distinguishes Australia from a conventional medicinal-authorisation model. Therapeutic vapes lawfully supplied are generally unapproved therapeutic goods rather than products fully evaluated and included in the Australian Register of Therapeutic Goods. As of July 2026, the Therapeutic Goods Administration stated that no vape for smoking cessation or nicotine-dependence management had been included in the register and that no such product had undergone full TGA assessment for quality, safety, efficacy or performance. Sponsors instead notify the TGA that their goods comply with applicable minimum standards, after which qualifying goods appear on the notified vape list. The distinction matters. Pharmacy supply and therapeutic classification can create an impression of pharmaceutical approval, yet notification is based substantially on sponsor declaration, supported by compliance monitoring and the possibility of civil or criminal penalties for false or misleading information.

Australia's product standards became substantially more demanding from 1 July 2025. Strengthened requirements under the therapeutic vaping goods standard and the medical-device standard apply to substances, cartridges, pods, devices and accessories. Permitted formulation ingredients are tightly restricted to nicotine, propylene glycol, glycerol, water and limited mint, menthol or tobacco flavouring. Nicotine concentration in products may not exceed 50 milligrams per millilitre in base form or equivalent base-form concentration, although non-prescription pharmacist supply remains limited to products containing 20 milligrams per millilitre or less. Menthol is restricted to a maximum concentration of 20 milligrams per millilitre. Vaping-substance containers may contain no more than 60 millilitres, while substance accessories such as pods or cartridges are limited to 5 millilitres. These limits produce a product class resembling a controlled therapeutic formulation rather than the diverse flavour market found in many consumer systems.

Packaging and presentation reinforce that therapeutic identity. Products must use plain pharmaceutical-style packaging, include prescribed information leaflets and comply with restrictions on product names. Devices and accessories are subject to plain-design and labelling requirements intended to prevent visual appeal from operating as a consumer marketing tool. The strengthened standards also require greater attention to medical-device quality management, risk management, battery and electrical safety, design and construction, instructions for use and toxicological risk assessment. This is scientifically significant because Australian regulation addresses the liquid and the aerosol-generating hardware as interacting parts of one therapeutic system. A compliant formulation is not sufficient if the device overheats, leaks, delivers nicotine inconsistently or introduces unacceptable material-derived emissions.

The sponsor-notification process provides the regulatory gateway. Importers, manufacturers and sponsors must notify the TGA of compliance with the relevant standards before importing, manufacturing or supplying therapeutic vaping goods, unless a specific exemption applies. The notified list identifies products that may enter lawful therapeutic pathways, but the TGA expressly warns that listing does not guarantee the accuracy, completeness or currency of sponsor-supplied information and does not constitute approval. Ongoing compliance assessment remains possible, and a sponsor that notifies a non-compliant product may face serious sanctions. The model therefore resembles notification in administrative form but operates within a much narrower market and a more medicalised legal context than the European system.

Advertising is heavily restricted because the lawful product is framed as a therapeutic intervention rather than a lifestyle commodity. The 2024 reforms prohibited advertising, promotion and sponsorship of vaping goods except where expressly authorised in limited circumstances. Pharmacy supply does not permit broad consumer advertising, influencer promotion, colourful point-of-sale campaigns or ordinary brand-building. This reduces youth-directed commercial exposure and supports the pharmaceutical presentation of the category. It also constrains the ability of manufacturers and retailers to communicate differences between products or to reach smokers who are not already seeking clinical or pharmacy assistance. The model relies more heavily on healthcare consultation and public-health communication than on competitive consumer marketing.

Importation controls are equally strict. The staged reforms began with a prohibition on importing disposable vapes from 1 January 2024, followed by broader controls over other vaping goods. Personal importation is no longer permitted, and commercial importation requires the appropriate licences, permits and conformity with therapeutic requirements. Australian Border Force officers may seize unlawful shipments, while the TGA can pursue escalated action for import offences. Removing the personal-importation route closes a pathway previously used by consumers with prescriptions and reduces the capacity for overseas suppliers to bypass domestic standards. It also makes the effectiveness of the pharmacy channel more important, because lawful consumers cannot compensate for limited domestic availability by ordering directly from foreign vendors.

Enforcement is organised through a national framework involving the TGA, Australian Border Force, Australian Federal Police, state and territory health departments and police services. Commonwealth bodies focus on border control, therapeutic-goods offences and advertising, while states and territories lead wholesale and retail enforcement. Authorities can investigate, seize and destroy unlawful goods, issue infringement notices and pursue civil or criminal proceedings. Maximum penalties can be severe, including imprisonment and multimillion-dollar financial exposure for corporations. The law does not criminalise genuine personal possession by individual users; prohibitions on possession are directed principally towards commercial dealers and unlawful supply chains. This distinction allows enforcement to target market actors without converting consumers into the primary offenders.

The principal strength of the Australian model is its attempt to remove vaping from ordinary youth-accessible retail while retaining a controlled route for adults using it therapeutically. Pharmacy consultation creates opportunities for age verification, discussion of established cessation treatments, dosage advice, interaction checking, informed consent and referral to support services. Restricted ingredients and strengthened device standards reduce formulation complexity and make the lawful product class more technically manageable. A notified list, defined sponsors and a traceable pharmacy channel also create clearer accountability than an open market containing rapidly changing brands, anonymous importers and products of uncertain composition.

Its principal weakness is that medicalisation does not automatically eliminate demand for consumer-style products. People who vape may seek flavours, prices, device formats or retail convenience that the therapeutic market does not provide. Pharmacists may decline to stock products, consumers may resist clinical consultation, and the limited permitted flavour range may not reproduce the products through which some smokers previously moved away from cigarettes. Where lawful supply does not meet existing demand, economic incentives for illicit importation, informal retail and organised distribution remain. Australia's own decision to establish a multi-agency national enforcement framework demonstrates that product prohibition and pharmacy restriction require substantial continuing action at borders and within domestic markets.

Early supply data illustrate both the existence and the limited scale of the lawful channel. The TGA estimated that more than 2,200 pharmacies supplied over 72,000 therapeutic vaping goods during 2024 and more than 220,000 during 2025, although those figures do not capture every prescription supply and should not be interpreted as numbers of individual patients. They show that pharmacy distribution can operate nationally, but they do not establish whether access matches the size or geographical distribution of demand. The figures also reveal why notification data need careful interpretation: a supply notification may include several cartridges, while prescription pathways are recorded differently. Market evaluation therefore requires pharmacy transactions, smoking and vaping prevalence, illicit seizures, quit outcomes and consumer behaviour to be examined together. A fall in legal retail visibility may reflect successful control, displacement into pharmacies, movement into illicit channels or some combination of these effects. Australia's framework is unusually capable of observing the lawful therapeutic pathway because pharmacist supply generates structured records, yet the unregulated market remains harder to quantify. The evidence needed to judge the model must therefore extend beyond the notified list and include whether consumers obtain compliant goods, abandon vaping, return to smoking or continue purchasing outside the legal system over time nationally.

The model also creates a scientific contradiction. Lawful therapeutic vapes are classified and supplied within a healthcare framework, yet they remain unapproved goods that have not undergone complete TGA evaluation. Minimum product standards can control ingredients, packaging, electrical safety and manufacturing expectations, but they do not prove clinical efficacy or long-term safety. Pharmacy consultation can support more informed use, but it cannot convert a sponsor-notified product into an authorised medicine. The TGA therefore requires consumers to be told that the goods are unapproved and continues to recommend registered nicotine-replacement products and behavioural support as first-line cessation options. Therapeutic status defines the legal purpose and supply channel more clearly than it establishes a completed pharmaceutical evidence package.

Federal and state interaction adds further complexity. Commonwealth law governs importation, therapeutic standards, sponsor notification and major advertising restrictions, while states and territories retain rules affecting prescribing, possession, pharmacy practice and supply. A product that satisfies federal standards may still encounter local limitations, and pharmacists must comply with both levels. National consistency is supported through cooperation, but complete uniformity is not guaranteed. For manufacturers and sponsors, lawful market access requires not only TGA notification but an understanding of scheduling, pharmacy distribution, local medicines law, logistics and post-market responsibilities across several jurisdictions.

The Australian system is therefore neither a complete ban nor a conventional consumer market. It is a controlled-access experiment that treats vaping as a potentially therapeutic but insufficiently proven intervention, permits pharmacy supply under defined conditions and criminalises most commercial activity outside that channel. Its success cannot be measured solely by the disappearance of vapes from lawful convenience retail. The meaningful outcomes are whether smoking cessation is supported, youth use declines, compliant products remain practically accessible, adverse events are detected and illicit supply is contained. Australia demonstrates how far a government can separate vaping from normal commerce, but it also demonstrates that legal classification cannot remove consumer demand, scientific uncertainty or the need for sustained enforcement.

New Zealand

New Zealand has developed a clear consumer harm-reduction model for vaping, but it has also tightened that model in response to youth uptake, retail proliferation and disposable products. The system does not treat vaping as an ordinary commodity, yet it does not confine access to prescriptions or pharmacies. Nicotine-containing and nicotine-free vaping products can be sold lawfully to adults through a regulated retail market, provided that manufacturers, importers and sellers comply with notification, product-safety, packaging, flavour, advertising and age-of-sale requirements. Its central policy assumption is that vaping can assist adults who smoke to move away from combustible tobacco, while commercial practices likely to recruit young people should be constrained. That dual purpose is embedded in the Smokefree Environments and Regulated Products Act 1990, as amended in 2020 and subsequently strengthened.

The 2020 vaping amendments transformed legislation originally designed around second-hand smoke and tobacco promotion into a broader regime for regulated nicotine and inhalation products. Vaping substances, devices and components became "notifiable products", creating a specific legal category rather than forcing them into medicines law. The legislation imposed age restrictions, advertising prohibitions, product-notification duties and retail controls while allowing adult consumer access. The state accepted that a lawful vaping market could contribute to smoking reduction, but required the market to operate under rules reflecting product risk and nicotine dependence. A technically compliant liquid cannot be sold by an unauthorised outlet in every flavour, and an approved retailer cannot lawfully sell an unnotified or prohibited product merely because its premises satisfy retail requirements.

Manufacturers and importers must notify the Ministry of Health before supplying vaping products in New Zealand. Notifications are made through the Health Advisory and Regulatory Platform, known as HARP, and attract a fee of NZ$50 plus goods and services tax for each product, renewed annually. The notifier supplies information identifying the product and declares that it complies with statutory requirements. Retailers are not expected to repeat manufacturer or importer notifications, but they must ensure that products they sell remain validly notified. It is nevertheless a notification system rather than full pre-market authorisation. The manufacturer or importer remains responsible for truthfulness, conformity and withdrawal where later evidence shows that the product does not meet legal standards.

The distinction became visible in 2025 when regulatory testing identified products exceeding the legal limit for diacetyl and other requirements. New Zealand specifies maximum levels for selected substances and emissions-related contaminants, including diacetyl, formaldehyde, acetaldehyde and certain metals. The diacetyl limit is 22 parts per million, reflecting concern about respiratory toxicity associated with inhalation. When a notified product exceeds a statutory threshold, its prior presence in HARP does not protect it from prohibition. The Ministry can publish warnings, identify products that must not be sold and require notifiers and retailers to remove them. It provides traceability and a responsible party, but scientific assurance depends on accurate declarations, competent supplier control, post-market testing and enforcement.

For vaping substances containing nicotine only in salt form and intended for reusable devices, the concentration may not exceed 28.5 milligrams per millilitre. For other vaping substances, the limit is generally 20 milligrams per millilitre. These numerical limits do not determine actual dose by themselves. Aerosol output, coil resistance, power, airflow, puff duration and consumer behaviour influence nicotine delivery, while salts can alter sensory harshness and inhalation patterns. From a compliance perspective, manufacturers must ensure that formulation calculations, nicotine assays, labels and notifications use the correct basis. Confusion between salt mass and nicotine equivalent, or between nominal and measured concentration, can turn a formulation error into a legal breach.

Flavour policy is structured through retailer type rather than a universal ban. General retailers, including dairies, supermarkets and service stations, may sell only tobacco, menthol or mint flavours. Approved specialist vape retailers can sell a wider range of approved flavours from authorised premises and websites. Colourings are prohibited in notifiable products, and flavour descriptions are controlled to reduce names or presentation likely to appeal to children. This division attempts to preserve flavour choice for adults who use specialist channels while limiting impulsive access and youth-facing variety in ordinary retail environments.

Specialist vape retailers require approval from the Ministry of Health and must satisfy conditions demonstrating that vaping products form the principal part of their business. Approval allows broader flavour sales and specialist advice, but carries stricter obligations concerning premises, online operations and access by minors. General retailers do not require the same approval, although they must submit regulated-product seller notifications and remain within their narrower product range. The structure also places greater responsibility on specialists, because their commercial privileges depend on continuing compliance.

It is unlawful to sell or supply vaping products to anyone under eighteen, and businesses face substantial penalties for breaches. Online sellers must use age-verification systems capable of doing more than asking customers to tick a box. The penalty framework was strengthened because repeated unlawful sales showed that nominal age limits were insufficient without meaningful commercial consequences. Enforcement operations can test compliance through controlled purchase exercises, while infringement notices and prosecutions create accountability for businesses rather than treating the shop assistant as the only responsible actor.

From 17 June 2025, New Zealand prohibited the manufacture, sale, supply and distribution of disposable vaping devices. The ban was framed to catch devices that could not be refilled with liquid or a replacement pod, or recharged by the user. Its environmental rationale was substantial: disposable vapes combine plastics, electronics, metals and lithium batteries in products used briefly and often discarded through waste streams. The ban retained access to rechargeable and refillable systems, thereby targeting a format rather than eliminating vaping. A product marketed as reusable may still function commercially like a disposable if refilling is impractical, components are designed for replacement after minimal use or the device is sold cheaply enough to encourage rapid disposal.

Following regulatory review, the Government removed the requirement for all vaping devices to have removable batteries from 1 September 2025, while retaining the disposable-vape prohibition. Child-safety mechanisms remain required and must not be capable of being overridden or permanently disabled by users. A removable battery may facilitate replacement and recycling, but it can also create engineering, sealing and consumer-handling problems. Requiring rechargeability, refillability and effective child resistance may address environmental and accidental-use concerns more directly than mandating one battery architecture.

Vaping products became subject to display controls intended to reduce their presence around children and young people, including restrictions affecting storefronts and retail interiors. Discounts, giveaways, rewards, rebates, competitions and promotional price mechanisms were prohibited across retailers and online stores. Specialist vape retailers lost an earlier exemption that had allowed promotional communications to existing customers. These restrictions also narrowed one of the original distinctions between specialist and general retailers: specialists may retain broader flavour availability, but not unrestricted marketing privileges.

Advertising restrictions extend beyond conventional paid advertisements. Communications that encourage the use, purchase or notified-product brand recognition can fall within the prohibition, and enforcement penalties have increased. This creates a difficult boundary between prohibited promotion and factual information required for informed adult choice. Specialist retailers need to explain device compatibility, nicotine strength, operating instructions and product availability, yet they must avoid lifestyle messaging, inducements or communications that function as advertising. The strength of New Zealand's approach lies in separating access from promotion; its weakness is that excessive caution can suppress accurate comparative-risk information and leave smokers with an undifferentiated impression that cigarettes and vaping present equivalent hazards.

Packaging and labelling requirements support product identification and risk communication. Packs must carry prescribed warnings and information, while prohibited features and flavour-naming rules limit presentation capable of increasing youth appeal. The label should correspond with the notified formulation, nicotine concentration and responsible operator. This sounds straightforward, but the market contains imported products, frequent brand revisions and multiple flavour variants, making reconciliation essential. A product may be notified under one name, advertised under another and sold in packaging using an abbreviated strength description. Compliance therefore depends on stable product codes and controlled artwork, not merely attractive front-panel design. Retailers also need enough information to verify that stock matches a current notification and has not been prohibited following testing or enforcement action.

New Zealand's regime includes continuing reporting obligations. Sellers of notifiable products must submit annual sales returns, giving the Ministry data on the volume and type of products supplied. Manufacturers, importers and retailers must retain records supporting compliance, while product notifications require annual renewal. These obligations allow authorities to see more than a static list of product names. Sales information can identify market concentration, shifts between formats and the significance of products associated with complaints or test failures. The usefulness of the data depends on consistent product identifiers and accurate reporting. A rapidly changing market can generate duplicate, expired or superficially different entries that obscure the real number of formulations and devices. Regulatory intelligence requires the Ministry to connect notification, sales, retailer, surveillance and enforcement datasets rather than treating them as separate administrative collections.

Compliance monitoring has become more visible as reforms have expanded. Ministry reporting in 2026 showed increased infringement activity following stronger monitoring of retail visibility and other requirements. Enforcement officers inspect premises, review advertising, conduct controlled purchase operations and investigate prohibited or non-compliant products. Published lists of products failing nicotine or contaminant requirements help retailers remove affected stock and demonstrate that notification is not a permanent shield. The enforcement problem remains practical scale. Thousands of products, online sellers, imported devices and rapidly changing brands can outpace laboratory and inspection capacity. Responsible firms bear notification fees, testing costs and retail restrictions, while unlawful suppliers may seek advantage through hidden sales or product substitution. The credibility of the framework depends on enforcement reaching non-compliant operators rather than concentrating solely on businesses already visible in HARP.

New Zealand's public-health context gives the model particular importance. Vaping was integrated into a national ambition to reduce daily smoking below five per cent, and policy has acknowledged that alternative nicotine products can contribute to quitting. This is not equivalent to declaring vaping harmless or appropriate for everyone. The intended population is adults who smoke, especially those who might otherwise continue using combustible tobacco. Evaluation should therefore consider complete switching, relapse, dual use, youth initiation and inequities between population groups. Māori communities have historically experienced higher smoking prevalence and tobacco-related harm, so a regulation that reduces overall smoking while leaving disparities unchanged would remain incomplete. Equally, restrictions that suppress lawful vaping without improving cessation support could have unequal consequences for populations carrying the greatest burden of smoking.

The model's greatest strength is proportionality. It allows a consumer market, differentiates general from specialist retail, controls nicotine and selected toxicants, requires product notification and restricts youth-oriented promotion. It has also shown capacity to evolve by banning disposable devices, tightening displays and adjusting an impractical battery rule. Its weakness is cumulative complexity. Manufacturers must navigate annual notifications, product standards and changing presentation rules; retailers must understand flavour permissions, visibility, promotions, seller notifications and sales returns; consumers may struggle to distinguish notified, compliant and prohibited products. Complexity can improve control only when guidance, databases and enforcement make the system intelligible. Otherwise, it can burden compliant operators while illicit trade remains comparatively simple.

New Zealand therefore represents a regulated-access model rather than either medicalisation or prohibition. It preserves the fundamental toxicological distinction between combustion and aerosol while rejecting the idea that lower risk removes the need for product control. The framework treats adult availability, youth protection, environmental impact and regulatory traceability as simultaneous objectives. Those objectives will sometimes conflict: stronger flavour restrictions may reduce youth appeal but weaken switching for some smokers; tighter promotion rules may reduce exposure while limiting comparative-risk communication; disposable bans may reduce waste while shifting demand towards cheaply replaceable pod systems. The quality of the model will depend on whether future decisions are guided by measured outcomes rather than symbolic severity. Its success should be judged by whether smoking falls, young non-smokers are protected, lawful products become more reliable and the regulated market remains capable of competing with both cigarettes and illicit supply.

Canada

Canada regulates vaping through a layered national federal model that combines tobacco-control legislation, consumer-product safety law, mandatory industry reporting, bilingual labelling, promotion restrictions and excise taxation. It does not require the product-by-product premarket notification used in the European Union, nor the affirmative marketing authorisation demanded by the United States. Instead, manufacturers and importers may place compliant products on the market while remaining responsible for meeting federal requirements and supplying prescribed information to Health Canada. Provincial and territorial rules then add controls over age, flavours, retailing, display, use in public places and taxation. The result is a lawful consumer market governed by several overlapping legal systems.

The federal centre is the Tobacco and Vaping Products Act, which was expanded in 2018 to regulate vaping products alongside tobacco. Its purposes include protecting young people and non-users from inducements to use vaping products, restricting access, preventing misleading promotion and enhancing public awareness of health hazards. The Act preserves a legal distinction between vaping and combustible tobacco. Vaping products can be sold to adults without prescription, provided that they are not represented as therapeutic products and comply with the applicable rules. A product promoted for treating nicotine dependence or making medicinal claims may enter a different legal pathway, but the ordinary Canadian vape remains a regulated consumer nicotine product.

Canada's model is unusual because legal market entry does not depend on a central register showing that each flavour, nicotine strength and device has completed a six-month notification or scientific review. Compliance is enforced through prohibitions, prescribed standards, reporting duties, inspections and laboratory testing. This reduces the administrative barrier to launching products, but transfers substantial responsibility to the manufacturer or importer. The absence of premarket authorisation does not permit unrestricted sale. A product exceeding the nicotine limit, carrying deficient labels, using unsafe packaging or promoted unlawfully is non-compliant from the moment it enters commerce, regardless of whether an authority has previously examined it.

Nicotine concentration is controlled nationally through the Nicotine Concentration in Vaping Products Regulations. Since July 2021, vaping products manufactured or imported for sale in Canada may contain no more than 20 milligrams of nicotine per millilitre, and packaging may not display a concentration above that limit. The rule applies to measured concentration rather than marketing intention, making analytical verification essential. Salt formulations require particular care because suppliers may describe nicotine as salt mass, nicotine equivalent, percentage strength or nominal formulation input. Manufacturers must ensure that calculations, certificates, finished-product assays and labels use the same chemical basis and remain within specification throughout shelf life.

The 20 milligram limit is legally clear but scientifically incomplete. Nicotine delivery depends on aerosol mass, device power, coil resistance, airflow, puff duration, formulation acidity and user behaviour. Two products containing the same liquid concentration can produce markedly different systemic exposure. Canada's approach therefore controls one important determinant without establishing a complete dose standard. It also influences product engineering: manufacturers may increase aerosol generation or optimise nicotine salts to produce satisfactory delivery within the ceiling. Regulatory assessment must consequently examine the liquid and device as an integrated exposure system rather than assuming that concentration alone predicts dependence potential or smoking-substitution performance.

The Vaping Products Labelling and Packaging Regulations create detailed national requirements. Products containing nicotine must display the concentration in milligrams per millilitre, prescribed health warnings and toxicity information. Ingredient lists are required, and information must generally appear in both English and French. The regulations control placement, legibility, minimum type size, contrast and presentation so that warnings cannot be technically present yet practically invisible. Products without nicotine are also subject to labelling rules designed to prevent confusion. Bilingual compliance requires more than literal translation because scientific terminology, flavour descriptions, first-aid statements and responsible-party information must remain accurate and consistent across both official-language panels.

Packaging rules also address accidental exposure. Legal vaping products containing nicotine at or above the specified threshold must use child-resistant containers under the Canada Consumer Product Safety Act and associated requirements. This is especially important for refill liquids, where a small volume can contain enough nicotine to cause poisoning if swallowed or absorbed. Closures must remain functional during ordinary use, transport and storage rather than merely passing an initial design review. Leakage, damaged seals, unsuitable dropper assemblies and inconsistent cap torque can defeat an otherwise compliant package. Manufacturers should therefore validate the complete container-closure system and monitor complaints involving leakage or child access.

The consumer-product safety framework extends beyond nicotine toxicity. Batteries, chargers, electrical components, plastics and mechanical design may create fire, burn, choking or chemical hazards. Health Canada can investigate products that present a danger to human health or safety and can use powers including seizure, corrective measures and recall. A vape is therefore regulated simultaneously as a nicotine product and as an electrical consumer article. Compliance teams must connect formulation, hardware and packaging records because a product may satisfy the Tobacco and Vaping Products Act while failing general safety obligations through battery instability, defective charging control or component breakage.

Promotion is tightly controlled at federal level. Advertising that could be seen or heard by young people is restricted, while lifestyle advertising, sponsorship, testimonials, endorsements, giveaways and youth-appealing themes are prohibited. Required health information must accompany permitted advertising in prescribed circumstances. These rules recognise that a lawful adult product can create population risk through its presentation. They also create a difficult distinction between promotion and factual communication. Retailers and manufacturers need to explain nicotine strength, device compatibility and operating instructions without converting technical information into aspirational marketing or implying that Health Canada has approved the product.

Flavour regulation illustrates the division between federal and provincial authority. Federal law restricts promotion of certain flavour categories and allows schedules to identify prohibited flavour representations, but Canada has not implemented a universal national prohibition confining all vaping products to tobacco flavour. Several provinces and territories have adopted stronger restrictions, producing substantial regional variation in what may be sold and where. A formulation lawful at federal level may therefore be prohibited in a particular province, while a descriptor acceptable on one market version may be unlawful elsewhere. National distribution requires market-specific product lists, artwork control and warehouse segregation rather than one Canadian label applied universally.

The minimum federal age is eighteen, but provinces and territories may establish higher ages, commonly nineteen and in some places twenty-one. Retailers must comply with the rule applicable where the sale occurs, including online transactions delivered across provincial boundaries. Simple website declarations provide weak assurance because the buyer's identity, age and delivery recipient may differ. Effective systems use documentary or third-party verification and age-controlled delivery. Federal enforcement expectations operate alongside provincial licensing, inspection and penalty systems, meaning that the same transaction can engage several authorities. Age restriction becomes credible only where verification is routine and commercial penalties outweigh the value of unlawful sales.

Mandatory reporting has moved Canada towards a more data-rich model. Under the Vaping Products Reporting Regulations, manufacturers and importers must provide Health Canada with prescribed sales and ingredient information electronically. Sales reports are submitted twice yearly for the preceding six-month periods, while ingredient information allows the regulator to understand the composition of products circulating nationally. These data support surveillance of product categories, flavour trends, nicotine strengths and regional sales. They also provide a foundation for targeted laboratory sampling and policy evaluation. The system is not a premarket dossier, but it reduces regulatory blindness.

The scientific value of reporting depends on data quality. Ingredient names must be sufficiently precise to distinguish individual chemicals from proprietary mixtures, and product identifiers must remain stable across sales, formulations and packaging versions. A flavour concentrate described only by a trade name cannot support meaningful toxicological analysis. Changes in suppliers, nicotine forms or constituent concentrations need to remain traceable to the affected products and reporting periods. Health Canada's plan to modernise and potentially consolidate tobacco and vaping reporting reflects the need to transform submitted information into usable regulatory intelligence rather than accumulating disconnected spreadsheets that cannot be reconciled with products found at retail.

Excise duty has become another defining layer. Canada imposes federal vaping duty on packaged vaping substances, with rates calculated by liquid volume or, for solids, by weight. Products intended for sale in participating specified provinces are subject to an additional coordinated duty of the same structure. Manufacturers generally require a vaping-product licence, must file monthly returns and must apply prescribed excise stamps before products enter the duty-paid market. The stamp identifies fiscal compliance, not scientific approval, and helps distinguish duty-paid goods from unlawful stock.

Volume-based taxation is administratively measurable but only indirectly related to risk. A large bottle of low-strength liquid may attract more duty than a small, highly efficient pod delivering comparable nicotine exposure. Tax can influence consumer movement between refill systems, prefilled cartridges and illicit products, while additional provincial duty creates regional price differences. A strong fiscal model must preserve sufficient price advantage over cigarettes to support switching while preventing tax evasion from becoming the main competitive advantage. Regulatory, customs and tax data should be connected because an unstamped product may also be mislabelled, unreported or imported through an unauthorised supply chain.

Federal compliance monitoring combines inspections, website reviews, sampling and laboratory analysis. Health Canada's report for April 2024 to March 2025 found non-compliance during a substantial proportion of manufacturer inspections and reported that many analysed samples failed nicotine-concentration requirements. Common retail problems included prohibited flavour promotion, testimonials or endorsements and deficient warnings. These findings show why post-market testing is central to the Canadian model. A framework without product-by-product authorisation can work only where regulators sample real products, compare measured composition with labels and take action through warning letters, seizures, stop sales, recalls or prosecution.

The enforcement findings also expose a limitation. A 20 milligram label does not establish that the liquid actually complies, and an excise stamp does not verify ingredients or aerosol performance. Retailers may assume that commercially distributed stock has already been cleared by government when the legal system places responsibility on manufacturers and importers. Better public databases, traceable product identifiers and publication of enforcement outcomes can improve due diligence, but no visible marker currently represents complete regulatory conformity. Each layer confirms only its own requirement, leaving businesses to integrate safety, labelling, reporting, promotion and duty obligations.

Provincial variation is both a strength and a source of fragmentation. Local governments can respond to youth prevalence, retail density and community priorities by restricting flavours, specialist outlets, displays and public use. They can also generate inconsistent requirements that complicate national manufacture and encourage cross-border purchasing. Consumers may travel or order from another province where products are available, while distributors must manage different ages, taxes and permitted ranges. The Canadian market is therefore federal in scientific and labelling fundamentals but regional in practical access. Effective compliance requires a jurisdiction matrix maintained as carefully as the master formulation database.

Canada's public-health challenge is to protect young people without obscuring relative risk for adults who smoke. Federal reviews recognise that vaping products are harmful and addictive but generally less harmful than combustible tobacco when smokers switch completely. Communication must avoid presenting vaping as harmless, medicinally approved or appropriate for non-users. It must also avoid equating aerosol with smoke in a way that removes the reason an adult smoker might change products. Policy outcomes should be measured through youth initiation, complete switching, dual use, smoking relapse, illicit supply and socioeconomic differences rather than through legal sales or vaping prevalence alone.

The Canadian model's principal strength is its layered adaptability. National rules control nicotine, labels, packaging, promotion, reporting and fiscal marking, while provinces can impose additional retail and flavour restrictions. Its weakness is that responsibility is distributed across laws, authorities and levels of government without a single market-access decision. This can preserve competition and product availability, but it demands active surveillance and sophisticated compliance management. Canada will succeed where its growing ingredient, sales, tax and enforcement datasets are connected to the physical products consumers use. The model must make lawful supply more transparent than illicit supply while retaining a regulated alternative capable of displacing combustible cigarettes.

Asia

Asia cannot be described through a single vaping regime because the region contains nearly every regulatory model applied to vaping products. It includes state-controlled legal markets, pharmaceutical restrictions, consumer-product regulation, excise-led systems and complete prohibitions covering manufacture, importation, sale, possession or use. They coexist with major differences in smoking prevalence, income, healthcare access, enforcement capacity and domestic tobacco industries. A product manufactured in one Asian country may be prohibited nearby, taxed as tobacco elsewhere and treated as an unapproved medicine in another market. Regional comparison therefore begins with fragmentation rather than convergence.

The region also occupies an unusual position in the global supply chain. Much of the world's vaping hardware has historically been manufactured in China and surrounding industrial networks. Asia is therefore not merely a collection of consumer markets; it is the engineering and production centre behind products regulated elsewhere. Factories produce market-specific versions differing in liquid volume, nicotine concentration, firmware, labelling and flavour. This separates domestic policy from export capability: a jurisdiction may impose restrictive internal controls while supporting production for foreign markets.

China demonstrates this duality most clearly. Electronic cigarettes have been brought within the tobacco-monopoly framework, placing licensing, production, wholesale distribution, retailing, importation and export activity under strong state supervision. Product standards and technical evaluation requirements have created a controlled domestic pathway rather than an unrestricted consumer market. Domestic products are subject to tighter flavour and presentation limitations than many export products, while manufacturers serving overseas customers must still meet destination-country specifications. Industrial capacity remains extensive, but lawful domestic commerce is channelled through licences, approved products, traceable distribution and central oversight.

This model allows government to observe production and distribution more directly than regimes depending on thousands of independent notifications. It also aligns vaping with an established tobacco-administration structure, taxation system and retail network. The scientific limitation is that monopoly control does not itself establish product safety. Technical evaluation must still examine nicotine accuracy, aerosol emissions, material transfer, battery behaviour and manufacturing consistency. A centralised market may improve traceability, yet innovation can be shaped by administrative permission rather than comparative-risk evidence. Export production adds another complication because products made to foreign specifications may differ substantially from those permitted within China.

Japan illustrates a different form of restriction. Nicotine-containing e-liquids are generally treated through pharmaceutical controls, while nicotine-free devices and liquids occupy a different legal position. Limited personal import may occur, but ordinary domestic sale of nicotine liquid differs sharply from open specialist retail in Britain or New Zealand. This classification has helped heated tobacco products become more commercially prominent than nicotine vaping. The distinction matters because heated tobacco and vaping have different thermal processes, emissions and architectures, yet regulatory availability can determine which alternative smokers adopt.

The Japanese example shows how classification can redirect innovation without formally choosing one technology over another. Where nicotine e-liquid faces medicinal barriers, companies and consumers may move towards products that fit existing tobacco law. This can produce rapid substitution away from cigarettes while narrowing consumer access to independent vaping systems. It also shows why prevalence data cannot be interpreted without regulation. Low use of nicotine vaping may reflect legal access constraints rather than low consumer interest, while high uptake of heated products may reflect commercial availability, established distribution and regulatory fit as much as intrinsic preference.

South Korea occupies a more commercially accessible but heavily fiscal position. Nicotine products can be affected by tobacco classification, national health policy, taxation and local restrictions, while the market contains cigarettes, heated tobacco and vaping systems competing within the same nicotine economy. Taxes and product definitions can influence whether consumers choose refill liquids, closed pods, synthetic nicotine or imports. Chemical origin becomes legally significant where legislation distinguishes tobacco-derived nicotine from other forms. Such distinctions may encourage reformulation without changing pharmacological exposure, demonstrating how tax and legal language can alter product chemistry for regulatory rather than toxicological reasons.

Singapore applies comprehensive controls to electronic vaporisers. Importation, distribution, sale, purchase, possession and use are prohibited, and enforcement extends to travellers, online transactions and social-media promotion. The policy prevents a legal consumer market and treats vaping as avoidable nicotine dependence rather than a regulated smoking alternative. Strong border administration and penalties make this more enforceable than prohibition where borders are porous or inspection capacity is limited. Even so, repeated seizures and enforcement campaigns show that legal exclusion does not remove demand or eliminate illicit products.

Singapore also illustrates an emerging risk of prohibited supply: products may contain undeclared psychoactive or pharmaceutical substances because manufacture and distribution occur entirely outside lawful oversight. When consumers cannot obtain regulated nicotine products, illicit devices may become delivery systems for compounds unrelated to ordinary vaping. This changes the risk profile from controlled nicotine exposure towards uncertain toxicology, adulteration and criminal supply. Prohibition may reduce population availability, but the residual market can become more hazardous per product because there are no legitimate manufacturers, ingredient disclosures or recall mechanisms. Enforcement data should therefore distinguish ordinary nicotine devices from adulterated products rather than treating all seizures as equivalent.

India adopted a national prohibition covering production, manufacture, import, export, transport, sale, distribution, storage and advertisement of electronic cigarettes. The legislation sought to prevent widespread uptake before the market became entrenched, particularly among young people. It provides a clear legal position and avoids the administrative burden of building notification or authorisation systems. The trade-off is that adult smokers cannot access a lawful vaping market even though combustible cigarettes and other tobacco products remain available. This creates a risk hierarchy in which the most hazardous nicotine product may remain legal while a non-combustible substitute is excluded.

Thailand has similarly maintained strong restrictions on importation and sale, with enforcement affecting residents, retailers and visitors. Such policies can create apparent market simplicity because there are no lawful product standards, notifications or retail categories to administer. In practice, tourism, online commerce and cross-border movement sustain availability outside formal channels. Consumers may obtain products with no reliable information on nicotine strength, battery safety or ingredients, while authorities focus resources on interception rather than product quality. The regulatory question is therefore not merely whether prohibition is legally coherent, but whether it produces lower total harm than a tightly controlled market would under local conditions.

The Philippines represents a contrasting regulated consumer approach. National legislation created rules for vaporised nicotine and non-nicotine products, including product standards, age restrictions, packaging, health warnings, sales controls and administrative responsibilities. The framework has been politically contested because it attempts to preserve adult access while addressing youth use and product quality. Regulatory responsibility has also shifted between agencies, illustrating how institutional design affects implementation. A law can specify standards, but laboratories, customs officers, local authorities and retailers must understand which body registers products, verifies conformity and removes non-compliant goods from sale.

Malaysia has moved from a fragmented position towards a more comprehensive statutory framework. The Control of Smoking Products for Public Health Act 2024 brought tobacco, electronic cigarettes, vaping liquids and substitute products within dedicated legislation. Registration, laboratory documentation, advertising restrictions, age controls, packaging requirements, retail-display rules and prohibitions on online and vending-machine sales create a layered model. Implementation dates have been phased, allowing businesses time to register products and adapt labels. This transition shows the difficulty of regulating an established market after years of partial control: authorities must formalise legitimate operators without allowing transitional arrangements to become permanent loopholes.

Indonesia represents another important pattern in which vaping develops within a large tobacco economy and is influenced strongly by excise policy. Rather than relying only on premarket scientific assessment, government control can operate through taxation, customs, manufacturing rules and product classification. This may generate revenue and bring producers into formal systems, but fiscal registration should not be mistaken for toxicological evaluation. An excise stamp can identify duty-paid liquid without confirming ingredient suitability, aerosol emissions or device compatibility. Where cigarettes remain socially and commercially dominant, vaping policy also interacts with employment, agriculture, domestic tobacco manufacturing and political resistance to measures perceived as threatening established industries.

Across Asia, nicotine concentration limits vary widely or are absent because some countries regulate the product through prohibition rather than compositional standards. Where limits exist, enforcement requires competent analytical laboratories and clear rules for nicotine salts, synthetic nicotine and measurement uncertainty. Labels may state nominal concentrations that do not match finished-liquid assays, particularly in informal markets. Device performance further complicates interpretation because identical concentrations can produce different delivered doses. Countries importing finished products need methods capable of testing both liquid and aerosol, while manufacturing jurisdictions need controls over raw nicotine, blending, filling and component compatibility.

Flavour policy is equally diverse. Some governments restrict products to tobacco-like profiles, others prohibit selected descriptors, and others allow broad flavour ranges under age-controlled retail. The scientific issue is not solved by choosing between unrestricted flavours and universal prohibition. Individual compounds differ in inhalation toxicity, thermal degradation and concentration, while flavour systems influence adult switching and youth appeal. Effective regulation should separate chemical acceptability from marketing presentation. A flavour may be toxicologically supportable but described in a child-oriented manner, or legally permitted despite inadequate inhalation evidence. Combining these questions into one political category prevents precise risk management.

Enforcement capacity may matter more than legislative severity. Wealthier city-states can monitor borders, online platforms and retailers intensively, while large archipelagic or land-border countries face different logistical realities. A prohibition copied from Singapore may operate very differently where informal trade is extensive and customs resources are limited. Similarly, a notification system imported from Europe may generate data that the receiving authority cannot analyse. Regulatory models should therefore match institutional capability. Requirements that cannot be verified may reward paperwork rather than compliance, while simple standards supported by regular sampling can sometimes produce better control than elaborate but unenforced dossiers.

Cross-border commerce intensifies these problems. Products can move from Chinese factories through regional distributors, free-trade zones, online marketplaces and small-parcel networks before reaching consumers in prohibited or restricted markets. Packaging may display false nicotine strengths, invented certification marks or regulatory identifiers belonging to unrelated products. Market-specific versions can be diverted, and genuine export goods can become unlawful when sold domestically or in neighbouring countries. Traceability therefore requires cooperation between manufacturers, customs authorities, platforms and destination regulators. National law remains essential, but no Asian jurisdiction can control the modern vape supply chain through domestic retail inspections alone.

Asia also exposes the relationship between vaping regulation and combustible tobacco most sharply. Several countries with restrictive vaping laws retain high smoking prevalence, powerful cigarette industries or widely available low-cost tobacco. Evaluating policy solely through vaping prevalence can therefore be misleading. A decline in vaping may appear successful while cigarette use remains unchanged, and a rise in vaping may reflect harmful initiation or beneficial substitution. The relevant measures include smoking displacement, dual use, youth uptake, illicit purchasing, cessation outcomes and product-related harm. Regulation should be assessed against the nicotine market it actually creates, not the one described in legislation.

The region is unlikely to converge rapidly on one model because political systems, tobacco markets and public-health priorities differ too greatly. Nevertheless, technical harmonisation remains possible. Shared laboratory methods, ingredient identifiers, battery standards, contaminant limits, manufacturing expectations and reporting formats could improve safety without requiring identical policies on sale or flavour. Mutual recognition of credible testing would reduce duplication and help smaller regulators use evidence generated elsewhere. Regional customs cooperation could also jointly target falsely declared or adulterated products more effectively than isolated national campaigns, particularly where the same suppliers serve several markets.

Asia ultimately demonstrates that regulation is an active determinant of product evolution. It decides whether consumers encounter refillable systems, tobacco-flavoured closed pods, heated products, illicit disposables or no lawful alternative to cigarettes. It influences nicotine chemistry, device design, price, retail access and the quality of evidence available after sale. The strongest future frameworks will avoid copying foreign rules without regard to local conditions. They will distinguish combustion from non-combustion, control genuine product risks, protect young people and recognise that prohibition, taxation, notification and authorisation each create different unintended markets. Scientific regulation begins by measuring those consequences honestly.

Middle East

The Middle East does not present a single regulatory philosophy for vaping. It contains tightly controlled legal markets, standards-based import systems, tobacco-style taxation, pharmaceutical restrictions and complete prohibitions. Products can therefore move from lawful retail to prohibited possession after crossing one border, even though their chemistry and hardware remain unchanged. This fragmentation is intensified by regional travel, free-trade zones, online commerce and supply chains passing through Gulf ports. The Middle Eastern regulatory question is consequently not only whether vaping is permitted, but which authority controls it, which standard defines conformity and whether enforcement can distinguish lawful goods from diverted or counterfeit stock.

The region's approach has been shaped by several overlapping concerns. Governments seek to prevent youth nicotine use, control imported consumer goods, protect public spaces, collect excise revenue and avoid repeating the health burden created by cigarettes and waterpipe tobacco. At the same time, combustible tobacco remains widely available in many markets, and adult smokers increasingly encounter vaping, heated tobacco and oral nicotine products as alternatives. This creates a policy tension between excluding unfamiliar nicotine technologies and regulating them sufficiently to compete with established smoking products. Where authorities permit vaping, they usually place it within tobacco-control structures rather than recognising a separate harm-reduction category.

The United Arab Emirates represents the region's clearest standards-based consumer model. Electronic nicotine products can be sold lawfully when they comply with mandatory national requirements, including UAE.S 5030, and with wider tobacco legislation governing importation, packaging, warnings and commercial supply. Compliance is linked to conformity assessment, product registration, approved labelling and responsible importation, giving authorities a route to identify lawful products before retail sale.

This system directly reflects the UAE's wider use of technical regulations to control imported products. A vape is assessed not merely as a branded consumer article but as an integrated nicotine-delivery system containing liquid, heating components, electrical parts and packaging. Manufacturers must consider nicotine accuracy, restricted substances, emissions, leakage, child resistance, battery safety and label presentation. Market access therefore depends on documentary and technical conformity rather than simple customs clearance. The model can support product quality, but only where certificates correspond to the item actually manufactured and where post-market sampling detects substitutions, oversized reservoirs or formulations differing from registered specifications.

The UAE also illustrates the importance of distinguishing legal availability from unrestricted promotion. A product may satisfy a technical standard while remaining subject to age controls, public-use restrictions, excise requirements and limitations on advertising. This layered approach recognises that product safety, market behaviour and population exposure are different regulatory questions. Scientific evidence may establish that a device emits fewer combustion-related toxicants than cigarettes, yet the government may still restrict how it is displayed or described. Conversely, commercial legality cannot be treated as evidence that the product is harmless or suitable for people who do not already use nicotine.

Saudi Arabia uses a similarly formal but more centrally supervised approach. The Saudi Food and Drug Authority has issued technical requirements for e-liquids and heated tobacco products used in electronic nicotine-delivery systems, alongside conditions governing tobacco-product clearance. Importers must operate through defined regulatory and customs processes, while products are also affected by packaging, taxation and market-control rules.

For manufacturers, Saudi compliance requires close alignment between the submitted technical file and the imported consignment. Product names, nicotine concentrations, flavour descriptions, package artwork, warning statements and quantities must remain consistent across regulatory, customs and commercial records. A change considered minor by a foreign factory may create a different regulatory product if it alters formulation, device performance or labelling. This is especially important where export manufacturers frequently revise disposable formats, puff-count claims and flavour portfolios. Supply-chain control must prevent unapproved variants from being packed into shipments intended for the Saudi market.

Bahrain provides another regulated pathway based on prior interaction with health and customs authorities. Before importing new tobacco or electronic nicotine products, businesses must submit product artwork and, for relevant processes, product samples for review. Customs services also recognise import procedures for electronic nicotine products, while excise measures apply to e-cigarette flavours. The system is consequently built around licensing, package review, customs inspection and fiscal control rather than a broad consumer notification database comparable with EU-CEG.

These Gulf models share a practical advantage: imported products can be controlled at identifiable commercial gateways. Domestic markets depend heavily on overseas manufacturing, allowing customs, conformity bodies and national distributors to become central points of accountability. The weakness is that high-volume ports, free zones, re-export operations and small parcels can create diversion opportunities. Goods manufactured for one destination may enter another without the required warnings, registrations or tax marks. A package appearing legitimate in Dubai, Riyadh or Manama may therefore represent a different product version beneath similar branding.

Qatar and Oman demonstrate the opposite regulatory choice. Qatar prohibits electronic-cigarette devices through tobacco-control and customs mechanisms, while Oman states that importing and using electronic cigarettes is illegal. These systems avoid the need to maintain product standards, notification portals or specialist retail categories because lawful consumer supply is excluded. The legal position is comparatively simple, but enforcement must address travellers, online orders, postal shipments and informal resale.

Prohibition changes the available evidence. Authorities receive no routine ingredient dossiers, sales reports or manufacturer vigilance data for illicit products. Consumers cannot distinguish regulated nicotine liquids from counterfeit or adulterated formulations because every commercial product exists outside the lawful framework. Seizures provide information on brands and quantities but rarely reveal actual exposure unless products are analysed. A prohibition may reduce visibility and accessibility, yet the remaining market can become scientifically opaque. Evaluation must therefore examine smoking, vaping, illicit supply and poisoning events together rather than treating the absence of legal sales as proof that use has disappeared.

The contrast between neighbouring Gulf states also creates regulatory displacement. Residents can encounter products during travel, purchase them through foreign websites or obtain stock diverted from legal markets. Tourism adds complexity because visitors may assume that rules resemble those of the country from which they departed. Airports and border authorities must communicate clearly whether devices are permitted, restricted or confiscated. Airlines separately regulate carriage because lithium batteries present fire risks, meaning that aviation safety rules and national nicotine laws can apply simultaneously to the same object.

Israel operates another distinct model: vaping products are legal but incorporated into a strict tobacco-control framework. Electronic cigarettes are covered by public-place restrictions, advertising controls, packaging and marketing rules, and a prohibition on products exceeding 20 milligrams of nicotine per millilitre. Uniform presentation, health warnings and reporting obligations extend tobacco-style controls to vaping while allowing adult access.

This approach produces regulatory parity in commercial controls without requiring toxicological parity between smoke and aerosol. The distinction is important. Applying common age, advertising and public-use rules can reduce youth exposure and simplify enforcement, but identical warnings or presentation may lead consumers to infer identical health risks. A scientifically coherent model should control nicotine dependence and marketing while preserving truthful information about combustion. Otherwise, smokers may receive strong warnings against switching but little explanation of why inhaling burnt tobacco remains uniquely hazardous.

Israel's experience also demonstrates the need to monitor adulterated liquids. The Ministry of Health has warned about e-cigarette liquids containing dangerous synthetic drugs, showing how a familiar device format can be repurposed for substances unrelated to ordinary nicotine vaping. This risk exists across the region wherever illicit supply develops. Regulators need analytical methods capable of screening unknown psychoactive compounds, not merely verifying nicotine and routine carbonyls. Product surveillance must follow the chemistry actually found in seized or reported devices rather than assuming every vape contains conventional e-liquid.

Egypt has moved towards recognising electronic cigarettes and heated products within taxation, import control and conformity-assessment structures. Its value-added tax legislation expressly captures liquids consumed by electronic cigarettes whether or not they contain nicotine, while the General Organization for Export and Import Control has developed testing and conformity functions covering tobacco products and alternatives. This creates a fiscal and border-control architecture even where the wider product-regulatory system remains less unified than European notification or American authorisation.

Tax recognition can formalise a market, identify importers and generate revenue, but it does not constitute scientific approval. Duty may be paid on a liquid with poor ingredient disclosure, inaccurate nicotine concentration or unsuitable aerosol performance. Conformity assessment must therefore connect tax status with product standards, laboratory capability and post-market action. Egypt's large population and established tobacco market make this especially important: a technically weak vaping market could introduce new harms, while an excessively restrictive one could leave combustible cigarettes with little lawful competition.

Across the Middle East, Arabic labelling presents a substantive compliance requirement rather than a translation exercise. Warnings, nicotine strength, ingredients, instructions, importer details and first-aid statements must remain chemically and legally accurate. Transliteration can obscure whether a flavour name is descriptive, promotional or misleading. Differences between Arabic and English panels may also create enforcement uncertainty. Artwork should therefore be controlled as regulatory data, with bilingual review performed before printing and the approved version linked to the exact formulation and device.

Excise taxation has become one of the region's most powerful regulatory levers. Several Gulf jurisdictions apply high rates to electronic-cigarette liquids or related products, often within broader selective-tax systems intended to discourage consumption. Tax stamps and customs declarations can improve traceability, but high fiscal burdens may also increase incentives for under-declaration, counterfeit packaging and cross-border diversion. Revenue policy should be assessed against cigarette prices because the relative cost of products influences whether smokers switch, continue smoking or purchase illicit goods.

The region's hot climate introduces technical issues that deserve greater regulatory attention. E-liquids, seals, batteries and plastics can be exposed to high temperatures during shipping, port storage, delivery vehicles and retail display. Heat can accelerate nicotine oxidation, flavour degradation, pressure changes, leakage and battery deterioration. Stability programmes designed for temperate markets may not represent Middle Eastern distribution. Manufacturers should generate data under relevant climatic conditions and validate packaging capable of maintaining performance throughout transport and shelf life.

Waterpipe culture also shapes how vaping is understood. In some markets, electronic devices are compared not only with cigarettes but with shisha, which has established social and hospitality contexts. Product names, flavours and device formats may deliberately borrow from waterpipe imagery. Regulators must therefore distinguish between technologies while recognising shared promotional cues. Public communication that discusses only cigarettes may fail to address consumers who move between shisha, vaping and heated products or who do not identify themselves as smokers.

Youth protection remains the most politically influential concern. Bright packaging, sweet flavours, compact disposables and social-media promotion can spread rapidly through urban markets even where formal advertising is restricted. Effective control requires age verification, retailer accountability, online-platform cooperation and penalties that reach importers and wholesalers. Restricting compliant shops while leaving informal delivery networks untouched can increase the market share of untraceable products. Enforcement should therefore follow supply chains upstream rather than treating individual possession as the principal problem.

Regional harmonisation could improve safety without requiring every state to adopt the same access policy. Shared methods for nicotine analysis, emissions testing, battery safety, child resistance and contaminant limits would allow laboratories and customs authorities to compare results. Common product identifiers and electronic certificates could reduce document fraud and simplify re-export control. Prohibition states could still reject legal sale, while regulated markets could use common evidence standards. Harmonising technical truth is more achievable than harmonising political attitudes towards nicotine.

The Middle East ultimately shows that regulation can make the same technology appear as a controlled consumer product, taxable tobacco substitute, prohibited import or public-health threat. The strongest systems will be those that connect legal classification with measurable product standards, realistic enforcement and honest comparison with combustible smoking. Severity alone is not enough. A prohibition without border control creates an opaque illicit market, while legalisation without scientific oversight creates a visible but unreliable one. Regional policy must be judged by the market it produces: which products consumers actually obtain, what those products contain and whether adult smoking declines without creating new patterns of youth dependence.

Emerging Markets

Emerging markets are not defined by geography alone. In vaping regulation, the term describes jurisdictions where product use, commercial supply and public concern are developing faster than the institutions responsible for controlling them. These markets may be located in Africa, Latin America, Central Asia, the Caribbean, the Pacific or parts of Eastern Europe, but they share a common regulatory condition: the product has arrived before a complete legal, scientific and enforcement architecture exists. Governments therefore face decisions under pressure, often with limited surveillance data, restricted laboratory capacity and competing priorities across tobacco control, customs, public health, taxation and consumer protection.

The first challenge is classification. A vaping product can be treated as tobacco, a nicotine-delivery system, a consumer electrical device, a chemical mixture, a medicine, an excisable commodity or a prohibited import. Emerging markets frequently inherit laws written before modern electronic cigarettes existed, leaving regulators to force new products into old definitions. This may produce inconsistent decisions between ministries or courts. Customs officers may regard the device as electronic equipment, health authorities as a tobacco product and medicines regulators as an unauthorised therapeutic good. Until classification is resolved, businesses cannot determine which licences, standards, warnings or taxes apply, and enforcement becomes selective rather than systematic.

Some governments respond by adopting legislation from larger jurisdictions. European nicotine limits, British warning language, American-style authorisation concepts or Gulf conformity procedures may be copied because they provide ready-made legal text. Borrowing can accelerate regulation, but legal transplantation is not the same as regulatory capacity. A notification system modelled on Europe requires databases, trained reviewers and competent authorities able to interpret ingredient and emissions information. An authorisation model resembling the United States demands toxicology, behavioural science and substantial administrative resources. Where those capabilities are absent, complex requirements can become ceremonial paperwork that lawful businesses complete while unregulated products continue to dominate the market.

A stronger approach begins with the market that actually exists. Regulators need to know which products are sold, where they originate, how much nicotine they contain, which age groups use them and whether consumers are switching from cigarettes, adding vaping to smoking or initiating nicotine use. These questions are often unanswered because national surveys do not separate product categories, import statistics use broad customs codes and informal retail escapes official reporting. Policy built without baseline data can overestimate one risk while missing another. A visible urban vape shop may attract political attention, while larger volumes move through social media, street markets, personal luggage and small parcels.

Informal supply is central to emerging-market regulation. Products may enter through undeclared imports, mixed consignments or neighbouring countries with different rules. Local distributors can repackage liquids, refill disposable devices or apply labels that do not correspond to the original formulation. Counterfeit branding further obscures responsibility. In such markets, the product described on the package may not match the liquid, nicotine strength, battery or coil inside. Regulation must therefore address supply-chain identity before expecting sophisticated toxicological compliance. Without traceability, even a well-designed standard cannot determine who should answer for a failed sample or adverse event.

Customs authorities often become the first practical regulators. They control import licences, tariff classifications, documentation and border inspection, but may have little access to specialist chemical information. A device can be declared as a battery, electronic accessory, atomiser or personal-care product depending on the code chosen by the importer. Liquids may be separated from hardware to avoid scrutiny. Effective border control requires clear commodity codes, risk profiles and rapid testing methods capable of identifying nicotine, container volume and obvious non-conformity. Customs databases should connect with health and tax authorities so that a suspicious shipment is not released merely because each agency sees only part of the product.

Laboratory capacity is another limiting factor. Full aerosol characterisation requires vaping machines, validated methods, chemical standards, calibrated equipment and experienced analysts. Many emerging markets do not have this infrastructure for routine enforcement. Requiring every possible emission measurement may therefore create dependence on foreign certificates that cannot be verified locally. A staged programme is more realistic. Initial surveillance can focus on nicotine concentration, prohibited ingredients, carbonyl screening, selected metals, fill volume and battery safety. Regional reference laboratories can then support more advanced testing, method validation and investigations involving novel compounds or suspected adulteration.

Standards should prioritise hazards that are both important and enforceable. Child-resistant packaging, leakage control, accurate nicotine labelling, electrical protection, ingredient disclosure and batch traceability provide immediate value. Prohibitions on oils, undeclared psychoactive substances or clearly unsuitable additives can address serious risks without requiring complete toxicological certainty for every flavour constituent. The objective should not be to create the longest rulebook, but to establish requirements that inspectors, laboratories and courts can apply consistently. An unenforceable threshold may appear scientifically sophisticated while contributing less protection than a simpler rule supported by routine sampling and meaningful penalties.

Manufacturing conditions vary greatly. Some emerging markets import finished products, while others develop local mixing, filling and assembly operations. Small-scale production can improve affordability and reduce dependence on imported stock, but it may occur without controlled raw materials, validated equipment or batch records. Nicotine can be handled in concentrated form by workers lacking appropriate protection, and flavour concentrates may be purchased through food channels without inhalation information. Regulation should distinguish responsible local manufacture from informal blending. Licensing, minimum premises standards, supplier documentation, training and batch release can raise quality without demanding pharmaceutical infrastructure that would eliminate every smaller producer.

Economic conditions strongly influence compliance. Testing, registration fees, specialist packaging and excise stamps may be manageable in wealthy markets but disproportionate where retail prices and business margins are low.

Excessive cost can remove compliant products while leaving cigarettes or illicit vapes more affordable. This does not justify weak standards, but it requires prioritisation and scalable fees. Product families can sometimes be assessed together where formulations and devices are genuinely related. Authorities can publish standardised templates, recognise accredited foreign laboratories and phase in requirements. The aim should be to lower unnecessary administrative cost while preserving scientific accountability.

Taxation is often introduced earlier than product regulation because revenue systems already exist. Excise can formalise importers, identify wholesalers and create visible tax-paid products. It can also generate perverse effects if rates are detached from risk or consumer behaviour. A high tax on vaping liquid may protect cigarette sales, encourage under-declaration or favour compact high-delivery devices. A low rate may improve substitution but attract criticism that government is encouraging nicotine use. Fiscal policy should therefore preserve a meaningful price advantage for non-combustible products while funding enforcement, cessation services and surveillance. Tax stamps should never be presented as proof of technical safety.

Smoking prevalence must remain the central comparator. Many emerging markets carry high burdens of combustible tobacco use, including cigarettes, bidis, waterpipe or locally produced tobacco. Vaping policy cannot be evaluated solely by whether vape sales increase or decrease. A rise may represent youth initiation, adult switching or both. A prohibition may reduce visible vaping while leaving smoking unchanged. A legal market may reduce cigarette consumption but widen nicotine use among non-smokers. Regulation must measure transitions between products, not merely count users within isolated categories. Complete substitution, dual use, relapse and initiation should be followed across age, income and geographic groups.

Health inequalities are particularly important. Urban consumers may access regulated specialist retailers while rural users rely on cigarettes or informal products. Imported premium devices can be unaffordable to smokers who bear the greatest disease burden. Medicalised access may exclude people without regular healthcare, while online sales may favour those with digital payment and reliable delivery. Policies that appear neutral can therefore distribute benefits and risks unevenly. Harm-reduction programmes should consider affordability, language, literacy and local smoking practices. Product warnings and cessation information must be understandable to the populations expected to use them, not copied mechanically from foreign packaging.

Youth protection requires more than a statutory age. Weak identity systems, informal retail and family-based commerce can make conventional age verification difficult. Bright packaging and social-media promotion can spread faster than official advertising controls. Enforcement should focus on retailer accountability, platform cooperation, wholesale supply and repeated breaches rather than isolated sales assistants. School surveys can identify trends, but responses should avoid assuming that every young person who experiments will become a long-term user. The severity of regulation should reflect frequency, dependence, nicotine exposure and progression, while prevention programmes should address smoking and vaping together.

Communication is a major regulatory tool. In markets where scientific literacy varies and misinformation circulates rapidly, official silence allows commercial claims and alarmist narratives to dominate. Authorities should state clearly that vaping is not harmless, nicotine can create dependence and products should not be used by children or non-users. They should also explain that combustion produces a different and generally more hazardous exposure profile than non-combustible aerosol. Without this distinction, smokers may believe there is no reason to switch, while young people may interpret prohibition as evidence of exceptional danger and seek products through illicit channels.

Environmental concerns are growing because low-cost disposable devices can enter markets without waste infrastructure capable of handling lithium batteries, plastics and residual liquid. Informal disposal, burning and landfill create hazards beyond nicotine exposure. Import rules can require rechargeable or refillable design, producer responsibility or collection arrangements, but these systems must be realistic. A nominal recycling obligation achieves little where no collection network exists. Environmental policy should consider durability, repairability, battery access and the economics of recovery. Product design standards can reduce waste before complex recycling systems become necessary.

Regional cooperation offers the greatest opportunity for emerging markets. Neighbouring countries often receive products from the same factories and distributors, yet investigate them separately. Shared alerts, testing protocols and supplier intelligence can identify repeated problems earlier. Regional economic communities can develop common definitions, labelling principles and laboratory methods while allowing national decisions on taxation, flavours or retail access. Joint training for customs officers, inspectors and analysts reduces duplication. Mutual recognition of credible evidence can make compliance more affordable, provided that authorities retain the power to sample products and challenge unreliable certificates.

A staged regulatory pathway is often more effective than immediate imitation of mature systems. The first phase can establish age restrictions, importer registration, nicotine limits, basic warnings, child resistance and a prohibition on clearly unsafe products. The second can introduce product notification, ingredient data, sales reporting and accredited testing. Later phases can add targeted emissions requirements, post-market vigilance and electronic traceability as capacity grows. Staging should not become indefinite delay. Each phase requires deadlines, responsible agencies and published criteria showing how the system will develop.

Regulatory success must be judged through outcomes rather than legislative appearance. Useful indicators include smoking prevalence, complete switching, youth regular use, product compliance rates, poisoning incidents, battery events, illicit-market share and enforcement response times. Registration totals, seizures or tax revenue describe activity but not necessarily health impact. Independent evaluation should test whether rules improve the quality of products people actually use and whether legal supply remains more attractive than illicit alternatives. Policies should be revised when evidence shows unintended movement back to smoking or towards unregulated products.

Institutional governance determines whether these measures remain coherent. One ministry should coordinate health, customs, tax, standards, trade and consumer-safety functions through a national plan. Regulatory ownership must be visible to businesses and the public, with published procedures for registration, testing, appeals, recalls and enforcement. Fragmented authority creates contradictory instructions, delayed decisions and opportunities for non-compliant suppliers to move between agencies without accountability or timely corrective action.

Emerging markets are not empty regulatory spaces waiting to copy rules from elsewhere. They are dynamic nicotine economies with their own tobacco histories, institutions, consumer behaviour and commercial pressures. Their opportunity is to avoid some mistakes made by earlier markets: uncontrolled product proliferation, data systems that collect more than authorities can analyse, standards detached from enforcement and restrictions that strengthen illicit supply. The strongest frameworks will be proportionate, staged and measurable. They will protect young people, raise product quality and preserve the toxicological distinction between combustion and non-combustion while building institutions capable of adapting as the market changes.

Towards Regulatory Harmonisation

Regulatory harmonisation in vaping is often presented as a technical objective: one set of definitions, one dossier, one testing protocol and one route to market. In practice, it is a political and scientific negotiation over what the product is, which risks deserve priority and how much national discretion should remain. Countries regulate vaping through tobacco law, medicines law, consumer-product law, customs controls, taxation or prohibition. These pathways reflect different histories and policy objectives. Harmonisation cannot therefore begin by forcing every jurisdiction into one legal model. It must begin by identifying which elements of product control require shared truth and which properly remain matters of domestic choice.

The strongest case for harmonisation lies in areas where disagreement creates no legitimate public-health benefit. Nicotine concentration should be measured using comparable methods. Chemical identities should be reported consistently. Device capacity, aerosol mass, battery safety, child resistance, leakage, emissions and product stability should be assessed against transparent technical standards. Laboratories should describe puffing regimes, calibration, uncertainty and limits of detection in ways that allow results to be compared. A carbonyl result generated under one method should not appear scientifically equivalent to a result generated under radically different power settings, puff durations or coil conditions. Harmonisation should reduce methodological noise before attempting to harmonise policy conclusions.

Shared terminology is the essential foundation. Terms such as electronic cigarette, vaping product, refill container, cartridge, pod, disposable, reusable device, nicotine salt, synthetic nicotine and heated tobacco product are used differently across jurisdictions. Ambiguous definitions create loopholes and make cross-border data unreliable. A product described as refillable in one country may be treated as disposable in another. A nicotine-free liquid may fall outside tobacco legislation while remaining chemically capable of being mixed with nicotine. International definitions should describe physical and functional characteristics rather than depend solely on branding. Clear terminology would improve customs classification, surveillance, research and enforcement without requiring governments to permit the same products.

Chemical identity requires similar discipline. Ingredient lists should use recognised names, CAS numbers where appropriate, concentration units and clear distinctions between pure substances, mixtures and proprietary flavour systems. Nicotine should be reported on a consistent basis, distinguishing base nicotine from salt mass and identifying the counterion. Suppliers should disclose enough composition for toxicological assessment while legitimate confidential information remains protected. A global data dictionary could specify mandatory fields for solvents, flavour constituents, acids, sweeteners, coolants, impurities and material-contact substances. This would not determine whether each ingredient is permitted, but it would ensure that regulators are evaluating the same chemical reality.

Testing standards offer a practical route towards convergence. International methods already exist for routine vaping-machine operation and selected emissions, but their regulatory use remains inconsistent. Harmonisation should define a core battery of methods while allowing justified product-specific additions. The core should include nicotine in liquid and aerosol, carbonyls, selected volatile compounds, metals, aerosol collected mass, fill volume, leakage and electrical safety. Results should be linked to device settings, coil age, sample conditioning and product version. A common minimum dataset would reduce duplicate testing and allow authorities to compare products across markets, provided laboratories operate under recognised competence standards and participate in proficiency testing.

Method harmonisation must not become method rigidity. Vaping technology evolves faster than many standards. A fixed regime developed for refillable tank systems may not represent high-output disposables, temperature-controlled devices or novel aerosol generators. Regulators should therefore accept scientifically justified alternative methods where the standard method is unsuitable. The objective is comparability, not mechanical conformity. International standards bodies, regulators, laboratories and manufacturers need a mechanism for updating methods when products change. Version control is crucial so that an old result is not compared uncritically with data generated under a revised protocol.

Product notification data could also be harmonised without creating a single global authority. Manufacturers now submit overlapping information in different formats, languages and portals. One jurisdiction may request ingredient concentrations, another broad ranges, another emissions, and another manufacturing details. Reformatting the same underlying evidence consumes resources without necessarily improving scrutiny. A modular international dossier could contain a common technical core covering identity, formulation, device, toxicology, testing, manufacturing and quality controls. National modules could then address local warnings, taxes, responsible operators, flavours, retail restrictions and legal declarations. This would preserve sovereignty while reducing pointless duplication.

Mutual recognition should be approached carefully. A laboratory result produced by an accredited laboratory using an accepted method should generally be usable across several jurisdictions. Requiring identical testing solely because the market changes wastes samples, time and money. Yet mutual recognition should not mean automatic acceptance of every foreign certificate. Authorities need confidence in laboratory competence, method suitability, sample traceability and data integrity. Shared audit principles, proficiency schemes and electronic verification could allow regulators to recognise credible evidence while rejecting unreliable or fraudulent documentation. Recognition should attach to the quality of the evidence, not merely to the country from which it originated.

Manufacturing expectations are another area suitable for alignment. Vaping products are produced through global supply chains involving nicotine suppliers, flavour houses, plastics manufacturers, battery producers, coil factories, filling sites and brand owners. National product rules cannot control this network effectively if each jurisdiction applies unrelated quality concepts. A shared baseline should include supplier qualification, traceability, change control, contamination prevention, batch records, deviation management, corrective action and complaint handling. These are not uniquely pharmaceutical requirements; they are fundamental controls for any inhaled nicotine product whose performance depends on both formulation and hardware.

Harmonised post-market surveillance could produce greater public-health value than increasingly elaborate premarket paperwork. Complaints, adverse events, battery incidents, leakage, poisoning, counterfeit reports and analytical failures often appear first in one country. At present, these signals may remain trapped within national systems or private company databases. A secure international alert mechanism could share product identifiers, batch information, failure modes and corrective actions. Regulators would retain control over national enforcement, but repeated problems could be recognised earlier. Shared signal detection is particularly important where the same device is sold under several brands or market-specific names.

Global product identifiers would make such surveillance possible. Brand names are unstable, translated inconsistently and easily copied. A structured identifier should link the manufacturer, formulation, device configuration, nicotine strength and market version. It should remain traceable through customs, notification, laboratory testing, wholesale distribution and recall. The identifier need not appear as a consumer-facing claim of approval. It would function as regulatory infrastructure, allowing authorities to determine whether a sampled product matches the submitted record. Counterfeiters can copy codes, so electronic validation and supply-chain records would still be necessary, but consistent identifiers would improve the starting point.

Customs harmonisation is equally important because many non-compliant products enter through misclassification rather than formal market channels. International commodity codes should distinguish devices, nicotine liquids, nicotine-free liquids, pods, cartridges and components more precisely. Commercial invoices should use standard descriptions linked to product identifiers. Customs officers need access to regulatory status, tax information and alerts without relying on paper certificates supplied by importers. Better integration between customs and health authorities would make it harder to declare regulated nicotine products as generic electronics or flavouring preparations. Border control is part of product regulation, not an administrative afterthought.

Taxation is less suitable for complete harmonisation because national fiscal systems and incomes differ, but shared principles would reduce distortion. Taxes should not inadvertently make combustible cigarettes more attractive than lower-risk alternatives. Rates based solely on liquid volume may favour concentrated products, while rates based on nicotine content may penalise effective smoking substitutes. Governments should evaluate price relationships, illicit trade and consumer switching rather than copying another country's duty structure. Regional coordination can reduce cross-border arbitrage, but fiscal convergence should preserve a meaningful economic incentive to move away from combustion.

Flavour policy is even more politically contested. Scientific harmonisation could identify ingredients presenting unacceptable inhalation risks, set impurity limits and standardise toxicological assessment. It cannot by itself determine whether fruit, dessert, menthol or tobacco flavours should be permitted. That decision involves youth appeal, adult switching, culture and enforcement capacity. A useful international framework would separate chemical safety from marketing presentation. A flavour could pass a toxicological screen while its name, imagery or packaging remains restricted. This distinction would allow regulators to target child-oriented promotion without pretending that every flavour compound has the same hazard.

Nicotine limits also require a more scientific approach than simple international copying. Concentration ceilings are easy to legislate but do not fully control delivered dose. Device efficiency, aerosol output, nicotine form and puffing behaviour all matter. Harmonisation should begin with accurate measurement and disclosure, then consider performance-based standards where evidence supports them. A universal concentration limit may be inappropriate across product types and smoking populations. What matters is whether products deliver nicotine consistently, avoid accidental poisoning and remain capable of substituting for cigarettes without creating excessive exposure or youth-oriented appeal.

Communication standards should converge around truthful comparative information. Every jurisdiction has reason to prevent claims that vaping is harmless, medically approved or suitable for non-users. Equally, public warnings should not erase the distinction between aerosol and combustion. International guidance could establish principles for communicating uncertainty, dependence, relative exposure and intended users. Governments would retain control over advertising, but consumers should not receive contradictory scientific messages merely because they cross a border. Consistent communication is essential for adult smokers making decisions and for preventing young people from interpreting lower risk as absence of risk.

Harmonisation must also account for regulatory capacity. A system requiring complex emissions dossiers, electronic portals and specialised review may overwhelm authorities with limited staff and laboratory access. International cooperation should therefore include training, shared reference laboratories, model legislation, data tools and technical assistance. Lower-resource jurisdictions should not be forced to choose between adopting unenforceable rules and leaving the market uncontrolled. A tiered framework could establish essential protections first, followed by more advanced requirements as capacity grows. Harmonisation should narrow protection gaps, not export bureaucracy without the institutions needed to support it.

Governance will determine whether convergence remains credible. Industry participation is necessary because manufacturers understand formulations, devices and supply chains, but standards cannot be written solely around commercial convenience. Public-health bodies contribute population evidence, laboratories contribute measurement expertise, consumers contribute experience of real-world use and enforcement agencies reveal what can be implemented. Conflicts of interest should be declared and evidence evaluated transparently. Decisions should explain why particular limits or methods were chosen, what uncertainty remains and when review will occur. Harmonisation without transparent governance risks becoming either industry self-regulation or symbolic restriction.

A realistic pathway would proceed in stages. The first stage would align definitions, identifiers, units, laboratory reporting and minimum safety principles. The second would establish a common technical dossier, recognised testing and shared surveillance alerts. The third could develop mutual recognition for selected evidence and coordinated responses to serious product failures. National governments would continue deciding whether products are notified, authorised, medically supplied, taxed or prohibited. Over time, evidence from comparable systems would allow policy differences to be evaluated more honestly because outcomes would no longer be obscured by incompatible data.

The purpose of harmonisation is not to create one global vaping law. It is to ensure that scientific facts remain stable while products move between legal systems. Nicotine concentration should not change meaning at a border. A battery failure should be recognisable everywhere. An ingredient should not acquire a different chemical identity because a portal uses another name. Comparable evidence would allow regulators to disagree openly about policy rather than unknowingly disagreeing about data. That distinction is essential.

Towards regulatory harmonisation therefore means building a common scientific language beneath diverse national choices. It requires aligned definitions, credible methods, interoperable data, traceable products and shared surveillance. It also requires restraint: not every political judgement can or should be standardised. The strongest international framework would preserve national authority while removing unnecessary inconsistency from the evidence on which that authority acts. Such a system would reduce duplication, improve enforcement, accelerate response to product failures and make lawful supply more accountable. Harmonisation succeeds when it creates common technical truth without pretending that every society must make the same final decision about nicotine globally.

CHAPTER 8

Industry, Politics and Public Health

Vaping regulation is often presented as though scientific evidence moves directly from the laboratory into law. In reality, evidence passes through institutions, professional cultures, political priorities, commercial interests, public anxieties and media narratives before it becomes policy. Chemical analyses may establish the constituents of an aerosol, toxicological studies may identify hazards, clinical research may examine smoking cessation and population surveys may describe patterns of use, yet none of these findings determines automatically how governments should respond. Regulation begins when evidence is interpreted through competing ideas about risk, responsibility and acceptable uncertainty. The resulting rules are therefore products not only of science, but of the relationships between the organisations and individuals authorised to speak on its behalf.

This matters particularly for vaping because the technology entered public life at the boundary between two powerful narratives. One described a non-combustible nicotine product capable of reducing exposure among people who would otherwise continue smoking. The other described a new commercial route into nicotine dependence, especially among young people, introduced before its long-term effects could be known. Both narratives can draw upon legitimate evidence, but they begin from different populations and different comparators. One asks what happens when an adult smoker substitutes vaping for cigarettes. The other asks what happens when a young non-smoker begins using a nicotine product. The physical device may be identical, yet its public-health meaning changes according to the person imagined holding it.

That difference has shaped the entire political history of vaping. Where the dominant comparator is cigarette smoking, the absence of combustion becomes the central scientific fact. Combustion generates the complex mixture of toxicants responsible for much of the disease burden associated with smoking, and replacing smoke with an aerosol can reduce exposure to many harmful constituents. Where the dominant comparator is non-use, any avoidable inhalation, nicotine dependence or uncertainty becomes more difficult to justify. Regulation must protect both populations, but the balance between them is not a mathematical calculation alone. It involves judgements about whose risks are most immediate, whose behaviour is most likely to change and which unintended consequences society is prepared to tolerate.

The organisations surrounding tobacco control do not approach this problem from neutral starting positions. Decades of litigation, concealed evidence, manipulative marketing and political interference by cigarette manufacturers created a justified culture of scepticism towards commercial nicotine interests. That history cannot be separated from modern debates, particularly where multinational tobacco companies now sell vaping and other non-combustible products. Suspicion is not irrational; it is rooted in documented conduct. Yet historical vigilance can become analytically limiting when every new product is interpreted exclusively through the behaviour of the cigarette industry. Independent manufacturers, consumer-led innovation, pharmaceutical-style product development and tobacco-company diversification may occupy the same market while presenting different conflicts, capabilities and incentives.

Public-health institutions face a related difficulty. Their authority depends on presenting evidence clearly enough to guide behaviour and justify intervention. Scientific uncertainty, however, rarely produces a simple message. Vaping can be less harmful than smoking without being harmless. It can support smoking cessation while also creating dependence among people who did not previously smoke. Flavours can assist adult switching and attract younger users. Product standards can improve safety while raising costs and concentrating the market. Restrictions can reduce lawful availability while increasing illicit supply. Each of these propositions can be true simultaneously, but public communication often rewards categorical positions more than conditional ones.

The political environment intensifies this pressure. Ministers and legislators are rarely asked to wait for decades of longitudinal evidence before acting. They respond to visible trends, public concern, electoral priorities, newspaper coverage, professional advice and the practical demands of enforcement agencies. A rise in youth experimentation can become politically urgent even when its long-term trajectory remains uncertain. A cluster of adverse events can alter public perception before causation or product identity has been established. A dramatic image of discarded devices can accelerate environmental regulation more rapidly than years of technical debate. Political systems are designed to respond to public salience, not solely to the maturity of the evidence base.

This creates a recurring mismatch between scientific timescales and policy timescales. Toxicological research may require validated methods, representative samples and repeated studies. Epidemiology requires sufficient exposure duration and population size. Regulatory decisions may need to be made within months. Authorities therefore act through provisional judgements, precautionary measures and indirect evidence. Such action is not inherently unscientific. Waiting can itself produce harm where risks are credible and exposure is expanding. The difficulty arises when provisional decisions become permanent despite later evidence, or when uncertainty is invoked selectively to support only one side of the policy argument.

Commercial actors operate under different pressures. Manufacturers and retailers seek market access, product differentiation and commercial survival. They may generate useful analytical, toxicological and behavioural evidence because regulators require it or because product improvement depends upon it. They may also present evidence strategically, emphasising reduced emissions, adult switching and consumer preference while minimising uncertainty, youth uptake or product failure. Commercial funding does not make data automatically false, but it changes the questions that must be asked about study design, interpretation, publication and control of the underlying information. Evidence should be examined according to its methods and transparency, while conflicts are disclosed rather than used as substitutes for scientific evaluation.

The same principle applies outside industry. Public bodies, universities, charities, advocacy organisations and professional groups also operate within institutional incentives. Funding priorities, organisational missions, political relationships and reputational commitments can shape which questions are investigated and which interpretations gain prominence. An organisation established to prevent tobacco use may naturally focus on initiation and dependence. A service working with smokers may prioritise cessation and substitution. A consumer organisation may emphasise autonomy and lived experience. None of these perspectives is complete, yet each contributes evidence unavailable to the others. Conflict of interest is therefore broader than direct financial payment; it includes intellectual, organisational and political commitments capable of influencing judgement.

Consumer experience occupies an unusual position in this system. Vaping developed partly through users modifying devices, exchanging information and identifying products that allowed them to replace cigarettes. Their experience revealed factors that laboratory studies and clinical programmes sometimes underestimated: nicotine satisfaction, flavour preference, ease of use, identity, ritual and the importance of rapid access during smoking transition. Consumers can also underestimate risk, defend preferred products and interpret criticism as an attack on their own choices. Their testimony is not a replacement for analytical science, but neither is it anecdotal noise. It provides evidence about behaviour, acceptability and unintended consequences that cannot be generated fully under controlled conditions.

The media acts as the principal translator between these communities and the wider public. Research findings rarely reach consumers in their original form. They are compressed into headlines, interviews, social-media posts and political statements. Relative risk becomes especially vulnerable to distortion. A study detecting a hazardous compound may be reported without its concentration, exposure context or cigarette comparator. A finding of lower emissions may be presented as proof of safety. An association between vaping and later smoking may be described as causation without adequate consideration of shared susceptibility. Once simplified claims circulate widely, corrections rarely achieve equivalent reach.

Media influence is not confined to inaccurate reporting. Selection itself shapes policy. A rare battery explosion, a child using a brightly coloured device or a shipment of illicit products provides a powerful image. Slow changes in smoking prevalence, improvements in manufacturing control or the statistical distribution of risk are less visually compelling. Public opinion consequently develops through memorable cases rather than representative evidence. Politicians then respond to the environment created by that coverage, and regulatory agencies may need to demonstrate action regardless of whether the proposed measure addresses the dominant source of harm.

Scientific advisory systems are intended to protect policy from such volatility, but they are not isolated from it. Committees must define their remit, select evidence, manage conflicts and translate uncertainty into recommendations. Their membership affects which disciplines and experiences are represented. A panel dominated by epidemiology may approach the evidence differently from one including aerosol chemistry, toxicology, behavioural science, clinical cessation, manufacturing quality and consumer research. Expertise is necessary, but no single discipline can describe the complete effect of a vaping product. The chemistry of an aerosol does not predict population uptake by itself, just as prevalence data do not establish the toxicological quality of the products being used.

The design of advisory processes therefore matters as much as the reputation of individual advisers. Evidence should be graded according to quality and relevance. Assumptions should be stated openly. Minority positions should not be erased where uncertainty remains genuine. Conflicts should be declared and managed consistently across commercial, professional and ideological interests. Recommendations should distinguish what is known, what is inferred and what is chosen as a policy preference. When these boundaries are blurred, political judgement can be presented as scientific inevitability, weakening both accountability and public trust.

Public consultation provides another route through which evidence and politics meet. In principle, consultation allows governments to understand how proposed controls will operate beyond the drafting room. Manufacturers can explain technical feasibility, retailers can quantify implementation costs, enforcement officers can identify loopholes and consumers can describe behavioural consequences. In practice, consultation responses vary greatly in quality. Large organisations may submit detailed legal and scientific analysis, while individual citizens provide personal views or standardised campaign text. The volume of responses does not necessarily reflect the strength of evidence, but neither should technically polished submissions automatically outweigh widespread lived experience.

The most valuable consultation evidence is often practical rather than ideological. A proposed packaging rule can be assessed through redesign times, write-off costs and the likelihood of counterfeit adaptation. A display restriction can be examined through store layouts and enforcement visibility. A flavour measure can be evaluated through product composition, adult switching patterns and cross-border purchasing. A tax proposal can be modelled against cigarette prices and illicit incentives. These details convert broad policy intention into an assessment of likely real-world effects. Without them, regulation can become symbolically attractive but operationally weak.

Industry influence becomes most controversial when access to policymakers is unequal or hidden. Technical engagement is necessary because authorities cannot regulate complex products without information from those who design and manufacture them. Yet engagement becomes problematic where commercial actors shape the agenda, withhold inconvenient evidence or use political relationships to delay proportionate controls. The answer is not to exclude all industry knowledge, but to structure participation transparently. Meetings, evidence submissions and declared interests should be recorded. Claims should be testable. Access should be balanced with independent science, enforcement experience and consumer perspectives.

Public-health advocacy carries its own responsibility. Campaigns can accelerate necessary protection, particularly where commercial markets move faster than legislation. They can also encourage policies whose apparent strictness exceeds their likely effectiveness. Banning a format, flavour or sales channel may attract support because it communicates decisive action. The actual outcome may be product substitution, illicit purchasing, smoking relapse or movement into less visible channels. Advocacy should therefore be judged not only by the moral clarity of its objective, but by the quality of its causal reasoning and willingness to examine unintended consequences.

The central challenge is that vaping policy concerns a market in motion. Products, users and commercial strategies adapt to regulation. When nicotine concentration is limited, devices may become more efficient. When one product format is prohibited, another may replace it. When lawful advertising is restricted, promotion can migrate to informal social networks. When notified products become expensive, illicit products gain a price advantage. Policy does not act upon a static object; it changes the conditions under which the object is produced, sold and used. Every intervention becomes part of the system it is attempting to control.

Together we will therefore examine the institutional life of scientific evidence. The question is not whether science or politics should prevail, because policy cannot exist without both. Science establishes what can be measured, what remains uncertain and which outcomes are plausible. Politics determines priorities, allocates authority and decides which trade-offs are acceptable. Industry produces products and information while pursuing commercial interests. Public-health organisations interpret population risk through their missions. Consumers experience the consequences directly. The media shapes which facts become visible. Regulation emerges from their interaction.

A credible system does not require these actors to agree. It requires their roles to be visible, their evidence to be scrutinised and their claims to be proportionate to what is known. It must resist the assumption that commercial involvement invalidates every finding, just as it must resist the assumption that public-health status guarantees neutrality. It must distinguish scientific disagreement from strategic doubt, lived experience from universal proof and political urgency from evidential certainty. Above all, it must remain capable of revision when the market, technology or evidence changes.

The regulation of vaping will always involve contested values because it concerns addiction, commerce, childhood, autonomy, uncertainty and the legacy of smoking. Those conflicts cannot be resolved by laboratory data alone. They can, however, be handled more honestly when the science is not simplified to serve predetermined positions. The quality of policy depends on whether institutions can preserve the distinction between protecting the public and controlling the narrative. Where evidence is selected primarily for political usefulness, trust deteriorates. Where political judgement is acknowledged openly and informed by complete evidence, regulation becomes more defensible, adaptable and capable of reducing harm in the world as it actually exists.

Figure 8.1. Industry, politics and public health: stakeholder influence map.

The diagram places **vaping regulation and public-health policy** at the centre of a circular stakeholder system. Surrounding the central policy outcome are six areas through which influence is translated into regulation: legislation, public messaging, product standards, market access, youth controls and risk communication. These functions show that policy is shaped simultaneously through legal authority, technical requirements, commercial permissions, behavioural controls and the way risk is communicated to the public.

Six stakeholder groups are arranged around the central regulatory system. **Industry** contributes product development, market knowledge, compliance data and commercial interests. Its influence is directed particularly towards legislation and market access, while its relationship with other stakeholders reflects both technical cooperation and commercial tension. Manufacturers and suppliers may provide essential information about formulations, devices, production systems and market behaviour, but they also seek outcomes that protect commercial viability and access.

Public-health organisations contribute population-level evidence concerning smoking, cessation, youth protection, prevention and patterns of nicotine use. Their influence is particularly visible in public messaging, age restrictions and the framing of regulatory objectives. Public-health bodies may support stronger controls where youth uptake or dependence is considered dominant, while other organisations may place greater emphasis on the potential role of non-combustible nicotine products in reducing smoking-related harm.

Media organisations influence the public and political interpretation of vaping through headlines, framing, selection of evidence and simplification of risk. The diagram connects media activity with public messaging and product standards because reporting can affect public concern, political urgency and the perceived need for regulatory intervention. Media coverage can elevate specific events or studies rapidly, sometimes before the underlying evidence has been evaluated fully.

Scientific advisory committees occupy the lower centre of the map and provide evidence review, expert interpretation, recommendations and analysis of uncertainty. Their position reflects their role as an intermediary between technical research and political decision-making. Advisory committees may assess toxicology, chemistry, epidemiology, behavioural evidence and population modelling, but their conclusions remain dependent on committee composition, terms of reference, evidence quality and the way uncertainty is managed.

Consumer advocacy groups contribute lived experience, adult-access concerns, harm-reduction perspectives and direct accounts of switching away from smoking. Their influence is linked closely to market access, youth controls and risk communication. Consumers can identify practical consequences that may not be visible in laboratory studies or policy modelling, including smoking relapse, illicit purchasing, flavour preferences, affordability and the usability of regulated products.

Lobbying and political influence represent the mechanisms through which stakeholders seek access to policymakers, shape legislation, participate in consultation and apply pressure to regulatory decisions. This influence may come from commercial organisations, public-health charities, professional bodies, campaign groups or organised consumers. The map therefore treats lobbying as a method of political engagement rather than as an activity confined exclusively to industry.

Solid arrows indicate direct influence on policy outcomes, while dotted arrows represent interaction, communication and information exchange between stakeholder groups. The two-way direction of many arrows emphasises that influence is dynamic rather than linear. Public-health organisations respond to media coverage, advisory committees receive evidence from industry and researchers, consumers influence political debate, and lobbying activity can amplify or resist proposals emerging from scientific or governmental bodies.

The diagram demonstrates that regulatory policy is formed through competing evidence, institutional authority, commercial incentives, public pressure and political judgement. It should be read not as a fixed hierarchy, but as a representation of a constantly changing system in which the relative power of each stakeholder depends on the issue, jurisdiction and political context.

Industry, Politics and Public Health

STAKEHOLDER INFLUENCE MAP

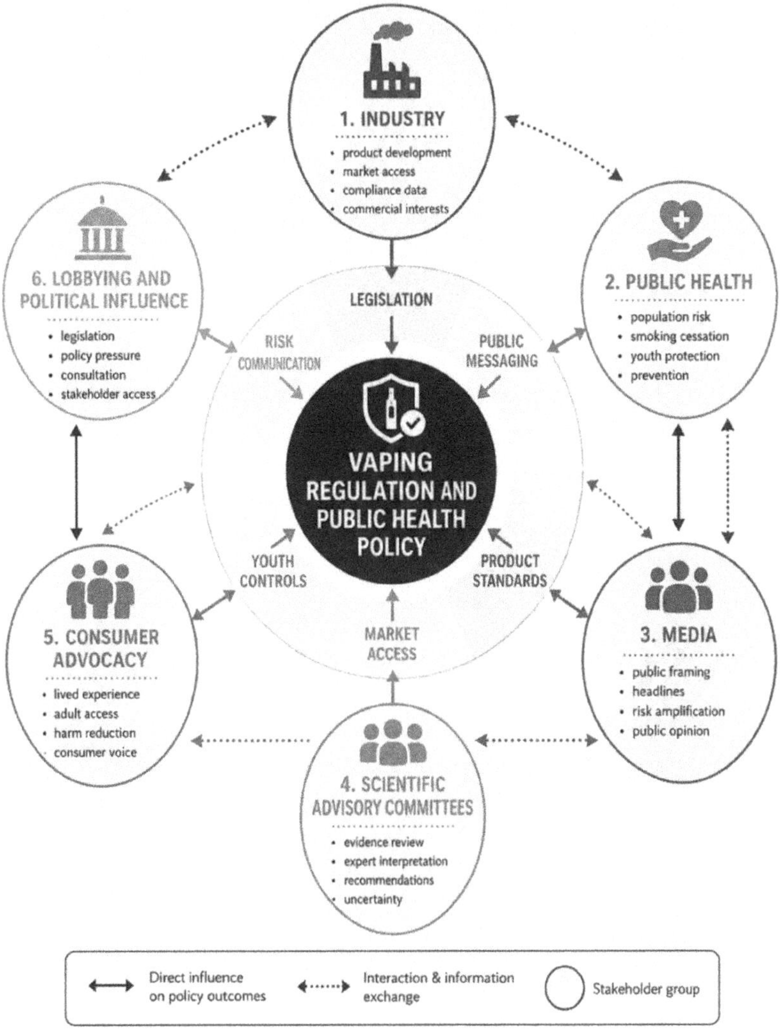

Stakeholder influence is dynamic and context dependent. Arrows indicate the direction of influence or information flow between actors and on policy outcomes.

Harm Reduction Philosophy

Harm reduction begins from a practical recognition that people do not always cease risky behaviour simply because the safest option is abstinence. Public health must therefore engage not only with ideal outcomes but with the conditions under which people actually live. In tobacco policy, this distinction is fundamental. Avoiding nicotine and inhaled products is the lowest-risk position, but millions continue smoking despite knowledge, quit attempts and cessation support. Harm reduction does not dispute that non-use is preferable. It asks whether a less hazardous substitute can prevent disease when non-use is not immediately achieved.

The philosophy developed across several areas of health policy before becoming central to debates over nicotine. Needle exchange, opioid substitution, safer-sex initiatives and protective equipment reflect the same reasoning. Each accepts that a behaviour may continue while attempting to reduce the probability or severity of harm associated with it. Critics sometimes portray this as moral surrender, yet the original risk remains central. It is concerned with outcomes rather than symbolic purity. A policy that condemns a behaviour but fails to reduce injury may be ethically weaker than one that tolerates an imperfect substitute and prevents measurable harm. The central question is whether the substitute is materially safer and improves health at individual and population levels.

Applied to smoking, the scientific basis of harm reduction rests on the distinction between nicotine and combustion. Nicotine can create dependence, affect cardiovascular function and present particular risks during pregnancy and adolescence, but it is not the principal cause of the cancers, chronic lung disease and vascular damage associated with smoking. Those harms arise largely from inhaling smoke containing carbon monoxide, particulate matter, carcinogens, oxidants and thermal degradation products. A non-combustible system can therefore retain dependence while removing the process responsible for much disease. This does not establish safety, but it creates a plausible and testable hierarchy of risk that regulation can use.

Vaping became politically important because it offered nicotine in a form that reproduced some of the behavioural and sensory features of smoking without burning tobacco. Hand-to-mouth movement, inhalation, flavour, throat sensation and rapid nicotine delivery can support substitution where other cessation products do not satisfy smokers. These characteristics are not incidental; they help displace cigarettes. A product that is chemically cleaner but behaviourally unacceptable will have little population effect. Assessment must combine toxicology with use, because reduced hazard becomes reduced harm only when smoking declines.

This distinction between hazard and harm is often misunderstood. Hazard describes the intrinsic capacity of a substance or product to cause injury, whereas harm reflects the realised outcome under actual conditions of exposure and use. A flavour compound may present inhalation hazard, yet population harm also depends on concentration, emissions, behaviour and smoking replacement. A low-emission product may generate little benefit if users continue smoking. Harm reduction requires comparative exposure, behavioural transition and net outcome. It asks not only what the product can do, but what happens when it enters a real nicotine market.

The comparator determines almost every conclusion. Comparing vaping with clean air emphasises avoidable exposure and supports caution for non-users. Comparing it with combustible cigarettes emphasises the absence of smoke and supports substitution for smokers. Both are valid, but answer different questions. Confusion arises when one invalidates the other. Evidence that vaping is not harmless does not demonstrate that it offers no benefit to smokers, just as evidence of lower exposure does not justify use among people who would otherwise avoid nicotine. A coherent philosophy must hold both propositions together and direct communication towards the relevant population.

The ethical argument for harm reduction is strongest where smokers have already tried and failed to stop. Dependence is not failure of will. It is maintained by pharmacology, cues, context, stress, habit and rapid reinforcement. Abstinence-only policies can leave people repeating quit attempts while smoke exposure continues. A less hazardous substitute may reduce immediate risk even if nicotine use persists. Denying access to that substitute because it does not represent complete cessation can place the moral appearance of purity above the physical consequences of continued smoking. Individuals bear that decision through continued exposure to combustion.

Autonomy also matters. Adults routinely make health decisions involving residual risk, including choices about alcohol, diet, travel, medication and sport. Nicotine use should not be exempt from regulation, but neither should adult smokers be treated as incapable of making informed comparative decisions. Respect for autonomy requires accurate information, reliable products and protection from deceptive marketing. It does not require government to endorse use. A harm-reduction framework allows adults to choose a lower-risk alternative while reserving stronger protections for children, non-users and vulnerable populations. The challenge is to preserve meaningful choice without allowing commercial freedom to override public-health safeguards.

Population-level assessment complicates this individual logic. A product may benefit many smokers while also attracting some people who would not otherwise have used nicotine. Public health must consider both pathways. If adult substitution is large and youth initiation remains limited, the overall effect may be favourable. If uptake among non-smokers becomes widespread, dependence persists and smoking displacement is weak, the balance may change. Chemistry alone cannot predict these outcomes. They require surveillance of who uses the product, how frequently, with what history and with what subsequent behaviour. Harm reduction is therefore conditional, not doctrinal. It depends on measured transitions rather than automatic approval of every non-combustible product.

Youth use presents the most difficult test because the interests of current smokers and future non-smokers can conflict. Features that make vaping acceptable to adults, including flavours, convenience and effective nicotine delivery, may also increase experimentation among young people. A simplistic response chooses one group and ignores the other. A more disciplined response examines how access, age verification, retail placement, packaging, product standards and communication can reduce youth uptake while preserving adult substitution. The objective is not universal attraction or inaccessibility, but a market shaped around populations with different risk-benefit balances and different regulatory protection needs.

Flavours illustrate this tension clearly. For many adults, non-tobacco flavours help break the sensory association with smoking and make continued substitution more acceptable. For regulators, the same flavours may raise concerns about youth appeal, trivialisation and rapid product proliferation. Harm reduction does not require unrestricted flavour markets, but it does require evidence before assuming that prohibition produces a net benefit. Restrictions may reduce experimentation, yet they may also encourage adults to return to cigarettes, purchase illicit products or mix unregulated liquids. The appropriate policy question is not whether flavours are good or bad in the abstract, but which formulations, descriptors and sales conditions support adult switching without creating disproportionate youth exposure.

Dual use creates another challenge. Smokers may begin vaping while continuing to smoke, sometimes for a brief transition and sometimes for years. Because cigarette risk is not reduced in direct proportion to cigarette count, prolonged dual use may deliver less health benefit than consumers expect.

Harm-reduction policy should therefore encourage complete switching rather than merely adding another nicotine product. At the same time, early dual use should not automatically be classified as failure. Behavioural transitions are often gradual, and partial substitution may precede cessation. The important questions are whether cigarette consumption continues to decline, whether complete switching becomes more likely and whether communication accurately explains the limits of partial reduction.

Risk communication sits at the centre of the philosophy because consumers cannot act on distinctions they are not permitted to understand. Messages that present vaping as harmless can recruit non-users and weaken caution. Messages that present it as equally harmful as smoking can deter switching and reinforce cigarette use. Both distort the evidence. Effective communication must state that vaping carries risk, that long-term uncertainty remains, that nicotine can sustain dependence and that complete substitution is likely to reduce exposure compared with continued smoking. Precision is difficult in mass communication, but simplification should not reverse the underlying hierarchy of risk. A public-health message that is memorable but materially misleading can produce harm even when issued with protective intent.

The precautionary principle is often invoked against harm reduction, yet precaution can point in more than one direction. Regulators may act to prevent uncertain long-term effects of vaping, particularly among young people. They must also consider the certain and immediate harms of continued smoking when alternatives are restricted. Precaution is not a command to prohibit every novel product; it is a framework for acting under uncertainty while considering the consequences of action and inaction. A policy that suppresses vaping but increases cigarette consumption is not precautionary in any meaningful health sense. The comparison must include the counterfactual market that regulation is likely to create.

Commercial involvement complicates acceptance of harm reduction because the nicotine market includes companies with very different histories and incentives. Tobacco companies may promote non-combustible products while continuing to sell cigarettes, creating justified scepticism about their objectives. Independent manufacturers may present themselves as challengers to smoking while still pursuing profit and market growth. The philosophy cannot depend on trusting either category. It requires rules that align commercial incentives with reduced harm: product standards, truthful claims, restrictions on youth marketing, surveillance and penalties for non-compliance. A useful product does not become useless because its seller profits, but profit must not determine how evidence is interpreted or how risk is communicated.

Equity strengthens the case for harm reduction. Smoking is often concentrated among people experiencing poverty, mental ill health, insecure housing, unemployment and other forms of disadvantage. These groups may face greater dependence, lower cessation success and higher cumulative exposure. Policies designed around idealised, well-resourced quitters can widen health inequalities if they remove alternatives used by those least likely to succeed with conventional support. Affordability, access and acceptability therefore matter alongside efficacy. A regulation that reduces vaping among affluent experimenters but pushes disadvantaged smokers back towards cigarettes may improve one indicator while worsening the distribution of preventable disease.

Harm reduction should not become a licence for regulatory complacency. Lower risk does not mean low-quality products should be tolerated, adverse events ignored or youth marketing accepted. The philosophy is strongest when paired with rigorous product control. Nicotine accuracy, ingredient assessment, emissions testing, electrical safety, manufacturing consistency, complaint handling and post-market surveillance all determine whether the theoretical reduction in risk is realised. Poorly manufactured products can narrow the margin between vaping and smoking, undermine public confidence and provide opponents with evidence that the market cannot govern itself. Proportionate regulation protects the credibility of harm reduction by ensuring that lawful products perform as represented.

The philosophy also requires willingness to revise conclusions. Devices, formulations and patterns of use change rapidly. Evidence supporting one generation of products may not transfer automatically to another. High-capacity disposables, synthetic coolants, novel nicotine analogues or increasingly efficient delivery systems can alter exposure and appeal. Harm reduction is not allegiance to a technology; it is commitment to reducing health damage through comparative assessment. Where a new product increases risk without meaningfully displacing smoking, the philosophy offers no reason to defend it. Where regulation removes a lower-risk option and strengthens combustible tobacco, it offers no reason to defend the regulation.

The ultimate measure is not whether vaping expands or contracts, but whether smoking-related disease and premature death decline without creating an unacceptable new burden of nicotine use. This demands patience, surveillance and intellectual discipline. Short-term prevalence figures, isolated toxicological findings and political declarations cannot settle the question alone. The philosophy must remain anchored to comparative risk, behavioural substitution and population outcomes. It recognises that perfection is rarely available in public health and that refusing an imperfect improvement can preserve a far greater harm.

Harm reduction therefore represents neither unconditional support for vaping nor indifference to nicotine dependence. It is a framework for making decisions where abstinence, substitution and continued smoking produce different probabilities of harm. Its integrity depends on scientific comparison, truthful communication, protection of non-users and realistic understanding of dependence. Properly applied, it asks the most demanding question in tobacco policy: not whether a product is free from risk, but whether the rules surrounding it are likely to leave people healthier than the alternatives those rules will produce.

Tobacco Control Organisations

Tobacco control organisations occupy a central position in the regulation of vaping because they provide the institutional memory of the long struggle against smoking. Their authority has been built through decades of epidemiology, litigation, smoke-free legislation, advertising restrictions and efforts to expose misconduct within the cigarette industry. They understand how commercial nicotine markets can normalise dependence, influence policy and adapt rapidly to regulation. This history gives them legitimate reason to approach new products with caution. It also means that their interpretation of vaping is often shaped by methods, assumptions and protective instincts developed against combustible tobacco, although aerosol products differ materially in chemistry, use and potential public-health function.

The term covers a diverse group rather than a single movement. It includes governmental agencies, national charities, international institutions, professional associations, academic networks, advocacy coalitions and locally focused public-health bodies. Some concentrate on cancer prevention, others on respiratory disease, cardiovascular health, children, addiction or health inequality. Their mandates affect the questions they ask and the outcomes they prioritise. An organisation focused on youth prevention may judge vaping primarily through initiation and dependence, while a cessation service may evaluate whether smokers switch completely from combustible products. Both perspectives are legitimate, but neither represents the whole regulatory problem. Its collective influence depends on whether these perspectives are integrated or allowed to compete as incompatible truths.

The movement established that tobacco-related disease is not simply the consequence of individual choice. Smoking behaviour is shaped by product design, nicotine delivery, pricing, marketing, social norms, retail availability and political influence. This insight remains relevant to vaping. Devices, flavours, package design, nicotine salts, advertising channels and retailer incentives all shape who uses a product and how. They are therefore correct to resist limiting regulation to consumer information while leaving the market untouched. Where commercial design can increase dependence or youth appeal, public institutions have a responsibility to intervene. The challenge is ensuring that intervention remains proportionate to the actual risk of the product and the market it replaces.

Experience with cigarette manufacturers has made conflict of interest a defining concern. Tobacco companies denied or obscured evidence, manipulated product design, targeted vulnerable populations and used political influence to delay regulation. Organisations that confronted this conduct learned that commercial assurances could not be accepted without independent verification. That scepticism continues when the same corporations market vaping, heated tobacco or oral nicotine products as part of a reduced-risk future. The concern is that these firms may use lower-risk products to rehabilitate corporate reputation, resist stronger cigarette controls, expand nicotine use or preserve dual consumption. These possibilities require scrutiny, transparency and clear separation between evidence, corporate communication and public policy.

The difficulty arises when justified distrust of particular companies becomes distrust of the entire concept of harm reduction. Vaping did not emerge solely from cigarette companies. Independent manufacturers, consumers, engineers and specialist retailers played major roles in its development. Many users adopted them specifically to move away from smoking. Treating every participant as an extension of historical tobacco strategy can obscure important differences in ownership, incentives and product function. It can also lead organisations to reject evidence because of its source before examining its methods. Funding and commercial interest must be disclosed, but scientific findings should still be judged through study design, reproducibility, data quality and relevance rather than through institutional identity alone.

Tobacco control organisations also differ in their approach to nicotine. Some treat the elimination of nicotine use as the long-term objective, while others distinguish nicotine dependence from the harms created by combustion. This distinction influences policy recommendations. An abstinence-oriented organisation may regard continued vaping as failure because dependence remains. A harm-reduction-oriented organisation may regard complete switching as substantial success even where nicotine use continues indefinitely.

Neither position is purely scientific because each contains a judgement about acceptable outcomes. Science can compare exposures and estimate risk, but cannot decide whether lower-risk dependence is morally or politically acceptable. That decision should be made openly rather than concealed within technical language.

International organisations exert particular influence because many governments lack capacity for comprehensive assessment. Global guidance can shape national legislation, donor priorities and professional opinion, especially in countries where vaping markets are new. Such guidance can promote minimum standards, youth protection and surveillance, but it can also encourage policy uniformity across very different smoking environments. A recommendation developed for a country with low smoking prevalence, strong cessation services and effective border enforcement may operate differently in a country where cigarettes remain cheap, smoking is widespread and illicit trade is extensive. International tobacco control should provide principles and evidence without assuming that one regulatory outcome will produce the same consequences everywhere.

National charities and professional bodies often hold greater trust than commercial actors or government departments. Their statements can influence media coverage, clinical advice and political debate. This authority creates a responsibility to communicate relative risk precisely. Describing vaping as harmful without explaining the cigarette comparator may be technically defensible but practically misleading. Conversely, presenting it as a straightforward solution can understate uncertainty, youth use and product variation. Organisations should tailor messages to different audiences: non-users need clear discouragement, young people need protection from initiation, and smokers need accurate information about substitution. A single undifferentiated warning cannot serve all three groups without distorting at least one decision.

Tobacco control organisations review broad evidence, but its weighting is often contested. Epidemiological associations, toxicological findings, clinical trials, behavioural surveys, market data and consumer testimony answer different questions. A study showing lower emissions does not establish population benefit. A survey showing youth use does not prove long-term dependence or smoking progression. A randomised cessation trial may not capture spontaneous switching outside clinical settings. Organisations should avoid treating one evidence type as decisive because it supports an established position. Robust assessment requires triangulation, explicit uncertainty and attention to the assumptions connecting laboratory findings with real-world outcomes.

Youth protection has become the strongest common ground across the movement. Few dispute that nicotine products should not be marketed or sold to children. Disagreement concerns which measures are effective and what collateral effects they create for adults who smoke. Product bans, flavour restrictions, display controls, retailer licensing and advertising prohibitions may reduce youth exposure, but they may also affect adult switching, lawful competition and illicit trade. Tobacco control organisations provide greatest value when they move beyond the language of urgency and examine these mechanisms carefully. Protecting children should be the objective, but interventions still require evaluation for proportionality, enforceability and wider market consequences.

Retail policy illustrates the need for precision. Restricting sales to specialist shops may improve age verification and staff knowledge, yet it may reduce access in rural or deprived areas. Allowing general retailers to sell vaping products can support cigarette substitution at the point of purchase, but it may increase visibility to young people. Pharmacy-only access may create professional oversight while medicalising a consumer product and limiting supply. Tobacco control organisations should analyse which channel best fits local conditions rather than treating one model as inherently protective. The design of the channel matters as much as its name: licensing, training, compliance testing, penalties and product verification determine actual performance.

The movement's relationship with consumers has sometimes been strained. Consumers may perceive tobacco control organisations as dismissive of lived experience or as willing to sacrifice adult access for symbolic restrictions. Organisations may view consumer groups as aligned with industry or insufficiently attentive to youth risk. Mutual suspicion weakens policy. People who have stopped smoking through vaping can provide important information about product acceptability, relapse, flavour, nicotine delivery and the practical effects of regulation. Their experience should not override population evidence, but excluding it produces blind spots. Consultation should distinguish independent consumer testimony from coordinated commercial campaigning while recognising that alignment on one policy question does not prove financial control.

Tobacco control organisations must also confront the possibility of unintended protection of the cigarette market. Combustible tobacco benefits whenever lower-risk competitors become less available, less acceptable or more expensive. This does not mean that every restriction on vaping serves cigarette interests, but the possibility should be included in policy analysis. A flavour ban may reduce youth use while also increasing smoking relapse. A tax may discourage initiation while narrowing the price advantage over cigarettes. A severe authorisation system may improve evidence while concentrating the market among tobacco companies with sufficient resources. The relevant question is not whether a measure appears tough, but how it changes competition between combustible and non-combustible products.

Funding relationships require consistent standards. Tobacco industry funding presents obvious concerns because of the sector's history and continuing cigarette sales. Pharmaceutical funding can also shape cessation narratives where companies market nicotine replacement or medicines. Government grants may encourage alignment with current policy, while charitable funding can reflect donor priorities. Intellectual commitments and organisational missions can influence interpretation even without direct financial payment. Tobacco control organisations should disclose relevant relationships, publish methods and separate advocacy from evidence review where possible. Transparency does not eliminate bias, but it allows others to assess how conclusions were reached and whether alternative interpretations were considered fairly.

Internal diversity within the movement should be treated as a strength rather than a public-relations problem. Genuine scientific disagreement is inevitable where products and behaviour evolve quickly. Organisations may differ over flavours, taxation, communication and the role of commercial products in cessation. Attempts to present a single unified position can suppress uncertainty and make later revision appear inconsistent or politically embarrassing. A more credible approach acknowledges areas of agreement, identifies contested assumptions and explains what evidence would change the recommendation. Public trust is strengthened when institutions demonstrate that conclusions are responsive to evidence rather than fixed by identity.

Their language has regulatory consequences. Terms such as epidemic, gateway, child-friendly and industry tactic can mobilise action, but they can also compress complex evidence into moral categories. Similarly, phrases such as safer alternative or reduced harm can be used so broadly that important distinctions disappear. Precision should not be abandoned for rhetorical impact. The frequency and intensity of youth use, the difference between experimentation and dependence, the distinction between complete switching and dual use, and the gap between hazard and realised harm all matter.

Advocacy is most durable when its language remains proportionate to the underlying evidence.

Enforcement is another area where they can add practical value. Passing legislation is easier than maintaining compliance across retailers, online platforms, importers and manufacturers. Tobacco control bodies can support mystery shopping, public reporting, surveillance and evaluation of whether penalties deter repeat offences. They can also identify when enforcement falls disproportionately on visible lawful businesses while organised illicit supply remains untouched. Effective advocacy should include resources, laboratory capacity, data systems and institutional responsibility, not merely demands for stronger statutory powers. A rule without credible enforcement can create the appearance of protection while rewarding operators willing to ignore it.

Their future role should preserve smoking-prevention achievements while adapting to a differentiated nicotine market. Combustible cigarettes remain the dominant source of tobacco-related death, but they now coexist with products presenting different exposure profiles and behavioural functions. Treating all products identically may simplify messaging, yet it risks weakening incentives to move away from combustion. Treating every alternative as beneficial would invite commercial expansion and youth uptake. The necessary position is demanding: rigorous control of products and marketing combined with accurate recognition of comparative risk. Their value lies in connecting historical vigilance with evidence suited to modern products.

Their legitimacy will ultimately depend on whether they remain focused on reducing disease rather than defending particular institutional positions. This requires evaluating policies by smoking prevalence, complete switching, youth regular use, illicit supply and health outcomes rather than by the number of restrictions introduced. It requires willingness to criticise both industry exaggeration and public-health overstatement. It also requires acknowledging when evidence changes. Tobacco control organisations possess experience, networks and moral authority capable of shaping the next phase of nicotine policy. That authority is strongest when scepticism is applied consistently, uncertainty is communicated honestly and the objective remains the reduction of preventable harm rather than the preservation of any single doctrine.

Public Health England

Public Health England became the institution most closely associated with the British interpretation of vaping as a potential instrument of tobacco harm reduction. Established in 2013 as an executive agency responsible for protecting and improving health in England, it entered the vaping debate when the evidence base was expanding but regulatory positions remained unsettled. Its significance did not arise from controlling market authorisations or enforcing product standards. It arose from its ability to commission evidence reviews, translate findings for practitioners and communicate a national public-health position. Through that role, it helped establish a distinction between the hazards of nicotine vaping and the far greater harms produced by combustible tobacco.

That distinction was politically consequential because public institutions had often discussed electronic cigarettes primarily through uncertainty. Early products varied widely in design, liquid composition, nicotine delivery and manufacturing quality, while long-term epidemiological evidence was necessarily unavailable. Public Health England did not deny those limitations. Its approach was to evaluate the evidence comparatively, asking whether continued vaping was likely to expose smokers to substantially less harm than continued cigarette use. This framing moved the debate away from the impossible demand that a new product be risk free before it could contribute to health improvement. It also placed smoking, rather than abstinence, at the centre of the relevant counterfactual for established smokers.

The agency commissioned expert work before its position became internationally recognised. A 2014 report examined electronic cigarettes as an emerging nicotine technology and considered their use, safety, quality and potential contribution to reducing smoking. The more influential 2015 evidence update concluded that vaping was substantially less harmful than smoking and could assist smokers who wished to stop. Its public communication stated that electronic cigarettes were around ninety-five per cent less harmful than smoked tobacco. That formulation travelled far beyond the report itself, becoming one of the most repeated and contested statements in the history of vaping policy.

The figure was never a direct measurement of lifetime disease incidence. No cohort had used modern vaping products for the decades required to calculate such a ratio epidemiologically. It represented an expert estimate based on the absence of combustion, the lower concentrations of major toxicants found in aerosol and the known causes of smoking-related disease. Public Health England's supporting explanation emphasised that most damage from cigarettes comes from smoke rather than nicotine. The estimate was intended to communicate a large order-of-magnitude difference, but its numerical precision encouraged readers to treat it as though risk had been measured to an exact percentage.

This created both communicative power and scientific vulnerability. A statement that vaping is substantially less harmful than smoking is accurate but easily diluted in public debate. The ninety-five per cent formulation was memorable, actionable and capable of correcting the belief that nicotine itself causes most smoking-related cancer. It could reassure smokers who were considering switching and give cessation practitioners confidence to discuss vaping. Yet opponents could challenge the apparent precision, the evidence underlying the estimate and the possibility that future findings might narrow the difference. A carefully qualified comparative judgement became a slogan that supporters and critics used for purposes extending beyond the original review.

Industry use of the statement intensified the controversy. Manufacturers and retailers repeated the estimate in advertising, political engagement and consumer communication, sometimes without the cautions that vaping was not harmless, product quality varied and non-smokers should not begin. The fact that a government health agency had issued the message gave it authority that commercial actors could borrow. This did not make the underlying comparison false, but it demonstrated how public-health language changes once it enters a market. Public Health England could control its report and press release, but not every later representation of its conclusion.

The agency responded by continuing rather than freezing the evidence-review process. Subsequent reviews examined prevalence among adults and young people, smoking cessation, health effects, nicotine, perceptions of harm and the development of heated tobacco products. The 2018 review reaffirmed that vaping was likely to pose only a small fraction of the risk of smoking and argued that complete switching would provide substantial health benefits. Later annual updates incorporated new survey data and changing patterns of use. This rolling approach recognised that one assessment could not permanently describe a rapidly evolving technology or market.

The reviews were generally commissioned from academic specialists rather than written solely by civil servants. This arrangement allowed Public Health England to draw upon expertise in tobacco dependence, epidemiology, behavioural science and cessation while retaining responsibility for commissioning and publishing the work. It also produced debate over what independence meant when a government agency selected the reviewers, framed the questions and promoted the conclusions. Independence should not be understood as absence of institutional context. The relevant safeguards are transparent methods, declared interests, reproducible searches, clear separation of evidence from recommendation and willingness to publish uncertainty.

Public Health England's role was often misunderstood as regulatory approval. It did not authorise individual devices, verify every notified formulation or certify that a particular product was safe. Consumer vaping products were governed through separate legislation and notification arrangements, with the Medicines and Healthcare products Regulatory Agency receiving notifications and other authorities handling enforcement. Public Health England assessed the category and its public-health implications. A favourable comparative conclusion about vaping could not guarantee the composition, emissions, battery safety or manufacturing consistency of every product available to consumers.

This distinction mattered because category-level evidence and product-level quality are not interchangeable. The absence of combustion supports a lower-risk expectation, but poor formulation, contamination, excessive thermal degradation or defective hardware can increase avoidable exposure. Public Health England's position functioned most coherently within a regulated market where nicotine limits, ingredient disclosure, packaging controls and post-market surveillance reduced variation. Its public message was therefore not an argument for an uncontrolled industry. It was an argument that proportionate regulation should preserve access to a lower-risk substitute while controlling products and commercial conduct.

The agency also influenced clinical and local practice. Stop-smoking services, healthcare professionals and local authorities needed guidance on whether vaping should be discussed with smokers, permitted in treatment pathways or distinguished from smoking in workplace and institutional policies. Public Health England's reviews gave practitioners a public-sector evidence base for supporting smokers who chose to vape, even though consumer products were not licensed medicines. This was especially important for people who had not succeeded with conventional cessation methods or who valued behavioural aspects of smoking that medicinal nicotine products did not reproduce.

Its position did not amount to claiming that vaping was suitable for everyone. The intended message was differentiated: smokers could benefit by switching completely, while people who did not smoke should not start and children should not vape. Maintaining that distinction became harder as youth use, disposable devices, sweet flavour descriptions and highly visible retailing generated greater concern. A framework developed during the rise of refillable products had to confront a market increasingly characterised by convenient, colourful and easily concealed devices. The public-health calculation remained comparative, but the populations requiring protection became more politically prominent.

Public understanding presented a persistent problem. Evidence reviews repeatedly reported that many smokers believed vaping was as harmful as, or more harmful than, smoking. Such misperception can preserve cigarette use by removing the perceived benefit of switching. Public Health England regarded correction of relative-risk misunderstanding as part of tobacco control, not promotion of nicotine use. Critics feared that strong reassurance could normalise vaping or weaken preventive messages. The dispute exposed a central difficulty in public-health communication: the same statement may reduce harm among smokers while reducing caution among non-smokers if audience, context and intended action are not made explicit.

The American lung-injury outbreak of 2019 intensified this communication challenge. News coverage frequently used the general language of vaping before investigators established the importance of illicit tetrahydrocannabinol products and vitamin E acetate. British consumers often encountered headlines without distinctions between regulated nicotine liquids and contaminated illicit cannabis cartridges. Public Health England argued that the outbreak should not be interpreted as evidence that ordinary regulated nicotine vaping had suddenly produced the same pattern in England. The episode showed why device format alone is an inadequate basis for causal explanation. Substance, source, formulation and supply chain determine exposure.

Institutional authority gave Public Health England's message considerable reach, but also made disagreement unusually polarised. Supporters treated the agency as evidence that Britain had adopted a uniquely rational approach. Critics portrayed it as excessively enthusiastic and insufficiently precautionary. Both readings simplified its actual position, which combined comparative reassurance with continuing surveillance and restrictions on youth access. The agency became symbolic because international debates needed recognisable institutional reference points. Its name was used to represent a broader British policy culture in which vaping could be regulated as a consumer product and incorporated into smoking cessation.

Public Health England formally ceased operating in 2021 as the government reorganised the public-health system following the coronavirus pandemic. Its health-protection functions moved principally to the UK Health Security Agency, while health-improvement responsibilities were transferred to the Office for Health Improvement and Disparities and other bodies. The closure did not represent a scientific reversal on vaping. The evidence-review programme continued under the Office for Health Improvement and Disparities, which published the comprehensive 2022 update on nicotine vaping, health risks and perceptions.

That transition illustrates how institutional structures affect continuity. A recognised agency can accumulate authority, a public identity and a coherent series of publications. When functions are divided, responsibility becomes less immediately visible even where staff, evidence and policy continue. Public Health England's name remains attached to the most influential British statements on vaping, while later work is associated with a less familiar successor. For public understanding, institutional reorganisation can therefore appear as policy change even when the underlying assessment remains broadly consistent.

The 2022 evidence update refined rather than abandoned the comparative approach. It concluded that, in the short and medium term, vaping posed only a small fraction of the risks of smoking, while acknowledging that vaping was not risk free and that long-term evidence remained limited. It examined biomarkers, toxicants, nicotine dependence, flavours, perceptions and prevalence among adults and young people. The language was broader and more systematic than the 2015 headline, reflecting a mature evidence base and greater awareness that product diversity, dependence and youth behaviour required sustained attention.

Public Health England's legacy should therefore not be reduced to one percentage. Its larger contribution was to establish comparative risk as a legitimate responsibility of a government health agency. It demonstrated that an institution could oppose youth use, support product regulation and still state clearly that smoking is more dangerous than vaping. That position challenged the idea that caution requires silence about relative harm. It also created an obligation to update conclusions, correct misuse and ensure that reassurance remained directed towards smokers rather than the population generally.

The limitations of its approach are equally instructive. Memorable numbers can outlive their evidential context. Category-level judgements can be mistaken for product approval. Government-backed communication can be appropriated commercially. Early confidence can become harder to recalibrate when products and patterns of use change. These are not reasons to avoid comparative assessment, but reasons to communicate its basis more carefully. Ranges, uncertainty, intended populations and conditions of benefit should accompany simplified messages, particularly where complete switching rather than dual use creates the expected reduction.

The current British position continues the basic architecture associated with Public Health England: smokers are encouraged to move away from cigarettes, people who do not smoke are advised not to vape, and children should never vape. Stronger controls on packaging, displays, flavours and promotion can coexist with that message if they preserve accurate risk communication and effective adult access. The enduring question is not whether Public Health England was perfectly correct in every formulation, but whether its intervention moved policy closer to the real distribution of harm. Its most important insight remains that public health cannot protect smokers by withholding the difference between smoke and aerosol.

That principle remains essential whenever simplicity threatens to replace disciplined comparison with undifferentiated warnings about nicotine.

Media Influence

Media influence on vaping regulation extends far beyond the accuracy of individual news reports. Media systems decide which events become visible, which experts are treated as credible and which risks are repeated until they appear settled. Most citizens, legislators and even professionals do not read toxicology papers, product standards or epidemiological analyses in full. They encounter compressed interpretations through headlines, television interviews, podcasts, campaign materials and social platforms. These interpretations shape public concern before formal policy analysis begins. In that sense, media coverage does not merely describe the regulatory environment; it helps create the conditions within which regulation becomes politically possible.

Vaping is especially vulnerable to distortion because its scientific meaning is comparative. Aerosol can contain harmful constituents while exposing users to fewer combustion products than cigarette smoke. Nicotine can sustain dependence without being the principal cause of smoking-related cancer. Youth experimentation can increase while adult smoking declines. Each statement requires a comparator, population, timeframe and measure of exposure. News formats frequently remove these qualifications because they complicate the story. A headline stating that a chemical has been detected may omit concentration, toxicological relevance and the level found in smoke. A report describing lower emissions may imply safety when the evidence supports only reduced exposure.

Agenda-setting is the first major mechanism of influence. Media organisations cannot cover every study, enforcement action or market development, so selection determines what the public regards as important. A battery explosion, hospital admission or school confiscation is immediate and visual. Gradual reductions in smoking prevalence, improvements in manufacturing control or changes in cessation behaviour are slower and less dramatic. The result is an asymmetry between rare events with compelling imagery and common outcomes represented by statistics. Policymakers then face pressure generated by the incidents receiving attention rather than by the complete distribution of risk across the nicotine market.

Framing is equally powerful. The same device may be presented as a smoking alternative, a youth epidemic, a consumer product, a medical aid, an environmental pollutant or a tobacco-industry strategy. Each frame activates a different moral and regulatory response. A cessation frame directs attention towards adult smokers and comparative risk. A youth frame directs attention towards initiation, flavours and access. An environmental frame centres batteries, plastics and disposability. None is inherently illegitimate, but each excludes other dimensions. Public debate becomes distorted when one frame dominates so completely that competing harms disappear from consideration.

Language strengthens these frames. Terms such as epidemic, gateway, crisis, toxic, safer and harmless carry implications beyond their technical meaning. "Epidemic" suggests rapid, widespread and severe harm, even where measures include occasional experimentation. "Gateway" implies a causal progression from vaping to smoking, although observed associations may also reflect shared susceptibility, social environment or prior risk-taking. "Safer" may be understood as safe, while "toxic" may imply unacceptable danger regardless of dose. Scientific communication requires language proportionate to evidence, yet media competition rewards certainty, novelty and emotional force.

The publication process itself contributes to simplification. Universities, journals, charities and government agencies issue press releases designed to attract coverage. These releases may emphasise the most dramatic finding, use stronger causal language than the underlying study or omit limitations that weaken the headline. Journal embargoes allow reporters to prepare stories, but tight deadlines still encourage reliance on summaries rather than independent appraisal. Once a press release establishes the frame, later articles frequently reproduce it with minor variation. The chain from study to public claim can therefore magnify interpretation at each stage without any single actor deliberately falsifying the evidence.

Observational studies create particular difficulty. A survey may find that young people who vape are more likely later to report smoking. Media accounts may convert this association into proof that vaping caused cigarette initiation. Yet the two behaviours share predictors including peer groups, family smoking, socioeconomic conditions, impulsivity and willingness to experiment. Statistical adjustment can reduce confounding but rarely removes it completely.

Conversely, industry communications may dismiss every association as meaningless. Responsible reporting should describe what the study establishes, what it cannot establish and how alternative explanations were addressed rather than choosing causation or irrelevance as the only options.

Laboratory studies are also vulnerable to decontextualisation. Researchers may expose cells to aerosol condensate, operate devices under severe conditions or identify constituents at trace concentrations. Such studies can reveal mechanisms and hazards, but they do not automatically predict disease risk under typical human use. News coverage may omit puffing conditions, dose, exposure duration and comparison with cigarettes. The opposite distortion occurs when lower emissions are reported without recognising product variability, long-term uncertainty or the difference between machine yields and absorbed dose. A useful account connects experimental findings to realistic exposure while preserving the distinction between hazard identification and risk estimation.

The 2019 outbreak of lung injury in the United States demonstrated how terminology can redirect global perception. Early reports referred broadly to vaping-related illness before evidence identified a strong association with illicit tetrahydrocannabinol cartridges and vitamin E acetate. Headlines often used images of nicotine e-cigarettes, and audiences outside the United States received little explanation of product source or substance. The episode showed that a delivery format is not a sufficient causal category. A regulated nicotine liquid and an illicit cannabinoid cartridge can share hardware while presenting different chemical risks. Once the broader association became established publicly, later clarification struggled to reverse it.

Social media accelerates this process because it collapses the distance between evidence, advocacy and reaction. Researchers, campaigners, companies, consumers and politicians can publish interpretations immediately, often before peer review or regulatory verification. Algorithms reward engagement, and anger, fear and certainty generally travel further than methodological caution. Short clips and screenshots detach findings from context, while repeated claims acquire credibility through familiarity. Social media also allows rapid correction and access to specialist commentary, but corrections compete at a structural disadvantage because they are less novel and less emotionally charged than the original allegation.

Influence does not flow only from journalism to the public. Public reaction feeds back into journalism through trending topics, comments, petitions and political statements. A local incident can become national when social engagement signals audience interest. Politicians may then demand action, generating further coverage and reinforcing the impression of escalating evidence. This feedback loop can transform a limited event into a policy crisis before prevalence, causation or enforcement context has been established. The speed of the cycle narrows the opportunity for regulators to distinguish between a genuine emerging hazard and an amplification event driven by attention dynamics.

Commercial actors operate within the same environment. Manufacturers may sponsor favourable content, brief journalists, promote cessation testimonials and publicise comparative emissions data. Some use public-health statements selectively, presenting category-level conclusions as validation of particular products. Retailers and influencers can blur advertising with personal experience, especially where sponsorship disclosure is weak. Tobacco companies possess substantial communications resources and established political networks, creating concern that reduced-risk narratives may serve corporate reputation as well as consumer information. Commercial participation does not invalidate every claim, but it requires transparent funding, precise product identification and independent verification.

Public-health organisations and advocacy groups also use media strategically. Campaigns may select vivid examples, emphasise youth appeal and use strong language to secure political attention. This can be effective where regulatory delay allows harmful practices to continue. It can also produce overstatement, particularly when occasional use is presented as dependence or when illicit and compliant products are combined in one category. Advocacy operates through persuasion, but institutions claiming scientific authority carry a duty to distinguish evidence from mobilisation. The credibility gained through urgency can be lost if later data reveal that claims were broader than the evidence supported.

Consumer communities provide a countervailing media force. People who switched from smoking often use online forums, videos and social networks to describe practical benefits, product preferences and the consequences of restrictions. These accounts humanise harm reduction and reveal outcomes that formal surveillance may miss, including relapse, illicit purchasing and difficulties with low-nicotine products. Yet personal success can be generalised too readily. A compelling testimony cannot establish population effect, just as a dramatic adverse event cannot define category-wide risk. Consumer media is most valuable when treated as behavioural evidence and policy feedback rather than as a substitute for controlled research.

Traditional ideas of journalistic balance can also mislead. Presenting two opposing speakers as equally authoritative may create false equivalence where evidence is uneven. Conversely, excluding dissenting experts because their conclusions challenge institutional consensus can conceal genuine uncertainty. The appropriate standard is not equal airtime but proportional representation of evidence, expertise and uncertainty. Reporters should examine methods, funding and relevance rather than categorising sources simply as pro-vaping or anti-vaping. Polarised labels encourage audiences to judge identity instead of argument and allow weak claims to survive through tribal alignment.

Regulatory agencies face a difficult communication task during uncertainty. Immediate silence may allow speculation to dominate, while premature certainty can damage trust when facts change. Effective crisis communication should identify what is known, what remains under investigation, which products or behaviours are implicated and what actions consumers should take. Product specificity is essential. Warnings should distinguish nicotine liquids, cannabinoid products, illicit sources, batteries and particular batches where evidence allows. Broad statements may appear safer institutionally, but they can unintentionally deter smokers from lower-risk products or direct consumers towards other unregulated channels.

Media coverage also affects enforcement priorities. Highly publicised youth sales, disposable waste or illicit imports can trigger inspections and legislative proposals. Visibility can mobilise resources that were previously unavailable. However, enforcement may then concentrate on easily photographed retail breaches while less visible wholesale networks, online sellers and fraudulent importers continue operating. The media logic of individual wrongdoing can obscure structural supply chains. Regulators should use public concern to strengthen investigation, but not allow coverage to determine which offences matter most scientifically or commercially.

Long-term trust depends on correction practices. Errors in vaping coverage often remain accessible online after evidence changes, continuing to influence search results and public belief. Corrections may be appended quietly rather than given equivalent prominence. Institutions should update summaries, clarify causal language and preserve transparent records of changes. Researchers should respond promptly when their findings are misrepresented, even where exaggeration favours their preferred policy. Trust is strengthened when organisations correct allies as readily as opponents and acknowledge uncertainty before it is forced upon them.

A healthier media environment would not require positive coverage of vaping. It would require disciplined comparison. Reports should identify the product, substance, user population, exposure conditions and relevant alternative. They should distinguish experimentation from regular use, dual use from complete switching, detection from meaningful dose and association from causation. They should state whether a finding concerns lawful regulated products, illicit products or the category as a whole. These details do not weaken journalism; they make the story more accurate and more useful to people making health and policy decisions.

For policymakers, the practical lesson is to treat media signals as evidence of public concern, not as direct measures of importance. A surge in coverage may justify investigation, communication or temporary precaution, but permanent rules should still rest on representative data, product-specific analysis and evaluation of likely substitution effects. Governments should publish accessible evidence summaries before controversy peaks, maintain spokespeople with competence and release underlying methods wherever possible. This reduces dependence on reactive briefing and makes selective quotation harder. The objective is not to control reporting, which would undermine scrutiny, but to improve the quality of information entering it. When institutions communicate early, precisely and consistently, the media is more likely to illuminate regulatory choices than to determine them through repetition alone.

Media influence is therefore neither inherently harmful nor merely external to regulation. Journalism can expose misconduct, identify emerging risks, challenge weak evidence and make technical decisions accountable. It can also amplify fear, simplify uncertainty and reward positions that fit existing narratives. The decisive issue is whether coverage preserves the relationships between chemistry, behaviour, comparator and population outcome. Vaping policy will always be contested, but contest should occur over evidence as it exists, not over slogans created by removing the conditions that give evidence meaning.

Scientific Advisory Committees

Scientific advisory committees occupy the space between evidence generation and political decision-making. They do not manufacture products, conduct every study or enact legislation, yet their assessments can determine how governments interpret risk, define uncertainty and justify intervention. In vaping policy, this intermediary role is unusually demanding because the evidence spans aerosol chemistry, toxicology, nicotine dependence, behavioural science, epidemiology, clinical cessation, engineering, economics and market surveillance. No single discipline can answer the complete regulatory question. Committees therefore exist to combine partial forms of knowledge into recommendations that are scientifically defensible, politically usable and sufficiently clear to support action.

Their influence begins with the question they are asked. A committee instructed to assess whether vaping is harmless will reach a different conclusion from one asked whether it is less harmful than smoking. A review centred on youth initiation will emphasise appeal, dependence and progression, whereas one focused on smoking cessation will examine substitution, relapse and treatment effectiveness. These are not merely differences of emphasis. The framing determines the comparator, evidence base and threshold for concern. Governments should therefore publish terms of reference that make the policy question explicit, because an apparently scientific conclusion may reflect the boundaries imposed before the committee begins its work.

Membership is equally consequential. A panel dominated by toxicologists may focus on intrinsic hazard and exposure, while one dominated by epidemiologists may prioritise prevalence and population association. Clinicians may emphasise cessation, engineers device performance, behavioural scientists user adaptation and regulators enforceability. Balanced membership does not mean assigning equal numbers to every discipline, but ensuring that the expertise matches the problem. Vaping products combine liquid formulation, heating systems, batteries, software, user behaviour and commercial presentation. A committee unable to examine interactions between these elements may assess fragments accurately while misunderstanding the product as a system.

The choice of chair can shape both deliberation and public confidence. An effective chair must manage disagreement, prevent dominant personalities from narrowing discussion and ensure that technical uncertainty is not concealed by consensus language. Chairs also mediate between committee members, civil servants and ministers, making procedural independence essential. They should not predetermine conclusions or treat dissent as institutional embarrassment. Where evidence is incomplete, a record of structured disagreement may be more scientifically honest than a unanimous statement produced through compromise so broad that its assumptions disappear.

Secretariats exercise quieter but substantial influence. They select papers, organise meetings, commission reviews, draft summaries and convert discussion into formal advice. Even where members approve the final text, the secretariat controls much of the information architecture through which evidence is presented. This role requires methodological competence and transparency. Search strategies, inclusion criteria, evidence tables and draft revisions should be documented. Without such safeguards, bias can enter through omission rather than explicit argument, especially when committees face large and rapidly changing literatures.

Evidence hierarchy presents a further difficulty. Randomised trials may provide strong evidence for cessation efficacy, but they often examine selected users, defined products and supported conditions that differ from ordinary markets. Observational studies capture real-world behaviour but remain vulnerable to confounding, selection and inaccurate self-reporting. Laboratory studies can identify emissions and biological mechanisms, yet may use conditions that do not reflect normal use. Surveys describe prevalence but can blur experimentation, regular use and dependence. Committees must resist ranking entire disciplines as inherently superior and instead judge whether each study answers the specific question under review.

Product heterogeneity makes synthesis particularly difficult. "Vaping" can describe low-powered refillable systems, closed pods, disposables, high-output devices and products containing different nicotine forms, flavours and thermal characteristics. Evidence generated with one design cannot automatically represent another. Committees should specify the products, formulations and usage conditions to which conclusions apply. Category-wide statements may be unavoidable for public communication, but the underlying assessment should identify variation and uncertainty. Otherwise, a favourable finding for regulated nicotine products may be extended to illicit or adulterated liquids, while a failure involving one device class may be generalised across the entire category.

Comparative risk requires particular discipline. The relevant benchmark for an established smoker is continued smoking, while the benchmark for a young non-user is non-use. A committee that merges these populations can produce advice that protects neither effectively. Its report should separate absolute risk, comparative risk and population impact. Absolute risk asks what harm vaping can cause. Comparative risk asks how that harm differs from smoking. Population impact asks how use patterns alter disease across smokers, former smokers and never-smokers. Each question uses different evidence and should not be collapsed into one simplified judgement.

Uncertainty should be expressed rather than hidden. Advisory reports often use verbal categories such as low confidence, moderate evidence or plausible risk, but these terms can be interpreted inconsistently. Committees should explain whether uncertainty arises from limited duration, product variation, small samples, measurement error, confounding or disagreement between studies. Different uncertainties imply different policy responses. Lack of long-term epidemiology may justify surveillance, whereas evidence of inaccurate nicotine labelling may justify immediate enforcement. Treating all uncertainty as one undifferentiated problem encourages either paralysis or excessive precaution.

Precaution itself requires balanced application. Committees may recommend restrictions when evidence suggests a credible threat, particularly to children or non-users. They should also consider the harms created by restricting access to lower-risk alternatives for smokers. Action and inaction both have consequences. A flavour prohibition, nicotine limit or authorisation burden can reduce one exposure while increasing smoking, illicit trade or market concentration. Scientific advice need not decide the political trade-off, but it should describe the plausible pathways through which each option could alter behaviour and health.

Conflicts of interest must be managed consistently. Financial relationships with tobacco, vaping, pharmaceutical or consultancy organisations can affect perceived and actual independence. Intellectual commitments, previous public statements, institutional missions and professional alliances can also influence judgement. These non-financial interests should not disqualify every experienced participant, because expertise often develops through sustained engagement. They should, however, be declared and considered when allocating roles. Exclusion rules should be proportionate, transparent and applied across competing interests rather than directed only at one category of stakeholder.

Industry evidence creates a recurring dilemma. Manufacturers often possess detailed information on formulations, emissions, stability, complaints and product performance that is unavailable elsewhere. Excluding these data may leave committees less informed, but accepting them uncritically invites selective reporting. A sound process requires full methods, raw or auditable data, product traceability and disclosure of study control. Committees should distinguish access to evidence from influence over conclusions. Commercial submissions can be considered without granting companies membership, editorial authority or privileged access to policymakers.

Consumer evidence deserves comparable care. People who have switched from smoking can identify barriers, product features and regulatory consequences that clinical trials may not capture. Their accounts may reveal smoking relapse after flavour restrictions, difficulties with low nicotine limits or the importance of device reliability. These experiences are not substitutes for population data, yet they are relevant to behavioural plausibility and policy implementation. Committees should hear independent consumer perspectives while identifying organised campaigning, sponsorship and selection bias. Lived experience becomes most useful when it informs questions and mechanisms rather than being treated as universal proof.

Transparency is central to legitimacy. Membership, declarations, agendas, evidence submissions, minutes and final recommendations should normally be public. Confidentiality may be necessary for personal data, commercially sensitive formulations or security matters, but secrecy should be limited and explained. Open meetings can improve trust, although they may also encourage performative positions and discourage candid exploration. A mixed model can preserve technical deliberation while publishing detailed records of evidence, reasoning and decisions. The objective is not theatrical openness but traceable judgement.

Minority opinions should be recorded where disagreement is material. Forced unanimity can conceal uncertainty and give ministers a false impression that science has resolved a contested question. A minority statement should identify the evidence or assumptions producing the divergence, not merely register objection. This allows future reviewers to determine whether disagreement was resolved by new data or suppressed by institutional pressure. It also protects committees from the expectation that every recommendation must represent scientific certainty.

Political independence does not mean political irrelevance. Committees advise elected governments, which must consider values, resources, enforcement and public acceptability alongside evidence. Problems arise when ministers present a preferred policy as scientifically required even though the committee offered several options, or when advice is ignored without explanation. Governments should distinguish scientific findings from political choices and publish reasons when departing from recommendations. This preserves democratic authority while preventing science from becoming a shield for decisions made on other grounds.

Timeliness is another challenge. Formal reviews can take months or years, while products and markets change quickly. By publication, the dominant devices, nicotine strengths or youth patterns may differ from those examined. Committees need mechanisms for rapid updates, horizon scanning and interim advice without abandoning methodological rigour. Living reviews, targeted technical notes and scheduled reassessment can reduce this lag. Advice should include an expiry point or review trigger where technology is evolving rapidly.

Post-market evidence should feed back into committee work. Notifications and premarket dossiers describe intended products, but complaints, enforcement samples, adverse events and sales data reveal how markets operate. Committees should examine whether products remain compositionally consistent, whether consumers modify devices and whether illicit substitutes emerge after regulation. Surveillance transforms advisory work from one-time judgement into adaptive governance. It also allows committees to test whether previous recommendations produced their intended effects.

Communication of findings requires precision. Headline summaries should not exceed the certainty of the underlying report. Numerical estimates can be useful, but apparent exactness may survive after qualifications are forgotten. Committees should state the comparator, population, timeframe and conditions attached to each conclusion. They should anticipate foreseeable misinterpretation by media, industry and advocacy groups. Clear communication is not simplification at any cost; it is the preservation of meaning while technical detail is reduced.

The performance of advisory committees should itself be evaluated. Governments rarely examine whether recommendations predicted outcomes accurately, improved policy or created unintended effects. Periodic review should consider disciplinary balance, timeliness, transparency, conflict management and the use made of advice. This does not mean judging committees solely by whether ministers followed them. It means asking whether their reasoning remained robust when confronted with later evidence and whether their processes supported legitimate decision-making.

Quantitative modelling can help committees connect individual exposure with population outcomes, but models are only as credible as their assumptions. Estimates of smoking displacement, youth initiation, relapse, dual use and long-term disease reduction may change substantially when transition rates or relative-risk values are altered. Committees should publish model structures, sensitivity analyses and alternative scenarios rather than presenting a single forecast as fact. Models are most useful when they reveal which variables drive the conclusion and which evidence would reduce uncertainty. They become misleading when political preferences are embedded invisibly within assumptions about behaviour, compliance or market response.

Committees also need a disciplined approach to evidence quality. Citation counts, institutional prestige and publication in a respected journal do not guarantee relevance or validity. Reviewers should examine preregistration, sample selection, comparator choice, exposure conditions, missing data, statistical power and reproducibility. Retractions, corrections and contradictory findings must be tracked after publication. Where several weak studies repeat the same methodological limitation, numerical volume should not be mistaken for independent confirmation. Conversely, one well-designed study should not be treated as conclusive when products, populations or outcomes vary. Explicit quality assessment protects the committee from both fashionable findings and strategic evidence production, while making it easier for outside readers to understand why apparently similar studies received different weight. This discipline is especially important where regulatory deadlines reward speed, selective publication and confidently stated preliminary results.

Scientific advisory committees are most valuable when they neither claim authority beyond evidence nor retreat into technical ambiguity. Their task is to organise uncertainty, integrate disciplines and show policymakers where facts end and judgement begins. In vaping regulation, this requires comparative analysis, product specificity and sustained attention to behaviour. A credible committee does not eliminate controversy. It makes disagreement more intelligible, exposes assumptions and ensures that political choices cannot be disguised as automatic conclusions of science.

Consumer Advocacy

Consumer advocacy occupies a place in vaping policy because it begins with the experience of people who use the products rather than with the institutions that regulate, manufacture or study them. Many vaping communities were formed by smokers who had struggled to stop using combustible tobacco and discovered that electronic cigarettes provided a workable alternative. Their knowledge developed through use: comparing devices, adjusting nicotine strength, identifying unreliable products, learning maintenance and describing which features supported complete switching. This practical expertise entered public debate before many health systems had established formal positions. Consumer advocacy therefore emerged not simply as defence of a market, but as an attempt to make personal experience visible within decisions that could determine whether smokers retained access to products they believed had changed their lives.

The contribution of consumer advocacy is its ability to explain the difference between theoretical availability and usable substitution. A product may satisfy regulatory requirements yet fail to replace cigarettes because nicotine delivery is inadequate, the device leaks, the flavour is unacceptable or the operating routine is too complicated. Laboratory evidence can describe emissions and clinical studies can measure cessation outcomes, but consumers reveal how products function in everyday environments. They identify the importance of convenience during work, battery life during travel, discreet use, rapid replacement of failed components and access to familiar retailers. These details may appear secondary beside toxicology, yet they determine whether lower-risk products are adopted, abandoned or used alongside smoking.

Consumer testimony also corrects the tendency to treat all nicotine users as a uniform population. Some people switch rapidly and cease smoking within days. Others reduce gradually, alternate between products or return to cigarettes during stress. Long-term smokers may require stronger nicotine delivery than occasional users. People with disabilities, low incomes or limited digital access may depend on local retailers rather than online supply. Advocacy groups can show how regulation affects these different pathways. A restriction that appears minor to policymakers may remove the only formulation, strength or retail channel that works for a particular group. Such evidence does not decide policy by itself, but it improves understanding of who bears the consequences.

Flavours illustrate this role clearly. Public debate often treats flavour as a marketing characteristic, while consumers may experience it as part of behavioural separation from smoking. Tobacco flavours can preserve familiar cues, but fruit, menthol, dessert or beverage profiles may help some former smokers detach nicotine use from the taste and smell of cigarettes. Advocates can explain why variety matters after the initial transition and why a narrow authorised range may increase dissatisfaction or relapse. Their evidence must still be weighed against youth appeal, misleading descriptors and product proliferation. The value of advocacy lies in demonstrating mechanisms and trade-offs that would otherwise remain hidden, not in asserting that every flavour should be protected.

Nicotine limits create similar concerns. Regulators may favour simple concentration ceilings because they are measurable and easy to enforce. Consumers can reveal how those limits interact with device efficiency, puffing behaviour and smoking history. A concentration that is adequate in one system may be ineffective in another. Users receiving insufficient nicotine may puff more intensely, consume more liquid or continue smoking. Others may prefer lower strengths after switching. Advocacy helps translate a numerical standard into behavioural consequences, reminding policymakers that concentration is not identical to absorbed dose or satisfaction. This practical perspective can prevent technically tidy rules from producing counterproductive outcomes.

Affordability is another area where consumer representation is essential. Product registration fees, taxation, packaging redesign and retail restrictions can raise prices even when each requirement appears proportionate in isolation. Consumers on lower incomes may respond by extending coil use, purchasing unverified liquids, mixing at home or returning to cheaper cigarettes. Advocacy groups can document these adaptations and challenge policies assessed only through compliance costs to businesses. They can also expose geographic inequalities where regulated products remain available in affluent urban areas but disappear from smaller towns. A harm-reduction policy that becomes inaccessible to the populations with the highest smoking burden may succeed administratively while failing socially.

Consumer advocates provide early warning of market problems. Online communities often identify leaking pods, defective batteries, incorrect labels, counterfeit packaging or unusual adverse effects before formal reporting systems detect a pattern. Users compare batch numbers, photographs and purchasing sources across regions, creating an informal surveillance network. Regulators and manufacturers can benefit from this information if channels exist to receive and verify it. Advocacy organisations can convert scattered reports into structured evidence, distinguish isolated complaints from repeated failures and direct concerns towards the responsible authority. Their role is strongest when they complement, rather than replace, formal vigilance and analytical testing.

Their independence is nevertheless a question. Consumer groups may receive funding, travel support, technical assistance or meeting access from manufacturers and trade associations. Such relationships can create real or perceived conflicts, particularly where organisations defend policies aligned with commercial interests. Financial support does not automatically invalidate consumer experience, but undisclosed dependence weakens credibility. Advocacy bodies should publish funding sources, governance arrangements and policies governing contact with industry. Representatives should distinguish positions developed from member consultation from arguments supplied by commercial sponsors. Transparency allows policymakers to evaluate evidence without dismissing consumers merely because their preferred products are sold for profit.

The opposite error is to assume that consumers who agree with industry must be controlled by it. Adults may independently oppose flavour bans, excessive taxation or pharmacy-only access because those measures affect their own behaviour and autonomy. Agreement between stakeholders does not prove coordination. Public-health organisations and governments should therefore assess the substance of consumer evidence, its representativeness and its supporting data. Labelling every dissenting user as an industry proxy silences legitimate participation and deepens mistrust. A democratic consultation process should be capable of hearing people whose lived experience conflicts with the preferred policy of established institutions.

Representation presents a second challenge. The most active advocates are not necessarily typical users. They may be experienced hobbyists, former heavy smokers, technically knowledgeable enthusiasts or individuals with strong political commitments. Their priorities can differ from those of casual users, recent switchers or people who buy simple disposable products. Effective organisations need methods for reaching beyond visible campaigners. Surveys, regional meetings, translated materials and partnerships with cessation services can broaden participation. Advocacy should acknowledge whose voices are missing and avoid presenting a self-selecting membership as the complete consumer population.

Youth interests require careful handling because adult consumer organisations cannot speak automatically for young people. Advocates have a legitimate interest in preventing underage sales, misleading promotion and products designed to resemble toys or confectionery. Their credibility suffers when every youth-protection proposal is treated as an attack on adults. At the same time, they can challenge measures that use youth concern as a broad justification without evidence of effectiveness. A mature position supports age verification, retailer accountability and proportionate marketing controls while scrutinising whether wider restrictions will reduce youth use or merely redirect it towards illicit supply.

Consumer advocacy is also connected to autonomy. Adults who understand that vaping is not harmless may still decide that it is preferable to smoking or to repeated unsuccessful abstinence attempts. Advocates defend the right to make that comparative choice, particularly where government communication exaggerates equivalence between products. Autonomy, however, depends on truthful information and dependable quality. It cannot justify deceptive claims, hidden ingredients or unsafe devices. The strongest consumer case is therefore not for an unregulated market, but for regulation that protects informed choice rather than eliminating it through paternalistic assumptions about what adults should prefer.

Risk communication is a central concern. Consumers who believe vaping helped them may react strongly to messages that appear to deny their experience. Overstated warnings can alienate former smokers and encourage distrust of health authorities. Advocacy organisations can test whether public messages are understood as intended and explain how wording affects behaviour. They can also help correct exaggerated commercial claims within their own communities. Credible advocacy should state that vaping carries residual risk, nicotine dependence may continue and complete switching is more beneficial than prolonged dual use. Defending relative risk does not require pretending that every pattern of use is desirable.

Public consultation offers the main formal route for consumer participation, but its design often favours organisations with legal and technical resources. Consultation documents can be lengthy, highly specialised and framed around predetermined options. Individual users may provide personal accounts that are emotionally powerful but difficult for officials to aggregate. Advocacy organisations can bridge this gap by translating proposals into practical questions, collecting structured responses and quantifying likely effects. They can distinguish between concerns affecting a small specialist group and those likely to alter behaviour across the market. This converts lived experience into evidence that can be evaluated alongside technical submissions.

The quality of that evidence matters. Policymakers need more than declarations that a regulation will cause relapse or illicit purchasing. Advocacy groups can strengthen their contribution through transparent surveys, clear sampling methods, anonymised case records and follow-up after policy changes. They can document price changes, product disappearance, smoking return, cross-border purchasing and home mixing. Partnerships with independent researchers may improve analysis without transferring ownership of the agenda. Consumer evidence becomes harder to dismiss when it is collected systematically and when limitations are acknowledged openly.

Digital platforms have expanded advocacy while creating new vulnerabilities. Social media allows rapid mobilisation, international coordination and direct challenge to misleading claims. It also rewards anger, certainty and confrontation. Advocacy can become polarised, with public-health professionals treated as enemies and any restriction interpreted as prohibition by stealth. Aggressive online behaviour may reinforce stereotypes that consumers are unwilling to consider youth risk or product control. Effective advocacy requires strategic discipline: challenging weak evidence firmly while maintaining accuracy, civility and willingness to revise a position when facts change.

Relationships with retailers are complex. Specialist vape shops often provide practical support that consumers value, including device selection, nicotine guidance and troubleshooting. Retailers may therefore become informal advocates and sources of market intelligence. Their commercial interest must remain visible, particularly when policies affect sales. Consumer organisations should not allow retail priorities to substitute for user priorities. A shop may favour product variety or higher margins, while consumers may prioritise affordability, reliability and continued access to a small number of familiar products. Maintaining organisational independence requires boundaries even where interests frequently overlap.

Advocacy can also expose unintended consequences after legislation is enacted. Authorities may count registered products, inspections or seizures without measuring whether smokers have returned to cigarettes, whether compliant retailers have closed or whether illicit products have become more common. Consumers experience these effects immediately. Structured feedback can identify where implementation differs from policy design and where guidance is confusing. This makes advocacy part of adaptive regulation rather than a one-time campaign against proposed rules. Governments should create continuing channels for consumer reporting, not limit participation to consultations conducted before consequences are observable.

The wider legitimacy of consumer advocacy depends on its willingness to address responsibility as well as rights. Users seeking access to lower-risk products should support measures that reduce sales to children, improve disposal, prevent battery misuse and remove demonstrably unsafe products. Advocacy is more persuasive when it recognises that the market creates external costs and that public confidence depends on visible standards. Defending every device, claim or retailer weakens the distinction between principled representation and commercial resistance. A credible movement can support strict enforcement against non-compliance while opposing rules that unnecessarily damage adult substitution.

Consumer advocacy is most valuable when it prevents policy from becoming detached from behaviour. Regulators can control ingredients, packaging and sales channels, but consumers decide whether products are used, modified, rejected or replaced. Their responses determine whether intended benefits are realised and whether restrictions create displacement towards smoking or illicit supply. Including consumers does not guarantee the correct decision, and lived experience cannot resolve every scientific uncertainty. It does ensure that policy is tested against the people expected to live with it. In a contested nicotine market, that is not an optional gesture of consultation; it is a necessary component of evidence-based regulation.

Industry Lobbying

Industry lobbying is contested in vaping policy because it sits between legitimate participation and attempted regulatory control. Manufacturers, distributors, retailers, trade associations and investors possess information governments need, yet have financial interests in those decisions. Their engagement can improve technical rules, reveal implementation problems and identify unintended consequences. It can also delay intervention, narrow the policy agenda or present commercial priorities as public-health necessity. The challenge is not to decide whether industry should be heard, but to determine how its evidence, access and influence should be structured.

The vaping sector is politically diverse. It includes multinational tobacco companies, independent device manufacturers, e-liquid producers, pharmaceutical businesses, specialist retailers, convenience chains, logistics companies and technology suppliers. A tobacco company may support strict authorisation requirements that smaller competitors cannot afford. An independent manufacturer may favour product notification but oppose rules designed around pharmaceutical evidence. Retailers may prioritise continued access to flavours and affordable stock, while device producers focus on technical standards and battery regulation. Treating these interests as one voice conceals the competitive strategies operating inside the industry itself.

Tobacco-company lobbying is historically sensitive. Cigarette manufacturers used political access, commissioned research, third-party organisations and legal pressure to weaken tobacco control. That record justifies scepticism towards claims aligning commercial interests with health. When the same corporations promote non-combustible products, policymakers must distinguish genuine product transition from reputation management, market expansion and defence of cigarette profitability. The existence of a potentially lower-risk product does not erase the history of the company selling it, but neither does corporate history determine the chemical or behavioural performance of the product.

Independent vaping businesses argue that they are not extensions of the tobacco industry. Many were created to compete with cigarettes, and some have no involvement in combustible tobacco. That distinction is relevant, particularly when access rules favour companies with large regulatory budgets. It does not establish neutrality. Independent firms still seek profit, may resist burdensome standards and may overstate the benefits of their products. Political analysis should therefore examine ownership, market position, evidence quality and policy incentives rather than relying on labels such as independent, innovative or reduced risk.

Technical lobbying can be constructive. Regulators drafting rules for refill mechanisms, coil materials, nicotine concentration, emissions or child-resistant packaging may lack manufacturing knowledge. Industry can explain device operation, reproducible test methods and conflicts between proposed limits and product physics. It can show how formulation changes alter aerosol generation or how packaging requirements affect leakage and stability. Excluding this information may produce rules that are impossible to implement or easy to circumvent. The important safeguard is that technical access must not become control over the regulatory objective or the interpretation of health evidence.

One method is agenda setting. Industry actors may seek to define the problem before rules are discussed. They may frame vaping primarily as smoking cessation, consumer choice, innovation, tax revenue or illicit-market control. Each frame directs attention towards favourable policy outcomes. A cessation frame may support broad product access, while an illicit-trade frame may be used against taxation or flavour restrictions. These concerns may be valid, but the selected frame can exclude youth initiation, dependence, product failure or environmental harm. Policymakers should ask which relevant questions are absent as well as which are emphasised.

Evidence submission is another central lobbying tool. Companies can provide toxicology reports, market data, consumer research, economic modelling and compliance assessments. Such information may be unavailable elsewhere, especially for proprietary formulations and sales patterns. The risk lies in selective disclosure. Firms may publish favourable findings while withholding failed studies, adverse events or internal analyses showing weaker outcomes. Regulators should require declarations of commissioning, study protocols, access to underlying data and disclosure of results relevant to the same question. Evidence should be judged through method and completeness rather than polished presentation.

Economic arguments are particularly influential because regulation has visible costs. Lobbyists may quantify product withdrawals, testing expenditure, shop closures, job losses and tax effects. These figures can improve impact assessment where assumptions are transparent. They can also be inflated by treating every affected product as economically essential or ignoring adaptation. Conversely, governments sometimes underestimate compliance cost because they assess each requirement separately. The strongest analysis distinguishes transitional expense from continuing burden, large companies from small businesses and genuine safety costs from avoidable administrative duplication. Economic impact should inform proportionality without becoming a veto over health protection.

Small-business lobbying deserves careful interpretation. Specialist retailers and local manufacturers may lack direct access to ministers and therefore rely on associations or coordinated campaigns. Their concerns can reveal how regulation affects market diversity and consumer access. Severe fees, repeated testing or short implementation periods may eliminate compliant smaller operators while leaving illicit sellers untouched. Yet the language of small business can also be used strategically by larger interests seeking a more sympathetic public face. Decision-makers should verify who funds representative groups, how membership positions are determined and whether submissions reflect the sector broadly.

Trade associations can aggregate technical expertise and reduce administrative burden by providing governments with a single point of contact. They may develop codes of practice, training programmes and standardised data. Their authority, however, depends on governance. Associations dominated by a few major members may present their commercial preferences as industry consensus. Voluntary codes may be promoted as alternatives to enforceable regulation even where non-members or low-compliance operators remain unaffected. Policymakers should therefore examine membership, voting structures, funding and enforcement mechanisms before treating an association as representative or self-regulation as sufficient.

Lobbying often extends beyond formal meetings. Companies commission opinion polling, sponsor conferences, support research centres, place commentary in the media and build relationships with professional groups. These activities can shape the intellectual environment in which policy is made without appearing as direct political pressure. Funding may influence which questions are studied, which speakers receive platforms and which narratives gain repetition. Disclosure should therefore cover more than registered meetings with officials. It should include commissioned research, event sponsorship, grants, advisory arrangements and third-party communication intended to influence public policy.

Third-party advocacy presents a particularly difficult problem. Industry may support consumer groups, retailers, think tanks or grassroots campaigns whose arguments appear independent. The views expressed may still be genuine, but undisclosed financial or organisational support changes how the evidence should be interpreted. Manufactured grassroots activity can create the appearance of spontaneous public opposition or support. Transparent funding does not silence these groups; it allows policymakers and the public to distinguish independent mobilisation from coordinated commercial strategy. The same standard should apply to public-health campaigns supported by foundations, pharmaceutical interests or government funding.

Direct access is distributed unevenly. Large corporations can employ specialist lobbyists, legal teams, economists and former officials, while small businesses and consumers rely on limited voluntary capacity. This imbalance affects not only the number of meetings but the quality and timing of information reaching policymakers. Early access can shape options before consultation begins, leaving later participants to respond within boundaries already established. Governments should publish meeting records, agendas and submitted materials, and should create structured opportunities for smaller stakeholders to contribute before proposals become fixed. Transparency after decisions are effectively made is not meaningful equality of participation.

Revolving-door relationships can intensify concerns about regulatory capture. Former ministers, civil servants, advisers or regulators may join companies or consultancies, while industry professionals may enter public appointments. Movement between sectors can bring useful expertise, but it can also create privileged networks, expectations of future employment and reluctance to impose unpopular decisions. Cooling-off periods, conflict declarations and restrictions on representing clients in matters previously handled can reduce these risks. The objective is not to prohibit expertise from crossing institutional boundaries, but to prevent private access from being purchased through public service.

Legal pressure is another form of lobbying. Companies may warn that proposed rules breach trade law, property rights, procedural fairness or proportionality. Litigation can protect businesses from arbitrary government action and force regulators to justify evidence. It can also delay implementation, increase public cost and discourage ambitious policy. Threats of legal challenge are most influential where governments lack specialist capacity or fear compensation claims. Robust legislation requires clear statutory authority, documented reasoning, consultation and evidence capable of surviving judicial scrutiny. Legal defensibility is part of good regulation, not an argument for avoiding regulation.

The tobacco-control principle of limiting industry influence raises difficult questions when applied to vaping. Governments have strong reasons to protect policy from organisations whose interests conflict with public health, particularly companies continuing to profit from cigarettes. Yet technical regulation cannot be designed intelligently without access to information about products and supply chains. A workable distinction separates participation from partnership. Industry may submit evidence, answer technical questions and comment on feasibility without setting public-health objectives, selecting advisers or negotiating policy privately. Engagement should be necessary, bounded, recorded and open to scrutiny.

Industry lobbying frequently invokes illicit trade. Firms argue that excessive taxes, flavour restrictions, packaging rules or product bans will transfer demand to unregulated sellers. This possibility is real and should be modelled, especially where enforcement is weak. It can also become a universal objection to almost any control. Credible claims require data on price differentials, consumer substitution, border routes, online supply and enforcement capacity. Industry should explain why a specific measure would change behaviour and provide evidence that can be tested. Policymakers should neither dismiss illicit-market warnings automatically nor accept them as proof that regulation is futile.

Innovation is used similarly. The vaping sector changes quickly, and rigid rules can freeze outdated designs or prevent safer technology from reaching consumers. Industry can identify where approval systems discourage battery improvements, reduce device reliability or make formulation changes excessively costly. Yet innovation is not inherently beneficial. Greater nicotine delivery, concealed use, disposable formats and youth-oriented design may also be described as innovation. Regulation should assess the direction and consequence of technological change rather than protect novelty as an end in itself. Lobbying claims should specify the public or consumer benefit that innovation is expected to deliver.

International lobbying adds another layer. Global companies may promote different positions across jurisdictions according to local opportunity. They can support stringent entry requirements where these protect established market share and oppose similar controls where they threaten expansion. Trade agreements, investment arguments and harmonisation proposals may be used to challenge national restrictions. At the same time, multinational supply chains make some cross-border alignment necessary. Governments should compare corporate submissions internationally, examine whether claimed principles are applied consistently and distinguish genuine technical harmonisation from attempts to secure the most commercially favourable rule.

Effective safeguards begin with disclosure. Policymakers should know who requested contact, whom they represent, what interests are affected and which evidence has been supplied. Minutes should record substantive arguments rather than merely the existence of a meeting. Consultation submissions should identify funding and authorship. Drafting assistance from outside parties should be visible. Officials should record significant changes made following stakeholder representations. These measures do not prevent influence, but they allow influence to be examined and contested.

Regulators also need internal capacity. Transparency alone achieves little if agencies lack scientists, economists, lawyers and enforcement specialists able to challenge sophisticated submissions. Dependence on industry information increases where public institutions cannot test claims independently. Investment in laboratory capability, market surveillance and data analysis is therefore an anti-capture measure as well as a technical necessity. Competent authorities can engage with industry without becoming dependent upon it, request better evidence and recognise when uncertainty is being used strategically.

Industry lobbying should ultimately be assessed by the quality of the policy process it enters. Commercial actors have legitimate rights to explain products, costs and operational consequences. They do not have a right to convert economic power into hidden political authority. Governments should hear evidence without surrendering objectives, distinguish technical knowledge from policy preference and test claims against independent data and affected populations. The most defensible system neither excludes industry reflexively nor treats access as partnership. It allows scrutiny, preserves institutional independence and ensures that decisions about nicotine, smoking and public health remain accountable to the public rather than to the organisations best equipped to influence them.

Public Consultation

Public consultation is the formal mechanism through which governments expose proposed regulation to those expected to implement, enforce, comply with and experience it. In vaping policy, consultation is especially important because legislation often touches several systems at once: product design, toxicology, retail practice, advertising, taxation, customs, youth protection, environmental management and smoking cessation. No department possesses complete knowledge of all these effects. Consultation allows evidence to enter the process before rules are fixed, but its value depends on design. A poorly framed exercise can collect large volumes of opinion while revealing little about how the proposed measures will operate in practice.

The purpose of consultation is not to conduct a referendum. Governments are not required to adopt the position supported by the greatest number of responses, because organised campaigns can generate thousands of identical submissions without adding new evidence. Nor should consultation be treated as a ritual performed after decisions have already been made. Its proper function is to test assumptions, expose unintended consequences, identify implementation barriers and improve regulatory design. The process is strongest when ministers publish the problem they are trying to solve, the evidence supporting intervention, the options considered and the uncertainties that remain.

Vaping consultations frequently begin from legitimate public concerns: youth use, disposable waste, illicit products, misleading promotion or inconsistent retail compliance. The difficulty arises when the consultation document presents only one causal explanation. Rising youth use may be attributed entirely to flavours, packaging or displays when price, social media, peer behaviour, product convenience and weak age verification also contribute. If the problem is framed too narrowly, respondents are asked to choose between preselected restrictions rather than examine which combination of measures would address the actual causes. Consultation then validates a preferred intervention instead of improving it.

Question design can determine the apparent result. Closed questions such as whether government should protect children from attractive vape products invite near-universal agreement while revealing nothing about the effectiveness of a specific rule. Technical questions may be so specialised that only large organisations can answer them. Leading language can associate opposition with indifference to harm, discouraging respondents from challenging assumptions. A well-designed consultation separates objectives from mechanisms. It asks whether the evidence establishes the problem, how each proposal would alter behaviour, what alternatives exist and which measurable outcomes should determine success.

Meaningful participation requires sufficient information. Respondents need draft definitions, proposed thresholds, implementation dates, enforcement responsibilities and the evidence used in impact assessment. Vague proposals produce speculative answers. A manufacturer cannot estimate redesign time without knowing whether restrictions apply to brand names, flavour descriptors, colours, device surfaces or outer packaging. A retailer cannot calculate display changes without understanding what must be concealed and whether specialist advice remains permitted. Precision before consultation allows stakeholders to provide operational evidence rather than general support or opposition.

Implementation periods deserve particular attention. Governments may underestimate the time required to reformulate liquids, validate stability, redesign artwork, manufacture packaging, amend notifications, clear existing stock and distribute compliant products. Businesses may exaggerate these demands to delay regulation, but their claims can be tested through documented production cycles, supplier lead times and inventory records. Consultation should distinguish the time needed for unavoidable technical work from time requested for commercial convenience. Transitional arrangements can then be matched to the complexity of the change rather than selected arbitrarily.

Stock write-off is another practical issue often dismissed as a private business cost. Unsold products represent more than lost revenue. Their disposal can create environmental waste, encourage discounting before a deadline or push stock into secondary and illicit channels. Small retailers may hold inventory purchased months earlier under lawful conditions and lack the financial capacity to absorb immediate prohibition. Consultation evidence should quantify affected units, wholesale values, expiry periods and disposal routes. Governments can then decide whether sell-through periods, returns schemes or phased restrictions reduce disruption without undermining the policy objective.

Product reformulation creates consequences beyond changing a flavour name or ingredient. Removing sweeteners, coolants or particular flavour compounds can alter aerosol generation, nicotine perception, stability and consumer acceptability. Changing nicotine concentration may require a different device configuration or coil resistance. A regulatory proposal that appears limited to marketing can therefore affect chemistry, emissions and user behaviour. Manufacturers should submit evidence on these interactions, while regulators should require sufficient detail to distinguish genuine technical complexity from strategic claims that every change demands extensive delay.

Retailers contribute a different form of knowledge. They understand store layouts, age-verification practices, purchasing patterns, consumer questions and the practical visibility of products. Display restrictions may operate differently in a specialist vape shop, supermarket, petrol station and convenience store. A rule that is simple in a large retail chain may be difficult in a small premises with limited storage. Retail evidence should include photographs, measurements, staff procedures, transaction data and compliance costs. This allows policymakers to design rules around real environments rather than an idealised shop floor.

Consumers can reveal behavioural consequences that commercial submissions may not capture credibly. They can describe why they chose particular nicotine strengths, flavours, devices or retailers and what they are likely to do if these options disappear. Personal testimony alone cannot establish prevalence, but structured consumer research can identify plausible pathways: complete switching, dual use, smoking relapse, home mixing, cross-border purchasing or illicit acquisition. Consultation should ask not merely whether consumers like a product, but how removing it would alter nicotine use and what substitutes are realistically available.

Youth perspectives also matter, although they require careful methods. Young people can explain how products are acquired, which features attract attention, how social media shapes perceptions and why school enforcement succeeds or fails. Their participation should not be reduced to campaign imagery or assumptions made by adults. Surveys, focus groups and school-based research can provide evidence about access routes and frequency of use. Safeguards are necessary, but excluding young people from consultation on policies intended to protect them leaves important behavioural mechanisms unexamined.

Public-health organisations contribute epidemiological evidence, cessation experience and understanding of health inequalities. Their submissions can identify where commercial arguments omit population effects or where consumer preference conflicts with prevention. They should nevertheless quantify expected benefits where possible. A proposal to restrict flavours, displays or packaging should explain the pathway through which the measure is expected to reduce initiation, the scale of change anticipated and how adult smoking outcomes will be monitored. Moral force strengthens an objective, but it does not substitute for causal analysis.

Enforcement bodies are essential participants because a rule that cannot be inspected, tested or prosecuted will not deliver its intended protection. Trading standards officers, customs authorities, laboratories and local government can identify ambiguous definitions, evidential burdens and resource gaps. They can explain whether officers need specialist equipment, whether samples require chemical analysis and how online sellers can be traced. Consultation should require government to publish an enforcement plan and funding assumptions.

Creating new offences without capacity to detect them transfers risk from non-compliant operators to those already willing to obey.

The illicit market must be examined without allowing it to become a universal argument against regulation. Importers, retailers, enforcement agencies and consumers may all possess relevant evidence on illicit supply, but their estimates can differ greatly. Consultation should distinguish counterfeit products, non-notified products, tax evasion, underage sales and lawful products diverted through unauthorised channels. Each requires a different response. Claims that restrictions will expand illicit trade should be supported by price comparisons, supply routes, previous market behaviour and enforcement data rather than repeated as an automatic prediction.

Economic impact assessment should examine distribution, not only aggregate cost. The same rule can affect multinational manufacturers, independent liquid producers, specialist shops and general retailers very differently. High fixed fees may favour large firms, while complex packaging changes may disproportionately affect small product ranges. Market concentration can reduce administrative burden but also weaken competition and consumer choice. Consultation should identify which businesses are likely to exit, which will adapt and whether the resulting market structure serves public health. Regulation should not protect inefficient business models, but neither should it create monopolistic advantage accidentally.

Confidential commercial information creates a procedural tension. Companies may need to disclose formulations, sales data, manufacturing costs or internal research to explain regulatory effects. Publishing all details could damage legitimate commercial interests, while excessive confidentiality prevents public scrutiny. Consultation systems should allow protected submission of sensitive evidence alongside publishable summaries. Officials should explain how confidential material influenced decisions without revealing proprietary content. Anonymous claims unsupported by accessible reasoning should carry limited weight, particularly where they are central to the final impact assessment.

Response analysis must be transparent. Governments should distinguish unique evidence from duplicated campaign responses, identify major themes and explain how conflicting claims were evaluated. Merely reporting that most respondents supported or opposed a proposal can be misleading where participation is self-selecting. The final response should show which evidence altered definitions, timelines, exemptions, enforcement or monitoring. Where government rejects a substantial technical objection, it should explain why. This does not require agreement with stakeholders, but it demonstrates that consultation was capable of influencing the outcome.

Consultation fatigue can weaken participation. Vaping businesses, health organisations and consumer groups may face repeated exercises across product rules, taxation, advertising, waste and youth policy. Smaller organisations lack teams able to respond continuously, while large institutions can recycle professional submissions. Governments can reduce this inequality by coordinating related consultations, publishing accessible summaries, allowing adequate time and offering standard data templates. Workshops and technical roundtables may help clarify proposals, but they should supplement rather than replace the public record.

Accessibility determines whose evidence reaches government. Consultation documents written in legal or technical language may exclude ordinary users, small retailers, people with limited literacy and communities with high smoking prevalence. Online-only responses may disadvantage those without reliable digital access, while English-only materials can miss populations directly affected by tobacco-related inequalities. Accessible summaries, translated documents, alternative response formats and community outreach are therefore substantive safeguards rather than administrative courtesy. They broaden the evidence base and reduce the risk that policy reflects only organisations already equipped to navigate government processes. Participation should also be geographically distributed, because urban specialist markets, rural retail networks and border regions can experience the same proposal differently.

Consultation should never be used to outsource governmental responsibility. Stakeholders may identify consequences, challenge assumptions and supply data, but ministers and officials remain responsible for deciding what evidence is credible, what trade-offs are acceptable and how competing rights are balanced. A large commercial submission cannot replace independent analysis, just as a large campaign response cannot establish effectiveness. Government must test claims, commission additional research where evidence is weak and acknowledge when decisions rest partly on values rather than settled science. The legitimacy of consultation depends on this separation. Participants contribute knowledge and perspective; public authorities retain accountability for the final rule and its consequences.

Responsibility cannot be delegated through procedural formality.

Post-consultation evaluation is as important as the consultation itself. Predictions made by government and stakeholders should be recorded so they can be tested after implementation. If a flavour restriction is expected to reduce youth use without affecting adult switching, surveys and sales data should examine both outcomes. If industry predicts widespread closure or illicit trade, those claims should also be measured. Evaluation prevents consultation from becoming a contest of unaccountable forecasts. It creates institutional learning and improves the quality of future submissions by rewarding evidence that proves reliable.

Public consultation works best when it is treated as part of regulatory science rather than political theatre. Its purpose is to connect policy intention with product chemistry, commercial systems, enforcement capacity and human behaviour. It should reveal where evidence is strong, where interests conflict and where practical detail determines whether a rule succeeds. Consultation cannot remove political judgement, and it should not grant any stakeholder a veto. It can ensure that judgement is made with visible assumptions, quantified consequences and a realistic understanding of the market. In vaping regulation, that discipline is essential because every intervention changes not only products, but the choices available to smokers, non-smokers, retailers, manufacturers and young people.

Conflicts of Interest

Conflicts of interest arise when a secondary interest has the capacity to influence, or appear to influence, a primary duty. In vaping policy, the primary duty may be scientific accuracy, protection of public health, impartial regulation, clinical judgement or faithful representation of consumers. The secondary interest may be financial gain, institutional reputation, career advancement, political alignment, commercial access or commitment to a previously stated position. A conflict does not prove misconduct, falsification or bad faith. It identifies a condition in which judgement may be vulnerable to distortion and therefore requires disclosure, scrutiny and, where necessary, restriction.

The subject is unusually sensitive because modern nicotine policy developed against the documented conduct of the cigarette industry. Manufacturers concealed evidence, manipulated scientific uncertainty and used political relationships to delay controls. This history created justified safeguards around tobacco industry participation and funding. Vaping complicated that architecture because the market includes tobacco companies, independent manufacturers, pharmaceutical interests, consumer organisations, charities, universities and public bodies. Their interests overlap without becoming identical. A rule that treats every commercial relationship as equivalent can obscure important differences, while a rule that accepts claimed independence without examining ownership and funding can create avoidable blind spots.

Financial conflicts are the most visible. Researchers may receive grants, consultancy fees, speaking payments, travel support, equipment or access to proprietary data from manufacturers. Clinicians may work with companies producing cessation medicines or nicotine products. Advocacy groups may receive donations from foundations, governments, retailers or industry associations. Regulators may later seek employment within sectors they previously supervised. These relationships can influence topic selection, study design, interpretation and communication even without explicit pressure. The effect is often subtle: favourable assumptions seem reasonable, inconvenient questions receive less attention and uncertainty is described differently depending on whose interests are affected.

Direct funding is only one form of influence. In-kind support can be equally important. A company may supply devices, liquids, laboratory standards, market data, software or technical staff. Such assistance may enable research that would otherwise be impossible, but it can also narrow the study to products chosen by the sponsor or create dependence on information that cannot be independently verified. Data-access agreements may restrict publication, delay release or prevent researchers from examining commercially sensitive variables. Proper disclosure must therefore describe not only who paid, but who selected products, controlled protocols, held the data and possessed authority over publication.

Institutional conflicts deserve equal attention. A university may depend on a research centre financed by a commercial donor. A charity may have built its public identity around a particular policy position. A government agency may be expected to defend legislation it previously recommended. A journal may benefit from attention generated by dramatic findings. These institutions can influence individuals through promotion, access, funding and reputational expectations. An investigator may have no personal payment yet still work within a structure that rewards one conclusion more than another. Focusing solely on personal declarations can therefore understate the environment in which scientific judgement occurs.

Intellectual conflicts are more difficult to manage because expertise itself requires sustained engagement. Researchers publish hypotheses, give evidence to committees and develop professional identities around particular interpretations. They may become known as supporters or critics of harm reduction, flavour restrictions or youth-focused regulation. Later evidence can threaten not only an argument but a career narrative. Previous statements should not disqualify participation, yet they should be visible where they create a strong commitment to a contested conclusion. Intellectual consistency is valuable, but refusal to reconsider assumptions should not be mistaken for scientific integrity.

Political conflicts arise when evidence assessment becomes tied to governmental objectives. Ministers may seek findings that support a promised ban, tax or public campaign. Civil servants may frame advisory questions narrowly to fit an established programme. Public agencies can emphasise evidence that demonstrates success and minimise indicators suggesting unintended consequences. Researchers dependent on government grants may understand which conclusions are institutionally welcome without receiving direct instruction. Political funding is not inherently less influential than commercial funding. The relevant question is whether sponsors can shape questions, methods, interpretation or access to results.

Conflicts also affect consumer advocacy. People who have stopped smoking through vaping may hold strong personal commitments because the issue concerns their health and autonomy. Their experience is legitimate evidence, but it can make criticism of products feel like denial of their success. Consumer organisations may receive support from retailers or manufacturers while maintaining genuine independent beliefs. The appropriate response is neither automatic dismissal nor unquestioning acceptance. Funding, governance, membership and decision-making should be transparent, and claims should be evaluated according to representativeness, method and relevance to the policy under consideration.

Public-health organisations are not free from conflicts merely because their objectives are non-commercial. Funding bodies, institutional missions and campaign priorities can shape which risks receive attention. An organisation established to prevent youth nicotine use may judge success through declining prevalence even if adult smoking cessation also changes. A body committed to tobacco endgame strategies may view continued nicotine use as failure regardless of reduced exposure. These positions may be ethically coherent, but they contain value judgements. Declaring the organisational objective helps distinguish scientific findings from the policy preferences built upon them.

Media relationships create further complications. Researchers and organisations gain visibility, influence and future funding through coverage. Dramatic claims are more likely to produce interviews, citations and political attention than careful statements of uncertainty. Press offices may strengthen language beyond the underlying paper, while authors accept the publicity because it advances their work. Commercial actors similarly use favourable coverage to build market legitimacy. Disclosure should therefore extend to media partnerships, sponsored content and communication support where these relationships could affect how evidence is framed for public consumption.

The presence of a conflict does not determine the validity of evidence. A well-designed industry-funded chemical analysis may be more reliable than a poorly designed independent study. Conversely, methodological sophistication cannot compensate for withheld results or sponsor control. Evidence assessment should examine protocol registration, product selection, comparators, analytical methods, statistical plans, missing data, access to raw results and publication rights. Source is a reason for scrutiny, not a substitute for scrutiny. Rejecting data solely because of funding can remove useful information, while accepting it without safeguards allows selective evidence to shape policy.

Disclosure is the first control, but it is not sufficient. Long declarations can create an illusion of transparency while leaving readers unable to judge materiality. Disclosures should identify the nature, value, timing and relevance of each relationship. Payments made years earlier may carry less weight than current funding, but repeated or strategically important relationships remain relevant. Institutions should define reporting periods and thresholds while allowing declaration of interests that fall outside formal categories. Ambiguity should favour openness, particularly where public trust is central.

Management should be proportionate to the risk. Some conflicts can be addressed through disclosure and independent review. Others require recusal from voting, exclusion from drafting, restricted access to confidential material or appointment of an independent chair. A person with unique technical expertise may provide evidence without determining the recommendation. A researcher funded by a manufacturer may present data while another group controls synthesis. Complete exclusion should be reserved for circumstances where the conflict is direct, substantial and incapable of mitigation. Overly rigid rules can remove knowledgeable participants and leave committees less capable of detecting weak technical claims.

Consistency is essential. Standards that scrutinise tobacco funding but ignore pharmaceutical, governmental or philanthropic influence appear selective. Historical conduct justifies heightened caution around cigarette companies, especially where they continue to sell combustible products, but other interests should still be declared and managed. Equal treatment does not mean pretending all conflicts have equal magnitude. It means applying a common analytical framework: what duty is owed, what secondary interest exists, how direct it is, what decisions it could affect and whether safeguards reduce the risk adequately.

Revolving-door appointments require particular attention. Movement between regulators and industry can improve mutual understanding, but it can also create privileged access and expectations of future employment. Officials may hesitate to impose requirements on organisations that could later employ them, while former regulators may sell knowledge of internal processes. Cooling-off periods, restrictions on lobbying former departments and publication of post-employment appointments can reduce these concerns. Equivalent safeguards should apply when industry personnel enter regulatory roles, including management of shareholdings, previous clients and confidential information.

Ghostwriting and undisclosed authorship represent more serious failures. A company or advocacy organisation may prepare analyses, consultation responses or academic manuscripts that are presented under apparently independent names. The problem is not assistance itself but concealment of who framed the argument and controlled the evidence. Contributions to drafting, statistical analysis, data ownership and editorial decisions should be stated. Third-party agencies should not be allowed to hide behind nominal authorship. Where independence is claimed, contracts and publication rights should support that claim.

Advisory committees need formal conflict procedures before members are selected. Declarations should be reviewed by an independent secretariat and published in accessible form. Chairs should decide whether an interest requires recusal for a particular agenda item rather than treating participation as permanently permitted or prohibited. Meeting records should identify recusals and explain how evidence from conflicted sources was handled. These procedures protect both the committee and the individual by replacing improvised accusations with predictable governance.

Regulatory consultation also requires disclosure. Trade associations should identify major funders, commissioned experts and organisations involved in drafting submissions. Consumer and public-health groups should state material financial support relevant to the issue. Governments should publish meetings and substantive evidence received outside the formal consultation window. Hidden access can influence options before the public is invited to respond, making later transparency incomplete. Recording who shaped the initial question is as important as recording who answered it.

Data transparency offers the strongest protection where conflicts cannot be removed. Protocols, analytical methods, code and sufficiently detailed results should be available for independent examination, subject to legitimate privacy and commercial protections. Regulators may need confidential access to formulations or sales data that cannot be published fully, but they can describe how those data affected conclusions. Replication by independent laboratories and reanalysis by separate statisticians reduce reliance on trust. The more consequential the policy claim, the stronger the case for verifiable evidence.

Conflict management should also address enforcement. Regulators funded through industry fees may face allegations that revenue dependence weakens oversight. Fee-funded systems are not inherently compromised, because charges can provide the resources needed for competent review, but governance should separate payment from decision outcomes. Inspectors, laboratories and assessors should not benefit from approving more products or imposing more failures. Published performance indicators, audit and appeal mechanisms can protect impartiality.

Public confidence depends on acknowledging that no institution is entirely without interests. The objective is not to locate a perfectly neutral observer, but to construct processes in which competing influences are visible and evidence can be challenged. Plural participation can reduce domination where industry, public health, consumers, scientists and enforcement bodies are all heard under common rules. Diversity alone is insufficient if one group possesses disproportionate resources or private access, so institutional design must also address power.

Conflicts of interest become most damaging when they are used selectively as political weapons. Accusations can discredit inconvenient evidence without examining its substance, while allies receive lenient treatment. This converts governance into tribal sorting. A credible system applies the same questions to every participant, recognises differences in seriousness and distinguishes conflict from misconduct. Misconduct requires evidence of deception, suppression or breach of duty. Conflict requires management before such failure occurs.

The purpose of conflict-of-interest policy is therefore not purification but accountability. Vaping regulation inevitably relies on people with experience, commitments and institutional relationships. The task is to ensure that those interests do not operate invisibly. Clear declarations, proportionate recusals, independent review, transparent data and consistent standards allow expertise to contribute without granting any actor unexamined authority. When conflicts are managed openly, disagreement can return to evidence and policy consequences. When they are concealed or applied selectively, even sound conclusions become vulnerable to distrust. That distrust ultimately weakens both science and governance.

Balancing Science with Politics

Balancing science with politics is not a matter of choosing one over the other. Regulation cannot be produced by evidence alone because evidence does not decide which risks society should tolerate, whose interests should receive priority or how quickly government should act. Politics cannot operate credibly without evidence because authority unsupported by reality creates ineffective rules, unintended consequences and declining trust. The difficulty lies in preserving the integrity of scientific assessment while acknowledging that public policy is necessarily shaped by values, institutions, resources, public opinion and electoral judgement. In vaping, this balance is especially demanding because the product sits between smoking prevention, adult harm reduction, youth protection, commercial innovation and unresolved long-term uncertainty.

Science contributes measurement, comparison and explanation. It can identify constituents in e-liquid, characterise aerosol emissions, assess nicotine delivery, examine cellular responses, measure patterns of use and model transitions between smoking, vaping and abstinence. It can estimate how product standards alter exposure and how population behaviour may affect disease. Yet scientific evidence does not arrive as a single answer. Different studies use different products, populations, methods and endpoints. Their findings must be interpreted, weighted and connected. The resulting advice always contains assumptions. Political systems become unstable when those assumptions are concealed and scientific uncertainty is presented as certainty merely to strengthen a preferred policy.

Politics contributes legitimacy, prioritisation and implementation. Elected governments decide how to distribute limited regulatory attention, which harms require urgent intervention and what constraints should be placed on individual choice and commercial conduct. They must consider fairness, enforceability, economic effects and public acceptability alongside toxicological or epidemiological evidence. A scientifically plausible measure may be politically impossible, administratively unaffordable or socially counterproductive. Conversely, a politically attractive measure may be scientifically weak yet command immediate support because it responds to visible concern. Good governance does not remove this tension. It makes the trade-offs explicit and subjects them to reasoned scrutiny.

The first requirement is to separate facts from values. Whether an aerosol contains a particular carbonyl is a scientific question. Whether the concentration is acceptable in a consumer product is partly a regulatory judgement. Whether flavours should be restricted involves evidence about chemistry, youth appeal and adult switching, but also a value judgement about how to balance competing populations. Whether nicotine use without smoking is an acceptable public-health outcome depends on the objective chosen. Governments should not present these decisions as though laboratories have dictated them. Scientific evidence constrains responsible policy, but political authority remains accountable for the final choice.

Comparators are central to this distinction. Vaping appears harmful when compared with non-use and substantially less harmful when compared with smoking. Policymakers who emphasise only one comparator can produce apparently coherent but incomplete policy. Youth protection naturally begins from non-use. Adult harm reduction begins from continued smoking. A balanced framework must consider both simultaneously and identify which group each intervention is intended to influence. Failure to state the comparator allows political rhetoric to move between populations opportunistically, using evidence about young non-smokers to justify restrictions affecting adult smokers without examining the resulting substitution effects.

Time also separates science from politics. Long-term epidemiology develops slowly, while governments face immediate demands. Waiting for complete certainty can allow avoidable harm to continue, but acting too quickly can entrench a poorly designed response. The appropriate standard is not certainty but proportionality. Strong evidence of serious and irreversible harm may justify rapid restriction. Limited evidence of a manageable risk may support surveillance, product standards or targeted controls rather than prohibition. Political urgency should determine the speed of review, not the desired conclusion. Temporary measures should include review dates so that precaution does not become permanent merely through administrative inertia.

Scientific advice should therefore present options rather than a single command wherever the evidence permits more than one reasonable response. Advisers can describe the expected benefits, uncertainties and risks attached to different regulatory pathways. They can identify which assumptions drive each outcome and what data would allow future revision. Ministers can then choose openly among those options. This approach protects science from being blamed for political priorities and prevents politicians from claiming that contested decisions were technically inevitable. Advice becomes more useful when it clarifies consequences rather than pretending to eliminate judgement.

The political use of numbers requires particular caution. Risk percentages, prevalence estimates and economic forecasts can create an appearance of precision that exceeds the underlying evidence. A single figure is easy to repeat in Parliament or the media, but its assumptions may be forgotten. Relative-risk estimates depend on product quality, duration and patterns of use. Youth prevalence depends on definitions of experimentation, regular use and frequency. Economic models depend on consumer response, enforcement and illicit supply. Scientific advisers should explain ranges and sensitivity, while politicians should resist selecting only the number that supports the strongest headline.

Evidence can also be politicised through selective timing. Governments may announce a dramatic finding quickly while delaying data that complicate the message. Advisory reports may be published alongside policy decisions, leaving little opportunity for independent scrutiny. Consultation may begin after ministers have committed publicly to a course of action. These practices do not necessarily falsify evidence, but they convert scientific work into strategic communication. Credible policy requires publication of methods, sufficient time for review and clear separation between evidence assessment and political announcement. The sequence matters because public commitment can make later revision appear as weakness.

Public opinion cannot be ignored, yet it should not be mistaken for scientific evidence. Citizens may reasonably demand action when products are visible in schools, discarded in public spaces or associated with aggressive marketing. Their concern gives political weight to the issue, but it does not establish which intervention will work. Government must translate concern into a properly defined problem and test possible responses against evidence. A policy can acknowledge public anxiety without reproducing every assumption contained within it. Leadership sometimes requires explaining why a popular measure would create greater harm or why a less dramatic intervention is more likely to succeed.

Media pressure further compresses decision-making. Ministers are asked for immediate responses to new studies, incidents and campaigns. Scientific uncertainty rarely fits the format of a short interview. There is a temptation either to overstate danger to demonstrate control or to dismiss concern to defend existing policy. Both approaches are fragile. Public communication should identify what is known, what is uncertain and what action is being taken while evidence develops. Credibility depends less on appearing certain than on showing that uncertainty is being managed competently.

Industry influence complicates the balance because companies possess relevant technical information while seeking favourable outcomes. Political systems need access to data on formulations, manufacturing, costs and market behaviour, but private access can distort priorities. Engagement should therefore be structured, recorded and tested against independent evidence. Policymakers should distinguish a technical claim about feasibility from a policy preference about market access. Industry should be allowed to challenge impractical rules, but not to define public-health objectives. Exclusion may produce ignorance; unrestricted access may produce capture. Transparent boundaries allow knowledge without surrendering authority.

Public-health organisations can exert similar pressure from a different direction. Their objectives may align with population protection, but advocacy can still simplify uncertainty or promote measures whose effectiveness has not been demonstrated. Political leaders may find it easier to adopt the language of protection than to question whether a proposed ban, tax or restriction will deliver the promised outcome. Respect for public-health expertise should not remove the need for evidence on causation, implementation and unintended effects. Institutional virtue is not a substitute for analytical quality.

The treatment of uncertainty is therefore political as well as scientific. Uncertainty can be exaggerated to delay regulation or minimised to justify intervention. Tobacco companies historically used doubt strategically, making regulators suspicious of calls for more evidence. That history matters, but it does not make every uncertainty claim illegitimate. Some evidence gaps are material. Long-term disease outcomes, patterns of dual use and the effects of product restrictions may genuinely be unresolved. The correct response is to identify who benefits from delay, what information is missing and whether interim safeguards can reduce risk while evidence improves.

Regulation should also recognise that markets respond. A flavour restriction may reduce lawful variety but encourage informal supply. A nicotine ceiling may alter device design or user behaviour. A costly authorisation system may improve documentation while concentrating the market among the largest companies. A disposable ban may reduce waste but stimulate technically compliant substitutes with similar environmental effects. Political debate often treats regulation as an instruction and compliance as the only response.

Scientific assessment must model adaptation, because real outcomes depend on how consumers, manufacturers and illicit suppliers react.

Evaluation closes the gap between political intention and scientific reality. Every major intervention should specify measurable objectives, baseline data and review points. If a display restriction is intended to reduce youth uptake, surveillance should examine exposure, regular use and purchasing routes. If a tax is intended to preserve adult switching while discouraging initiation, price relationships, smoking relapse and illicit sales should be monitored. Policies should be revised when outcomes differ materially from predictions. Without evaluation, political success becomes defined by enactment rather than effect.

Institutional design can support this discipline. Independent advisory committees, published impact assessments, transparent consultations and accessible post-implementation reviews create friction against impulsive decisions. Friction is valuable when it requires government to explain evidence and alternatives. It becomes obstructive when procedures are so slow that emerging harm is ignored. The goal is not maximal process, but a structure capable of acting rapidly while retaining traceability. Emergency action should remain exceptional and subject to later scrutiny.

Scientists also bear responsibility for how their work enters politics. They should avoid presenting personal policy preferences as direct outputs of data. Advocacy is legitimate, but roles should be clear. A scientist may conclude that a restriction is justified, yet that conclusion incorporates values about acceptable risk and distribution of harm. Transparency strengthens rather than weakens authority. Experts who acknowledge uncertainty, competing evidence and the limits of their discipline are more useful than those who offer certainty beyond what the methods can support.

Politicians, in turn, should not demand impossible certainty or convenient simplicity. They should be prepared to defend value choices openly, including decisions that prioritise youth protection, adult harm reduction, environmental goals or market freedom. They should explain why one risk has been given greater weight and what safeguards protect those disadvantaged by the choice. Political accountability is weakened when ministers attribute every difficult trade-off to "the science". Science can inform responsibility, but it cannot absorb it.

The balance is most credible when no stakeholder is permitted to monopolise the definition of evidence. Laboratory scientists, clinicians, epidemiologists, economists, enforcement officers, consumers and manufacturers each see different parts of the system. Their contributions should be evaluated through transparent methods and conflicts managed consistently. Inclusion does not mean equal authority on every question. It means that assumptions can be challenged by those who understand product performance, behaviour and implementation from different positions.

Institutional memory is essential because regulatory debates repeatedly revisit the same uncertainties under new technologies and political pressures. Officials should preserve the assumptions, evidence and predicted consequences attached to earlier decisions, allowing later reviewers to see why a measure was adopted and whether its foundations remain valid. Without that record, policy change can resemble inconsistency and policy continuity can persist without justification. Memory enables learning, prevents convenient reinvention of history and makes revision an expected feature of governance.

Balancing science with politics ultimately means creating decisions that are evidence-constrained rather than evidence-disguised. The best policy may not satisfy every scientific ideal or political demand. It should, however, state its comparator, acknowledge uncertainty, explain trade-offs and remain open to revision. In vaping regulation, the central danger is not disagreement. It is the conversion of disagreement into fixed camps where evidence is valued only when it supports prior commitments. A mature system accepts that science and politics perform different functions and that legitimacy depends on keeping those functions connected without allowing either to impersonate the other.

CHAPTER 9

Regulation in Practice

Regulation acquires meaning only when it changes what happens in the market. Legislation may define nicotine limits, reservoir capacities, packaging requirements, notification duties, age restrictions and producer responsibilities, but none of those provisions protects a consumer merely because it appears in a statutory instrument or regulatory guidance document. Protection arises when the lawful product supplied through a retailer corresponds to the product described in the regulatory submission, when the importer can demonstrate where it came from, when the distributor preserves its identity and integrity, when the retailer refuses unlawful sales, when enforcement authorities can identify non-compliance and when defective or unsafe products can be removed quickly enough to prevent further exposure. The distance between a legal requirement and its practical effect is therefore the decisive space in which regulation succeeds or fails. It is also the space in which the strengths and weaknesses of vaping regulation become most visible, because modern nicotine products move through complex supply chains, cross national borders easily, change rapidly in response to demand and can be sold through physical shops, websites, social-media accounts, online marketplaces and informal networks that do not respond equally to conventional regulatory control.

The preceding chapters have considered how regulatory systems are formed, how products are designed for compliance, how toxicological and analytical evidence is generated, how quality systems maintain consistency, how notifications are constructed and how different jurisdictions select their preferred model of control. Those processes create the legal and technical architecture of regulation, but they do not guarantee that the product held by a consumer is lawful, accurately labelled or manufactured according to the information supplied to the regulator. A technically complete notification can coexist with a poorly controlled manufacturing process. A compliant brand can be copied by counterfeiters. A lawful product name can be applied to an unauthorised formulation or an oversized device. An importer can receive goods that differ from the samples previously assessed, while a distributor can separate products from the records needed to establish their origin. A retailer may assume that anything supplied by a wholesaler is compliant, and an online seller may operate from a jurisdiction in which enforcement authorities have little practical reach. Regulation in practice begins where these assumptions are tested against the physical product and the commercial conduct surrounding it.

The regulated object is not merely the formulation, device or package considered in isolation. It is the complete chain through which the product is made, transported, declared, stored, advertised, offered for sale and delivered to the user. Every point in that chain can preserve compliance or weaken it. Manufacturing determines whether the product matches its approved or notified specification. Importation determines whether a responsible economic operator can be identified within the jurisdiction. Distribution determines whether batches remain traceable and whether products are stored and handled appropriately. Retail determines what is actually presented to consumers and whether age restrictions, warnings, product controls and sales conditions are observed. Online commerce determines whether national restrictions can be applied to sellers, platforms and fulfilment networks that may operate across several territories. Enforcement determines whether violations produce consequences substantial enough to alter commercial behaviour. Border control determines whether unlawful products are intercepted before they become dispersed through thousands of outlets. Withdrawal and recall systems determine whether a known problem can be contained after distribution has begun. These functions are often governed by different bodies, yet the market experiences them as one regulatory system.

Retailers occupy a particularly exposed position within that system. They are the point at which regulatory policy encounters everyday consumer demand, commercial pressure and practical judgement. A retailer may handle hundreds of rapidly changing products supplied by multiple wholesalers, carrying similar brand names, flavour descriptions and device formats. Determining compliance cannot reasonably depend upon visual confidence alone, because packaging can be copied, regulatory identifiers can be misused and illegal capacities may be concealed within devices labelled as lawful. Retailers therefore require access to reliable product records, identifiable suppliers, invoices, batch information and clear regulatory guidance. They must also understand that purchasing from an apparently established wholesaler does not remove their own obligations. At the same time, regulation must recognise the limitations of the retail environment. A shop assistant cannot reproduce the work of an analytical laboratory or regulatory assessor, and a compliance system that expects individual retailers to verify hidden technical properties without providing usable tools transfers responsibility without creating control.

The effectiveness of retail regulation depends upon the quality of the upstream supply chain. Importers and distributors determine which products reach shops, how quickly new variants appear and whether records exist that connect the goods to a responsible manufacturer. An importer is not simply a transport intermediary. Where the manufacturer is located outside the market, the importer may become the principal economic operator available to regulators. It may be expected to confirm that required submissions have been made, that labelling and packaging are appropriate, that supporting documentation exists and that the products supplied correspond to the declared specification. This responsibility becomes difficult when goods are produced through remote contract manufacturers, international trading companies and layered purchasing arrangements in which the commercial entity named on the invoice has limited knowledge of the factory or formulation. A low-cost supply chain may move products efficiently while remaining incapable of answering elementary regulatory questions about ingredients, manufacturing controls, test reports or batch identity.

Distribution can appear less scientifically significant than formulation or toxicology, yet it determines whether compliance remains attached to the product after importation. A distributor that maintains accurate records can identify which retailer received a particular batch, isolate affected stock and support a targeted withdrawal. One that purchases mixed consignments, relabels outer packaging, divides batches or fails to preserve supplier documentation can destroy that visibility. Traceability is therefore not an abstract quality-system principle but a practical enforcement capability. When a product fails testing or becomes associated with a safety concern, the response depends upon knowing how many units entered the market, where they were sent and whether further stock remains in warehouses or shops. Without those records, regulators may issue a general warning while the affected goods continue to circulate. The commercial convenience of rapid, fragmented distribution can consequently conflict with the regulatory need for stable product identity.

Online sales extend this difficulty beyond the physical marketplace. A website can display products to consumers in one country while the seller, payment processor, warehouse, marketplace operator and delivery service are located in several others. Product listings can be changed rapidly, removed after complaints and restored under a new seller identity. Age-verification systems vary greatly in reliability, while social-media promotion can direct consumers towards private messaging services or informal payment channels outside conventional retail oversight. The digital market also weakens the connection between what is advertised and what is delivered. Images may show compliant packaging while the supplied device differs in capacity, nicotine strength or formulation. Reviews and promotional claims can be generated by affiliates who are not clearly identified as advertisers. A national prohibition or product standard may therefore be clear in law while remaining porous in practice because the transaction is distributed across platforms that deny responsibility for the underlying goods.

The practical regulation of online trade requires more than action against individual listings. Marketplaces, hosting services, payment providers, fulfilment businesses, couriers and advertising platforms each control part of the commercial infrastructure. Their cooperation can make illegal sales more difficult, while their indifference can allow removed sellers to reappear almost immediately. Platform governance therefore becomes part of product regulation even where the platform does not manufacture or formally own the goods. This raises legitimate questions concerning proportionality and responsibility. An online marketplace cannot conduct a complete toxicological review of every product offered through it, but it can require sellers to provide verifiable identities, regulatory records and evidence of lawful market status. It can remove repeat offenders, preserve transaction data and respond promptly to enforcement notices. The practical challenge lies in converting those capabilities into consistent obligations rather than relying on voluntary action that varies according to commercial priority and public pressure.

Enforcement is the mechanism that connects all these responsibilities. It must identify non-compliance, establish evidence, determine the responsible party and impose a response that protects the public and discourages repetition. This is considerably more demanding than discovering that a product appears suspicious. The authority may need to purchase or seize samples, verify notification status, measure liquid volume or nicotine concentration, assess packaging, obtain laboratory analysis, establish the route of supply and determine whether the offence lies with the manufacturer, importer, distributor, retailer or several parties simultaneously. The evidence must be sufficiently reliable to support administrative action, civil penalties or criminal proceedings. Where legal definitions are ambiguous, analytical methods are contested or the responsible company disappears, enforcement can become slow and expensive. Products may be sold through much of their commercial life before formal action is completed.

Resources therefore determine the practical reach of regulation. Local enforcement teams may be responsible for vaping products alongside food standards, product safety, weights and measures, age-restricted sales and numerous other statutory duties. Laboratory testing is costly, particularly where a product requires chemical, electrical and physical assessment. Border authorities must inspect enormous volumes of goods while identifying consignments that may be incorrectly declared, divided into small parcels or imported through rapidly changing companies. National regulators may maintain product databases without possessing the personnel required to compare every market sample against the corresponding submission. The existence of extensive legal powers cannot compensate for inadequate intelligence, inspection capacity and technical expertise. Regulation becomes selectively real: highly visible to responsible businesses that prepare submissions and maintain records, but less consequential to traders whose commercial model assumes that only a small proportion of unlawful stock will be detected.

This enforcement asymmetry can distort the market. Compliant manufacturers incur costs for ingredient assessment, analytical testing, quality systems, notifications, packaging and lifecycle management. Responsible importers examine documentation and may reject questionable consignments. Legitimate retailers purchase through traceable channels and accept restrictions on the products they sell. Illegal operators avoid those costs and may offer larger capacities, higher nicotine concentrations, lower prices or prohibited presentation. Where detection is infrequent and penalties are limited, non-compliance becomes commercially rational. The lawful market then bears the burden of regulation while the unlawful market captures demand created by the restrictions. This does not justify weakening appropriate standards, but it means that every additional obligation should be accompanied by an enforcement plan capable of preventing evasion from becoming the more profitable business model.

Counterfeit products intensify this imbalance because they exploit consumer confidence in established brands. A counterfeit device may reproduce logos, colours, packaging and authentication features while containing an unknown liquid, inferior battery, altered reservoir or poorly controlled heating element. It may copy a product that has been properly notified, creating the impression that regulatory status extends to the counterfeit unit. The legitimate producer can suffer reputational damage, retailers may be unable to distinguish genuine and false stock, and regulators may initially associate complaints or test failures with the lawful product family. Counterfeiting therefore creates more than an intellectual-property problem. It breaks the relationship between the regulatory dossier and the physical item bearing the product name. Authentication technologies can assist, but codes and labels can themselves be copied unless linked to secure databases, controlled distribution records and active investigation.

The wider illegal market includes more than counterfeits. It contains genuine products diverted from another jurisdiction, unauthorised versions made by the original factory, products deliberately designed beyond legal limits, falsely declared nicotine strengths, unnotified formulations, untaxed goods and devices assembled from components that individually appear lawful. Some products enter through conventional commercial imports, while others arrive in small parcels, passenger luggage or informal wholesale networks. The distinction between lawful and unlawful supply may become difficult for consumers to recognise, particularly where the illegal product is sold openly from an established shop or professional-looking website. Visible availability can create an assumption of legality, while inconsistent enforcement can normalise non-compliance until unlawful products become a routine part of the market rather than an exceptional breach.

Illegal markets are not created by regulation alone, but regulatory design influences their scale and profitability. Demand persists when consumers value features unavailable through lawful channels, when duties create large price differences, when product restrictions are introduced without adequate transition or when prohibited goods remain easy to obtain. Some consumers will accept lawful substitutes, while others will seek familiar products through informal routes. Suppliers respond to that demand. A credible regulatory assessment must therefore examine not only whether a restriction is justified in principle, but how consumers, retailers and importers are likely to react. The risk of evasion does not confer a veto over public health policy, yet ignoring predictable substitution can allow a measure to move exposure from a controlled market into a less controlled one.

Border control is frequently expected to prevent this movement, although the border is only one point in a dispersed supply chain. Authorities must identify products among vast volumes of legitimate trade, often using customs declarations that provide limited technical detail. Nicotine products may be described generically as electronic goods, flavouring liquids, samples or components. Consignments can be divided to reduce the likelihood of inspection or routed through intermediate countries to obscure their origin. Even when suspect goods are detected, officers need clear legal powers, accessible product information and technically defensible criteria for detention or seizure. A device that appears to exceed lawful capacity may require destructive examination or laboratory confirmation. A liquid labelled as nicotine-free may contain nicotine. Packaging may show a valid product identifier while the internal specification differs from the notified version. Border enforcement therefore depends upon intelligence and risk profiling rather than inspection of every shipment.

The strongest control systems connect border information with domestic market surveillance. Repeated imports by the same company, abnormal product volumes, prior test failures and links to non-compliant retailers can guide inspection. Samples seized at the border can reveal emerging product formats before they become widely distributed. Retail discoveries can be traced backwards to import declarations and freight records. Regulatory databases can confirm whether a product identity exists, while tax and customs information can reveal whether the declared trade is consistent with the goods found in the market. Such integration is technically possible but institutionally difficult because information may be held by separate agencies operating under different legal powers, priorities and data systems. Fragmentation allows each authority to perform its own function while the complete commercial pathway remains unseen.

Product withdrawal is the final practical test of this pathway. When a defect, non-compliance or safety concern is identified, the responsible business must determine the affected product and batch, stop further distribution, inform customers, recover stock where necessary and report the action to the relevant authority. A withdrawal removes products from the supply chain before they reach consumers, while a recall may require action involving products already supplied. The distinction is operationally important, but both depend upon traceability, communication and decisive management. A business that lacks accurate batch records may withdraw too little and leave affected products in circulation, or withdraw too broadly and create unnecessary disruption. A company that fears reputational damage may delay notification, while one without sufficient financial resources may disappear rather than fund recovery and investigation.

Withdrawal and recall should not be interpreted automatically as evidence that a regulatory system has failed. Defects can occur even within well-controlled industries, and the ability to detect and correct them is itself a sign of functioning oversight. Failure arises when warning signals are ignored, when affected products cannot be located, when responsibility is disputed or when identical problems recur without effective corrective action. Complaints, laboratory failures, adverse-event reports, retailer observations and enforcement intelligence should feed into a structured investigation capable of establishing root cause. The objective is not merely to remove one consignment but to determine whether the problem originated in formulation, manufacturing, component substitution, labelling, storage, counterfeiting or deliberate non-compliance.

Regulatory casework exposes the limitations of treating compliance as a binary label. A product may be notified but incorrectly manufactured, correctly manufactured but sold in unlawful packaging, lawful in one jurisdiction but diverted into another, compliant when originally assessed but altered through an uncontrolled component change, or genuine in appearance but counterfeit in origin. The response must correspond to the actual failure. Administrative correction may be appropriate for a minor documentary error that creates no material exposure. Immediate withdrawal may be necessary where nicotine concentration is seriously incorrect, batteries are unsafe or prohibited ingredients are present. Deliberate evasion, falsified documentation and repeated sale of illegal products require sanctions capable of removing the financial benefit of non-compliance. Proportionality does not mean leniency. It means directing the strongest intervention towards the conduct and products that create the greatest risk.

The legitimacy of vaping regulation ultimately depends upon whether this practical system can distinguish responsible commerce from unlawful supply. A framework that imposes extensive obligations but fails to act against obvious evasion loses credibility with manufacturers, retailers and consumers. Responsible businesses begin to view compliance as a competitive disadvantage. Consumers become uncertain about which products can be trusted. Enforcement authorities face growing markets that exceed their resources, while political pressure produces further restrictions without resolving the underlying operational weakness. The answer is not simply more law. It is better connection between product data, supply-chain records, customs intelligence, market sampling, laboratory capacity, retail oversight and corrective action.

Regulation in practice is therefore where scientific competence, administrative design and enforcement reality meet. The product placed in a submission portal is an electronic record; the product placed in a consumer's hand is a manufactured object moving through a commercial system. Effective regulation must keep the two connected. It must know who made the product, who imported it, who distributed it, who sold it, what it contained, whether it matched its specification and how it can be removed when something goes wrong. Where that chain remains intact, regulation can protect consumers while allowing lawful harm-reduction products to compete. Where it breaks, extensive legislation may coexist with a market in which compliance is uncertain, counterfeit goods are common and illegal operators respond more quickly than the authorities intended to control them.

The task of practical regulation is not to create the appearance of strictness. It is to make lawful conduct easier to verify, unlawful conduct harder to profit from and regulatory intervention fast enough to affect real exposure. That requires technically informed retailers, accountable importers, traceable distribution, controlled online commerce, coordinated enforcement, intelligent border surveillance and withdrawal systems capable of acting before a local defect becomes a national problem. It also requires restraint in the design of obligations, because a system overwhelmed by low-value administrative breaches may have insufficient capacity to address products presenting genuine risk. The measure of success is not the number of notices issued, products listed or powers created, but whether the market becomes more transparent, more accountable and materially safer for the adults who depend upon it as an alternative to combustible tobacco.

Figure 9.1. Regulation in Practice: Enforcement Pathway.

This diagram shows how regulatory control follows a vaping product from manufacture and export through importation, distribution, physical retail and online sale. Each commercial stage is matched with the corresponding compliance responsibilities, including product notification, technical documentation, importer due diligence, supply-chain traceability, age-of-sale controls, online seller verification and record retention. The lower sections illustrate how market surveillance, border inspections, online monitoring, intelligence sharing and laboratory testing identify suspected non-compliance and move it through risk assessment, investigation and formal enforcement decision-making.

The diagram also shows the possible regulatory outcomes, including advisory action, improvement notices, penalties, product seizure, licence suspension and prosecution. Where a product must be removed from the market, the pathway continues through withdrawal or recall, root-cause investigation, corrective action, preventive controls and follow-up verification. The side panel identifies the principal threats encountered in practice: counterfeit products, illegal markets, diverted goods, misleading claims and safety hazards. Feedback loops emphasise that enforcement should not end with the removal of one product, but should strengthen future surveillance, supply-chain controls and regulatory intelligence.

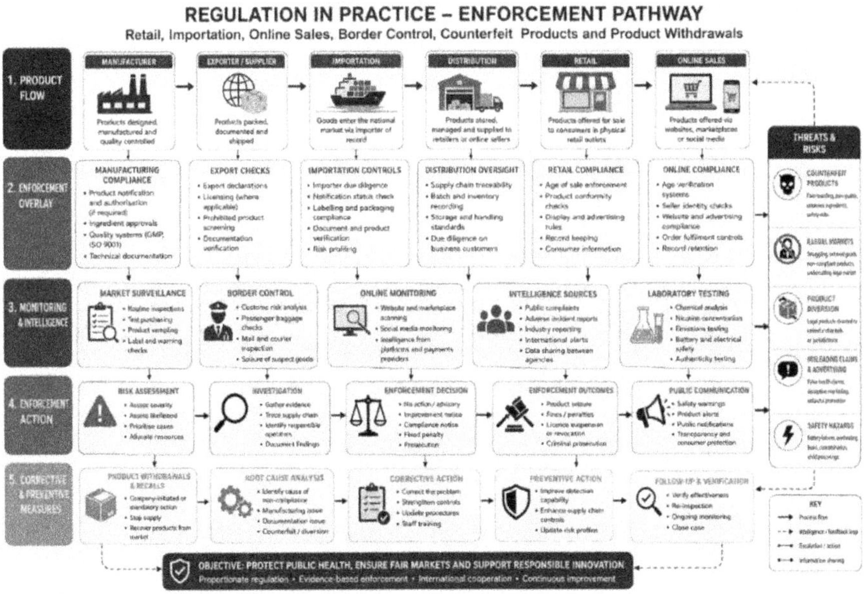

Retail compliance

Retail compliance is the point at which the regulatory system becomes visible to the consumer. Legislation, product notifications, laboratory reports, supplier declarations and quality systems may all exist upstream, but the retail transaction determines which product is actually placed into a consumer's hands, how it is presented, whether its legal status can be demonstrated and whether the seller observes the restrictions governing nicotine products. Retailers occupy the final commercial position before use, yet they often operate with less scientific information and fewer technical resources than manufacturers, importers or regulators. This creates a difficult allocation of responsibility. A retailer cannot be expected to reproduce a toxicological assessment, verify a formulation independently or dismantle every device to confirm liquid capacity, but it cannot rely blindly on the appearance of professional packaging or the assurances of a wholesaler. Effective retail compliance therefore depends on proportionate due diligence, traceable purchasing, competent staff, accurate records, responsible presentation and a willingness to reject products whose legal status or origin cannot be established.

The retail environment is diverse. Specialist vape shops, convenience stores, supermarkets, petrol stations, pharmacies, online sellers, market stalls and temporary outlets may all sell vaping products, but their knowledge, commercial priorities and control systems differ considerably. A specialist retailer may understand coil resistance, nicotine strengths, refill systems and consumer switching behaviour in detail while still maintaining weak documentary controls. A national chain may possess formal compliance procedures and centralised purchasing but rely on frontline staff with limited product knowledge. A small independent shop may receive stock from several wholesalers, each supplying rapidly changing brands and flavour variants. Regulation must operate across all these settings without assuming that one model of retail competence applies universally. The core obligations may be common, but the systems needed to meet them must reflect the scale, complexity and risk profile of the business.

The first retail responsibility is to know the supplier. A lawful product should arrive through an identifiable commercial chain supported by invoices, delivery records and contact details for the wholesaler, distributor or importer. Cash purchases from informal traders, stock acquired through messaging applications or products supplied without proper invoices create immediate compliance concerns because the retailer may be unable to establish where the goods originated or who is responsible if a problem emerges. Supplier familiarity is not enough. A wholesaler may appear established while distributing products that are unnotified, incorrectly labelled, counterfeit or intended for another jurisdiction. Retailers should therefore maintain an approved-supplier process proportionate to their business, checking company identity, address, tax and registration details where relevant, product documentation, recall capability and willingness to provide evidence of lawful market status.

Product status must then be verified. In Great Britain, nicotine-containing vaping products intended for consumer sale should correspond to products notified through the applicable regulatory process and published by the competent authority. Retailers should be able to compare the brand, product type, nicotine strength, flavour, submitter and other identifying details against the official record. This is not always straightforward. Product names may be entered inconsistently, packaging may use abbreviations, and a manufacturer may market numerous closely related variants. A listing under a similar name does not necessarily cover every strength, flavour or device configuration. The retailer must avoid treating the presence of one product from a brand as proof that the entire range is lawful. Where the product cannot be matched confidently, clarification should be obtained from the supplier before sale.

Notification status is only one part of compliance. A product may be correctly notified yet sold in a form that no longer matches the submitted specification. Packaging, reservoir capacity, nicotine concentration, device components or formulation may have changed after notification. Counterfeiters may copy the name and appearance of a notified product, while unauthorised manufacturers may produce visually similar versions. Retail checking must therefore combine documentary verification with physical inspection. The label should identify the product clearly, state the nicotine content accurately, display required warnings and include the details needed to identify the responsible producer or importer. Packaging should be intact, tamper-evident where required and free from obvious alteration. Devices and refill containers should not appear inconsistent with legal volume limits, although visual inspection alone cannot confirm hidden capacity. Suspicious differences between batches, unusual spelling, poor print quality, missing inserts or altered security codes should be investigated rather than dismissed as minor presentation defects.

Nicotine concentration is a particularly important retail control because products may be mislabelled, diverted from another market or deliberately supplied above permitted limits. Retailers are not expected to perform chemical analysis, but they should understand the legal maximum applying to the products they sell and recognise labels that exceed it. Products described through percentages rather than milligrams per millilitre may create confusion, especially where staff have not been trained to convert between units. A liquid marked as 5 per cent nicotine is not equivalent to a 5 milligram-per-millilitre product, and failure to understand that distinction can allow unlawfully strong products to be sold. Training should therefore cover common concentration formats, nicotine salts, zero-nicotine products and the difference between the declared strength of a liquid and the total quantity of nicotine contained in the package.

Volume limits require similar attention. Refill containers, tanks, pods and disposable devices may be subject to different requirements, and product design can obscure the amount of liquid actually present. Retailers should be cautious where claimed performance appears incompatible with the stated volume or where devices are materially larger than comparable compliant products. A high claimed puff count is not proof of unlawful capacity because puff duration, power and aerosol output vary, but it can provide a reason to request supporting information. Retail staff should not be expected to make engineering judgements from appearance alone, yet businesses should have an escalation process through which questionable products are withheld from sale pending supplier confirmation or regulatory advice.

Packaging and labelling controls are not decorative obligations. They communicate product identity, nicotine content, warnings, use instructions, storage conditions and the responsible economic operator. Retailers should ensure that products are supplied in the packaging intended for the market rather than separated from mandatory leaflets, outer cartons or warning information. Multipacks should not be broken down where individual units lack the required labelling. Imported stock should not be sold with foreign-language warnings or instructions where domestic requirements demand otherwise. Stickers applied to correct missing information may not be acceptable if they obscure original text, can be removed easily or fail to satisfy format requirements. The retailer must resist the commercial temptation to treat packaging defects as harmless where the product itself appears functional, because the package forms part of the regulated product and may contain information necessary for safe use and traceability.

Retail presentation also falls within compliance. Products should not be displayed or described in ways that mislead consumers about safety, medicinal status, environmental performance or regulatory approval. Claims such as safe, harmless, healthy, approved or medically proven require particular caution. A product may have been notified without being authorised as a medicine or certified as risk-free. Retailers frequently repeat promotional language supplied by manufacturers, but responsibility for misleading presentation does not disappear because the words originated upstream. Shelf labels, websites, staff recommendations and social-media posts should be reviewed to ensure that factual product information is distinguished from unsupported health claims. Relative-risk communication may be appropriate in the context of adult smoking substitution, but it must remain accurate, balanced and consistent with the applicable advertising and consumer-protection rules.

Flavour names, imagery and brand presentation have become increasingly important regulatory concerns. Retailers may not control the original packaging, yet they control which products they stock, how they display them and whether additional promotional material amplifies child-oriented themes. Confectionery references, cartoon imagery, imitation branding and language associated with sweets or youth culture may create legal, reputational and public-health risk even where the underlying formulation is otherwise compliant. Retailers should assess presentation as part of purchasing rather than assuming that a notified product is automatically suitable for every display or promotional context. The obligation to protect children is not satisfied solely by refusing a transaction at the till if the wider retail environment presents nicotine products as toys, collectibles or ordinary soft drinks.

Age-of-sale compliance is one of the most visible retail duties and one of the most frequently tested. The law prohibits sale to persons below the minimum age, but the effectiveness of that prohibition depends on staff behaviour, store systems and management culture. A written policy is insufficient if employees are pressured to prioritise sales, are uncertain about acceptable identification or fear challenging customers. A robust system normally includes a clear age-verification policy, recognised forms of identification, refusal procedures, incident records, periodic training and management review. Challenge 25 or an equivalent approach provides a practical margin by requiring identification from anyone who appears younger than the legal threshold. The policy should apply consistently regardless of whether the customer appears familiar, is accompanied by an adult or claims to be purchasing for someone else.

Proxy purchasing presents a more complex problem. An adult may attempt to buy a vaping product for a minor after the young person has selected the item, provided money or waited nearby. Retailers should train staff to recognise behavioural indicators without assuming wrongdoing solely from association. Conversations between customers, repeated entry and exit, payment transfers, requests made immediately after a refusal and the involvement of school-age individuals can justify declining a sale. Staff need management support because proxy-sale decisions may provoke confrontation and are more difficult than simple identification checks. The business should record significant incidents and, where appropriate, share intelligence with local enforcement authorities or neighbouring retailers.

Staff competence extends beyond age checks. Employees should know which products the business is authorised or willing to sell, how to identify questionable packaging, how to respond to complaints and what to do when a safety concern or regulatory notice arises. Training should be role-specific and documented. A cashier may need concise guidance on age verification and refusal, while purchasing managers require deeper knowledge of notification status, supplier approval, product limits and recalls. Specialist staff who advise smokers on nicotine strength and device selection should understand the boundary between practical consumer support and medical advice. Training should be refreshed when law, product categories or store procedures change, and records should show who completed it, when and with what outcome.

Refusal logs are useful when they support management rather than becoming paperwork completed without purpose. They can identify repeated attempts by particular individuals, times when underage demand is greatest, products most frequently requested and staff who may require additional support. The records can demonstrate a culture of compliance during inspection, but their value lies in the patterns they reveal. A store reporting no refusals despite high youth footfall may not necessarily have perfect compliance; it may indicate that checks are not being made or incidents are not recorded. Managers should therefore review logs critically and compare them with test-purchasing results, CCTV, complaints and staff observations.

Storage conditions also belong within retail compliance. E-liquids and devices should be protected from excessive heat, direct sunlight, moisture and physical damage. Products should be rotated so that older stock is sold first, while expiry or best-before information is respected. Damaged, leaking or swollen products should be quarantined rather than discounted for rapid sale. Lithium-battery devices require particular care because crushing, puncture, overheating or unsuitable charging can create fire risk. Returned goods should not be placed back into saleable stock without assessment, especially where seals have been broken or the consumer reports a defect. The retail environment is the final opportunity to prevent visibly compromised goods from reaching another user.

Inventory control creates the link between purchasing, sale and corrective action. Retailers should be able to identify what products they hold, when they were received and from whom. Batch or lot information should be recorded where available, particularly for liquids and prefilled products. Small businesses may not require complex enterprise software, but they do need records capable of supporting a targeted withdrawal. If a supplier reports that one batch is affected, the retailer should be able to determine whether it remains in stock and whether units have already been sold. Without batch-level visibility, the business may have to remove an entire product range or be unable to act confidently at all.

Product complaints are an important source of regulatory intelligence. Retailers may be the first to hear about leakage, burnt taste, battery failure, unexpected effects, incorrect nicotine strength or packaging discrepancies. Staff should not dismiss repeated complaints as ordinary customer dissatisfaction, nor should they make unsupported causal claims. A complaint procedure should capture the product identity, batch, purchase date, nature of the problem, consumer description and any remaining sample. Serious concerns should be escalated promptly to the supplier or responsible producer, and products should be quarantined where continued sale could expose others to the same problem. Where required, the relevant authority should be informed.

Returns and refunds can reveal patterns that are invisible upstream. A high return rate for one device may indicate manufacturing variation, while repeated reports of harshness or unusual colour may suggest formulation or storage problems. Retailers should preserve defective samples where safe to do so and avoid disposing of them before investigation. The commercial relationship with the supplier should include a route for technical feedback rather than treating returns solely as credit transactions. A wholesaler that repeatedly replaces defective stock without examining cause does not provide an adequate corrective system.

Withdrawals and recalls test the retailer's records and responsiveness. Notices should be received through reliable communication channels and acted upon immediately. A retailer should remove affected stock from sale, segregate it clearly, prevent accidental redistribution and follow instructions concerning return or destruction. Consumer-facing notices may be required where products have already been sold. Staff should understand that a recall is not a discretionary commercial request. Failure to act can extend exposure after a known problem has been identified. Businesses should periodically test their recall procedure through a simple traceability exercise, confirming whether they can locate specified products and document the action taken.

Inspection by Trading Standards or another enforcement body should not be treated as an exceptional confrontation. A compliant retailer should be able to provide supplier invoices, product records, training evidence, refusal procedures and access to stock. Officers may examine labelling, capacity, nicotine declarations, notification status and age-control systems, and may purchase or take samples for testing. Cooperation does not require accepting every interpretation without question, but obstruction, missing records or inconsistent explanations weaken the retailer's position. Where an officer identifies a defect, the business should establish whether the concern affects one unit, one batch, one supplier or the wider product range.

Test purchasing is particularly important because written policies cannot demonstrate how staff behave under real conditions. An underage volunteer may attempt to buy a product while officers observe the transaction. Failure can lead to warnings, penalties, licence consequences where applicable or prosecution, but the wider value of test purchasing lies in identifying weaknesses before they become routine. Businesses should conduct their own internal checks or mystery-shopping exercises, ensuring that these are designed to improve behaviour rather than to trap employees. Where failure occurs, management should examine staffing, training, supervision, store layout and commercial pressure rather than attributing the event solely to one individual.

The relationship between lawful and illicit retail remains central. Shops selling oversized, counterfeit or untaxed products may compete directly with businesses that follow the rules. Consumers may prefer the illegal product because it is cheaper, stronger or available in a prohibited format. Enforcement that focuses mainly on documentary errors among compliant retailers while visible illegal sales continue will undermine confidence in the system. Risk-based inspection should therefore distinguish between minor correctable deficiencies and deliberate commercial evasion. Resources should be directed towards products and businesses presenting the greatest combination of exposure, youth access, falsification and market scale.

Retail compliance is strongest when it is embedded in ordinary commercial management rather than treated as a folder prepared for inspection. Purchasing, stock control, staff training, age verification, complaints, recalls and supplier review should operate as connected processes. Information from one area should influence another. A complaint pattern should trigger stock review. A supplier's failure to provide documentation should affect approval status. A test-purchase failure should alter training and supervision. A regulatory alert should be matched against inventory immediately. This integration allows a relatively small business to exercise meaningful control without pretending to possess the capabilities of a regulator or laboratory.

The retailer's role is therefore neither passive nor unlimited. It is passive only in the sense that the retailer does not design the product or generate the original scientific dossier. It is active because the retailer chooses suppliers, selects stock, controls presentation, verifies age, observes consumer behaviour and provides the final opportunity to intercept obvious non-compliance. The standard should be reasonable competence: know the legal boundaries, retain traceable records, inspect what can be inspected, question what appears inconsistent and escalate matters that require technical assessment.

A well-regulated retail market depends on regulators making those duties practicable. Official product registers must be searchable and current. Guidance must explain how retailers can verify products without specialist knowledge. Alerts and recalls must reach businesses quickly. Enforcement expectations should be consistent enough that retailers understand what evidence will be accepted. Small shops should not be left to interpret complex regulatory databases unaided, while large chains should not be permitted to reduce compliance to central policies that are poorly implemented at store level.

Retail compliance ultimately determines whether upstream regulation survives contact with the market. A product may have been formulated responsibly, tested competently and notified correctly, yet still be sold to a child, separated from its warnings, stored badly, misrepresented or replaced by a counterfeit. Conversely, a vigilant retailer can identify doubtful stock, refuse an unlawful sale, preserve traceability and provide intelligence that prevents wider harm. The retail stage is therefore not the end of regulation but an active control point where product law, consumer protection and public health are applied through every day commercial decisions.

Importation

Importation is the point at which a vaping product crosses from international manufacture into the legal and enforcement system of the destination market. That transition is often treated as a logistical event involving freight, customs declarations and warehouse receipt, but in regulatory terms it is more significant. The importer may become the first economic operator within the jurisdiction capable of being identified, inspected and held responsible for the product. Where the overseas manufacturer has no domestic establishment, the importer is the practical link between the factory, regulator, distributor and consumer. Its obligations therefore extend beyond arranging transport. It must understand what has been purchased, whether the product is lawfully marketable, whether the supporting evidence is credible, whether the goods received correspond to the goods described and whether the supply chain remains traceable after customs clearance.

The first requirement is the clear identification of the importer and its legal role. Commercial arrangements can obscure responsibility because products may be ordered through trading companies, agents, freight forwarders, fulfilment businesses or distributors whose names differ from those shown on packaging and regulatory submissions. A company may believe that it is merely purchasing stock from an overseas supplier while the law regards it as the importer because it first places the goods on the domestic market. That distinction matters. The importer may be expected to verify notification or authorisation status, ensure that the product carries the correct labelling, retain supporting records, cooperate with enforcement authorities and organise corrective action where a defect is discovered. Responsibility cannot be avoided by describing the transaction as agency, drop shipping or private-label supply if the commercial reality shows that the business caused the product to enter the market.

Due diligence must begin before an order is placed. Price, flavour range, device appearance and promised delivery time are not sufficient bases for supplier approval. The importer should establish the legal identity of the manufacturer, the location of production, the relationship between the factory and any trading company, the product specification, the formulation owner and the party responsible for quality release. It should obtain current technical documents rather than generic certificates assembled for marketing. These may include product specifications, ingredient information, certificates of analysis, emissions data, safety assessments, quality-system evidence, battery documentation, packaging files and confirmation of applicable notifications. Documents should be checked for internal consistency. A test report referring to one coil, nicotine strength or product code cannot automatically support a different configuration. Likewise, a factory certificate does not prove that every batch manufactured at that site conforms to the relevant market requirements.

Private-label arrangements create additional risk because the importer may control the brand without controlling the underlying formulation or manufacturing process. A supplier may offer a catalogue product that can be relabelled rapidly, encouraging the belief that compliance transfers automatically with the product. In reality, a change in brand name, flavour description, nicotine concentration, device component or responsible operator can affect notification, labelling and technical documentation. The importer must know whether it is buying an existing, properly documented product or creating a new market variant that requires its own regulatory treatment. It should also understand whether the same factory produces visually identical goods for jurisdictions with different nicotine limits, reservoir capacities or warning requirements. The possibility of mixed production makes batch segregation and destination control essential.

Notification or authorisation status must be verified independently. Supplier assurances that a product is "registered", "approved" or "compliant" may be ambiguous or false. A submission made in one country may not permit sale in another, and a notification covering one flavour or nicotine strength may not extend to the entire range. The importer should match the exact product identity, including brand, type, flavour, strength and configuration, against the applicable register or regulatory record. It must also confirm that the party named in the submission corresponds to the responsible operator and that any required waiting period has expired before market placement. A regulatory identifier printed on packaging should not be accepted without verification because counterfeiters and careless suppliers can copy genuine numbers or apply them to products that differ from the original submission.

The physical product must be assessed against the documentary record. Importers should use pre-shipment samples, approved artwork and agreed specifications, but they must recognise that samples can be manufactured more carefully than ordinary production. Goods received should therefore undergo incoming inspection based on risk. Checks may include nicotine declaration, liquid volume, product dimensions, packaging integrity, warning text, batch coding, manufacturer and importer details, instructions, tamper evidence and security features. Where the product category presents a higher risk, independent analytical or functional testing may be justified. Sampling plans should reflect shipment size, supplier history and the consequences of non-compliance. Inspecting one unit from a large consignment provides only limited confidence where variation can occur across cartons, production lines or filling runs.

Nicotine concentration and liquid capacity are among the most common import concerns because both can be misstated deliberately or through poor manufacturing control. A device labelled within the legal limit may contain more liquid than declared, while a formulation intended for another market may exceed the permitted nicotine concentration. High claimed puff counts, unusual device dimensions or inconsistent weights may provide warning signals, but they do not substitute for measurement. Importers should establish acceptance criteria and commission testing where reasonable doubt exists. The laboratory method must be appropriate and the sample chain documented. A result showing a significant breach should trigger investigation of the consignment, not merely removal of the sampled unit, because the failure may represent the entire production batch or a broader supplier practice.

Customs compliance is related to product compliance but does not replace it. Correct commodity classification, valuation, origin and import declarations are necessary. However, customs clearance is not evidence that the product satisfies all health, consumer or nicotine-specific requirements. Border systems process enormous volumes of goods and frequently rely on information supplied by the importer or freight agent. A consignment can be released without detailed inspection, and an inaccurate declaration may remain undetected. Importers must therefore resist the assumption that clearance confers regulatory approval. They remain responsible for ensuring that the goods placed on the market comply with the relevant product rules, even where the border authority has taken no action.

The use of freight forwarders and customs agents can improve administrative accuracy, but responsibility for the underlying information remains with the importer. Agents may prepare entries based on descriptions, invoices and codes provided by the client. They are not ordinarily positioned to assess whether a liquid has been notified, whether flavour ingredients are acceptable or whether the device matches the submitted specification. Importers should provide precise product descriptions, maintain records supporting classification and review declarations before or after submission. Repeated use of vague descriptions such as electronic accessories, flavouring products or samples can create enforcement suspicion. Transparent declarations reduce the risk of seizure, delay and allegations of deliberate evasion.

Storage and transport conditions during importation can affect product integrity. Extended exposure to heat, freezing, sunlight, humidity or physical shock may alter liquids, damage seals or compromise batteries. Containers can remain in ports, vehicles and unconditioned warehouses for longer than expected. The importer should define suitable transport conditions, require appropriate packaging and assess whether excursions have occurred. Temperature monitoring may be warranted for sensitive or high-value shipments. Damaged cartons, leakage, swelling batteries, strong odours or staining should prompt quarantine and investigation. Goods should not be released merely because replacement would be expensive or delivery commitments have already been made. Commercial urgency is one of the principal pressures capable of overriding good import control.

Batch identification is essential from the moment the goods arrive. Each consignment should be linked to purchase orders, invoices, shipping records, customs entries, factory batch codes, quantities and downstream customers. Where manufacturers use weak or duplicated batch coding, the importer should require improvement or apply a controlled supplementary system without obscuring original information. Traceability should allow the business to identify which shipment contained a particular batch and where units were distributed. This capability supports targeted withdrawal, complaint investigation and enforcement cooperation. Without it, a problem affecting one production run may require removal of an entire range, or affected products may remain in circulation because their destination cannot be established.

The importer must also control changes. Overseas manufacturers may substitute components, flavour suppliers, battery cells, plastics, coil materials or packaging without recognising the regulatory significance. A change that appears minor to the factory can alter emissions, nicotine delivery, stability, safety or legal status. Supply agreements should therefore prohibit unapproved changes and require prior notification. The importer should compare incoming goods with approved specifications and investigate unexplained differences in colour, weight, dimensions, performance or packaging. Periodic requalification is necessary because a supplier that performed acceptably during initial assessment may decline as volumes increase, ownership changes or cost pressures intensify. Long commercial familiarity is not a substitute for ongoing oversight.

Counterfeit and unauthorised production present a particular challenge where legitimate factories operate alongside brokers and subcontractors. Goods may be produced after hours, made with rejected components or assembled at an undisclosed site while carrying the branding and documentation of the approved product. The importer should understand the manufacturer's control over tooling, artwork, labels and security features. Serialisation, authentication codes and tamper features can help, but they are only effective when supported by secure data and controlled issuance. Codes generated in predictable sequences or verified through easily copied websites provide limited protection. Sudden price reductions, changes in payment destination, inconsistent cartons or unexplained shipping routes should be treated as possible indicators of diversion or counterfeit supply.

Importers are also responsible for responding to intelligence after market entry. Complaints from retailers and consumers may reveal defects that were not detected during incoming inspection. Reports of leakage, incorrect nicotine strength, unusual taste, battery overheating or packaging differences should be linked back to the relevant shipment and supplier. The importer should retain reference samples where proportionate and maintain access to documentation needed for investigation. Serious concerns require prompt quarantine of remaining stock and communication with distributors, retailers and regulators. Delay increases the number of consumers exposed and can transform a manageable withdrawal into a national recall.

Corrective action must address the cause rather than the immediate consignment alone. If testing identifies excessive nicotine concentration, the importer should determine whether the problem arose from formulation calculation, raw-material assay, mixing, filling, labelling or deliberate substitution. If capacity exceeds the limit, the device specification, tooling and production records should be examined. Supplier explanations should be supported by evidence, and repeat testing may be necessary. Continued purchasing should depend on credible corrective and preventive action. A supplier that replaces stock without explaining the failure remains a regulatory risk. Commercial dependence on one factory can make suspension difficult, but that dependence does not justify exposing the market to repeated non-compliance.

Enforcement authorities may require importers to provide records, samples, test reports and details of downstream supply. A competent importer should be able to respond quickly and coherently. Missing documents, inconsistent product names or inability to identify the manufacturer can suggest that the business lacks effective control. Cooperation should include preserving evidence and preventing further distribution while questions are resolved. Where goods are detained at the border, the importer may challenge the decision through appropriate procedures, but it should not attempt to reroute or re-declare the same products to evade scrutiny. Deliberate circumvention can convert a technical dispute into evidence of dishonest conduct.

The most effective importer combines commercial knowledge with regulatory discipline. It verifies exact product status, qualifies factories, controls specifications, inspects incoming goods, preserves customs and batch records, monitors changes and acts decisively when evidence suggests a defect. This does not require every importer to maintain a laboratory, but it does require access to competent testing and the judgement to know when it is needed. Importers cannot guarantee that every unit is perfect, yet they can ensure that uncertainty is managed rather than ignored. Their role is decisive because the border between overseas production and domestic sale is where responsibility must become visible.

Distribution

Distribution is the regulatory bridge between importation or manufacture and the point of sale. Once a vaping product has entered the domestic market, it may pass through several intermediaries before reaching the consumer. Each transfer creates an opportunity to preserve product identity, documentation and traceability, but also an opportunity for those controls to weaken. A product that was correctly manufactured, notified and imported can become difficult to verify if cartons are split, outer packaging is discarded, batch details are not recorded or stock is mixed with similar goods from other sources. Distribution therefore cannot be treated as a neutral movement of boxes. It is a controlled stage within the product lifecycle in which lawful market status must remain attached to the physical goods.

The distributor's first responsibility is to know what it is receiving and from whom. Stock should arrive through an approved supplier supported by invoices, delivery records, product identifiers, batch information and contact details for the responsible manufacturer or importer. Vaping markets change quickly, and legitimate wholesalers may introduce new ranges faster than their internal compliance systems can manage. Distributors should therefore confirm that each product variant is intended for the jurisdiction, carries the required packaging and warnings, corresponds to the relevant notification or authorisation record and has not been altered after regulatory submission. A product family may contain lawful and unlawful variants under nearly identical branding, making precise identification essential.

Incoming-goods control should be proportionate to risk and volume. A distributor is not normally expected to repeat the full scientific assessment performed by the producer, but it should inspect consignments for obvious inconsistencies before stock is released. This includes checking brand, flavour, nicotine strength, package language, warning statements, declared capacity, batch coding, importer details and packaging integrity. Cartons that differ from approved artwork, products with missing identifiers, mixed nicotine strengths or inconsistent security features should be quarantined pending clarification. Distributors handling large quantities should use documented sampling procedures rather than relying on casual visual checks. Where a supplier has a history of errors, the level of inspection should increase, and repeated failures should affect approval status rather than being managed indefinitely through credit notes and replacement stock.

Traceability is the defining distribution control. Every product received should be linked to the supplier, purchase order, date of receipt, quantity, batch or lot code and downstream customer. If a regulator identifies an unsafe batch, the distributor should be able to determine how many units were received, how many remain in stock and which retailers obtained the rest. Without that information, corrective action becomes either incomplete or unnecessarily broad. A system that records only product names and quantities may be inadequate where multiple batches, suppliers or specification versions circulate under the same brand.

Batch coding can be problematic because some manufacturers use codes that are difficult to read, duplicated between production runs or applied only to outer cartons. Once cartons are opened and individual units are redistributed, the connection to the original batch may be lost. Distributors should therefore preserve outer packaging information and, where necessary, record batch details at unit, tray or case level. They should avoid relabelling products in ways that obscure the manufacturer's code or create confusion over origin. Where supplementary warehouse labels are used, these should support rather than replace the original identity. Poor batch discipline is especially dangerous in high-volume operations where similar flavours, strengths and device formats are stored close together.

Stock segregation prevents legal and operational errors. Products intended for different jurisdictions may have different nicotine limits, warnings, tax status, packaging or notification requirements despite looking almost identical. Goods awaiting clearance, under investigation, returned by retailers, damaged in transit or subject to recall should be physically and electronically separated from saleable stock. Quarantine status must be clear enough that warehouse staff cannot release affected goods by mistake. This requires controlled locations, restricted system access and defined authorisation for release. A handwritten note on a pallet is not a reliable control where stock moves rapidly, temporary staff are used or several shifts operate.

Storage conditions influence whether the product supplied remains the product originally assessed. E-liquids can change through heat, light, oxygen exposure and prolonged storage, while batteries and electronic components may be damaged by temperature extremes, moisture, crushing or impact. Distributors should define acceptable warehouse conditions, monitor them where necessary and protect goods from direct sunlight, freezing, excessive heat and physical damage. Inventory should be rotated using first-expiry-first-out or an equivalent system where shelf-life information is available. Products approaching expiry, showing leakage, discolouration, swelling or damaged seals should be reviewed before dispatch.

Order fulfilment presents another opportunity for compliance failure. Similar product names, flavours and nicotine strengths can lead to picking errors, especially where packaging differs only in small text or colour. Supplying the wrong strength is not a trivial warehouse mistake because it can expose consumers to an unintended nicotine concentration and create inaccurate retail labelling. Barcode systems, clear location coding, independent checks and scan verification can reduce these risks. Manual processes require particular care, including line clearance, separation of look-alike stock and verification before dispatch. Error rates should be measured and investigated rather than accepted as an inevitable feature of high-volume distribution.

Distributors also influence which products become commercially prominent. Their purchasing decisions determine what reaches retailers, how quickly new brands expand and whether questionable suppliers gain market access. A distributor that prioritises low price and novelty without examining product status can introduce non-compliant stock across a wide retail network within days. Conversely, a competent distributor can act as an effective gatekeeper by refusing products with incomplete documentation, implausible specifications or irresponsible presentation. This gatekeeping role is especially important for small retailers that rely heavily on wholesaler assurances and may lack the resources to investigate every product independently.

Commercial pressure can undermine that role. Rapidly selling products generate demand from retailers, and distributors may fear losing customers if they delay supply while compliance questions are resolved. Competitors may offer the same goods immediately, creating an incentive to accept supplier assurances without verification. The regulatory consequence of this pressure is market acceleration without control. Once stock has been divided among hundreds of shops, recovery becomes more difficult and expensive. A short delay before release is therefore often less damaging than a later withdrawal. Distribution procedures should give compliance personnel authority to block stock without requiring them to prove definitively that a breach has occurred.

Returns require controlled handling. Retailers may send back unsold stock, damaged units, customer complaints, recalled products or goods supplied in error. Returned products should not automatically re-enter saleable inventory. The distributor must identify why they were returned, whether seals remain intact, whether storage conditions are known and whether the batch is subject to investigation. Products associated with leakage, battery damage, unusual taste, incorrect labelling or suspected counterfeiting should be quarantined and escalated. Repeated returns from different retailers may reveal a systemic problem that would not be visible if each case were processed only as a commercial credit.

Complaint information should therefore be aggregated and reviewed. Distributors occupy a valuable position because they receive feedback from multiple retailers across a broad market. One shop may report a leaking pod, another a burnt taste and a third a device that overheats. Considered separately, these may appear isolated; considered together, they may indicate a batch defect or design problem. Complaint systems should record product identity, batch, customer, date, nature of failure and any sample retained. Significant trends should be reported to the importer or manufacturer, and serious concerns should trigger immediate stock review. The distributor should not wait for absolute proof where continued supply could increase exposure.

Product withdrawals and recalls depend heavily on distribution capability. When instructed to stop supply, the distributor must identify affected stock, block further dispatch, notify customers and preserve records of the action taken. A recall notice sent by email is insufficient if the business cannot confirm that retailers received and understood it. Follow-up may be necessary, particularly where products have been supplied to small independent outlets with limited administrative capacity. The distributor should reconcile quantities received, held, dispatched, returned and destroyed. Any discrepancy should be investigated because missing units may remain available to consumers or be diverted into informal channels.

Destruction must also be controlled. Nicotine liquids, batteries and electronic devices cannot simply be discarded as ordinary waste. Recalled or non-compliant goods should be handled through authorised waste routes appropriate to their chemical and electrical components. Records should identify the quantity, product, reason for destruction, contractor and date. Where enforcement authorities require evidence, certificates or witnessed destruction may be necessary. Unsaleable stock should not be resold through secondary markets, exported casually to another country or transferred to unknown brokers. Moving a regulatory problem elsewhere is not corrective action.

Counterfeit and diverted products present a distinctive distribution risk. A distributor may receive goods that appear genuine but entered through an unauthorised channel, were manufactured outside the brand owner's control or were intended for another jurisdiction. Price anomalies, inconsistent packaging, altered authentication codes, missing invoices or unusual payment arrangements should trigger scrutiny. Products sourced from liquidation sales, informal brokers or overseas surplus markets require particular caution. Genuine branding does not guarantee lawful status. A genuine product can still be non-compliant if it was not intended, notified or labelled for the destination market.

Tax and duty controls increasingly intersect with distribution. Where vaping products become subject to excise, stamps, warehouse requirements or movement controls, distributors must distinguish duty-paid stock from goods held under suspension or imported unlawfully. Fiscal non-compliance can coexist with product compliance, and both affect market legitimacy. Records must allow authorities to trace quantities, movements and tax status. The introduction of duty also increases the incentive for diversion, false declarations and illicit wholesale supply. Distribution systems therefore need to integrate product identity with fiscal identity rather than treating tax as a separate accounting matter.

Online fulfilment has blurred the distinction between distributor and retailer. A warehouse may store stock for multiple sellers, pick orders automatically and dispatch directly to consumers without owning the goods or controlling the website listing. Nevertheless, its operations can enable unlawful supply at scale. Fulfilment businesses should know their commercial customers, retain product and transaction records and respond to enforcement notices. They may not be responsible for every claim made by a seller, but they should not continue shipping products known to be illegal, recalled or associated with false identities. The practical ability to stop dispatch makes them part of the enforcement chain.

Regulatory inspections of distributors should examine more than the warehouse floor. Authorities may review supplier approval, notification checks, traceability, batch records, quarantine controls, complaints, recalls and customer lists. Sampling may compare products with declared nicotine strength or capacity, while documentary review can reveal whether goods came through legitimate importers. Distributors should be able to produce records promptly and explain discrepancies. Missing invoices, retrospective paperwork or inconsistent quantities may indicate weak control or deliberate concealment. Cooperation is particularly important because the distributor's records can expose the wider network through which illegal goods have moved.

The standard expected should remain proportionate. A small regional wholesaler may not require the same software or staffing as a national distribution centre, but both must preserve product identity, control stock and support corrective action. Paper records can be acceptable if accurate and retrievable; complex digital systems are ineffective if data are incomplete. The essential test is whether the business can demonstrate what it received, where it came from, what happened to it and how quickly it can stop supply when necessary.

Distribution is therefore not a passive interval between importation and retail. It is the stage at which products are multiplied across the market, and small failures can become widespread exposure. Competent distributors protect the integrity of lawful products, filter out doubtful stock, preserve traceability and convert recalls into practical action. Weak distributors obscure origin, fragment batches and allow non-compliance to spread faster than regulators can respond. The quality of distribution control consequently determines whether upstream compliance remains connected to the products consumers actually encounter.

Online Sales

Online vape sales have transformed the commercial structure of the vaping market by separating the point of purchase from the physical location of the seller, the stock and, in many cases, the jurisdiction responsible for enforcement. A consumer can view a product on a website hosted in one country, pay through a processor based in another, receive goods from a fulfilment warehouse elsewhere and deal with a seller whose legal identity is difficult to establish. This fragmentation creates convenience and broad consumer access, but it also weakens many of the controls that operate naturally in physical retail. A shop can inspect identification, observe suspicious behaviour, display warnings, retain local stock records and be visited by enforcement officers. An online seller depends on digital systems to perform equivalent functions, while regulators must identify the commercial actors behind listings that can be altered, removed or recreated rapidly. Online compliance must therefore be treated as a complete commercial and regulatory system rather than as a website attached to an ordinary retail business.

The first requirement is the clear identification of the seller. A compliant website should disclose the legal business name, trading address, contact details and other information required by consumer and electronic-commerce law. These details allow customers to understand who is supplying the product and give regulators a point of accountability if the goods are unsafe, unnotified or otherwise unlawful. Anonymous websites, disposable email addresses, payment requests to unrelated individuals and the absence of a verifiable business address are warning signs that the seller may be operating outside normal regulatory controls. Social-media accounts and private messaging services intensify this problem because a commercial operation can present itself informally, move between accounts and accept payment without any durable public record. A seller that cannot be identified cannot support meaningful recall, complaint investigation or enforcement.

Age verification is the most visible online compliance challenge. In a physical shop, staff can observe the customer and inspect identification at the point of sale. Online systems must establish age without direct contact and without creating an easy route for minors to enter false information. A simple tick box confirming that the purchaser is over the legal age is weak because it relies entirely on self-declaration. Entry of a date of birth provides little more protection if no independent check follows. Stronger systems compare personal information against reliable data sources, require recognised identification, use payment or identity verification and apply further checks where the information does not match. The process should occur before the order is completed rather than merely when the customer enters the website, because an age-gate screen alone does not prevent purchase.

Age assurance must also extend to delivery. An online seller may conduct a competent digital check and still supply the product to a minor if the parcel is left unattended, delivered to an alternative address or accepted by another person without verification. Age-verified delivery can provide an additional control, but its effectiveness depends on the courier, the instructions attached to the parcel and the behaviour of the delivery driver. Systems that allow redirection to lockers, neighbours or safe places can undermine the original check. Retailers should therefore understand how their carrier handles age-restricted goods, whether proof of age is requested and how failed deliveries are recorded. Delivery is not separate from the sale; it is the final stage of the age-control process.

Proxy purchasing remains possible online. An adult can place an order for a minor using genuine identification, and no digital system can eliminate that risk completely. The appropriate response is to reduce obvious vulnerabilities rather than claim perfect prevention. Unusual purchasing patterns, repeated orders to school-related addresses, multiple accounts using the same payment method or a sudden concentration of youth-oriented products may justify review. Retailers must avoid discriminatory or arbitrary profiling, but they can use transaction monitoring to identify behaviour inconsistent with ordinary adult purchasing. Clear terms prohibiting proxy supply, refusal of suspicious orders and cooperation with enforcement authorities can strengthen the system, particularly where the same customer repeatedly attempts to circumvent controls.

Product verification is equally important online because consumers cannot inspect the physical package before purchase. The listing becomes the principal source of information and must correspond accurately to the product supplied. Brand, flavour, nicotine strength, liquid volume, device type, warnings, package contents and responsible operator should be described clearly. Stock photographs reused across several variants can mislead where the delivered product differs in strength, capacity or packaging. Sellers should avoid presenting one image for a product family when individual versions have different regulatory status. The exact product offered should be traceable to an applicable notification or authorisation record, and a general claim that the brand is registered should not be used to imply that every flavour and configuration is lawful.

Online descriptions create particular risk around health and regulatory claims. Terms such as approved, certified safe, harmless, medical, clean or healthy may give consumers an inaccurate impression of regulatory assessment. A notified product is not necessarily approved in the sense applied to a medicine, and inclusion on a regulatory list does not establish the absence of risk. Sellers often copy language supplied by manufacturers or distributors, but publication on a retail website is a fresh commercial communication for which the seller may carry responsibility. Relative-risk information should be accurate, contextual and directed towards adult smokers rather than presented as a general lifestyle benefit. Claims concerning smoking cessation, therapeutic effect or disease reduction require especially careful control because they may cross into medicinal presentation or unsupported advertising.

Flavour names, product imagery and digital promotion deserve close scrutiny because online platforms allow highly visual marketing to reach audiences beyond existing adult consumers. Bright graphics, animation, confectionery references, cartoons, influencer content and short-form video can make nicotine products appear ordinary, fashionable or youth-oriented. Even where the product itself is lawful, the method of presentation may attract regulatory concern. Online retailers should assess the combined effect of product names, page design, promotional banners, discounts and social-media content rather than examining each item in isolation. A statutory warning placed in small text does little to counter a page dominated by imagery associated with sweets, gaming or youth culture.

Advertising restrictions apply differently across media and jurisdictions, making online compliance particularly complex. A retailer may lawfully provide factual information necessary for a consumer to make a purchase while being restricted from using broader promotional communications. The boundary between a product listing and advertising can become blurred when websites use countdown offers, affiliate links, competitions, influencer endorsements, referral bonuses or targeted social-media campaigns. Sellers should distinguish between making a product available and actively promoting nicotine consumption. Commercial affiliates should be subject to written rules, approval processes and monitoring because the retailer may suffer regulatory and reputational consequences from claims made by third parties acting on its behalf.

Cross-border distance sales create another layer of responsibility. A product lawful in the seller's home market may be prohibited, restricted or subject to a different notification process in the customer's country. Nicotine limits, flavours, tax, packaging, language, age requirements and product classifications vary considerably. A website visible internationally does not automatically create the right to sell everywhere. Sellers should define the territories they serve, restrict checkout where lawful supply cannot be demonstrated and maintain jurisdiction-specific product catalogues where necessary. Shipping a domestic product into another market without checking local requirements can turn an otherwise compliant business into an unauthorised importer or distance seller.

Marketplaces complicate responsibility because the platform, seller and fulfilment operator may be separate. A marketplace may describe itself as a neutral intermediary while controlling search rankings, payment, advertising, warehousing and delivery. Individual sellers can disappear after enforcement action and reappear under new names, while identical products continue to circulate through other accounts. Platforms should require verified seller identities, evidence of lawful product status and rapid removal of recalled or illegal goods. They should preserve transaction and account data for legitimate investigations and prevent repeat offenders from opening new accounts using related details. Voluntary measures are useful, but the scale of marketplace commerce increasingly supports formal duties proportionate to the platform's practical control.

Dropshipping creates similar uncertainty. The seller may never handle the product and may rely entirely on an overseas supplier to select, pack and dispatch the order. This business model reduces inventory cost but weakens the seller's knowledge of the physical goods. Product specifications, packaging and even the identity of the manufacturer may change without warning. A domestic website can therefore present itself as a local retailer while the consumer receives an undeclared direct import from abroad. A seller using dropshipping remains responsible for understanding what is supplied, whether it is lawful and how complaints or recalls will be managed. Commercial distance from the product does not remove regulatory responsibility.

Payment providers and advertising platforms can influence online compliance by restricting access to the infrastructure required for unlawful trade. Sellers operating anonymously often depend on mainstream payment services, search advertising or social-media promotion to reach customers. When these services verify business identity and respond to regulatory notices, illegal supply becomes more difficult. Excessive reliance on private platform decisions can be problematic because lawful businesses may be suspended without clear appeal, but complete indifference allows repeat offenders to exploit the same services. Cooperation should therefore be based on transparent legal standards, reliable evidence and proportionate processes rather than informal pressure alone.

Record keeping is essential because online sellers generate detailed transaction data that can support traceability and enforcement. Orders should be linked to product identity, batch information where available, customer delivery details, payment, dispatch date and carrier. Privacy law requires appropriate protection and limited retention, but it does not prevent businesses from maintaining records necessary for legal compliance, complaints and recalls. If a batch must be withdrawn, the seller should be able to identify affected customers and contact them directly. This is a practical advantage over anonymous cash retail, provided the data are accurate and accessible.

Complaints and adverse events should be integrated into the online system. Consumers need a clear route to report leakage, battery failure, incorrect nicotine strength, damaged packaging or other concerns. Automated customer-service responses should not prevent technical escalation where several reports involve the same product. Returned products should be quarantined and assessed rather than placed back into stock. Trends across reviews, refunds and support messages can reveal defects earlier than formal regulatory reports, but only if the seller analyses them rather than treating each case as an isolated service issue.

Enforcement of online sales requires coordinated action. Authorities may use test purchases, website monitoring, payment records, parcel interception and platform notices to establish breaches. A listing can be captured as evidence before it is removed, while the delivered product can be compared with the claims made online. Action against the website alone may be insufficient if the seller continues through social media, marketplaces or a replacement domain. Effective enforcement follows the business identity, stock source, payment flow and fulfilment chain rather than focusing solely on one web address.

Cybersecurity forms part of responsible online operation because identities, age-verification records, payment details and order histories are sensitive data. Weak systems can expose consumers to fraud and undermine confidence in retailers. Businesses should minimise collected data, restrict access, maintain secure platforms and prepare for breaches. Compliance technology should support lawful sales without creating surveillance, while third-party verification providers should be selected and monitored with the care applied to product suppliers.

Online vape sales can support adult access, particularly for consumers who lack specialist local retailers or require products not stocked nearby. They can also provide detailed information, broad choice and direct recall communication. Those benefits depend on regulatory equivalence with physical retail rather than exemption from it. A compliant online seller must identify itself, verify age, control delivery, describe products accurately, restrict claims, observe jurisdictional boundaries, retain records and respond to safety concerns. The central principle is that digital convenience must not dissolve responsibility. The route to market may be virtual, but the product, exposure and public health consequences remain entirely real.

Enforcement

Enforcement is the mechanism through which regulatory requirements become more than statements of intention. Product notifications, ingredient restrictions, nicotine limits, packaging rules, age controls, manufacturing obligations and online sales requirements only protect the public when authorities can detect breaches, identify the responsible operator, secure evidence and impose consequences quickly enough to change behaviour. In the vaping market, this task is difficult because products evolve, supply chains cross jurisdictions, retailers range from major chains to informal sellers, and unlawful goods can move through shops, websites, marketplaces, messaging services and small-parcel imports. Enforcement must therefore operate as an integrated system combining intelligence, inspection, laboratory capability, legal authority and commercial understanding. A framework that lacks any one of these elements may appear strict while remaining weak in practice.

The first challenge is identifying what should be enforced. Vaping products can fail in many different ways. A product may be unnotified, incorrectly labelled, over the permitted nicotine concentration, larger than the legal capacity, supplied in defective packaging, sold to a child, advertised unlawfully, manufactured outside specification or imported without a responsible economic operator. Some failures are documentary, others technical, commercial or deliberate. Effective enforcement must distinguish between them because the appropriate response depends on the nature and seriousness of the breach. A missing document may require correction, while falsified records, dangerous batteries or deliberate youth sales may justify seizure, prosecution or business closure. Treating every failure as identical either wastes resources on minor defects or allows serious misconduct to be absorbed into routine administrative action.

Detection begins with intelligence. Complaints from consumers, retailers, manufacturers, schools, healthcare professionals and competitors can reveal products or businesses requiring attention. Market surveillance data, online monitoring, customs records, product registers, social-media advertising and test-purchase results can provide signals. No single source is sufficient. Competitor complaints may be commercially motivated, consumer reports may be incomplete and online listings may not correspond to the product actually delivered. Authorities must therefore corroborate information and identify patterns. Repeated reports concerning the same brand, importer, retailer or product feature are more significant than isolated allegations. Intelligence-led enforcement allows limited resources to be directed towards areas where the combination of scale, exposure and deliberate evasion is greatest.

Inspection remains the most visible enforcement activity. Officers may visit retailers, warehouses, distributors and importers to examine stock, records, labelling, supplier information and age-control systems. A competent inspection should go beyond surface appearance. Professional packaging does not prove lawful status, and a product carrying familiar branding may be counterfeit or intended for another market. Officers need access to current product registers, guidance on legal limits and practical tools for identifying suspicious goods. They should be able to distinguish between nicotine concentration, total nicotine content, tank capacity, refill-container volume and claimed puff count. Without this technical understanding, inspections risk focusing on obvious presentation defects while missing more significant non-compliance concealed within the product.

Sampling and laboratory testing are often necessary because many breaches cannot be established visually. Nicotine concentration, liquid capacity, undeclared ingredients, metals, carbonyls and battery performance may require measurement. The evidential quality of testing is therefore critical. Samples must be obtained through documented procedures, sealed, identified and transported in a manner that preserves integrity. Laboratories should use validated or otherwise defensible methods and report uncertainty clearly. A result that exceeds a legal limit only marginally may require careful interpretation where analytical uncertainty overlaps the threshold. Conversely, gross breaches should not be obscured by unnecessary technical debate. Enforcement science must be sufficiently rigorous to withstand challenge without becoming so slow or complex that unlawful products remain on sale throughout the process.

The legal pathway following detection should be proportionate, transparent and capable of escalation. Authorities may begin with advice, warning letters, improvement notices or voluntary withdrawal where the business is cooperative and the breach is limited. Stronger action may include formal seizure, suspension, fixed penalties, licence consequences, injunctions or prosecution. Escalation should reflect risk, intent, history and response. A retailer that unknowingly receives one defective batch and acts immediately is not equivalent to a trader repeatedly selling oversized products after warnings. Proportionality protects fairness, but it should not become a reason for endless informal engagement with operators whose business model depends on non-compliance. Repeated warnings without consequence can teach the market that breaches are commercially tolerable.

Speed is central to enforcement effectiveness. Vaping products can be sold rapidly, rebranded quickly and replaced before an investigation concludes. A slow process may establish liability only after the stock has disappeared and the company has dissolved. Authorities therefore need powers to detain suspect goods, stop supply and preserve evidence while technical assessment continues. Interim action should be used carefully because it can harm legitimate businesses, but delay also carries public-health costs. The decision should consider the plausibility and seriousness of the risk, the scale of distribution and the ease with which the product could continue moving. Fast containment followed by disciplined investigation is often more effective than waiting for complete certainty before acting.

Local variation creates another difficulty. Enforcement responsibilities may be distributed among national regulators, local Trading Standards teams, customs authorities, tax bodies, advertising regulators and environmental agencies. Each may control a different part of the market. A product can therefore be compliant under one area of law and unlawful under another, or several agencies may possess partial information without seeing the complete pattern. Coordination is essential. Product identifiers, batch data, importer records, seizure information and test results should be shared through compatible systems. Where one authority identifies a problem, others should know whether the same goods are appearing elsewhere. Fragmentation allows unlawful operators to exploit gaps between institutional mandates and geographical boundaries.

Resource inequality is one of the most persistent weaknesses. Large markets can contain thousands of products and retailers, while enforcement teams may be small and responsible for many unrelated duties. Laboratory analysis, legal proceedings and specialist training are expensive. As a result, enforcement may become complaint-driven rather than systematic, with action concentrated on the most visible outlets while online sellers, informal wholesalers and cross-border networks remain harder to reach. This produces an asymmetry in which compliant businesses are easy to inspect because they have stable premises and records, while deliberate offenders are more elusive. Risk-based strategy must therefore avoid equating accessibility with priority. The businesses easiest to visit are not always those causing the greatest harm.

The growth of illegal products makes sanction design particularly important. Where profits are high and detection rates low, modest fines may be treated as a business cost. Penalties must remove the financial advantage of evasion and account for the scale of offending. Seizure of stock, recovery of proceeds, director accountability and restrictions on future trading may be necessary for organised or repeated breaches. At the same time, sanctions should not be so indiscriminate that minor procedural failures threaten otherwise responsible businesses disproportionately. The credibility of the system depends on visible distinction between error and deception. Severe penalties are most defensible where evidence shows falsification, concealment, repeated youth sales, dangerous products or deliberate circumvention of prior enforcement action.

Online enforcement requires different methods from physical inspection. Authorities may use test purchases, capture website content, trace payment flows, identify hosting and fulfilment providers and request platform cooperation. Removing one listing is rarely sufficient because sellers can reappear under new accounts or domains. Enforcement must follow the underlying business identity, stock source and transaction infrastructure. Marketplaces and social-media companies should preserve relevant data, verify sellers and prevent repeat offenders from reopening accounts through minor changes in identity. Payment providers, couriers and fulfilment warehouses can also support disruption where lawful authority exists. This networked approach recognises that online trade depends on infrastructure even when the visible seller is difficult to locate.

Border enforcement is similarly dependent on intelligence rather than universal inspection. Vaping products may be misdeclared as electronics, flavourings, samples or accessories, while consignments are divided into small parcels or routed through intermediate countries. Customs officers need risk profiles based on importer history, product type, unusual values, repeated seizures and known supply networks. When suspect goods are found, they require rapid access to product rules and technical support. A device may appear oversized but need measurement; a nicotine-free label may require chemical confirmation. The border should connect to domestic surveillance so that findings inform later inspections and retail discoveries can be traced back to import activity.

Evidence management determines whether enforcement survives challenge. Photographs, samples, invoices, product records, website captures, witness statements and laboratory reports must be preserved in a coherent chain. Poor documentation can undermine otherwise obvious cases. Officers need procedures that are legally sound but practical enough for routine use. Businesses should also have a fair opportunity to understand the allegation and present relevant evidence. Transparency strengthens legitimacy and reduces the risk that enforcement becomes arbitrary. However, procedural fairness should not allow delay tactics to defeat action where risk is clear and stock continues to circulate.

Public communication is another part of enforcement. Alerts, recalls and published actions can inform consumers and deter businesses, but they must be accurate. Naming a product before identity is confirmed can damage a legitimate brand, particularly where counterfeits are involved. Conversely, vague warnings may fail to help consumers recognise affected goods. Communications should identify the product, batch, risk, action required and responsible contact wherever possible. Authorities should distinguish between a notified genuine product and a counterfeit or unauthorised variant. The purpose is to reduce exposure and support informed action, not merely demonstrate institutional activity.

Enforcement should also produce learning. Each case can reveal weaknesses in legislation, product definitions, supply chains or surveillance methods. Repeated discovery of the same circumvention may indicate that the rule is poorly drafted or that sanctions are inadequate. Frequent mislabelling may show that supplier guidance is unclear. Persistent illegal capacities may reveal weak border controls or strong consumer demand that policy has not addressed. Case data should therefore feed back into regulatory design, technical standards and resource allocation. Enforcement is not only the final stage of regulation; it is a source of evidence about how the market responds to the law.

The relationship with responsible industry is important but must remain controlled. Manufacturers, distributors and retailers often possess information about counterfeit products, suspicious suppliers and emerging evasion techniques. Authorities can benefit from this intelligence, particularly where criminal networks move faster than formal systems. Commercial reports must still be verified because businesses may seek action against competitors. Transparent channels for reporting, combined with independent assessment, can improve detection without allowing enforcement priorities to be privately dictated.

Consumer participation also matters. People who encounter leaking products, unexpected effects, illegal sales or misleading websites may provide the first warning of a problem. Reporting routes should be simple and should capture sufficient detail to support investigation. Consumers should not be expected to determine which law has been breached. Their role is to describe what happened and identify the product or seller. Authorities can then assess whether the report indicates a wider pattern.

Effective enforcement ultimately depends on credibility. Businesses must believe that serious breaches are likely to be detected and punished, while compliant operators must believe that the system recognises their investment. Consumers must be able to distinguish lawful from unlawful products and trust that alerts are meaningful. Regulators must possess enough technical competence to challenge false documents, interpret laboratory evidence and understand how products are modified around legal boundaries. Enforcement that is sporadic, slow or focused mainly on paperwork will not control a market characterised by rapid innovation and profitable evasion.

The strongest system is intelligence-led, scientifically competent, coordinated and proportionate. It directs resources towards the products and conduct presenting the greatest risk, acts quickly enough to prevent continued distribution, preserves evidence properly and escalates sanctions where behaviour does not change. It also reviews outcomes, because seizure numbers and prosecution totals do not by themselves prove improved public health. Success lies in reducing unlawful availability, protecting children, removing dangerous products and ensuring that responsible businesses are not undercut by those avoiding the rules. Regulation becomes real only when enforcement consistently changes what reaches the market.

Border Control

Border control is the point at which national product regulation encounters the physical movement of goods. Vaping products arrive in shipping containers, air freight, courier consignments, postal packets, passenger luggage and mixed commercial loads. Components may be imported separately and assembled domestically, while liquids, devices, packaging and batteries may travel under different commodity descriptions. A product can therefore cross the border without appearing in documentation as a complete vaping product at all. Effective border control depends less on inspecting every item than on identifying risk, connecting declarations to product intelligence and ensuring that goods released into the market remain traceable to a responsible importer.

The difficulty is scale. Border authorities process vast quantities of legitimate trade and cannot examine every parcel, pallet or container. Inspection must be selective, which means that risk assessment becomes more important than physical presence alone. Importer history, declared origin, product description, shipment value, route, frequency, previous seizures and known associations with non-compliant suppliers can all influence targeting. A newly formed company importing unusually large quantities of low-value electronic devices may warrant closer examination than an established operator with a consistent compliance record. Equally, a familiar importer should not be treated as permanently low risk, because suppliers, product ranges and commercial pressures can change. Risk profiling must remain dynamic and informed by domestic market findings rather than relying only on customs data.

Accurate declaration is central to this system. Goods may be described broadly as electronic accessories, flavouring liquids, atomiser parts, batteries or samples, even where their intended use is within a regulated nicotine product. Some vague descriptions result from poor understanding, while others are designed to avoid scrutiny, duty or product-specific controls. Border authorities need access to commercial invoices, packing lists, product images and supporting documentation sufficient to determine what the goods actually are. Where descriptions are incomplete or inconsistent, the importer should be required to clarify them. Repeated use of misleading codes, implausible valuations or declarations that omit nicotine content may indicate deliberate concealment rather than administrative error.

Commodity classification alone cannot establish product compliance. A consignment may be declared under the correct customs heading and still contain products that exceed legal capacity, carry excessive nicotine concentration, lack notification, use prohibited presentation or omit required warnings. Customs systems are designed primarily to control importation, valuation, origin and revenue, whereas vaping regulation also involves health, product safety, labelling and market-status requirements. The release of goods by customs therefore does not amount to regulatory approval. Importers remain responsible for compliance after clearance, and border officers require routes to consult the agencies holding product registers and technical expertise where a shipment raises concerns beyond ordinary customs matters.

Information sharing is consequently fundamental. Border authorities may detect a suspicious consignment but need confirmation from a national regulator or Trading Standards body concerning notification status, legal nicotine limits, product capacity or packaging requirements. Domestic enforcement teams may discover illegal products in shops but lack visibility over how they entered the country. When these systems operate separately, intelligence becomes fragmented. A seizure at the border may be treated as an isolated event even though identical goods are already circulating nationally. Conversely, repeated retail discoveries may not influence border targeting because the product names, importer details and shipment routes have not been entered into a shared intelligence system.

Product identifiers can help connect these records, but only when they are reliable. Brand names, model numbers, flavours and nicotine strengths may be inconsistent across packaging, notifications and customs documents. Counterfeiters can copy genuine identifiers, while traders may alter names slightly to create the appearance of a different product. Border control therefore requires more than a name search. Officers may need to compare packaging, responsible-operator details, batch codes, device dimensions and technical characteristics with the product record. A product that resembles a notified item may still be an unauthorised variant, a counterfeit or a version intended for another jurisdiction. Exact identity is necessary before lawful status can be inferred.

Small-parcel traffic has weakened traditional inspection methods. Online sellers and overseas suppliers can ship individual products directly to consumers or retailers, dividing what would once have been a commercial consignment into hundreds of packets. Each parcel has a low value and may attract little attention, yet the total market impact can be substantial. High-volume small-parcel imports are difficult because the sender, purchaser and product description may vary, while automated sorting systems prioritise speed. Effective control requires digital screening, platform cooperation and data analysis capable of identifying repeated patterns across apparently separate parcels. Focusing only on large freight allows illicit trade to migrate towards channels where inspection probability is lower.

Passenger baggage and informal carriage create another route. Individuals may bring products across the border for personal use, resale or supply to local businesses. Distinguishing reasonable personal quantities from commercial importation can be difficult, especially where products are distributed among several travellers. Controls should therefore consider quantity, packaging, repetition, payment records and evidence of onward sale rather than relying solely on what the traveller claims. Personal-use allowances should not become a mechanism for structured commercial evasion. At the same time, enforcement must remain proportionate and avoid treating ordinary travellers as organised smugglers where there is no evidence of trade.

Physical examination is sometimes necessary because documentation may conceal the decisive breach. A device labelled as containing a lawful volume may hold substantially more liquid. A product described as nicotine-free may contain nicotine. Packaging may display a valid warning while the internal reservoir, formulation or battery differs from the product on record. Officers need practical methods for preliminary assessment, including weighing, measurement, visual comparison and portable screening where available. Suspect goods may then require laboratory testing or technical dismantling. The chain of custody must be documented carefully because detention, seizure and later prosecution may depend on proving that the tested sample came from the identified shipment and remained intact.

Laboratory capacity can become a bottleneck. Nicotine analysis, liquid-volume determination and ingredient identification require appropriate methods, trained analysts and time. If every suspicious consignment must wait weeks for confirmation, storage costs rise and products may remain unresolved while importers challenge detention. Risk-based testing is therefore needed. Grossly oversized devices, obvious foreign-market packaging or absent responsible-operator details may justify action without full chemical analysis, while borderline nicotine or ingredient questions require stronger evidence. Authorities should establish clear protocols indicating which findings support immediate refusal, which require laboratory confirmation and how uncertainty around legal thresholds will be interpreted.

Detention powers must be effective enough to prevent rapid release but constrained enough to protect legitimate trade. Goods should be held where there are reasonable grounds to suspect non-compliance, where distribution could disperse them quickly. Importers should receive clear reasons, evidence requirements and a route to provide clarification. Delays caused by institutional uncertainty should not become an indefinite commercial penalty. At the same time, incomplete paperwork produced after detention should not automatically overcome substantive concerns. The purpose of due process is to test compliance fairly, not to provide time for records to be reconstructed retrospectively around the goods.

Where non-compliance is confirmed, authorities need a range of outcomes. Goods may be refused entry, seized, destroyed, re-exported under control or released subject to corrective action where the defect is limited and lawful correction is genuinely possible. Relabelling at the border may be appropriate for a minor packaging issue but not where the product itself is unnotified, oversized or falsely declared. Re-export also requires caution because unlawful goods may simply be routed into another market or returned later through a different channel. Destruction may be necessary, but nicotine liquids, batteries and electronic components require controlled waste handling rather than ordinary disposal.

Penalties must address the economics of evasion. If an importer risks only losing one intercepted shipment while most consignments pass through, non-compliance may remain profitable. Enforcement should consider repeated behaviour, false declarations, use of shell companies, links to prior seizures and attempts to reroute detained goods. Financial penalties, recovery of costs, director accountability and restrictions on future imports may be justified where conduct is deliberate. Minor first-time errors should still be distinguishable from organised evasion, but repeated administrative explanations cannot excuse a pattern that consistently places unlawful products into the market.

Shell companies and rapidly changing importers present a major challenge. A business may be incorporated, used for several shipments and dissolved or abandoned when enforcement begins. The same individuals can then continue through another company. Border intelligence should therefore look beyond the legal entity to directors, addresses, contact details, payment accounts, freight agents and supplier relationships. Where enforcement follows only the name on one customs declaration, organised operators can remain ahead of the system by changing the visible importer.

Freight forwarders, customs agents and warehouses can provide valuable intelligence because they see repeated patterns across clients and consignments. They are not substitutes for regulators, yet they should conduct reasonable customer due diligence and avoid facilitating obviously misleading declarations. Warehouses should not release detained or recalled goods without authorisation. Where service providers repeatedly support the same non-compliant network, authorities may need to examine whether their role is passive, negligent or knowing.

Counterfeit detection is especially difficult at the border because copied packaging may appear professional. Brand owners can assist by providing genuine samples, authentication features and intelligence on authorised factories and shipping routes. Their technical knowledge can help distinguish genuine goods from imitations. Secure digital verification, serialisation and controlled code issuance may support inspections, although counterfeiters adapt quickly. Authentication must therefore be linked to shipment records, manufacturer data and market intelligence rather than treated as a single decisive test.

Border control also intersects with taxation. Once vaping products become subject to excise duties, the incentive to under-declare, misclassify or divert goods increases. Product legality and fiscal compliance may overlap but should not be confused. A correctly notified product can still be imported without proper duty, while a duty-paid product can still breach capacity or nicotine rules. Customs, tax and product-safety authorities need compatible data so that one form of compliance does not create a false assumption about another. Duty stamps, importer registration and movement records can strengthen traceability if they are integrated with product identity.

Environmental obligations add a further dimension. Imported devices contain batteries, plastics, metals and liquids that may engage waste, producer-responsibility and recycling requirements. An importer who places such goods on the market may acquire environmental duties regardless of whether the product satisfies nicotine regulation. Border control is not necessarily the primary enforcement point for all these obligations, but missing producer registration or implausible waste arrangements can indicate a wider lack of compliance.

The effectiveness of border control should be measured by more than the number of seizures. High seizure totals may demonstrate active enforcement, but they may also indicate a large underlying flow of unlawful goods. Success should include disruption of repeat networks, reduction in illegal availability, improved importer compliance and faster intelligence transfer to domestic authorities. Data should identify which products, routes and operators generate the greatest risk.

Border control ultimately functions as one part of a wider regulatory chain. It can intercept unlawful goods before distribution, but it cannot guarantee that every product entering the country is compliant. Some goods will evade inspection, some will be assembled domestically from imported components and some will become non-compliant through later modification or mislabelling. Domestic market surveillance, retailer inspection and supply-chain traceability remain essential. The strongest system uses border findings to guide inland enforcement and uses inland findings to refine border targeting.

The central objective is not to create an impermeable frontier, which is unrealistic in commerce, but to make unlawful importation difficult, detectable and commercially unattractive. That requires accurate declarations, identifiable importers, intelligence-led targeting, access to technical expertise, proportionate detention powers, reliable testing and sanctions capable of changing behaviour. When these elements operate together, the border becomes an effective regulatory control point rather than a symbolic barrier through which compliant operators pass openly and illegal traders merely search for the least supervised route.

Counterfeit Products

Counterfeit products represent one of the most disruptive forms of non-compliance because they sever the relationship between the product presented to the consumer and the scientific, technical and regulatory record attached to the legitimate brand. A genuine manufacturer may have developed a formulation, qualified suppliers, completed analytical testing, submitted product information, implemented quality controls and established systems for complaints and corrective action, yet a counterfeit product can reproduce the name, colours and external appearance of that lawful product while containing entirely different materials, nicotine concentrations, batteries, heating elements or liquids. The consumer sees a familiar package and assumes continuity, but the regulator, retailer and brand owner may have no reliable knowledge of what is inside. Counterfeiting therefore creates an untraceable product carrying borrowed credibility and can convert the reputation of a compliant business into a shield for uncontrolled manufacture.

The distinction between a counterfeit and other forms of illegal product must remain clear. A counterfeit product falsely presents itself as originating from, or being authorised by, the legitimate brand owner. An unauthorised product may use its own branding but enter the market without notification, testing or lawful importation. A diverted product may be genuine but intended for another jurisdiction, while an altered product may begin as genuine stock before being refilled, relabelled or modified. A product bearing a copied trade mark may also exceed legal capacity, contain unapproved ingredients or evade duty, yet its counterfeit character arises from the false representation of identity. Classification matters because the response may involve product-safety law, customs controls, intellectual-property rights, fraud and consumer protection simultaneously.

Modern vaping products are particularly vulnerable because their packaging is visually distinctive, their components are compact and their supply chains are international. Counterfeiters can reproduce cartons, labels, holograms and device casings at relatively low cost, while contract manufacturing allows technically similar products to be produced by factories with access to comparable materials and tooling. A copied product only needs to appear convincing enough to pass through wholesalers, retailers and online marketplaces before discrepancies are detected. High consumer demand for established brands gives counterfeiters an immediate market, and frequent changes in flavours, designs and packaging can make unusual variations appear plausible. Retailers may assume that a new edition is legitimate, while consumers may interpret differences as ordinary redesign.

The routes through which counterfeit goods enter the market are varied. Some are produced by factories with no legitimate connection to the brand. Others may originate from subcontractors, rejected production runs, unauthorised shifts or genuine manufacturing sites operating outside the brand owner's controls. Components, packaging and labels can be sourced separately and assembled in another location. Goods may be imported in commercial consignments, divided into small parcels or supplied through informal wholesale networks. Online marketplaces and social-media sellers allow counterfeit products to reach consumers without passing through conventional distribution, while physical retailers may purchase them unknowingly from brokers offering attractive prices and rapid delivery.

Price is often the first warning sign, but it is not decisive. Counterfeit products are frequently sold below normal wholesale or retail levels because the producer has avoided testing, notification, duty and quality-control costs. However, some are priced close to the genuine product precisely to avoid suspicion. Unusually favourable payment terms, pressure to buy quickly, requests for cash, cryptocurrency or transfers to unrelated accounts, and reluctance to provide invoices should increase concern. A supplier who cannot explain the origin of stock, identify the importer or provide evidence of lawful market status should not be treated as credible merely because the goods look professional.

Packaging inspection remains useful, although counterfeit quality has improved considerably. Poor print definition, spelling errors, inconsistent colours, misaligned warnings, missing batch codes, low-quality seals or incorrect manufacturer details can reveal obvious copies. Differences between genuine and false products can appear in typeface, carton dimensions, foil texture, barcode placement, leaflet quality, device weight or the shape of small moulded components. Retailers and enforcement officers need current reference material because counterfeiters adapt when detection guides become public.

Authentication codes, serial numbers, holograms and tamper features can strengthen control, but none is infallible. Codes may be copied from genuine products, generated in plausible sequences or attached to websites designed to imitate the legitimate verification system. A code that returns a valid result may already have been used hundreds of times. Secure systems should therefore detect repeated verification, unusual geographic patterns and sequences inconsistent with authorised production. Consumers should reach verification systems through trusted channels rather than links printed on potentially counterfeit packaging. Authentication is strongest when it connects the individual unit to manufacturing, shipment and distribution records.

The physical product may provide stronger evidence than the packaging. Counterfeit devices can differ in battery capacity, circuit protection, coil construction, reservoir volume, seals, plastics and metal components. Liquids may use different nicotine sources, solvent ratios, acids, flavourings or colourants. The aerosol generated may therefore bear little resemblance to that of the genuine product. Consumers may report unusual taste, excessive harshness, leakage, weak performance, overheating or rapid battery failure. These symptoms do not prove counterfeiting, but repeated differences associated with one supply route should trigger investigation.

Analytical testing is often required to establish the seriousness of the risk. Nicotine concentration may be higher or lower than declared, ingredients may be substituted and contaminants may arise from poor raw materials or uncontrolled manufacturing. Metals, carbonyls and other emissions can differ because of heating-element quality, device power and material selection. Testing should compare the suspect product with authenticated genuine samples where possible, using documented methods and preserving chain of custody.

Counterfeiting damages post-market surveillance because complaints may be attributed initially to the legitimate brand. A consumer experiencing a battery incident or unexpected reaction may report the name printed on the package, and the regulator may search the product record associated with that name. The genuine manufacturer may then be asked to investigate goods it did not produce and cannot trace. If the counterfeit is not recognised, adverse-event data can distort the apparent safety profile of the lawful product. Brand owners should therefore maintain procedures for examining suspect samples, comparing serialisation and reporting counterfeit findings to regulators. Regulators should recognise that a lawful name does not necessarily identify the lawful product.

Retailers are central to prevention because counterfeit goods gain legitimacy when sold from established premises. Retail purchasing should therefore be limited to approved suppliers, with invoices and batch details retained. Goods offered by travelling sales representatives, informal brokers or liquidation sellers require heightened scrutiny. Retailers should compare incoming stock with authenticated examples and quarantine unusual products. Returning doubtful goods without recording the concern may simply move them elsewhere.

Distributors and importers possess greater responsibility because they can spread counterfeit stock across hundreds of outlets rapidly. Supplier qualification should include confirmation of manufacturing authority, brand-owner relationships and shipping routes. Importers should examine whether factories are authorised to produce the brand and whether the specific product variants are genuine. A distributor that relies only on the visible product risks becoming the mechanism through which counterfeit goods acquire national reach.

Online marketplaces face a particular challenge because sellers can open accounts quickly, use copied images and conceal their real location. Removing one listing does little where the same operator reappears under another name.

Platforms should verify seller identity, preserve transaction records, respond to brand-owner and regulator notices, and prevent repeat offenders from returning through related accounts, addresses or payment details. Automated systems can detect copied imagery, suspiciously low prices, repeated product descriptions and sudden clusters of complaints, but human review remains necessary. Counterfeit detection should not depend entirely on brand-owner monitoring.

Border authorities can intercept counterfeit products before distribution, but visual identification at the border is difficult. Rights holders can support control by registering intellectual-property information, providing genuine samples and identifying authorised manufacturers, importers and routes. Customs officers may detain suspicious consignments while authenticity is checked. Intelligence from domestic seizures should therefore feed back into border targeting, while border findings should alert inland enforcement to brands, suppliers and retailers requiring inspection.

Counterfeiting is frequently connected to broader criminal conduct. False invoicing, tax evasion, money laundering, identity misuse, labour exploitation and organised smuggling may sit behind apparently ordinary retail stock. Enforcement should not assume that every counterfeit transaction is controlled by sophisticated criminal groups, but repeated large-scale supply, shell companies and coordinated import routes require investigation beyond routine product compliance. Agencies responsible for customs, tax, fraud, intellectual property and product safety may need to work together. Action against individual retailers will not dismantle an upstream network that can replace stock rapidly.

The legal response should remove the financial incentive. Seizure and destruction protect consumers, but if suppliers retain profits from previous consignments, the trade may continue. Penalties should reflect scale, intent, repetition and the risks created by the product. Directors and individuals controlling disposable companies should not escape responsibility merely by dissolving one entity and forming another. Brand owners may pursue civil remedies, while authorities use criminal, customs or product-safety powers. Cooperation must not allow private interests to dictate enforcement priorities, although legitimate rights holders possess essential evidence and technical knowledge.

The evidential threshold for establishing authenticity should also be defined carefully. A packaging discrepancy may justify detention or quarantine, but conclusive action may require comparison with verified production records, expert examination or confirmation from the rights holder. Authorities should avoid allowing commercial authentication alone to replace independent judgement, particularly where disputes concern parallel imports or legitimate manufacturing variation. Equally, businesses should not exploit uncertainty over authenticity to delay action when multiple indicators point towards false origin and continuing sale would expose consumers to an unidentified product without traceability.

Consumer communication requires care. Alerts should describe how to identify affected goods without implying that every product under the brand is unsafe. Where counterfeit and genuine versions coexist, the warning should explain verified differences, purchase routes and authentication steps. Overly broad statements can damage the lawful manufacturer and confuse users, while vague advice provides little practical protection. Consumers should be encouraged to retain packaging, receipts and suspect devices rather than disposing of them immediately, because those materials may support investigation. They should also know where to report concerns.

Product recall is unusually difficult where the counterfeit supplier does not maintain records or acknowledge responsibility. Authorities may know that suspect goods are circulating without knowing how many were imported or where they were sold. Retailers and distributors must then search their own records and identify stock obtained through the relevant route. Public notices may be needed because direct consumer contact is impossible. Once identity is uncertain, every invoice, batch code and transaction record becomes evidence.

Counterfeit prevention should be designed into the legitimate supply chain. Controlled artwork, secure component sourcing, factory oversight, serialisation, restricted access to labels and regular market monitoring can reduce opportunity. Brand owners should investigate unexplained sales patterns, duplicate codes and products appearing in markets they do not supply. Contract manufacturers should account for rejected units, excess components and destroyed packaging. Tooling and digital files should be protected, and subcontracting should require approval. These controls cannot eliminate copying, but they can expose leakage from legitimate facilities.

The market also needs affordable lawful products. Counterfeit demand increases where genuine goods are scarce, heavily restricted or substantially more expensive. This does not excuse deception, but enforcement strategy should recognise the commercial conditions that support it. Tax, product bans and supply constraints can increase margins available to illegal traders.

Regulation must therefore combine strong action against counterfeits with a lawful market capable of meeting adult demand through controlled products.

Counterfeit vaping products represent a direct attack on regulatory identity. They imitate the appearance of compliance while avoiding the systems that give compliance meaning. Their principal danger lies in uncertainty: the formulation, components, manufacturer and supply history cannot be trusted. Effective control requires coordinated work by brand owners, importers, distributors, retailers, platforms, border authorities, laboratories and regulators. The objective is not merely to defend trade marks, but to restore the connection between the name on the package and the product that was actually assessed, manufactured and placed on the market.

Illegal Markets

Illegal markets emerge when demand, product restrictions, taxation and weak enforcement combine to create a supply chain outside lawful control. In the vaping sector, the illegal market is not a single organised system but a spectrum ranging from small-scale resale of unauthorised products to structured importation, counterfeit distribution, tax evasion, false declarations, online supply and repeated retail sale through businesses that also trade in compliant goods. Some operators specialise in illicit products, while others mix lawful and unlawful stock so that the appearance of legitimacy protects the activity. The result is a market in which consumers may purchase goods from shops, websites or social-media sellers without knowing that the product has not been notified, may exceed legal capacity or nicotine limits, may avoid duty, may carry false warnings or may lack an identifiable manufacturer.

The distinction between an illegal product and an illegal transaction matters. A product may be technically compliant in its country of manufacture yet become illegal when supplied in a jurisdiction where it has not been notified, labelled or taxed correctly. A genuine product can be diverted from an authorised supply chain and sold outside the market for which it was intended. A compliant device may be sold unlawfully to a minor, while a lawful liquid may be advertised through prohibited claims. Conversely, a product can be illegal in itself because its nicotine concentration, reservoir volume, ingredients, construction or presentation falls outside the applicable rules. Enforcement must therefore systematically examine both the characteristics of the goods and the conduct surrounding their sale. Focusing only on the object can miss unlawful marketing, tax evasion and age-of-sale offences, while focusing only on the retailer can fail to identify an upstream network distributing unsafe or deliberately misdeclared products.

Demand is the principal force sustaining illegal supply. Consumers do not necessarily stop seeking a product when legislation removes it from lawful sale. They may switch to an alternative, reduce use, return to smoking or purchase through informal channels. The outcome depends on price, availability, perceived risk, product preference and the strength of enforcement. Where consumers place high value on large-capacity devices, flavours, higher nicotine strengths or low prices, restrictions can create a profitable gap. Illegal suppliers enter that gap because they can offer features unavailable in the compliant market while avoiding the costs of notification, testing, duty, quality control and responsible disposal. Regulation does not create all illicit trade, but poorly designed or weakly enforced rules can enlarge the commercial reward available to those willing to ignore them.

The economic advantage of non-compliance can be substantial. A lawful manufacturer may pay for formulation assessment, laboratory testing, quality systems, packaging development, product notification, insurance, excise administration and environmental obligations. An illegal supplier can bypass most of these expenses, purchase low-cost stock, underdeclare value and sell rapidly through cash or informal payment channels. Even when seizures occur, the loss may be absorbed if shipments reach the market. Small penalties may then function as an operating cost rather than a deterrent. The illegal market becomes especially resilient where businesses can dissolve companies, reopen under new names, move stock between premises or use third parties to separate the visible retailer from the importer and financial beneficiary.

Legal and illegal supply frequently coexist within the same commercial premises. A retailer may stock notified refill liquids and devices alongside oversized disposables, foreign-market products or unverified nicotine strengths. This mixed model reduces suspicion because invoices, registered business details and compliant stock create an appearance of trade. It also allows retailers to respond selectively during inspection, removing questionable products temporarily or presenting lawful invoices that do not correspond to all goods held. Effective enforcement therefore requires product-level traceability rather than assumptions based on the status of the business. A licensed or established shop is not automatically compliant, just as an unfamiliar seller is not necessarily unlawful. The decisive questions concern origin, specification, notification, tax status and the route by which the individual product entered the market.

Wholesale networks are central because a single distributor can place illegal products into hundreds of outlets before authorities detect the pattern. Goods may be promoted through trade messaging groups, temporary showrooms, social-media accounts or travelling representatives offering cash discounts and delivery. Retailers may be told that the products are registered, awaiting publication, permitted because they are rechargeable or lawful under an alternative interpretation of capacity. These explanations can sound plausible to businesses that lack technical expertise, particularly where competitors are already selling the same products openly. Once widespread availability creates the impression that enforcement accepts the product, hesitation declines and unlawful stock becomes normalised across the market.

Online trade expands this reach further. Sellers can operate through websites, marketplaces, social platforms and encrypted messaging services while holding little or no stock themselves. Orders may be fulfilled directly from overseas suppliers or domestic warehouses that serve multiple storefronts. Accounts can disappear after complaints and reappear under new names, while payments move through personal accounts, cryptocurrency, vouchers or processors with incomplete seller verification. Online listings can show compliant images even when the delivered product differs, and age controls may consist of little more than self-declaration. Enforcement focused on removing individual listings is therefore unlikely to be sufficient. Authorities must follow seller identities, payment flows, fulfilment addresses, import records and associated accounts to disrupt the commercial infrastructure rather than merely the most visible webpage.

Illegal markets also exploit consumer uncertainty. Many purchasers do not understand notification systems, capacity limits, nicotine declarations or duty arrangements, and some assume that anything sold openly must be lawful. Professional packaging, copied regulatory identifiers and familiar retail premises reinforce that assumption. Others knowingly choose illegal products because they prefer the capacity, flavour, strength or price and perceive enforcement as a matter for businesses rather than consumers. Risk communication should therefore explain why lawful status matters without implying that every non-compliant product is equally dangerous. The central concern is that unregulated goods lack reliable evidence, traceability and accountability, meaning that problems cannot be assessed or corrected with the same confidence available in the lawful market.

The relationship between illegal vaping products and combustible tobacco deserves careful consideration. Restrictive measures may be justified by youth protection, product safety, environmental concerns or taxation, yet their consequences depend partly on what consumers do next. Some adult users may move to compliant alternatives, while others may return to cigarettes or enter illicit channels. Young people may shift between vaping products, nicotine pouches and tobacco. An assessment that counts removed products without examining substitution provides an incomplete picture. Illegal markets can preserve nicotine demand in less visible forms, and enforcement success should be measured through changes in availability, exposure and behaviour rather than seizure totals alone.

Youth access is one of the most serious consequences because illegal sellers may disregard age restrictions alongside product rules. Cheap devices, informal delivery, social-media promotion and peer resale can make nicotine products available outside supervised retail. School-based networks and local resellers may purchase larger quantities online or from wholesalers and divide them among younger users. Inspection of licensed shops will not reach these routes fully. Intelligence from schools, parents, youth services, parcel data and social platforms may be necessary, but intervention should distinguish between young users and the adults or businesses profiting from supply. Punitive responses directed mainly at children risk missing the upstream commercial structure.

Taxation can intensify illicit incentives when duties create a substantial price difference between lawful and untaxed products. Excise systems can support traceability and provide resources for enforcement, but they also increase the value of smuggling, false declarations and diversion. Duty stamps, registrations and movement records help only when they are difficult to counterfeit and integrated with product identity. A stamped product may still be technically non-compliant, while a compliant product may be sold without duty. Tax and product enforcement must therefore share information rather than treating fiscal and safety compliance as separate worlds. Where penalties for tax evasion are stronger and better resourced, fiscal intelligence may become an important route into wider product investigations.

Organised criminal involvement varies by market and should not be exaggerated, but profitable illicit supply naturally attracts networks experienced in smuggling, fraud and money movement. Compact size, high unit value and rapid turnover of vaping products make them suitable for concealed importation and distribution. The same routes may handle counterfeit goods, tobacco or other contraband. Shell companies, nominee directors, false invoices and multiple storage sites can obscure control. Product regulators may lack the powers and intelligence needed to address these structures. Cooperation with customs, tax, fraud, financial investigation and law-enforcement bodies becomes necessary where evidence indicates coordinated activity rather than isolated retail breach.

Enforcement against illegal markets must be selective enough to use resources effectively and strong enough to alter incentives. Minor documentary errors should not consume the same effort as deliberate importation of large quantities of falsely labelled products. Risk assessment should consider scale, youth access, product hazard, previous warnings, falsification, tax loss and the operator's response. Advice and corrective action may be appropriate where a responsible business identifies a limited error and cooperates. Seizure, prosecution, licence consequences, recovery of proceeds and director accountability may be necessary where non-compliance is repeated or organised. The objective is not to maximise punishment but to make unlawful supply less profitable and less reliable than compliance.

Intelligence-led enforcement should connect border seizures, retailer inspections, online purchases, laboratory results, complaints and financial records. A single product discovery may reveal a common importer, warehouse or distributor serving several regions. Shared identifiers, batch details and company relationships allow agencies to recognise patterns that remain invisible within separate case files. Rapid communication matters because illegal products can be rebranded and redistributed before formal investigations conclude. Authorities need systems capable of warning other regions, platforms and retailers while preserving evidential standards and avoiding premature claims that could damage legitimate businesses.

Laboratory testing remains essential because illegal status is not always visible. Products may contain more nicotine or liquid than declared, use unexpected ingredients or differ materially from genuine versions. Testing must be targeted, timely and linked to enforcement decisions. Long delays reduce practical value because stock may sell through before results arrive. Portable screening, weight comparison and physical measurement can support initial decisions, while accredited analysis confirms chemical breaches. Authorities should publish clear methods and tolerances so that businesses understand the basis of action and cannot exploit technical ambiguity indefinitely.

The lawful industry has a role in reporting suspicious goods, emerging brands and unusual supply offers. Manufacturers and distributors often identify counterfeits or illegal variants before regulators, while retailers can describe demand and local wholesale activity. This intelligence should be welcomed but independently verified because commercial competitors may use complaints strategically. Transparent reporting channels, evidence requirements and feedback improve trust. Industry cooperation should support enforcement without allowing private firms to determine which rivals are targeted or to obtain confidential regulatory information.

Reducing illegal markets also requires a lawful market that remains usable. Compliance obligations should be strict where they address genuine risk, but unnecessarily complex, slow or expensive pathways can push responsible operators out while leaving demand intact. Consumers need access to products that are acceptable enough to compete with cigarettes and attractive enough to displace illicit alternatives. This does not justify retaining every flavour, format or strength, but it requires policymakers to consider cumulative burden, price differentials and behavioural response. A system that makes lawful products uncompetitive and then relies on enforcement alone is likely to struggle.

Illegal markets are therefore both a regulatory failure and a market response. They reveal weaknesses in border control, retail oversight, online governance, taxation, product design and consumer communication. Their existence does not prove that regulation should be abandoned, but it does show that law cannot be assessed only through the conduct of compliant businesses. Effective control requires coordinated intelligence, proportionate sanctions, rapid testing, traceable products, platform cooperation and review of demand. The objective is not merely to seize unlawful stock, but to reduce the commercial conditions that allow illegal supply to become normal and more responsive than the market created by regulation.

Product Withdrawals

Product withdrawal is the controlled removal of a vaping product from the supply chain when evidence indicates that it is defective, non-compliant, incorrectly described, or unsuitable for continued sale. It is distinct from routine stock rotation, commercial delisting or a retailer choosing not to reorder a product. A withdrawal is a corrective regulatory action directed towards goods that have entered distribution but may not yet have reached consumers. Where products have already been supplied to consumers and must be recovered or the public must be warned, the action may become a recall. Both depend on traceability, rapid decision-making, accurate communication and the ability to identify the affected product precisely enough to remove the right stock without creating unnecessary confusion across the wider market.

The need for withdrawal may arise from many sources. A laboratory result may show that nicotine concentration falls outside the permitted or declared range. Market surveillance may identify excessive liquid capacity, prohibited ingredients, incorrect health warnings or packaging that fails to meet legal requirements. Complaints may reveal leakage, battery overheating, unexpected taste, device failure or repeated variation between units. A supplier may disclose that the wrong flavour concentrate, coil, battery cell or label was used during manufacture. Border authorities may identify that goods were imported under false declarations, while regulators may determine that the product was not properly notified or differs materially from the version described in the submission. A counterfeit investigation may also require immediate removal because the product's origin and composition cannot be trusted, even where no specific toxicological defect has yet been demonstrated.

One damaged unit does not necessarily justify withdrawal of an entire range, while one confirmed analytical failure may indicate a batch-wide or process-wide defect. The responsible business must define the scope from evidence rather than convenience. Batch records, production dates, component lots, formulation records, filling lines, packaging runs and distribution data should be examined to identify the units potentially affected. Where records are incomplete, the scope may need to be widened because the business cannot prove that other stock is unaffected. Conservative action is justified when uncertainty concerns a serious hazard, but unnecessarily broad withdrawal can create avoidable disruption, financial loss and consumer alarm. The objective is to remove all affected product and no unaffected product wherever the evidence allows that distinction.

The assessment should consider the defect, likelihood and severity of exposure, affected population, distributed quantity and whether consumers can recognise or stop using the product. A minor typographical error has a different significance from undeclared nicotine, severe concentration error, unsafe batteries or contamination. The fact that vaping products are generally lower risk than combustible cigarettes does not reduce the need to address avoidable defects within the category. At the same time, risk assessment should remain proportionate and distinguish safety-critical failures from administrative defects capable of prompt correction.

Decision-making authority must be clear in advance. Businesses should define who can place stock on hold, stop dispatch, notify regulators and authorise a withdrawal. Delays often arise because commercial, legal and quality teams debate responsibility while products continue moving. A competent system gives designated personnel authority to act on credible information before complete certainty. Initial quarantine can be reversed if investigation shows that no wider problem exists, whereas units sold during delay may be impossible to recover. The decision should be documented, including available information, rationale, scope, affected markets and required actions. These records also demonstrate whether the business controlled the incident with urgency and discipline. Documentation provides accountability and allows later review of whether the response was timely and proportionate.

Once withdrawal is initiated, all stock under the business's control should be blocked physically and digitally. Warehouse systems must prevent further picking, dispatch or transfer, while quarantined goods should be clearly labelled and segregated from saleable inventory. Stock held by distributors, wholesalers, fulfilment centres and retailers must then be identified. Communication should specify brand, flavour, nicotine strength, device type, batch or serial range, packaging and reason. Vague notices such as "remove affected products" create mistakes where several similar variants are sold. Images can assist recognition, but written identifiers remain necessary where packaging has changed or counterfeits coexist. Recipients should understand the required action, deadline and confirmation method.

Traceability determines whether this process succeeds. The manufacturer or importer should know how many units were produced or received, which batches they belonged to and where they were supplied. Distributors should be able to identify downstream customers, while retailers should locate stock and, where possible, sales records. Where products have passed through cash wholesalers, informal brokers or mixed consignments, the chain may break. The business may then be unable to establish how much product remains in circulation. This is why traceability is not merely a quality-system formality. It is the operating mechanism that converts a withdrawal decision into physical removal. A product without reliable distribution records may require public warning because targeted commercial recovery is no longer possible.

If the defect is unlikely to affect safety and remaining stock can be removed before sale, a trade-level withdrawal may be sufficient. Where consumers may possess affected units, the response may require direct contact, notices, website alerts, retailer signage, platform notifications or communication through health and enforcement channels. The message should explain the product identity, the nature of the concern, what consumers should do and how refunds, returns or replacements will be handled. Minimising the issue can prolong exposure, whereas exaggerated language may damage confidence in unaffected products and in vaping as a regulated alternative to smoking.

Communication with regulators should occur according to seriousness and legal obligations. The responsible operator should not wait until every detail is resolved before informing the competent authority of a potentially significant safety or compliance concern. Early notification allows authorities to coordinate market surveillance, border action and public communication. The initial report can be updated as investigation progresses. Regulators may require quantities, distribution lists, test reports, risk assessments and evidence that customers have been contacted. They may also determine that voluntary action is insufficient and impose formal measures. Cooperation is generally more effective than defensive delay, but businesses should still ensure that information is accurate and clearly distinguish confirmed facts from provisional hypotheses.

Retailers play a critical part because they hold stock close to the consumer and may receive the first complaints. A withdrawal notice should trigger immediate removal from shelves, online listings and back-room storage. Staff must know that affected products cannot be discounted, returned casually to general stock or sold after a customer asks for them. Retailers should record quantities held, sold, returned and destroyed, then report these figures to the supplier. Where consumers are likely to return products, staff need clear handling instructions, especially for leaking liquids or damaged batteries. Returned goods should be isolated safely and not tested informally in store. The retailer's ability to respond consistently depends on prior training and on notices that are practical rather than written solely in legal or technical language.

Online sales require additional controls because stock may be listed across several websites, marketplaces and social-media accounts. The seller should suspend the affected listing immediately, stop automated fulfilment and identify customers from transaction records. Marketplaces and fulfilment providers must be informed separately where they control inventory or dispatch. Digital records can make direct consumer notification easier than in cash retail, but only if product variants and batches were recorded accurately. Generic stock-keeping units that combine several batches weaken this advantage. Search advertising, affiliate links and cached pages may continue directing customers towards a withdrawn product even after the main listing is removed, so the business should review its wider promotional network and ensure that partners cease activity.

Recovered stock must be reconciled. The business should compare the quantities manufactured or imported with units held, distributed, returned, sold and unaccounted for. Complete recovery is rarely possible once consumers have used or discarded products, but the reconciliation reveals how much potential exposure remains. Low response from retailers may indicate that notices were ineffective or records were poor. Follow-up contact, site visits or enforcement assistance may be needed. Completion should not be declared merely because the first communication was sent. Effectiveness checks should confirm that recipients understood the instruction, removed the correct goods and prevented further sale. A withdrawal is a process with measurable outcomes, not an email event.

Investigation must continue alongside recovery. The purpose is to establish root cause and prevent recurrence. A nicotine error may result from incorrect raw-material assay, calculation, weighing, mixing, sampling, analytical release or label selection. Leakage may arise from component tolerances, material incompatibility, filling volume, transport damage or storage conditions. Battery incidents may involve cell quality, circuitry, charger compatibility or counterfeit substitution. Root-cause analysis should test competing explanations against evidence rather than accept the supplier's first account. Where contract manufacturers are involved, the brand owner or importer must retain sufficient access to production records and samples to investigate properly. Commercial distance from the factory cannot excuse an inability to determine what went wrong.

Corrective and preventive action should address the system that allowed the defect to occur and escape detection. Corrective action deals with the immediate cause, such as replacing a faulty component, revising a formulation or correcting artwork. Preventive action strengthens controls through supplier qualification, revised specifications, additional testing, improved line clearance, staff training, enhanced incoming inspection or better change control. The adequacy of the action should be verified after implementation. A promise from the supplier is not evidence that the problem has been solved. Follow-up batches may require increased sampling, independent analysis or audit. Repeated withdrawal for the same cause demonstrates that the earlier response was ineffective.

Financial and reputational pressures can distort withdrawal decisions. Businesses may fear lost sales, disposal costs, retailer claims and damage to brand confidence. These concerns are real, particularly for small companies, but delay usually increases eventual cost. More stock reaches consumers, enforcement action becomes more likely and trust deteriorates if the business appears to have concealed the problem. Product liability and recall insurance may reduce financial exposure, although policies depend on accurate disclosure and compliance with notification requirements. Contracts with suppliers should allocate responsibilities for investigation, replacement, transport and destruction, but contractual disputes must not delay public protection.

Recovered vaping products require appropriate handling and disposal. Nicotine liquids, lithium batteries, electronic circuits, plastics and metals create chemical, electrical and environmental hazards. Products should not be placed in ordinary waste, resold through secondary channels or exported casually to another market. Destruction should use authorised contractors and preserve evidence where investigation or legal proceedings remain active. Quantities, batch identities, dates and disposal certificates should be retained. Where rework is legally and technically possible, it must be controlled through documented assessment and release. Relabelling cannot correct an unsafe formulation, and component replacement cannot be assumed to restore compliance without verification.

Authorities should evaluate withdrawals as part of market surveillance. Repeated events involving one manufacturer, importer, component or flavour supplier may reveal a wider pattern. Data should inform inspections, laboratory priorities and future guidance. Publication of significant withdrawals can protect consumers and encourage industry learning, but communication should distinguish genuine products from counterfeits and affected batches from the wider brand. Transparency should not become indiscriminate reputational punishment. The strongest system encourages early voluntary action while retaining powers to compel withdrawal when businesses fail to act.

Product withdrawal is ultimately a test of whether regulatory records remain connected to the goods in circulation. A business may possess extensive technical documentation, yet that documentation has limited value if it cannot identify affected batches, locate customers or stop supply. Effective withdrawal depends on preparation before the incident: accurate product identity, batch control, distribution records, designated authority, communication templates and tested procedures. When those elements are present, a defect can be contained, investigated and corrected. When they are absent, uncertainty spreads through the market and regulators may be forced to issue broad warnings or remove entire ranges. Withdrawal is therefore not an admission that regulation has failed, but evidence that a functioning system can recognise failure within a product and act before it becomes wider harm.

Regulatory Case Studies

Regulatory case studies are valuable because they reveal what legislation does after it leaves the page. A notification requirement, capacity limit, age restriction or import prohibition may appear clear in isolation, yet the practical outcome depends on intelligence, sampling, laboratory methods, legal powers, supply-chain records and the speed with which authorities can act. Individual cases also expose the difference between apparent and actual compliance. Packaging may declare one nicotine strength while analysis finds another; a product may display a familiar brand while differing from the notified specification; an importer may provide documentation while the physical device fails a basic safety requirement. The most useful case studies are therefore not selected merely because they produced large seizures or dramatic headlines. They are selected because they show where the regulatory chain worked, where it failed and what changed afterwards.

Operation Joseph provides a relevant British example of coordinated market surveillance. The programme brought local Trading Standards services together around illegal vaping products, underage sales and evidence gathering. One of its most instructive findings came from testing products sold as nicotine-free across Devon, Somerset, Torbay, Plymouth, Salford and Berkshire. Of seventy-six samples, ten, or 13.2 per cent, contained nicotine, with measured concentrations ranging from 0.06 to 27.02 milligrams per millilitre. All ten also exceeded the permitted liquid-volume limit, and two exceeded both the volume and nicotine-strength limits. The case demonstrated that packaging claims could not be accepted as evidence and that nicotine-free products could fall outside the nicotine-notification framework while still exposing consumers to nicotine. It also showed why surveillance must include products presented as exempt from tighter controls rather than concentrating only on openly nicotine-containing devices.

The practical lesson from that exercise was broader than the failure rate. Retailers purchasing products labelled zero nicotine could not identify the breach by ordinary visual inspection, and consumers seeking to reduce nicotine use could unknowingly continue exposure. Laboratory sampling converted suspicion into evidence that could be communicated to regulators, suppliers and policymakers. It also revealed an enforcement vulnerability: a regulatory system organised around declared product identity can be defeated where the declaration itself is false. Future control therefore requires selective chemical verification, clear responsibility for nicotine-free formulations and a route for tracing failed samples back through wholesalers and importers. Testing only the products already expected to contain nicotine would have missed the precise conduct that made these goods commercially attractive.

A second Operation Joseph example illustrates how intelligence can move from reports of youth supply to physical seizure. Enfield Trading Standards raided three premises in January 2024 after receiving reports that age-restricted products, including vapes, were being supplied to children. Officers seized 521 illegal disposable devices. Some claimed capacities of up to fourteen millilitres and around 9,000 puffs, approximately seven times the permitted liquid capacity applying to the products then on sale. The goods were valued at £6,252 and designated for destruction. This was not simply a capacity case. The initial intelligence concerned sales to children, while the inspection uncovered product illegality. It shows why enforcement officers should examine the complete business rather than limiting an investigation to the complaint that opened it.

The Enfield case also exposes the limitations of seizure as an endpoint. Removing 521 devices protected consumers from those particular units, but it did not necessarily identify the importer, wholesaler, payment route or other retailers supplied from the same source. A shop-level intervention becomes strategically valuable only when invoices, messages, delivery records and company relationships are used to move upstream. Destruction prevents seized goods returning to sale, but disruption requires action against the commercial network capable of replacing them. The case therefore illustrates the difference between product removal and market control. Both are necessary, but the second depends on intelligence sharing, financial investigation and follow-up inspections rather than the visual impact of confiscated stock.

A particularly clear example of border control, product assessment and corrective redesign involved the Hayati Twist 5000+ Puffs Juicy Peach electronic vape. The Office for Product Safety and Standards reported the product as presenting a high chemical risk because its ten-millilitre nicotine-liquid cartridge was not locked robustly to the device. The cartridge could be removed easily, allowing nicotine liquid to leak and creating a human-health risk. The import was rejected at the border, and the reported corrective action was redesign by the manufacturer so that the cartridge locked effectively. The case is useful because enforcement addressed the actual engineering failure rather than relying only on branding, puff count or declared composition. It also connected border action with product improvement instead of ending solely in confiscation.

This example demonstrates why legal compliance cannot be reduced to nominal component separation. A manufacturer may construct a device around a detachable reservoir and argue that its parts fit within a particular interpretation of capacity or reuse. The regulator must examine how the product functions physically, whether the consumer can access nicotine liquid and whether child-resistance, tamper evidence and leak protection remain effective. The rejection prevented distribution before the defect became dispersed through wholesalers and retailers, making intervention less costly and more complete than a later recall. The redesign also provides a model of effective corrective action: identify the mechanism of failure, alter the engineering control and verify that the amended product addresses the risk. Repackaging or relabelling would not have corrected the underlying defect.

The United Kingdom's single-use vape ban provides a case study at the scale of an entire product category. From 1 June 2025, businesses were prohibited from selling, supplying, offering to sell or supply, or holding for sale single-use vapes, whether or not they contained nicotine and whether supplied online or in shops. Remaining stock intended for disposal had to be separated from saleable goods and recycled appropriately. The measure extended practical responsibility beyond nicotine regulation into environmental product design and waste management. It also required retailers and enforcement officers to distinguish genuinely reusable products from devices given superficial rechargeable or refillable features principally to avoid the prohibition.

The ban illustrates the importance of definitions and transition planning. A rule aimed at disposability can be weakened if a product is technically rechargeable but unlikely to be reused, or if replacement components are unavailable. Enforcement must therefore examine whether the device is designed and intended for continued use, not simply whether a charging port is present. Retailers required time to stop purchasing, manage residual stock and arrange recycling, while online sellers and fulfilment centres had to remove listings and block dispatch. The case shows how legislation can redirect design rapidly, but also how manufacturers adapt around the wording. Post-implementation evaluation must measure waste, youth use, illegal sales and the durability of replacement devices rather than assuming that removal of products labelled disposable proves that the policy objective has been achieved.

The United States offers a contrasting case in which a demanding premarket authorisation system coexists with extensive enforcement against unauthorised products. In July 2024, the Food and Drug Administration issued warning letters to eighty physical retailers in fifteen states for selling unauthorised e-cigarettes, including Elf Bar and Lost Mary products, and filed civil-money-penalty complaints against eight additional retailers that had failed to correct earlier violations. In the same month, it warned five online retailers selling unauthorised disposable products marketed under brands including Geek Bar, Lost Mary and Bang. These actions demonstrate an escalating pathway from identification and warning to financial sanction, while also showing that unauthorised products had achieved substantial retail and online distribution despite the legal market-entry gate.

The American example shows that the strictness of premarket review and the effectiveness of market control are separate variables. Requiring a marketing order may create a clear legal boundary, but that boundary has limited practical value if unauthorised goods remain widely available and retailers consider warnings tolerable. Enforcement must connect manufacturers, importers, distributors, shops, websites and payment infrastructure. In January 2025, the FDA updated import alerts to reinforce that unauthorised e-cigarettes could be detained without physical examination, strengthening the border component of the same strategy. The approach allows officers to act on regulatory status and identified risk patterns rather than examining every shipment individually. It also places considerable importance on accurate product identification, since legitimate and unauthorised variants can circulate under closely related names.

Australia provides a further contrast because it moved vaping goods into a tightly controlled therapeutic framework and combined domestic enforcement with border action. The 2024 reforms prohibited the importation, manufacture, commercial possession, supply and advertising of disposable single-use and non-therapeutic vapes, with the central legislative changes commencing on 1 July 2024 after the disposable-import prohibition began on 1 January. The Therapeutic Goods Administration, Australian Border Force and state and territory agencies adopted a coordinated enforcement model. By October 2025, the TGA reported that more than 13.6 million illicit vaping products, with an estimated street value of approximately A$684 million, had been seized and kept out of the community since January 2024.

The Australian figures demonstrate enforcement scale, but they also require careful interpretation. Large seizure totals show operational activity and substantial attempted illegal supply; they do not by themselves prove that consumer demand or unlawful availability has been eliminated. In February 2026, a targeted operation in Burwood, New South Wales, seized more than 57,000 illegal vaping goods, while another operation reported in April 2026 removed more than 30,000 goods from sites in Chipping Norton and Casula. These cases show the need for repeated domestic action even after strong border and market prohibitions. They also illustrate how restrictive access models can require sustained policing of warehouses, retailers and distribution networks rather than relying on import rules alone.

European Safety Gate notifications provide a different kind of case study: cross-border communication after a dangerous or non-compliant product has been identified. A January 2026 alert concerned an electronic cigarette declared as containing thirty millilitres of liquid at fifty milligrams of nicotine per millilitre, both substantially beyond the limits applied under the European framework. The value of the alert system lies not merely in recording one failed product but in enabling authorities in other states to recognise the same brand, model or supplier and take corresponding action. Where products move across several national markets, a local laboratory result should become shared regulatory intelligence rather than remain confined to the authority that commissioned the test.

Taken together, these cases show that effective regulation depends on a sequence rather than a single intervention. Operation Joseph demonstrates the importance of sampling products whose labels appear to remove them from nicotine control. Enfield shows how intelligence concerning youth sales can expose wider product illegality. The Hayati border rejection shows how physical design assessment can prevent distribution and produce meaningful redesign. The British single-use ban demonstrates the difficulty of regulating a category through functional definitions. FDA actions show that a sophisticated authorisation pathway still requires retailer, online and import enforcement. Australia demonstrates the resources needed when access is restricted severely, while Safety Gate shows the value of international alert exchange. No case proves that one regulatory model is universally superior. Each identifies a different control point and a different vulnerability.

The common lesson is that regulatory success should be judged by what changes after the case. Seizures should lead upstream to importers and distributors. Analytical failures should alter surveillance priorities and supplier controls. Border rejections should produce verified corrective design. Warning letters should escalate where conduct continues. Product-category bans should be reviewed against waste, youth use, lawful substitution and illicit supply. International alerts should prompt coordinated searches rather than passive publication. Case studies become useful regulatory evidence only when authorities preserve the chain from discovery through investigation, corrective action and verification. Without that feedback, the same breach reappears under another product name, company or route, and enforcement becomes a repeated removal exercise rather than a system capable of learning. The strongest regulatory case is therefore not the largest seizure, but the one that identifies cause, reaches the responsible operator, protects consumers promptly, changes future conduct and generates evidence capable of improving the wider regulatory system over time.

CHAPTER 10

The Future of Regulation

The future of vaping regulation will not be determined by one new Directive, one national statute or one decisive scientific conclusion. It will emerge through a continuing contest between technological change, public health objectives, political pressure, environmental responsibility, commercial adaptation and the practical limits of enforcement. The first generation of regulation established legal categories, notification requirements, product limits and minimum responsibilities. The second extended those controls into manufacturing systems, market surveillance, taxation, youth protection and restrictions on particular product formats. The next generation will have to do something more difficult: regulate a mature but rapidly changing nicotine market without allowing yesterday's rules to become obstacles to tomorrow's evidence.

Modern nicotine technology does not remain still while legislation is debated. Devices become smaller, more efficient and more electronically controlled. Formulations change in response to nicotine limits, flavour policy and consumer demand. Manufacturers redesign products around legal definitions, environmental requirements and taxation structures. Retail channels move between physical stores, websites, social platforms and direct fulfilment. Artificial intelligence is beginning to influence literature review, toxicological screening, regulatory intelligence, document preparation and market monitoring. Digital identification can connect products to batches, submissions, import records, duty status and recalls. At the same time, illegal suppliers use many of the same technologies to copy packaging, automate sales, obscure commercial identities and move products across borders faster than conventional enforcement systems can respond.

This difference in speed presents the central problem of future regulation. Law develops through evidence gathering, consultation, drafting, parliamentary scrutiny, implementation and legal challenge. These processes protect legitimacy and reduce arbitrary government action, but they can take years. Product development and commercial adaptation can occur within months. By the time a rule reaches the market, the product that originally prompted it may have disappeared or been modified into a technically different form. A framework based too heavily on fixed physical characteristics will therefore remain vulnerable to circumvention, while one based only on broad principles may create uncertainty and inconsistent enforcement. Future systems must combine clear legal boundaries with technical mechanisms capable of changing as products, evidence and patterns of use evolve.

Adaptability does not mean allowing regulators to alter obligations without scrutiny. Businesses need sufficient certainty to invest in product development, laboratories need stable requirements against which to validate methods, and enforcement authorities need definitions capable of supporting legal action. Consumers also need confidence that a product considered compliant today will not become unlawful tomorrow without explanation or transition. Adaptive regulation must therefore operate within a disciplined structure. Technical standards may be updated more quickly than primary legislation, but changes should remain transparent, evidence-based and open to challenge. Temporary measures should have review points. Restrictions introduced in response to emerging concerns should be reassessed when stronger evidence becomes available. Flexibility without accountability becomes regulatory unpredictability; rigidity without review becomes institutional stagnation.

The need for adaptability is particularly clear where regulation relies on simple numerical limits. Nicotine concentration, reservoir volume and container size provide measurable boundaries, but they do not capture the full performance of a modern vaping product. Nicotine exposure depends on formulation, device efficiency, aerosol production, puffing behaviour and frequency of use. A lower-concentration product may deliver nicotine effectively through improved engineering, while a stronger formulation used in a low-output device may produce a different exposure pattern. The same limitation applies to liquid volume. Capacity can be defined and measured, yet consumption, device lifetime and environmental burden depend on how the product is designed and used. Future regulation will need to decide whether fixed limits remain sufficient, whether they should be supplemented by performance measures or whether more sophisticated exposure-based controls can be made practical enough for enforcement.

Scientific sophistication must not produce rules that only highly resourced organisations can understand or obey. A theoretically precise exposure model may be difficult to apply across thousands of device and formulation combinations. Regulators must balance scientific relevance with administrative usability. Requirements that cannot be tested consistently, interpreted transparently or enforced at reasonable cost may create uncertainty without improving protection. The challenge is to select measures that represent meaningful risk closely enough while remaining reproducible across laboratories and understandable to producers, importers and courts. Better science should reduce unnecessary regulation, not merely generate more elaborate documentation.

Artificial intelligence may help manage this complexity. Regulatory systems already depend on large volumes of ingredient data, scientific literature, analytical results, product submissions, complaints and market intelligence. Human review remains essential, but no authority or business can examine every document manually at the speed required by a global product market. AI-assisted tools may identify inconsistencies in submissions, compare ingredient identifiers, screen scientific literature, detect unusual emissions results, recognise repeated packaging or trace suspicious seller networks. They may assist with toxicological read-across, predict potential hazards and prioritise products for expert assessment. These capabilities could make regulation more targeted by directing limited human attention towards the information most likely to matter.

The use of artificial intelligence also creates new regulatory risks. An automated system may reproduce weaknesses in the data on which it was trained, overlook novel hazards, misunderstand confidential formulations or present uncertain predictions with unjustified confidence. Proprietary models may produce conclusions that regulators, manufacturers or courts cannot examine fully. A rejected product or enforcement action cannot rest responsibly on an unexplained algorithmic output. AI should therefore support professional judgement rather than replace it. Its methods, training data, limitations and validation must be understood sufficiently for the output to be challenged. Human responsibility must remain identifiable. Efficiency is valuable, but accountability cannot be delegated to software.

Digital product passports offer another possible change in the relationship between products and regulators. The traditional regulatory dossier is held separately from the physical item. A notification record sits in a database, while the product moves through factories, ports, warehouses, retailers and consumers. The connection between the two depends on names, codes and documents that may be inconsistent or copied. A digital passport could connect an individual product or batch to its manufacturer, importer, formulation record, regulatory status, test information, duty position, environmental obligations and recall history. Enforcement officers could verify identity more quickly, retailers could confirm lawful status and consumers could obtain reliable information without depending entirely on packaging claims.

The usefulness of such a system would depend on governance rather than technology alone. A digital code is only as trustworthy as the information behind it. Counterfeiters can copy visible identifiers, businesses can upload inaccurate data and obsolete records can remain online after products change. Secure authentication, controlled access, version management and independent verification would be necessary. Confidential formulation details must be protected while safety-relevant and market-status information remains accessible. Regulators would need compatible systems across product notification, customs, taxation and market surveillance. A digital passport that creates another isolated database would add administrative burden without solving the fragmentation it was intended to address.

Environmental responsibility will increasingly shape these decisions. Vaping regulation began primarily as a question of nicotine exposure, product quality and consumer protection. The rise of small electronic devices brought batteries, plastics, metals, packaging and disposal into the same policy field. A product may present comparatively lower toxicological risk than smoking while still creating avoidable environmental damage. Regulation will therefore need to consider the full product lifecycle, including raw materials, manufacturing, transport, product longevity, repairability, collection, recycling and final disposal. Environmental performance cannot be assessed solely through whether a device carries a charging port or whether one component is technically replaceable. The relevant question is whether products are designed and supported for meaningful continued use.

This shift will change commercial responsibility. Manufacturers and importers may be expected to finance collection, disclose material composition, design products for disassembly and demonstrate that replacement components remain available. Retailers may become collection points, while waste operators require better information about nicotine residues and lithium batteries. Digital identification could connect product sales with producer-responsibility obligations and help prevent businesses from placing large quantities of electronic goods on the market before disappearing. Environmental requirements should nevertheless remain coordinated with nicotine regulation. Separate systems that define products differently, demand incompatible identifiers or impose overlapping reporting will create unnecessary complexity without improving recycling.

Disposable products have already shown how quickly environmental and public health concerns can converge. Their convenience lowered barriers for adult smokers but also encouraged rapid turnover, visible litter and widespread youth use. Regulatory responses have increasingly treated the product format itself as the problem, yet manufacturers can alter designs to satisfy legal definitions while preserving much of the same commercial behaviour. Future policy will need to distinguish genuine reuse from nominal reuse and assess product lifetime through realistic consumer practice. A device that can technically be recharged but is discarded after one short cycle may satisfy the wording of a rule while defeating its environmental purpose. Regulation must therefore examine function, durability and availability of replacement components rather than relying only on simple product labels.

Flavour restrictions will present a similar challenge because the regulatory object is difficult to define. A flavour can be described through ingredients, sensory character, product name, imagery or consumer perception. Banning named categories may encourage renaming. Restricting descriptors may leave the formulation unchanged. Prohibiting individual compounds may lead to substitutes with less toxicological evidence. A broad restriction may reduce youth appeal while also removing products that adults use to maintain separation from smoking. Future policy must therefore identify the mechanism it intends to control. If the concern is child-oriented marketing, presentation and retail enforcement may be more direct targets. If particular compounds create inhalation hazards, toxicological and analytical controls are required. If the policy objective is to reduce product variety generally, the effects on adult switching and illegal supply should be acknowledged openly.

Nicotine policy will require the same clarity. Governments may seek to reduce dependence, prevent initiation or standardise exposure, but concentration limits do not operate independently from device performance and consumer compensation. Reducing permitted strength may lead some users to consume more liquid or use higher-output devices. Increasing limits may support effective substitution for highly dependent smokers while raising concerns about inexperienced users. The appropriate regulatory question is therefore not simply whether nicotine is addictive, which is already established, but what product characteristics produce acceptable exposure for different populations and how those characteristics can be controlled without making the lawful market less effective than cigarettes or illegal alternatives.

International cooperation will become increasingly necessary because no national system can control a global nicotine market in isolation. Formulations may be developed in one country, devices manufactured in another, brands owned in a third and products sold online into many more. Scientific assessments, laboratory methods and product identifiers remain fragmented across jurisdictions. The same ingredient may be accepted, questioned or prohibited under different systems, while identical products require separate submissions and packaging. Some variation is justified by national law and public health priorities, but unnecessary divergence increases cost and encourages regulatory arbitrage. Manufacturers can direct products towards the least controlled market, while consumers and traders purchase across borders.

Harmonisation should not require every country to adopt the same political position on nicotine. Governments differ in smoking prevalence, healthcare systems, enforcement capacity and tolerance of consumer markets. Cooperation can begin with more practical matters: common chemical identifiers, interoperable data formats, recognised analytical methods, shared counterfeit intelligence and rapid communication of serious product failures. Authorities should be able to recognise the same product across customs, notification and recall systems even where the legal decision attached to that product differs. Scientific and technical compatibility can improve control without removing national sovereignty.

Future legislation must also recognise that vaping no longer exists as an isolated category. Heated tobacco, nicotine pouches, synthetic nicotine, medicinal products and emerging delivery technologies compete within the same broader market. Rules applied to one category alter demand in another. A flavour restriction on vaping may increase pouch use. A high duty on non-combustible products may preserve cigarette sales. A nicotine limit may encourage technological changes that alter aerosol exposure. Regulation organised entirely through historic product categories can therefore miss the relationships that determine population harm. A more coherent system would preserve product-specific controls while recognising that consumers move between categories and that relative risk remains central to the consequences of policy.

This does not require treating harm reduction as a commercial entitlement. Manufacturers should still demonstrate product identity, control quality, substantiate claims and accept post-market responsibility. Children and non-users should remain protected. Products presenting avoidable hazards should be corrected or removed. The central requirement is proportionality: the burden, restriction and enforcement priority should reflect the nature of the product, the evidence of harm and the consequences of available alternatives. Cigarettes should not gain regulatory protection by default merely because they are older, easier to classify or already integrated into taxation systems.

The future of regulation will therefore depend less on whether governments choose to intervene and more on whether they can build systems capable of learning. A learning system records why a rule was introduced, what outcome was predicted and how success will be measured. It links notifications to market samples, complaints to batches, imports to retailers and enforcement findings to legislative review. It distinguishes absence of evidence from evidence of absence and treats uncertainty as a reason for investigation rather than permanent political convenience. It also retires requirements that no longer serve their purpose, because regulation that only accumulates eventually becomes too complex to enforce coherently.

Evidence-based regulation is sometimes described as though evidence will produce one inevitable answer. It will not. Decisions about youth protection, adult access, environmental burden, consumer autonomy and acceptable uncertainty contain political and ethical judgements. Scientific evidence can clarify likely consequences, identify false assumptions and compare alternatives, but it cannot decide which social objective should dominate. Credible future regulation will make that distinction visible. Governments should state when a measure reflects precaution, public preference or political priority rather than presenting every decision as a direct command of science.

The final test will remain practical. Future systems may use artificial intelligence, digital passports, automated surveillance and sophisticated exposure models, but they will still fail if illegal products remain more accessible than lawful ones, if retailers cannot verify stock, if laboratories cannot reproduce results or if regulators cannot act quickly on credible evidence. Technology can improve information, but it cannot substitute for institutional competence, clear responsibility and sustained enforcement. The objective is not to create the most elaborate regulatory architecture. It is to create one capable of distinguishing products accurately, targeting genuine risk, preserving realistic alternatives to smoking and changing as the evidence changes.

The future of vaping regulation should therefore be neither unrestricted innovation nor permanent precaution. It should be controlled adaptation: strict where products or conduct create demonstrated harm, responsive where uncertainty requires monitoring, and flexible where technology can reduce exposure. The framework must be capable of protecting children without treating adult smokers as though their alternatives are irrelevant, controlling environmental waste without preserving combustion, and demanding evidence without allowing regulatory cost to become a substitute for scientific judgement. The next generation of law will be judged not by how much it prohibits or how many databases it creates, but by whether it produces a nicotine market that is more transparent, enforceable, proportionate and responsive than the one it replaces.

Figure 10.1. The Future of Regulation: Adaptive regulation framework.

This diagram presents future vaping regulation as a continuous adaptive cycle rather than a fixed body of rules. At its centre, the framework moves through five connected stages: monitoring emerging products and risks; assessing evidence, impact and proportionality; deciding on clear regulatory objectives; implementing rules, guidance and enforcement capacity; and reviewing outcomes so that weaknesses can be corrected and successful measures retained. The central principle is that regulation should remain evidence-based, proportionate and responsive as products, markets and scientific knowledge change.

The surrounding sections show the principal systems expected to support this future framework. AI-assisted compliance is used to screen submissions, identify unusual ingredients or emissions results, detect illicit products and support risk-based market surveillance, while preserving human regulatory judgement. Digital product passports connect individual products or batches to ingredients, analytical testing, compliance status, traceability and recall information. Environmental regulation extends control across product design, recyclability, repairability, producer responsibility, take-back systems and lifecycle impacts. Nicotine limits and delivery controls are presented as evidence-led measures that require regular review as device efficiency, consumer behaviour and scientific understanding develop.

The lower section connects the adaptive cycle to future law and policy. It emphasises clear legal definitions, technology-neutral drafting, enforceable rules, proportionate penalties, international cooperation and legislation capable of evolving with science and society. The enabling principles across the base of the diagram reinforce the wider objectives of protecting young people, preserving less harmful alternatives for adults who smoke, prioritising high-quality evidence, maintaining transparent stakeholder engagement, sharing international intelligence and ensuring public accountability.

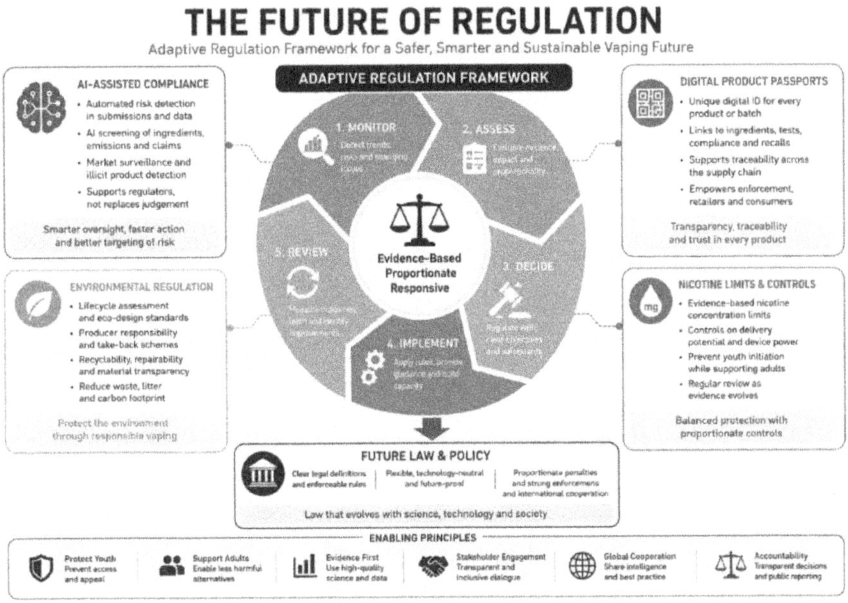

Adaptive Regulation

Adaptive regulation begins from the recognition that vaping products, nicotine markets and patterns of use change more quickly than conventional legislation. A rule written around one generation of devices may remain legally valid while becoming technically obsolete, commercially distortive or ineffective against the products that later dominate the market. Early electronic cigarettes were comparatively simple, yet subsequent systems introduced variable power, nicotine salts, compact pods, disposable formats, rechargeable hybrids and products designed around the narrow wording of capacity or refillability rules. The regulatory problem is therefore not merely that innovation continues, but that every fixed requirement creates incentives for manufacturers, retailers and illegal suppliers to redesign products around it. Adaptive regulation accepts that law must provide stability, but it also requires structured mechanisms through which evidence, technical standards and enforcement practice can be revised without waiting for complete legislative reconstruction.

The purpose of adaptation is not to make regulation uncertain or permanently provisional. Manufacturers need predictable requirements, laboratories need stable methods and enforcement bodies need legal definitions capable of supporting action. Consumers also need confidence that products considered lawful today will not become prohibited tomorrow through unpublished administrative interpretation. Adaptive regulation must therefore distinguish between the enduring principles that should remain stable and the technical controls that may need regular adjustment. Stable principles include identifiable responsibility, ingredient disclosure, product traceability, youth protection, accurate labelling, manufacturing control, post-market vigilance and proportionate enforcement. More adaptable elements include reporting formats, analytical methods, permitted technical specifications, warning presentation, digital identifiers and the evidence thresholds used to prioritise market surveillance. This division allows the law to preserve accountability while responding to scientific and technological development.

A functioning adaptive system begins with continuous monitoring. Product notifications, sales information, complaints, adverse-event reports, laboratory surveillance, border seizures, retailer inspections and published research should be treated as connected sources of regulatory intelligence rather than separate administrative records. Monitoring should identify not only individual breaches but wider shifts in the market. A rapid increase in one product format, unusual ingredient use, repeated failures involving a component supplier or a growing pattern of youth access may indicate that existing controls are no longer addressing the dominant risk. Regulators should be able to detect these changes early enough to investigate them before political pressure reduces the available options to prohibition or inaction. Monitoring is most useful when it produces defined signals, thresholds and questions rather than accumulating data that no institution has the capacity to interpret.

Assessment follows monitoring and requires more than confirming that a concern exists. The regulator must determine the seriousness, scale and plausibility of the risk, identify the affected population and compare the possible interventions. Detection of a hazardous chemical does not establish that exposure is sufficient to create a material health risk. Evidence of youth use does not by itself establish which product feature caused initiation. Discovery of illegal products does not prove that the lawful category should be restricted further. Adaptive assessment should separate hazard, exposure, behaviour and enforcement failure, because each points towards a different response. It should also examine the risk created by intervention itself, including reduced switching among smokers, market consolidation, higher prices, product substitution and movement towards illegal supply. Adaptation without comparative assessment can become a mechanism for repeated tightening rather than evidence-led correction.

Proportionality is therefore the central discipline. A moderate uncertainty may justify enhanced monitoring, targeted testing or a temporary reporting requirement. A well-characterised and serious hazard may justify immediate restriction or withdrawal. Persistent youth-oriented marketing may require controls on presentation and retail conduct, whereas repeated battery failures may require engineering standards and supplier intervention. The strength of the measure should correspond to the strength of evidence, the severity of potential harm and the feasibility of less restrictive alternatives. This approach avoids two opposite errors: waiting for complete certainty before acting, and treating every new concern as grounds for a permanent prohibition. Adaptive regulation should preserve the ability to escalate when evidence strengthens and to withdraw controls when anticipated harms do not materialise or when the measure causes greater unintended consequences.

Decision-making should be organised around explicit regulatory objectives. A policy intended to reduce youth initiation should define whether success means lower experimentation, lower regular use, reduced dependence or fewer underage sales. A measure intended to reduce environmental waste should identify whether the target is battery disposal, total device turnover, recyclability or litter. A nicotine control should specify whether it seeks to limit concentration, delivered dose, dependence potential or accidental exposure. Without this precision, regulators may choose controls that are politically visible but poorly connected to the intended outcome. Clear objectives also make review possible. If the authority cannot state what a measure is expected to achieve, it cannot later determine whether the measure should be retained, amended or abandoned.

Adaptive regulation requires a range of instruments rather than repeated reliance on primary legislation. Technical standards, guidance, implementing rules, licence conditions, data-reporting requirements and targeted market restrictions can sometimes respond more quickly than Acts or Directives. Their use must nevertheless remain bounded by legal authority and public accountability. Secondary mechanisms should not permit regulators to impose major commercial restrictions without consultation, evidence and review. The more significant the effect on market access or consumer choice, the stronger the procedural safeguards should be. Publication of reasoning, stakeholder evidence, impact assessment and implementation timelines helps distinguish legitimate adaptation from unpredictable rulemaking. Businesses can then prepare for change, while courts and the public retain the ability to examine whether the regulator acted within its powers.

Regulatory sandboxes may provide one controlled method for examining new technologies before full market entry. A sandbox permits a limited product, manufacturing process or data system to operate under defined conditions, enhanced reporting and close oversight. In vaping regulation, this could support evaluation of digital product passports, reusable device systems, automated age verification or novel nicotine-delivery controls. The objective is not to exempt participants from safety requirements, but to generate evidence under conditions that reduce uncontrolled exposure. Sandboxes should have clear entry criteria, limits, endpoints and publication arrangements. They should not become privileged routes available only to large firms, nor should participation imply endorsement. Used carefully, they can reveal practical problems before legislation is applied across the whole market.

Performance-based requirements offer another adaptive tool. Traditional rules often specify particular physical features, such as container size, reservoir volume or refill mechanism. Performance standards instead define the outcome that must be achieved, such as leak resistance, consistent nicotine delivery, child protection, electrical safety or meaningful reusability. This can allow multiple technical solutions and reduce the ease with which minor redesign defeats the purpose of the rule. Performance standards are only useful, however, where the outcome can be measured reproducibly. A requirement that a product be safe, proportionate or environmentally responsible is too vague unless supported by methods, thresholds and evidence expectations. Future-proof drafting depends on combining broad functional objectives with sufficiently precise technical criteria for laboratories, manufacturers and enforcement officers.

Review clauses are indispensable. Measures introduced under uncertainty should include dates or triggers for reassessment. The review should consider whether the original problem persisted, whether the intervention changed behaviour as expected and whether new evidence altered the risk assessment. Sunset clauses may be appropriate for temporary restrictions, although automatic expiry is not always suitable where removing a rule could create abrupt risk. An alternative is mandatory renewal based on published evidence. Review must be substantive rather than ceremonial. Authorities should be willing to conclude that a measure failed, caused displacement or became obsolete. Regulation that can only become stricter is not adaptive; it is cumulative.

Post-market surveillance provides the evidence needed for that review. Premarket submissions describe products before or at entry, but real-world use reveals manufacturing variation, consumer adaptation, misuse, counterfeit substitution and effects on smoking behaviour. Complaint trends, sales patterns, laboratory sampling and enforcement outcomes should therefore inform lifecycle control. Manufacturers and importers must contribute accurate post-market information, but regulators should not depend entirely on industry reporting. Independent sampling, consumer reporting and retailer intelligence provide necessary checks. Data should be linked to exact products, batches and responsible operators so that signals can be investigated rather than remaining general concerns attached to an entire category.

Institutional coordination is equally important because vaping regulation crosses health, consumer protection, medicines, customs, taxation, advertising and environmental law. Adaptive action by one authority can create unintended effects elsewhere. A new duty may increase illegal imports; an environmental requirement may alter device design; a flavour restriction may shift demand towards nicotine pouches; a packaging rule may affect authentication and counterfeit detection. Joint assessment should occur before major changes, with compatible definitions and shared implementation plans. Fragmented adaptation can produce contradictory obligations, duplicated reporting and enforcement gaps. The system must adapt as a whole rather than through isolated agencies pursuing separate objectives.

Stakeholder engagement should support adaptation without allowing regulatory capture. Manufacturers possess technical knowledge, retailers understand consumer demand, laboratories can explain method limitations and users can describe why products succeed or fail as substitutes for cigarettes. Public health organisations contribute evidence on population effects, youth use and prevention. These perspectives should be heard through transparent processes in which funding, interests and evidence quality are disclosed. Consultation should begin early enough to influence the problem definition, not merely after the preferred policy has been selected. The regulator must retain independent judgement, but excluding practical expertise can produce rules that are scientifically elegant and operationally unworkable.

Adaptive systems also require regulatory capacity. Constant data collection is useless without people able to interpret chemistry, toxicology, engineering, behaviour and market structure. Authorities need technical teams capable of distinguishing genuine product innovation from superficial circumvention, assessing laboratory uncertainty and understanding how consumers respond to restrictions. They also need legal and economic expertise to evaluate enforceability, market concentration and illicit incentives. Adaptation cannot be outsourced entirely to consultants or automated tools, because responsibility for public decisions must remain within accountable institutions. Investment in competence is therefore as important as investment in databases.

The treatment of uncertainty should remain explicit throughout the cycle. Regulators should state what is known, what remains uncertain and which assumptions support the chosen measure. This reduces the temptation to present political judgement as scientific inevitability. It also allows later reviewers to determine whether the assumptions proved correct. In vaping policy, uncertainty exists on both sides: the long-term effects of particular exposures may be incomplete, while the consequences of restricting products used by smokers may also be uncertain. Adaptive regulation should not apply precaution only to market access while ignoring uncertainty created by intervention. The relevant comparison is between available courses of action, not between regulation and an imaginary absence of consequences.

Data governance determines whether this cycle can operate credibly. Regulators need timely access to product, market and enforcement information, but collection should remain purposeful, standardised and proportionate. Reporting systems should use consistent identifiers, preserve version history and distinguish confidential formulation data from information necessary for public protection. Automated alerts may help identify anomalies, yet thresholds should be validated and reviewed to avoid overwhelming authorities with false signals. Data quality obligations should apply to regulators as well as industry: duplicate records, inconsistent terminology and obsolete submissions can distort priorities. Where evidence is shared internationally, common formats and clear legal safeguards are required. An adaptive framework cannot depend on databases that are extensive but unreliable, inaccessible or disconnected from the physical products moving through the market. Information architecture is therefore part of regulatory design, not a minor supporting administrative detail.

Successful adaptation should therefore improve the fit between regulatory objectives and market reality. It should identify emerging problems earlier, select controls more precisely, test whether those controls work and revise them when evidence changes. It should preserve stable responsibilities while allowing methods and technical requirements to evolve. Most importantly, it should prevent regulation from becoming detached from the products, behaviours and risks it was created to govern. A mature system does not treat amendment as an admission of failure. It treats the capacity to learn, correct and respond proportionately as the defining feature of competent regulation.

AI-Assisted Compliance

AI-assisted compliance is emerging as one of the most significant developments in modern regulatory practice because vaping regulation produces more information than any conventional review system can examine manually at sufficient speed. Product notifications contain ingredient identities, concentrations, toxicological summaries, emissions data, device specifications, manufacturing descriptions and market information. Post-market systems add complaints, adverse-event reports, laboratory findings, retailer intelligence, border seizures and online listings. Each source may be individually manageable, but the combined volume becomes difficult for regulators and businesses to interpret consistently. Artificial intelligence offers tools for sorting, comparing and prioritising this material, although its value depends entirely on the quality of the data, the transparency of the method and the continued involvement of competent human judgement.

The most immediate use of artificial intelligence lies in regulatory data screening. A submission system can apply automated checks to identify missing fields, inconsistent units, duplicated ingredients, implausible concentrations or identifiers that do not correspond with recognised chemical records. It can compare the product description with earlier versions, highlight unexplained changes and detect whether a purportedly new product appears materially identical to an existing submission. These functions do not require the system to decide whether the product is safe. They reduce administrative error and direct reviewers towards records requiring closer examination. In a market containing thousands of variants, automated triage can prevent expert time from being consumed by routine formatting problems while allowing more attention to be given to toxicological, analytical and engineering questions that cannot be resolved through simple validation.

Ingredient assessment provides a more technically demanding application. Artificial intelligence can search chemical databases, scientific literature and regulatory records for known hazards, structural alerts, respiratory effects, thermal degradation products and restrictions applied in other jurisdictions. It may identify inconsistencies between ingredient names, Chemical Abstracts Service numbers and supplier descriptions, or recognise that several trade names refer to the same substance. It can also assist in comparing related compounds where direct inhalation evidence is limited. Such screening may strengthen the initial review, particularly where flavour formulations contain many components. The output, however, remains a prioritisation tool. Structural similarity does not prove equivalent toxicity, and absence from a hazard database does not establish safety. Every automated signal requires interpretation in relation to concentration, exposure, device conditions and the quality of the underlying evidence.

Toxicological literature review may also become faster and more systematic. Conventional review depends on carefully constructed searches, selection criteria and expert interpretation, but the number of publications relevant to nicotine products continues to expand. AI-assisted tools can identify new studies, classify them by endpoint, extract product characteristics and compare methods across papers. They may help distinguish research involving realistic operating conditions from experiments conducted under severe thermal stress, or identify when conclusions are based on products no longer representative of the market. The benefit lies in improved coverage and faster detection of emerging evidence. The danger lies in false confidence. Automated summaries may omit methodological weaknesses, misunderstand context or reproduce errors contained in published abstracts. Reviewers must retain access to the original study and remain responsible for judging relevance, reliability and biological significance.

Analytical data offer another important area. Emissions testing generates large datasets containing nicotine, carbonyls, volatile compounds, metals and other measured constituents across different products and operating conditions. Artificial intelligence can compare results across batches, identify outliers and detect patterns associated with particular coil materials, formulations or power settings. It may reveal that one supplier's component is repeatedly linked to elevated metal emissions or that one flavour family produces unusual degradation products under defined conditions. These patterns can guide investigation and market surveillance. They cannot be treated as automatic findings of non-compliance unless the underlying methods are comparable. Differences in puffing regime, instrument calibration, sample conditioning and reporting limit can create apparent anomalies that reflect method variation rather than product risk.

Manufacturing compliance can benefit from predictive monitoring. Production equipment already generates information on temperatures, filling volumes, weights, mixing times, line speeds and rejection rates. AI systems can examine these data continuously and detect drift before a specification failure becomes widespread. They may identify combinations of variables associated with leakage, nicotine variation or device failure, allowing maintenance or process adjustment before defective goods are released. This is a stronger use of artificial intelligence than retrospective document generation because it is connected directly to process control. The system should nevertheless operate within a validated quality framework. Alerts, decision thresholds and automated interventions must be tested, documented and reviewed, while personnel retain authority to investigate causes and determine whether affected batches require quarantine.

Supplier management may become more evidence-led through automated comparison of certificates, audit findings, complaint histories and test results. An AI-assisted system can identify repeated documentation inconsistencies, changes in raw-material specifications or suppliers associated with a disproportionate number of failures. It may recognise that a flavour house has altered a formulation without updating the declared composition, or that a device component has changed dimensions despite being supplied under the same part number. These findings can support risk-based auditing and incoming inspection. They should not create unchallengeable supplier scores. Smaller suppliers may produce less data without being less competent, while large suppliers may appear reliable because their documentation is extensive. The model must distinguish quantity of information from quality of control.

Online market surveillance is likely to be one of the most visible applications. Artificial intelligence can scan websites, marketplaces and social-media content for products appearing to exceed legal capacities, use prohibited claims, imitate established brands or target young people. Image recognition can compare packaging with known notified products and identify copied artwork or altered warnings. Language models can detect medicinal claims, misleading safety statements and product descriptions associated with illegal strengths or formats. Network analysis can connect apparently separate seller accounts through shared contact details, payment information, images or fulfilment addresses. This enables enforcement to focus on commercial networks rather than remove isolated listings repeatedly.

Automated online surveillance requires strong safeguards because errors can affect lawful businesses. A product may appear oversized in an image because of perspective, while a seller may quote puff count without exceeding liquid limits. Shared photographs can arise from legitimate distribution rather than counterfeiting. Words associated with smoking cessation may appear in factual consumer information rather than unlawful medicinal promotion. Systems should therefore identify leads, preserve evidence and refer cases for human review. Platforms and authorities should not impose irreversible penalties solely because an algorithm assigns a high-risk score. Businesses need a route to understand the concern, provide evidence and challenge incorrect classification.

Border control can use artificial intelligence to improve risk profiling across import declarations, shipment histories, product descriptions and previous seizures. Models may identify unusual valuation, repeated changes in importer identity, routes associated with misdeclaration or consignments divided into patterns consistent with avoidance. They can compare declared products with notification records and alert officers when a brand, nicotine strength or device format appears inconsistent. This can make selective inspection more effective where universal examination is impossible. The system must be monitored for bias and adaptation. Illegal traders change routes and descriptions once controls become predictable, while legitimate importers can be delayed if historical associations are treated as permanent evidence of risk.

Complaint and adverse-event systems can also benefit from automated signal detection. Reports often contain incomplete product names, varied symptom descriptions and uncertain causal relationships. Language processing can group similar reports, recognise recurring device failures and identify clusters linked to one batch or retailer. It can distinguish a rising pattern from ordinary background complaints and prompt earlier investigation. Causation must remain a human scientific judgement. A report following product use does not prove that the product caused the event, and automated grouping may combine clinically different outcomes. The value lies in finding signals that deserve review, not manufacturing certainty from weak data.

Artificial intelligence can assist regulatory writing and document management, but this is also where superficial use may become most dangerous. Businesses may use generative systems to draft toxicological summaries, standard operating procedures, risk assessments and notification text. This can reduce repetitive workload and improve consistency where the system is grounded in verified company data. It can also produce fluent but inaccurate material, invented references, unsupported conclusions and generic statements that do not correspond to the product. A polished document may conceal the absence of genuine assessment. Organisations must therefore define which uses are permitted, require expert review and preserve evidence showing how conclusions were reached. Regulatory responsibility remains with the producer, not the software.

Data confidentiality and cybersecurity are central because AI-assisted systems may process proprietary formulations, supplier records, consumer complaints and enforcement intelligence. Information should be collected only for defined purposes, protected against unauthorised access and governed by clear retention and sharing rules. Cloud-based services may transfer sensitive data across jurisdictions or use submitted information to improve external models unless contracts prohibit it. Regulators and businesses need assurance concerning data location, model training, access control and incident response. A compliance tool that exposes confidential formulations or personal information creates a new regulatory failure while attempting to solve another.

Model validation should be treated with the same seriousness applied to analytical methods. The intended use must be defined, performance measured and limitations understood. A model used to detect missing fields requires a different standard from one used to prioritise safety investigations. Training datasets should represent the products, languages and market conditions in which the tool will operate. False-positive and false-negative rates should be assessed, and performance should be re-evaluated when products or data sources change. Version control is essential because model updates can alter outcomes without visible changes to the user interface. Significant decisions should remain reproducible, allowing reviewers to understand which model and data produced the result.

Explainability becomes especially important where AI output affects market access or enforcement. A regulator should not reject a submission merely because a proprietary system labels it high risk without identifying the underlying concern. A manufacturer should be able to respond to the ingredient, data inconsistency or evidence pattern that triggered review. Full mathematical transparency may not always be practical, but decision-relevant reasons must be available. Public authorities carry a higher obligation because their decisions affect rights, competition and lawful commerce. Automated systems should support accountable reasoning rather than create a technical barrier that prevents meaningful challenge.

Human competence remains indispensable. Artificial intelligence can identify patterns across more data than an individual reviewer can process, but it does not possess regulatory responsibility or contextual understanding equivalent to an experienced toxicologist, analytical chemist, quality professional or enforcement officer. It may recognise correlation without understanding causation, apply outdated thresholds or fail to notice that a product has changed in a way not represented in its data. Human reviewers must understand enough about the system to question its output rather than treating technology as neutral. Training should include both the regulatory subject and the limitations of automated analysis.

Governance should define who approves tools, who monitors performance, who can override recommendations and how errors are reported. Businesses require policies covering authorised data, validation, review and record retention. Regulators require public standards for the use of automated systems in submission assessment, surveillance and enforcement. Independent audit may be appropriate where models influence high-impact decisions. International cooperation could support common validation principles, reducing the risk that every jurisdiction develops incompatible or opaque systems.

AI-assisted compliance is therefore most valuable when it strengthens attention rather than substitutes for it. It can reduce administrative burden, reveal hidden patterns, accelerate literature review, improve manufacturing control and direct enforcement towards higher-risk products. It becomes dangerous when fluent output is mistaken for evidence, automated suspicion becomes automatic sanction or proprietary systems remove decisions from public scrutiny. The future regulatory system should use artificial intelligence as an instrument of disciplined analysis: validated for its purpose, governed transparently, protected against misuse and always connected to identifiable human responsibility. Its success will be measured not by how many tasks become automated, but by whether decisions become materially faster, more consistent, scientifically defensible and easier to correct when either the data or the model proves wrong.

Digital Product Passports

Digital product passports offer a way to connect the physical vaping product moving through manufacture, importation, distribution, retail and post-market control with the regulatory information that gives that product its lawful identity. Formulation details sit within a notification database, analytical reports remain in technical files, customs declarations are held by border authorities, batch records remain with manufacturers, duty information sits within fiscal systems and recalls are communicated through separate notices. The physical item reaching the consumer may display only a brand name, flavour, nicotine strength, warning and batch code. Once products are copied, diverted, modified or separated from their original cartons, the connection between the object and its evidence can weaken quickly. A digital product passport is intended to preserve that connection through a secure identifier linked to a structured record that can be accessed by authorised participants across the lifecycle.

The passport should not be confused with a marketing QR code or a website containing generic product information. Its regulatory value depends on whether it identifies the exact product, version or batch and whether the data behind it are controlled, current and verifiable. A code that directs every item in a range to the same promotional webpage provides little help when one nicotine strength, formulation or production batch is affected. A useful passport should distinguish the notified product family from the manufactured batch and, where proportionate, from the individual unit. Refillable liquids may require batch-level identification, while higher-value devices, duty-controlled products or components with safety relevance may justify serialised unit-level records. The identifier must remain connected to the original manufacturing and submission data throughout distribution rather than being recreated independently by wholesalers or retailers.

The passport could contain or link to the legal product name, brand, variant, nicotine strength, liquid volume, device model, formulation version, manufacturer, importer, responsible economic operator and markets for which the product is authorised or notified. This would allow retailers and enforcement officers to distinguish visually similar versions intended for different jurisdictions. A product lawful in one market may exceed the nicotine or capacity limits of another, use different warnings or fall under a separate tax system. Packaging alone may not reveal these differences reliably, particularly where brand families use common artwork. A trusted passport could show whether the item is recognised for the destination market and whether its status remains active, suspended, withdrawn or superseded by a later version.

The same record could support supply-chain traceability. Manufacturers would associate the product with raw-material lots, component batches, production dates, filling lines, test results and release decisions. Importers would add shipment, customs and receipt information. Distributors could record onward movements, while retailers could verify receipt and, where required, confirm the status of recalled stock. A retailer may need confirmation that the product is genuine and marketable without access to the proprietary formulation. An enforcement officer may need batch, importer and test information, while the consumer may need authenticity, ingredients of concern, instructions and recall status. The architecture must therefore support role-based access rather than assume that one public record can serve every purpose.

Counterfeit detection is one of the strongest potential benefits. Counterfeiters can copy packaging, regulatory numbers and visible codes, but secure serialisation combined with central verification can make duplication easier to detect. If the same identifier is scanned repeatedly in different locations or before the recorded product has left the factory, the system can generate a signal. Brand owners and regulators could identify abnormal verification patterns and focus investigation on the retailers, importers or online sellers involved. This is more useful than a simple valid-or-invalid response because copied genuine codes may appear valid individually. It should also provide an offline or alternative verification route where connectivity is poor, while preventing the offline function from becoming an easy method of bypassing central controls.

Digital passports could improve border control by allowing officers to compare the product physically presented with the record attached to the identifier. The system could show whether the named importer is authorised, whether the product has been notified, whether the shipment corresponds to expected trade movements and whether the batch has already appeared elsewhere. Customs declarations could be linked to the same product identity used by health regulators and tax authorities. This would reduce the ambiguity created when one agency identifies goods by commodity code, another by brand name and another by notification number. A common identity does not remove the need for inspection or testing, because false labels can still be attached to different goods, but it allows officers to detect inconsistencies more quickly and to trace suspect consignments into domestic distribution.

At present, retailers may need to search product registers manually, interpret inconsistent names and rely on supplier assurances. A passport-enabled system could confirm whether the exact item is recognised, whether its importer is identifiable and whether any alert or withdrawal applies. This would support due diligence without requiring retail staff to interpret complete regulatory dossiers. A green status should never imply that the product is harmless or that every unit has been independently approved. It should mean only that the identifier corresponds to a valid record and that no current restriction is known. The language used by the system must avoid turning administrative status into a misleading safety claim.

Product withdrawals and recalls would benefit substantially from the same infrastructure. When a batch is affected, its passport status could be changed centrally and communicated across wholesalers, retailers, marketplaces and consumers. Businesses could scan stock to identify affected units rather than removing an entire product family. Online sellers could block fulfilment automatically, while distributors could produce movement records showing where the batch had been supplied. Consumers scanning the product could receive a warning and instructions concerning return, disposal or continued use. This speed matters because conventional recall notices often depend on email chains, website updates and retailers matching written descriptions against stock manually.

A passport could contain material composition, battery type, repairability, replacement-component availability, recycling instructions and producer-responsibility information. Waste operators could identify whether a device contains a removable lithium cell, residual nicotine liquid or materials requiring specialist handling. Regulators could verify whether the manufacturer or importer responsible for placing the product on the market is registered within the relevant environmental system. Product durability claims could be linked to evidence concerning intended life, recharge cycles and replaceable parts. This would help distinguish meaningful reuse from devices designed to satisfy a legal definition while remaining functionally disposable. Environmental data should, however, be based on standardised measures rather than unverified sustainability claims supplied by the producer.

A passport could connect product identity with duty status, authorised production, importation and movement records. Duty stamps or fiscal identifiers could be incorporated into the same system while remaining legally distinct from health notification. Enforcement officers could determine whether a product is both technically lawful and correctly taxed, avoiding the assumption that compliance in one area establishes compliance in another. Serialised records could make diversion, duplicate stamps and unexplained stock movements easier to detect. The challenge is to avoid creating several overlapping codes for product notification, customs, duty, recycling and brand authentication. A coherent passport should act as a common gateway to distinct regulatory records rather than adding another isolated label.

Data quality will determine whether the system improves regulation or merely digitises existing errors. Ingredient names, CAS numbers, product versions and responsible-operator details must be standardised. Records should include creation dates, revision history and the authority responsible for each field. Changes to formulation, coil, battery, manufacturing site or packaging must be assessed and reflected promptly. If obsolete information remains active, the passport may falsely reassure users and enforcement officers. Validation rules can identify incomplete or inconsistent entries, but human review remains necessary where technical judgement is involved. The system should make clear which data were supplied by the manufacturer, which were verified by a regulator or laboratory and which represent market intelligence or enforcement findings.

Confidentiality requires careful design. Full formulations, supplier identities and analytical methods may contain legitimate trade secrets, while complaints and transaction records may include personal data. Consumers need meaningful product and safety information; regulators need access sufficient for oversight; businesses need protection against unnecessary exposure of proprietary knowledge. Role-based permissions, encryption, audit logs and legal limits on secondary use are therefore essential. Access should be traceable so that misuse can be investigated. The system must also comply with data-protection principles by collecting only what is necessary, defining retention periods and preventing commercial profiling of consumers through routine product scans.

Cybersecurity is not a secondary concern because a passport becomes valuable precisely when multiple decisions depend upon it. Attackers could attempt to create false records, alter recall status, harvest confidential formulations, generate valid-looking identifiers or disable verification services during enforcement action. The system requires resilient hosting, authentication, backup, incident response and independent security testing. Critical functions should not depend on one private supplier without contingency arrangements. Public authorities must retain control over regulatory status even where technology is provided commercially. A proprietary platform that cannot be audited, migrated or operated after the vendor fails would create a new form of regulatory dependency.

Governance must define who creates the record, who verifies it, who can change it and who is responsible when information is wrong. Manufacturers may enter technical data, but regulators should control legal status and enforcement alerts. Importers should not be able to overwrite manufacturer records without documented change control. Retailers should confirm movements or receipt without gaining access to confidential content. Consumers should be able to report discrepancies, but public reports should not alter product status automatically. Disputes concerning identity, notification or authenticity require a transparent review process so that legitimate businesses are not removed from the market through an unexplained digital flag.

Products move across borders, while jurisdictions use different legal categories, data fields and notification systems. A passport should not imply that one country's acceptance binds another. It should carry market-specific status and allow authorities to recognise the same product while applying their own law. Common identifiers, data standards and secure exchange protocols could reduce duplication without requiring identical regulatory policy. Manufacturers could maintain a core product record supplemented by jurisdictional modules covering warnings, nicotine limits, tax and market permissions. This would be more efficient than recreating disconnected records for every country, but only if governance prevents the lowest standard from becoming the default.

Requiring unit-level serialisation for every low-cost component immediately could impose substantial cost, exclude smaller firms and create systems too complex to operate reliably. Priority could begin with nicotine-containing finished products, high-risk devices, duty-controlled goods and categories associated with counterfeiting or illegal capacities. Pilot programmes should test scanning speed, data accuracy, recall functionality and retailer usability before national adoption. A passport that only large multinational companies can implement would reshape the market through technology cost rather than scientific merit.

Digital product passports cannot replace physical inspection, analytical testing or competent enforcement. A genuine identifier can be attached to a false product, data can be entered incorrectly and illegal sellers can avoid the system entirely. Their value lies in making identity, status and movement easier to verify, while creating evidence when the product and record diverge. Properly designed, they can connect notification, importation, distribution, taxation, environmental responsibility and recall through one controlled information architecture. Poorly designed, they will become another code on the package, another database for compliant businesses and another symbol copied by counterfeiters.

The strongest passport system will therefore be secure, interoperable, proportionate and transparent about the limits of what it proves. It should confirm product identity without pretending to certify safety absolutely, protect confidential data while making market status visible and support enforcement without replacing professional judgement. Its success will be measured by whether recalls become faster, counterfeits easier to detect, retailers better able to verify stock and regulators more capable of connecting the physical product with the evidence and responsibilities attached to it. Digital identity is not the end of regulation, but it may become the infrastructure that allows future regulation to remain connected to the products it is intended to control.

Environmental Regulation

Environmental regulation has become inseparable from the future governance of vaping because every device combines a nicotine-delivery function with a material lifecycle involving plastics, metals, electronic circuitry, lithium batteries, packaging, transport and eventual disposal. Earlier regulatory systems concentrated principally on ingredients, emissions, nicotine concentration, warning statements and consumer safety, while the environmental consequences of device sales remained secondary. That separation became difficult to defend as low-cost single-use products entered the market in large numbers and were discarded after short periods of use. A product could comply with the principal nicotine rules while still embodying avoidable material waste, poor recyclability and a battery that remained functional when the device was thrown away. Environmental regulation extends product responsibility beyond what the consumer inhales and asks how the device is designed, how long it remains useful, what resources it consumes and who bears the cost of recovering its components.

The United Kingdom's prohibition on the sale and supply of single-use vapes, which took effect on 1 June 2025 and applies to nicotine-containing and nicotine-free products sold both online and in shops, marked a shift from managing waste after disposal towards regulating the product format before sale. Businesses were also required to arrange appropriate recycling for remaining stock rather than treating unsaleable devices as ordinary refuse. The measure demonstrated that environmental policy can remove a product category even where it remains subject to separate health, consumer and nicotine rules. It also showed why definitions matter. A reusable product must be more than a single-use device fitted with a nominal charging port or refill feature. The design, replaceable components, availability of consumables and expected pattern of use must make repeated operation realistic rather than theoretical. Otherwise, manufacturers can preserve the disposable commercial model while satisfying the rule's wording.

Product longevity should become a central environmental performance measure. A device that survives hundreds of charging cycles, accepts replaceable pods or coils and remains supported by available components creates a different waste profile from one that is technically rechargeable but discarded when the liquid is exhausted or the coil deteriorates. Regulation should examine durability, repairability, battery life, replaceability and compatibility rather than through one physical feature. Manufacturers could be required to define the intended service life, demonstrate that replacement parts remain available for a reasonable period and avoid designs in which the battery, reservoir and heating element are permanently bonded without functional necessity. Such requirements would reduce waste more directly than broad sustainability claims and would encourage engineering decisions that extend useful life without compromising leak resistance, electrical safety or tamper protection.

Waste electrical and electronic equipment obligations already provide a framework for electrical products placed on the British market. Producers must register and meet responsibilities associated with the electrical equipment they supply, while distributors have take-back duties, including free like-for-like collection in relevant circumstances and record retention. Guidance specifically excludes vape retailers from using the Distributor Takeback Scheme, making direct take-back compliance important. Guidance also distinguishes the reporting of electrical equipment weight from the weight of incorporated batteries, which must be addressed under the separate waste-battery system. This division reflects the legal structure, but it can be confusing for businesses selling one item containing electronics and a battery. Future regulation should integrate these obligations operationally so that producers and retailers can report, collect and finance recovery through one coherent route while regulators retain the distinct data needed for electrical and battery waste.

Battery regulation is important because a discarded vape may retain electrical charge and nicotine residue, creating fire, chemical and handling risks during collection and treatment. British producer-responsibility rules require manufacturers and importers to record the tonnage and chemistry of batteries placed on the market, while larger portable-battery producers finance collection, treatment and recycling through approved compliance arrangements. Retailers and distributors supplying at least the specified annual quantity of portable batteries may also have free take-back obligations. These requirements were not designed specifically around vaping, yet the sector exposes their practical limitations. Consumers may not regard an integrated device as a battery, retail staff may be uncertain about appropriate collection, and waste facilities can receive products mixed with ordinary refuse. Clear labelling, accessible return points and training are necessary if producer responsibility is to translate into actual recovery.

Collection alone does not guarantee effective recycling. Vaping devices combine small batteries, plastics, wires, printed circuit boards, metal housings, absorbent materials and residual liquid within casings difficult or uneconomic to dismantle. A collection target can be met while recovered devices are processed inefficiently or exported without transparent treatment outcomes. Environmental standards should address design for disassembly, material identification and safe removal of batteries and nicotine-containing components. Producers should be required to provide treatment information to authorised recyclers and to avoid unnecessary adhesives, mixed materials or sealed structures that prevent component separation. Where disassembly would undermine consumer safety, the manufacturer should demonstrate how authorised treatment can still recover valuable materials and manage residues. Recyclability must be assessed through realistic treatment processes rather than laboratory possibility.

Extended producer responsibility should align financial incentives with the environmental performance of the product. If every producer pays the same contribution per unit or kilogram regardless of durability, repairability or recovery cost, better-designed systems receive little regulatory advantage. Modulated fees could impose higher costs on products that are difficult to dismantle, contain non-replaceable batteries or generate high quantities of mixed waste, while reducing charges for demonstrably durable and recoverable designs. Such modulation must be based on measurable criteria and protected against superficial compliance. A product should not qualify for a lower fee merely because it carries recyclable symbols or contains a small proportion of recycled plastic. Evidence should include service life, return rates, component accessibility, verified treatment performance and the continued availability of replacements.

Retailers should form part of the recovery network because they have direct contact with consumers and already supply the replacement products that create the waste stream. Take-back points can make disposal convenient and keep devices out of household rubbish, but implementation must recognise the realities of small premises, fire safety, staff training and hazardous residues. Containers should protect against short circuits, leakage and unauthorised access, while collection frequency must prevent excessive accumulation. Online sellers require equivalent arrangements rather than relying on physical retailers to bear the burden created by remote sales. Prepaid returns, courier collection or accessible local networks may be necessary. Environmental responsibility should follow the sale regardless of whether the transaction occurs in a shop, through a marketplace or by direct overseas fulfilment.

Online marketplaces and foreign sellers create an enforcement problem because products can be placed on the market without a domestic producer meeting registration and recycling costs. This creates free riding: compliant businesses finance recovery while unregistered sellers undercut them. The United Kingdom has already signalled reform intended to make online marketplaces and vape producers contribute more fairly to electrical-waste recycling. A future system should require platforms to verify environmental registration before listings, retain seller and product data, and assume defined responsibility where no compliant producer can be identified. Without this approach, domestic obligations will remain concentrated on visible businesses while direct imports continue to generate waste outside the financing system.

Digital product passports could strengthen environmental regulation by linking each product or batch to material composition, battery chemistry, responsible producer, repair information, recycling instructions and take-back arrangements. The European Union's Batteries Regulation points towards this wider digital architecture by establishing sustainability and lifecycle requirements for batteries and providing for QR-code information and battery passports for specified categories from 2027. Small batteries incorporated into vaping devices may not fall within every passport provision, but the direction is important: product identity is increasingly expected to carry environmental information throughout the value chain. A vape-specific passport could help waste operators identify construction, allow retailers to verify producer registration and enable regulators to compare units placed on the market with quantities recovered.

Environmental claims require the same evidential discipline as health claims. Terms such as eco-friendly, recyclable or carbon neutral can mislead when they describe only one feature of a product or depend on collection systems that consumers cannot access. A rechargeable device may still have a short service life; recyclable materials may remain inseparable; a take-back scheme may recover only a negligible proportion of units sold. Claims should therefore specify the basis, boundaries and verification method. Lifecycle assessment can compare raw-material extraction, manufacturing, transport, use and disposal, but its conclusions depend heavily on assumptions concerning device life, charging, consumer behaviour and recovery. Regulators should require transparent methodologies and prevent selective claims that highlight a reduced packaging weight while ignoring batteries, electronics or low return rates.

Packaging regulation should be integrated with product regulation rather than treated as a separate exercise in reducing cardboard or plastic. Packaging protects against leakage, tampering, accidental exposure and damage during transport, so environmental reduction cannot mean removing material without assessing safety. The objective should be right-sizing, material simplification, recycled content where suitable and elimination of unnecessary secondary layers. Refill liquids, pods and replacement coils generate recurring packaging streams even when the device itself is durable. Standardised collection or material requirements could reduce this burden, but they must not compromise nicotine containment or child resistance. The best design considers the device, consumables and transport packaging rather than improving one component while shifting waste elsewhere.

Regulation should also examine manufacturing and logistics. Device production consumes metals, plastics, energy and water, while global supply chains create transport emissions and make recovery more difficult. Producers could be required to report material inputs, recycled content, manufacturing waste and carbon intensity consistently. Such reporting should be proportionate and focused on information capable of changing design or procurement rather than becoming another unexamined database. Smaller firms may need standard tools and phased requirements, while larger producers should provide more detailed lifecycle evidence. Performance should be compared within product categories and against the function delivered, recognising that a durable system may use more material initially but generate less waste per period of use than repeated low-mass devices.

Enforcement must connect environmental status to the same product identity used for nicotine notification, customs, duty and market surveillance. An inspector should be able to determine whether the responsible producer is registered, whether the product qualifies as reusable, whether take-back information is accurate and whether claimed replacement components are genuinely available. Border authorities should identify imports lacking a responsible environmental operator, while online monitoring should detect products marketed as reusable despite designs inconsistent with repeated use. Sanctions should address both the physical goods and the advantage gained by avoiding recovery costs. Seizing one consignment will have limited effect if the seller can reopen through another marketplace account without assuming producer responsibility.

Environmental regulation must remain proportionate to the public-health role of vaping. A reusable product that assists an adult smoker to move away from combustible tobacco may create electronic waste while still contributing to a reduction in health risk. The appropriate comparison is not between vaping and an imaginary product with no material footprint, but among realistic nicotine-delivery options and patterns of use. Environmental policy should reduce avoidable waste without making lawful non-combustible products so expensive, inconvenient or technically weak that consumers return to cigarettes or illegal devices. This requires coordination between environmental departments, health regulators, manufacturers, retailers and waste authorities rather than rules developed around one objective.

The future framework should move from disposal management towards lifecycle accountability. Producers should design products for durability, disclose materials, finance recovery and verify treatment. Importers and marketplaces should ensure that a responsible operator exists before sale. Retailers should provide practical return routes, and consumers should receive clear instructions that match the collection infrastructure available to them. Regulators should measure units placed on the market, service life, return rates, recovery performance, illegal supply and behavioural substitution rather than relying only on the number of products labelled reusable. Environmental regulation will be effective when it changes design and recovery in practice, not when it merely transfers discarded vapes from one waste category to another.

Disposable Products

Disposable vaping products became one of the most influential and controversial formats in the modern nicotine market because they combined simplicity, low purchase price, strong sensory delivery and immediate availability in a form requiring almost no consumer knowledge. A user did not need to select a device, understand coil resistance, fill a reservoir, replace a pod or maintain a battery. The product was purchased, activated by inhalation and discarded when exhausted. That simplicity helped some smokers try vaping who might otherwise have rejected more complicated systems, but it also removed many of the practical barriers that had limited experimentation among younger and inexperienced users. The same characteristics that made disposables commercially successful therefore created regulatory pressure across public health, product safety, retail conduct, waste management and illegal trade.

Their significance lies in the way one product format altered the economics and visibility of vaping. Earlier reusable devices required a higher initial purchase, periodic maintenance and continued purchase of liquids or replacement components. Disposable products converted the experience into a low-commitment retail transaction similar to buying a confectionery item, soft drink or packet of cigarettes. Bright presentation, compact dimensions, sweet flavour profiles and prominent puff-count claims made comparison easy at the point of sale. Retailers could stock large numbers of variants without providing technical advice, while consumers could move between flavours and brands without becoming tied to one hardware system. Regulation designed around refillable products was therefore confronted by a format that changed consumer behaviour more quickly than the underlying law.

The rapid growth of disposables also exposed the weakness of treating technical compliance as sufficient evidence of responsible market conduct. A product might satisfy nicotine concentration, liquid volume, labelling and notification requirements while being presented in a manner likely to attract children or encourage frequent replacement. High sales volumes generated visible litter, schools reported widespread possession, and enforcement authorities encountered products claiming capacities far above permitted limits. These developments encouraged governments to consider format-based restrictions because existing controls appeared unable to address the combined effects of product design, marketing, retail ubiquity and disposal.

A format prohibition is a powerful regulatory intervention because it removes an entire design model rather than correcting individual defects. Its justification should therefore be examined carefully. The strongest arguments concern environmental waste, youth access, enforcement difficulty and the ease with which illegal variants circulate alongside lawful products. A single-use device contains a battery, circuit, heating element, plastics and residual nicotine liquid that are discarded after a comparatively short period. Collection and recycling systems struggle when products are small, distributed widely and placed in household waste. At the same time, the low unit price and simple operation make the format attractive to inexperienced users and informal resellers. Where oversized or high-strength products resemble lawful units closely, retail and consumer distinction becomes difficult.

Some users value the consistency, portability and absence of refilling. Others use disposables temporarily before moving to reusable systems. Removing the format does not guarantee that all users will adopt compliant reusable alternatives. Some may return to cigarettes, purchase illegal disposables, move towards other nicotine products or stop using nicotine altogether. The distribution of these responses determines the public-health effect. Regulation should therefore assess substitution rather than assuming that the disappearance of one product from lawful shelves represents a complete solution.

The definition of a disposable product is central to enforceability. A rule based only on whether a battery can be recharged is vulnerable to superficial redesign. Manufacturers may add a charging port while leaving the liquid reservoir non-refillable, the coil irreplaceable and the device economically unattractive to retain. A technically rechargeable product may still be discarded after one liquid cycle because the consumer has no practical reason to keep it. Similarly, a device may include a removable pod that is not sold separately or is difficult to replace. Regulation must therefore consider whether the product is designed and supported for repeated use, whether replacement components are available, whether the consumer can perform the necessary maintenance safely and whether the expected service life is materially longer than that of a single-use unit.

Functional definitions should be supported by objective criteria. The regulator should avoid relying solely on manufacturer intention because intention can be stated more easily than demonstrated. Evidence may include design drawings, component availability, retail listings, user instructions and real-world durability testing. A product that technically meets one criterion but fails the overall purpose of reuse should not be treated automatically as compliant. At the same time, criteria must be clear enough for manufacturers, retailers and enforcement officers to apply consistently. The resulting system should reward products that achieve repeated use in practice, not those that satisfy a narrow definition while preserving the commercial pattern, material turnover and consumer behaviour of disposability across the wider market.

Product design following a disposable ban is likely to evolve rapidly. Rechargeable pod systems, prefilled cartridges, larger reusable bodies and modular products may replace the original format. This transition could improve environmental performance if consumers retain the main device and discard only smaller consumables. It could also create new waste streams if low-quality batteries, proprietary pods and short-lived bodies continue to be replaced frequently. Regulators should therefore monitor the total material footprint rather than count only products classified as disposable.

The transition also creates opportunities for regulatory arbitrage. Suppliers may market products as reusable while designing them to be used briefly, or separate devices and consumables in ways that satisfy legal wording without changing consumer behaviour. Some products may be imported as components and assembled domestically to avoid controls applying to finished goods. Others may be described as empty devices while containing residual liquid or as refillable despite sealed construction. Enforcement must examine the physical product, commercial offering and intended use together.

Retail compliance becomes especially important during transition because lawful and unlawful formats may appear almost identical. Retailers need clear guidance on the features required for sale, the date from which restrictions apply, treatment of residual stock and evidence expected from suppliers. A vague assurance that a product is rechargeable or compliant should not replace due diligence. Retailers should confirm that replacement components are genuinely available, that the device has an identifiable responsible operator and that its market status can be verified. Where the law prohibits possession for sale as well as completed transactions, stockrooms and online listings must be controlled alongside shelves.

Residual stock presents a practical problem because large volumes may remain within warehouses and shops when a prohibition takes effect. Transitional periods should be long enough for orderly adjustment but not so long that suppliers accelerate imports to create a final sales window. Clear cut-off dates for manufacture, importation, wholesale movement and retail sale may be necessary. Unsold products should be quarantined and directed into authorised recovery systems rather than exported casually, relabelled or sold through informal channels. Responsibility for financing disposal should not fall entirely on retailers where manufacturers or importers created the stock and benefited from its placement on the market.

Online sales require particular scrutiny because sellers can continue offering prohibited products from overseas, through marketplaces or under altered descriptions. Search terms, images and product specifications can be changed faster than formal enforcement notices are issued. Platforms should verify seller identity, product status and domestic responsible operators before allowing listings. They should preserve transaction data, remove repeat offenders and prevent relisting through linked accounts. Payment processors, fulfilment centres and delivery companies may also hold information capable of identifying large-scale supply. Removing one webpage without disrupting the commercial infrastructure leaves the market largely intact.

Border control is another decisive point because domestic retail enforcement becomes increasingly inefficient once thousands of small consignments enter the country. Risk profiling should combine product descriptions, sender histories, importer identities, declared values and known brand patterns. Officers require clear legal powers to detain products whose construction or status cannot be verified. Small parcels and direct-to-consumer shipments remain difficult because inspection capacity is limited and traders can divide consignments. Cooperation between customs, product regulators, tax authorities and postal operators is therefore essential. A ban that is visible in domestic shops but weak at the border may shift supply towards less transparent channels without reducing overall availability substantially.

Illegal markets may expand when demand remains strong and lawful substitutes do not satisfy consumers. If reusable alternatives require a much higher initial cost or provide a noticeably different experience, some consumers may continue seeking prohibited formats. Illegal sellers can exploit established brand familiarity and social-media networks. The regulatory response should focus principally on importers, wholesalers and commercial sellers rather than adult consumers possessing individual products. Criminalising users may discourage reporting and do little to disrupt supply.

Youth access may change rather than disappear. A disposable ban can reduce the availability of the format most associated with experimentation, but young users may move towards refillable pods, nicotine pouches, cigarettes or illicit devices. Retail age controls, proxy purchasing, social supply and online verification therefore remain necessary. Evaluation should examine prevalence, frequency, dependence, product substitution and sources of access. A decline in one product category accompanied by stable overall nicotine use would indicate displacement rather than complete policy success.

Environmental outcomes should be measured through collection data, waste composition, battery recovery and product longevity. Reduced sales of disposables do not automatically prove reduced waste if replacement devices fail quickly or are discarded with each pod cycle. Producers should report units placed on the market, expected service life, return rates and component availability. Waste operators can provide evidence on the number and type of products entering treatment streams. Litter surveys may reveal whether visible disposal has declined.

Manufacturers have an obligation to support the transition responsibly. Redesign should aim at genuine durability, replaceable components, safe charging and clear recycling pathways rather than minimal technical compliance. Proprietary systems may ensure quality control, but excessive incompatibility can increase cost and waste. Standardisation of charging interfaces, material labelling and certain replaceable components could improve usability and recovery, although full interchangeability may create safety concerns where power and coil specifications differ. Regulation should encourage practical compatibility without requiring combinations that undermine product performance.

Confusing messages can lead users to assume that all vaping products are prohibited or that rechargeable devices are inherently safe. Retail staff should be able to identify compliant replacement systems and explain maintenance, charging and disposal. Public information should avoid overstating environmental certainty or ignoring the relative health risks of smoking. The purpose is to support informed transition, not to use one policy objective to obscure another.

The future treatment of disposable products will test whether regulation can distinguish symbolic action from effective market change. Removing a highly visible format may reduce litter, youth appeal and illegal capacity abuses, but only if definitions are robust, substitutes are genuinely reusable and enforcement reaches online and cross-border supply. The policy should be reviewed against real outcomes rather than protected from criticism because its intention was popular. Where circumvention appears, technical criteria should be updated. Where adult smokers return to cigarettes or illegal products, corrective measures should be considered.

Disposable products demonstrate how quickly one design can transform a regulated market and expose weaknesses across several legal systems at once.

Their rise was driven by convenience, affordability and sensory appeal; their restriction has been driven by youth protection, environmental burden and enforcement difficulty. The lasting regulatory lesson is not that simplicity must always be prohibited, but that product format can shape behaviour as strongly as formulation. Future law must therefore assess how products are actually purchased, used, reused and discarded. A successful framework will not merely replace one label with another. It will produce devices that remain accessible to adults, less attractive to underage users, harder to supply illegally and materially capable of continued use.

Nicotine Limits

Nicotine limits are a prominent vaping control because they translate a complex exposure question into a numerical rule. A concentration ceiling appears measurable and easy to communicate, yet nicotine delivery does not depend on concentration alone. Device power, aerosol generation, liquid composition, coil efficiency, puff duration, inhalation pattern and frequency of use all influence the dose reaching the consumer. A lower-concentration product can deliver substantial nicotine through an efficient device, while a higher-strength formulation used in a low-output system may produce a different exposure profile. Regulation based only on concentration therefore controls one variable within a wider system. The challenge is to retain enforceable boundaries without treating one number as a complete description of dependence, toxicity or risk.

Concentration limits originally offered administrative simplicity. Regulators could define a maximum, laboratories could test samples against it and businesses could formulate products within a clear boundary. This reduced uncertainty and created a common market threshold. The limit also addressed accidental exposure where concentrated liquids might be swallowed, spilled or handled unsafely. However, the same limit influenced product design. Manufacturers developed more efficient coils, tighter airflow systems and formulations that improved nicotine uptake within the permitted concentration. Nicotine salts reduced harshness and made higher delivery from compact devices more acceptable. The market adapted, demonstrating that numerical controls change technology rather than merely restricting it.

Future regulation should distinguish between concentration, delivered dose and use. Concentration describes the amount of nicotine present in a liquid. Delivered dose describes how much enters the aerosol under specified conditions. Systemic exposure describes how much is absorbed by the user, while behavioural exposure includes the number, duration and spacing of puffs across the day. These measures are related, not interchangeable. A concentration limit may be useful for formulation control and accidental poisoning prevention, but it does not necessarily predict dependence, satisfaction or exposure during real use. Regulation should avoid claiming that a product below the legal maximum is inherently low-dose or that one above it is always more hazardous.

The relationship between nicotine limits and smoking substitution is important. Cigarette smokers vary substantially in dependence, smoking intensity, inhalation behaviour and previous quit attempts. Some obtain sufficient satisfaction from low-strength products, while others require faster delivery to leave smoking completely. Where lawful vaping products deliver nicotine too slowly or weakly, users may compensate by puffing more frequently, consuming more liquid, using higher-powered devices or continuing to smoke alongside vaping. A precautionary product-level limit may therefore produce less favourable population behaviour. The relevant comparison is among nicotine products and the realistic choices available to people who smoke.

Compensation complicates exposure assumptions. When nicotine concentration falls, experienced users often adjust puffing intensity, duration or frequency to obtain the desired effect. This can increase liquid consumption and exposure to non-nicotine aerosol constituents. Compensation varies by device, formulation and user, but the principle is established. Regulators should therefore consider whether a lower concentration ceiling could increase total aerosol inhalation without reducing nicotine intake proportionately. Conversely, very high concentrations may allow satisfactory nicotine delivery with fewer puffs and less liquid consumption, although they can increase the consequences of accidental ingestion, leakage or misuse. Policy cannot assume that lower concentration always means lower overall risk.

Device performance matters because concentration limits can encourage engineering changes difficult to capture in law. Manufacturers may improve heating efficiency, airflow, aerosol particle characteristics or formulation chemistry to increase delivery from the same liquid strength. These innovations can support substitution but may also appeal to inexperienced users. A limit expressed only in milligrams per millilitre does not account for the amount of liquid vaporised per puff or the fraction of nicotine transferred into aerosol. Future systems may consider performance measures such as nicotine yield under defined conditions. Such measures require robust methods, realistic puffing regimes and manufacturing tolerances.

A nicotine-yield standard could better reflect exposure, yet introduces complexity. Machine-generated yield depends on the puffing protocol, device settings, coil condition, liquid level and user activation. No laboratory regime represents every use pattern. Manufacturers could optimise products for the regulatory test while performance differs under real conditions. Laboratories may produce inconsistent results if conditioning, puff duration or analytical recovery varies. A yield requirement should supplement concentration limits unless methods are validated across product types and predict meaningful exposure. The search for scientific precision should not create a rule too unstable to enforce.

Product categories may need different approaches. Refillable liquids, prefilled pods, closed systems and medicinal products do not present identical risks or usage patterns. Open systems allow users to combine liquids and devices, making delivered dose difficult to control solely through the product as sold. Closed systems offer greater control over hardware and formulation but may concentrate market power in proprietary platforms. Medicinally authorised products may justify different nicotine strengths where supervised or evidence-supported use requires them. A universal limit is simple, but category-specific limits may better reflect purpose. Multiple categories can create loopholes, encourage reclassification and confuse consumers. Any differentiation must rest on clear functional criteria rather than commercial labels.

Youth protection strongly supports restrictive nicotine limits. Higher-delivery products may establish dependence more quickly among inexperienced users, particularly where flavours, concealability and easy inhalation reduce barriers to experimentation. However, concentration is only one influence on youth uptake. Price, packaging, retail access, social supply, product visibility and flavour presentation may be equally important. A concentration limit cannot compensate for weak age verification or widespread illegal sales. Future policy should treat nicotine strength as part of broader youth protection, not a stand-alone solution. Enforcement should also verify declared strength because illegal suppliers may mislabel products or market high-strength liquids as nicotine-free.

The distinction between nicotine concentration and form deserves attention. Free-base nicotine and protonated nicotine salts can differ in sensory harshness, volatility and user acceptability. Products with the same labelled concentration may feel and perform differently. Acid choice, pH and formulation components influence aerosol transfer and absorption. A future rule might consider whether concentration limits should be interpreted alongside formulation characteristics, but this would require careful evidence.

Regulating pH or nicotine form without understanding consumer and exposure consequences could encourage substitutions with less established toxicological profiles. Complete disclosure, targeted testing and post-market monitoring may be more practical than premature formulation restrictions.

Labelling matters because consumers use nicotine strength to choose products and manage intake. Milligrams per millilitre, percentage notation and total nicotine content can be misunderstood, especially when packaging emphasises one value and obscures another. Standardised presentation would improve comparison between refill liquids, pods and devices. Labels should distinguish concentration from total content and avoid presenting puff count as a dose estimate. Digital product information may explain expected performance, but it should not overwhelm users with technical data. Disclosure should support informed selection, not transfer risk assessment to the consumer.

Nicotine-free products create an enforcement problem. Products labelled as containing no nicotine may escape parts of the regulatory system while still using similar devices, flavours and marketing. Testing has shown that undeclared nicotine can occur through contamination, poor manufacturing control or deliberate misrepresentation. Future regulation should require evidence for nicotine-free claims and permit surveillance across both categories. Tolerances must distinguish trace contamination from meaningful undeclared content, but the threshold should be scientifically justified and applied consistently. False zero-nicotine claims undermine trust and may expose users seeking to reduce or avoid nicotine.

Taxation can interact unexpectedly with nicotine limits. Duties based on liquid volume may encourage stronger formulations because consumers can obtain the desired nicotine from less liquid. Duties based on nicotine concentration may encourage larger-volume, lower-strength products and greater material use. A flat product tax may disadvantage refill systems or favour high-capacity devices. Fiscal design should be considered alongside concentration rules, environmental objectives and illicit incentives. A poorly aligned tax can reverse the behaviour intended by the health regulation. Policy should model consumer and manufacturer responses before combining nicotine limits with duty.

Illegal markets grow more attractive when lawful products do not meet demand. If experienced smokers find permitted strengths ineffective, they may import higher-strength liquids, purchase unnotified products or modify formulations themselves. This creates greater uncertainty than a controlled legal pathway. Enforcement alone may not eliminate demand, particularly where products are easily transported and sold online. A credible lawful market should provide products capable of replacing cigarettes across realistic dependence levels. This does not require unrestricted strengths, but it does require evidence that the permitted range is functionally adequate for the intended population.

Clinical and behavioural evidence should inform future limits. Randomised studies, pharmacokinetic research, real-world switching data and post-market surveillance can help determine which strengths support complete substitution and which patterns are associated with persistent dual use. Evidence should be product-specific because older-device results may not apply to modern systems. Population surveys can identify trends, but they often rely on self-reported strength and incomplete product information. Linking product identity, formulation and behaviour would improve assessment. Digital product passports and standardised sales data could support this work if privacy is protected.

Review is essential because nicotine delivery technology will change. A limit established for one generation of products should not remain immune from reassessment when device efficiency, smoking prevalence or evidence evolves. Reviews should ask whether the limit supports adult switching, whether it contributes to youth dependence, whether compensation increases aerosol exposure and whether illegal supply is expanding. The burden of proof should not fall on one side. Maintaining a limit requires evidence as much as changing it. A mature system should tighten, relax or differentiate requirements when the risk balance changes.

Manufacturers should demonstrate that products deliver nicotine consistently and remain within specification. Batch testing, formulation control, device compatibility and stability studies are necessary because labelled concentration can drift through poor mixing, oxidation, evaporation or measurement error. Where devices and liquids form a system, the producer should understand its delivery profile. Claims about satisfaction, rapid delivery or equivalence to smoking require evidence and may enter medicinal or advertising regulation. Compliance should not test one liquid sample while ignoring the hardware determining use.

Regulators must maintain analytical competence. Nicotine testing appears straightforward, but sampling, extraction, calibration, uncertainty and product heterogeneity can affect results. Enforcement thresholds should account for method performance without tolerances that weaken the limit. Laboratories should use harmonised methods and report uncertainty transparently. Where a product marginally exceeds a limit, the response should consider analytical confidence, manufacturing control and repeated evidence. Deliberate high-strength supply requires a different response from an isolated result close to the measurement boundary.

International divergence will remain challenging. Different jurisdictions may set different concentration limits, classify nicotine products differently or permit higher strengths through therapeutic pathways. This encourages cross-border purchasing, relabelling and confusion over lawful status. Complete harmonisation may be unrealistic, but common terminology, methods and data exchange would reduce friction. A product should not have different measured nicotine concentrations simply because laboratories apply incompatible methods. Shared standards can coexist with national policy choices.

Consumer education should accompany changes because numerical limits are easily misunderstood. Smokers may interpret lower strength as universally safer, while inexperienced users may assume that products below the legal ceiling cannot create dependence. Guidance should explain concentration, total content, delivery and compensatory use in plain language without presenting vaping as equivalent to smoking. Retailers and cessation services also need consistent information so that advice reflects device type and smoking history rather than one standard strength. Understanding will not replace regulation, but it can reduce misuse, support appropriate product selection and help users recognise when a product label, claim or delivered effect appears inconsistent.

Future nicotine limits should move beyond the assumption that one ceiling captures every risk dimension. Concentration remains a useful and enforceable control, particularly for formulation quality, accidental exposure and market clarity. It should be interpreted within a broader framework that considers device performance, nicotine form, delivered dose, compensatory behaviour, youth protection, smoking substitution and illegal supply. The strongest policy will not pursue the lowest number as an end in itself. It will seek the range and control system that reduce population harm, preserve effective alternatives to smoking and remain practical to test, explain and enforce as technology changes.

Flavour Restrictions

Flavour restrictions are likely to become one of the defining questions in the future regulation of vaping because flavour sits at the intersection of adult acceptability, youth appeal, toxicological uncertainty, commercial differentiation and political symbolism. Few regulatory issues are discussed with greater certainty while remaining so difficult to define precisely.

Governments often speak of restricting "flavours" as though flavour were a single product attribute, yet flavour can arise from named ingredients, mixtures of aromatic compounds, cooling agents, sweeteners, acids, product names, colours, packaging imagery and the expectations created by marketing. A rule directed only at flavour names can therefore leave the formulation unchanged, while a rule directed only at specific chemicals can encourage substitution with compounds that have less evidence. Effective regulation must identify which mechanism is causing concern and design the intervention around that mechanism rather than treating all sensory variation as one undifferentiated problem.

By 2015, I had already argued publicly that the industry should move towards a restricted palette of pharmaceutically controlled flavour systems and ingredients that had passed appropriate quality and safety assessment. The principle was not that an orally used pharmaceutical flavour was automatically proven safe for inhalation, because route of exposure remains fundamental, but that the sector should adopt the discipline of pharmaceutical excipient control: defined composition, controlled suppliers, traceable specifications, toxicological review, impurity limits and clear exclusion criteria. Had the industry established such a framework early, it could have demonstrated that flavour use was being narrowed and governed rather than expanded without restraint. Instead, much of the market treated flavour proliferation as a commercial race, increasing the number of variants faster than the evidence base, analytical capacity or regulatory systems could follow.

The failure to create an industry-wide positive list left regulators facing thousands of mixtures described through trade names that revealed little about their composition. One "strawberry" flavour could contain a very different set of compounds from another, while complex dessert or beverage profiles might contain dozens of constituents at low concentrations. Suppliers sometimes changed formulations without altering the commercial flavour name, and manufacturers could receive limited information where concentrates were treated as proprietary. This made toxicological assessment, notification maintenance and change control difficult. It also meant that political debate focused increasingly on flavour categories and consumer appeal rather than the quality and composition of the flavour system itself.

A future regulatory framework should distinguish three separate questions. The first is whether the ingredients used to create flavour present unacceptable inhalation hazards. The second is whether the sensory effect or product presentation increases initiation among children or non-users. The third is whether flavour availability helps adult smokers adopt and continue using lower-risk alternatives. These questions overlap, but they require different evidence and different controls. Toxicological concerns may justify ingredient restrictions, concentration limits or emissions testing. Youth-oriented presentation may justify rules on names, imagery, packaging and advertising. Adult substitution requires behavioural evidence concerning product acceptance, switching and relapse. Collapsing all three into a broad flavour ban risks selecting a politically simple response that does not address the underlying cause precisely.

The toxicological issue should begin with substance identity. Every flavouring ingredient should be identified through a recognised chemical name, CAS number where applicable, supplier specification and concentration range. Trade-secret protection should not prevent disclosure to regulators or responsible manufacturers. The composition of concentrates should be controlled through agreements requiring notification of any change. Ingredients should then be screened for known respiratory sensitisation, irritation, genotoxicity, developmental toxicity, carcinogenicity, thermal instability and the formation of harmful degradation products. Evidence from food use can support general characterisation but cannot substitute for inhalation assessment. Pharmaceutical use can provide stronger assurance of purity and manufacturing control, yet the route, dose and formulation context must still be examined.

A positive-list system would provide a more coherent future model than repeated bans on isolated compounds after they become controversial. Under such a system, only substances meeting defined identity, purity, toxicological and exposure criteria would be permitted for use in vaping products. Inclusion would not mean that a compound was harmless under every condition; it would mean that its use had been assessed within specified concentration and product parameters. The list could be revised as evidence developed, with conditions placed on maximum concentration, product type or thermal operating range. This would create a clear incentive for suppliers to generate data and would reduce the uncontrolled substitution that follows when regulators prohibit one substance without considering what will replace it.

The design of a positive list would require caution. If the criteria were so demanding that only a few large flavour houses could comply, regulation could consolidate the market without necessarily improving public protection proportionately. A transparent pathway should allow manufacturers, suppliers, laboratories and independent researchers to submit evidence. Decisions should explain the basis for inclusion, restriction or removal. Historical use alone should not be sufficient, but neither should absence of inhalation data lead automatically to permanent exclusion where exposure is low and targeted evidence can resolve uncertainty. The system should be adaptive, using post-market surveillance and analytical findings to refine the list rather than assuming that the initial assessment is final.

Negative lists would remain necessary for substances with established reasons for exclusion. Compounds associated with severe respiratory toxicity, prohibited pharmacological effects, unstable thermal behaviour or unacceptable impurities should not remain available merely because their sensory contribution is commercially valuable. Cooling agents, sweeteners and acids deserve the same scrutiny as conventional flavour chemicals because they shape sensory perception and may influence use. A product described as unflavoured may still contain cooling, sweetness or masking agents that alter appeal. Regulation must therefore define flavour functionally as well as linguistically, otherwise manufacturers can remove characterising flavour names while preserving the sensory effect through alternative additives.

Youth appeal is more difficult to regulate through chemistry alone. Children respond not only to taste but to colour, branding, novelty, social visibility, price and product concealability. A plain tobacco-named product could still be marketed through youth-oriented imagery, while an adult-oriented fruit flavour could be sold responsibly through controlled channels. Conversely, flavour names derived from confectionery, cartoons, energy drinks or exaggerated fantasy concepts can make products appear detached from nicotine and closer to ordinary consumer treats. Restrictions on presentation may therefore be justified even where the formulation itself remains permitted. The objective should be to prevent trivialisation and child-directed marketing without pretending that changing the label alters the underlying chemistry.

Naming rules should be clear enough to enforce and narrow enough to avoid arbitrary interpretation. Terms explicitly referencing sweets, children's characters or products strongly associated with minors can be restricted more readily than broad categories such as fruit or dessert. A complete ban on descriptive names could reduce consumer information and make it harder for adults to distinguish products. Standardised naming conventions may offer a compromise, allowing a limited sensory descriptor, nicotine strength and product identity without promotional exaggeration. Packaging, point-of-sale display and online presentation should be considered together because removing a name from the bottle achieves little if retailers continue using colourful digital imagery and informal descriptions.

Evidence on adult use must remain central. Many smokers report that non-tobacco flavours help them separate vaping from the taste and ritual of smoking. Over time, some users move away from tobacco flavours because they no longer wish to reproduce the sensory experience of cigarettes. This can strengthen product substitution and reduce relapse, although the magnitude and durability of the effect vary. A regulatory framework that permits only tobacco flavour may satisfy a simple narrative of adult targeting while reducing the practical attractiveness of the product for some smokers. The correct question is not whether adults can use tobacco flavour, but whether restricting alternatives changes complete switching, dual use, cessation attempts or return to smoking.

Population evidence should be interpreted carefully. Cross-sectional surveys can show associations between flavour use and behaviour, but they do not always establish causation. Young people may choose flavours because they are experimenting, while committed adult users may also choose broader flavour ranges because they have used vaping longer. Product categories change rapidly, and a flavour label may conceal very different formulations and marketing styles. Future policy should combine surveys with longitudinal studies, sales data, product-level information and natural experiments following regulatory changes. Outcomes should include youth initiation, regular use, adult switching, smoking relapse, illegal purchasing and movement towards other nicotine products.

Partial restrictions may provide more proportionate options than universal bans. Regulators could limit flavour sales to age-restricted specialist retailers, prohibit particular descriptors in general retail, restrict online promotion, or apply stronger verification to products with higher youth appeal. Such approaches would recognise that the same product may create different risks depending on how and where it is sold. However, channel restrictions must be enforceable and should not simply push sales towards unregulated websites or informal networks. Specialist retail can support adult advice and product matching, but it is not automatically compliant. Licensing, inspection and traceability would still be necessary.

Flavour restrictions also interact with illegal markets. When widely used products are removed from lawful sale while demand remains, unauthorised imports, home mixing and informal distribution can expand. Illegal suppliers may offer stronger flavours, larger devices and lower prices without ingredient disclosure or quality control. This does not mean that every restriction creates a large illicit market, but policymakers should assess the likelihood and prepare enforcement accordingly. A restricted lawful palette should be broad enough to remain acceptable to adult users while narrow enough to support meaningful toxicological control. The objective is not maximum variety, but a credible legal alternative that does not surrender demand entirely to uncontrolled supply.

Manufacturers should be required to justify each flavour system rather than relying on historical market presence. The technical file should describe ingredient function, concentration, supplier control, toxicological screening, stability and relevant emissions. Complex mixtures should face greater scrutiny because uncertainty increases with the number of constituents and possible interactions. This does not necessarily mean that every complex flavour is unsafe, but the evidential burden should reflect its complexity. Product stewardship should favour simpler, well-characterised formulations where they can achieve the intended sensory effect.

Pharmaceutical discipline remains the most useful model. It does not require vaping products to become medicines, nor does it assume that pharmacopoeial status proves inhalation safety. It requires the industry to behave as though ingredients matter: controlled specifications, qualified suppliers, documented changes, impurity limits, traceable batches and defensible exposure assessments. Had this principle been adopted collectively a decade earlier, flavour regulation might have developed through standards rather than repeated political crisis. The opportunity has not disappeared, but it now requires regulatory compulsion where voluntary restraint failed.

Sensory assessment should also be formalised. Regulators cannot control flavour solely through chemical lists because sensory character depends on combinations, concentration, device output and perception. Standardised panels, descriptors and testing conditions could help determine whether products fall within permitted categories or use masking strategies to evade restrictions. Sensory evidence should support, not replace, analytical composition data. Laboratories may confirm the presence of compounds, while trained panels describe the character under operating conditions. This combined approach would be useful where legislation restricts characterising flavours, cooling intensity or sweetness. Without agreed methods, enforcement will depend on subjective impressions that vary between officers and jurisdictions. Sensory protocols would improve consistency, allow businesses to test products before launch and provide courts with a defensible evidential basis.

Future flavour policy should therefore move away from the false choice between unrestricted variety and complete prohibition. A stronger system would combine a positive list of assessed ingredients, a negative list of excluded substances, limits on youth-oriented presentation, controlled naming conventions, supplier transparency, product-specific toxicology and continuous post-market review. It would examine whether restrictions reduce youth use without increasing smoking, illegal supply or uncontrolled formulation. Most importantly, it would regulate the composition and presentation of flavour with the same seriousness applied to nicotine and device performance. Flavour is not a decorative feature added after the science. It is part of the product's chemistry, behaviour, market identity and public-health effect, and it should be governed accordingly.

International Cooperation

International cooperation will become increasingly important as vaping products, nicotine formulations, digital commerce and regulatory evidence move across borders more quickly than national systems can respond. A device may be designed in one country, manufactured in another, filled with liquid produced elsewhere, branded through a company registered in a fourth jurisdiction and sold online into many more. The product reaching a consumer may therefore sit within several legal, commercial and scientific systems at once. National governments retain responsibility for protecting their own populations, yet many of the problems they face are generated beyond their territorial control. Counterfeit production, undeclared ingredients, illegal strengths, misleading claims and unsafe components cannot be addressed efficiently when each authority investigates the same product in isolation and communicates only after harm or market penetration has already occurred.

The central purpose of international cooperation should not be to force every country into one regulatory philosophy. Jurisdictions differ in smoking prevalence, healthcare systems, enforcement resources, political priorities and attitudes towards nicotine. Some treat vaping mainly as a consumer product, others as a tobacco-related product, a therapeutic good or a prohibited category. These differences are unlikely to disappear, and complete legal harmonisation may be neither realistic nor desirable. Cooperation should instead begin with the technical and operational areas where shared systems can improve control without removing national sovereignty. Common chemical identifiers, compatible product data, recognised analytical methods, shared alerts, coordinated border intelligence and clearer identification of responsible operators can strengthen national decision-making even where the final policy choices remain different.

Product identity is the most basic requirement. Authorities cannot cooperate effectively if the same device appears under different names, codes or corporate owners in each jurisdiction. Brand names alone are unreliable because they can be copied, translated, abbreviated or applied to several formulations. A common product identifier should connect the device, liquid, nicotine strength, formulation version, manufacturer, importer and market destination. Digital product passports could support this structure by allowing each jurisdiction to attach its own legal status while recognising the same underlying product. One authority may permit the product, another may restrict it and another may detain it, but all should be able to confirm that they are dealing with the same item. Without this shared identity, laboratory findings, recalls and enforcement alerts remain fragmented.

Chemical data require similar standardisation. Ingredient submissions should use consistent substance names, CAS numbers where available, concentration units and clearly defined functions. Regulators currently encounter trade names, internal codes and supplier descriptions that make comparison difficult. The same compound may appear under several synonyms, while one commercial flavour name may conceal changing compositions. International agreement on minimum data fields would allow authorities to compare formulations and recognise repeated substances of concern. Such agreement would not require a common permitted list, but it would ensure that decisions are based on comparable information. It would also reduce duplication for responsible manufacturers that currently reformat the same technical data repeatedly for separate national portals.

Analytical methods are another priority. A product may be considered compliant in one country and non-compliant in another because laboratories use different puffing regimes, extraction procedures, calibration standards or reporting conventions. Some variation reflects legitimate research questions, but enforcement requires reproducibility. Common methods for nicotine concentration, liquid volume, carbonyls, metals, battery safety and selected flavour constituents would allow results to travel across borders with greater confidence. Method validation, uncertainty and proficiency testing should be shared, while laboratories should disclose conditions sufficiently for others to reproduce findings. Mutual recognition of accredited results could prevent unnecessary retesting, although authorities should retain the right to confirm results where chain of custody, sample identity or local legal thresholds differ.

International cooperation is especially valuable when new hazards emerge. If one authority detects a serious contaminant, battery failure or undeclared pharmacologically active substance, delay in communicating that finding may allow the same product to remain on sale elsewhere. Rapid alert systems should therefore carry product identifiers, photographs, batch information, analytical evidence, responsible companies, distribution routes and the action taken. Alerts must distinguish confirmed findings from preliminary suspicion so that other authorities can respond proportionately. A weak alert can damage lawful businesses unnecessarily, while a delayed alert can permit avoidable exposure. The system should support follow-up updates as investigations develop, including correction where the original concern proves unfounded.

Border enforcement also depends on shared intelligence. Illegal suppliers often alter routes, declarations and company names when one country strengthens controls. Customs authorities can identify patterns across consignments, sender addresses, freight forwarders and payment structures that would be invisible within one national dataset. Cooperation should allow risk profiles to be updated rapidly and coordinated inspections to occur across connected ports or parcel hubs. Where one country seizes a large consignment, others should be informed about likely parallel shipments and associated importers. This approach moves enforcement upstream, disrupting networks rather than repeatedly removing retail stock after distribution. Safeguards are needed to ensure that intelligence remains accurate, lawfully shared and subject to review.

Online trade makes territorial enforcement particularly difficult. A website hosted abroad can sell products into a country whose rules it ignores, while social-media accounts and marketplace listings can reappear under new identities. Cooperation between regulators should include shared seller intelligence, evidence-preservation requests and coordinated engagement with platforms, payment processors, domain registrars and fulfilment providers. Platforms operating internationally should not have to interpret entirely different data formats for every authority. Common notice structures, product identifiers and minimum seller-verification requirements would make removal and investigation faster. National authorities should still apply their own legal tests, but they should not be forced to reconstruct the same commercial network repeatedly.

Taxation and product regulation should also be connected internationally. Divergent duties create incentives for diversion, underdeclaration and cross-border purchasing. A product may be genuine and technically compliant yet enter a market without the required tax, while an illicit product may display copied duty markings. Fiscal authorities, product regulators and customs services should share enough information to distinguish these cases. Track-and-trace systems may help, but they must not become incompatible national islands. Common standards for identifiers and movement records could support enforcement while preserving each country's ability to set its own tax rate. Cooperation is most effective when it follows the product and the responsible operator rather than treating health, customs and fiscal compliance as separate worlds.

Mutual recognition can reduce duplication, but it must be used selectively. A laboratory report, manufacturing audit or quality certification produced under one credible system may be accepted elsewhere if standards are equivalent and the evidence remains relevant to the local product. This can lower cost and accelerate lawful market access, particularly for smaller firms. Mutual recognition should not mean automatic acceptance of another country's policy decision or risk tolerance. A product authorised under one nicotine limit may still be unlawful under another. The strongest model recognises technical evidence where it is reliable while preserving national authority over legal classification and public-health judgement.

Shared scientific assessment could improve efficiency where evidence gaps are common. Regulators repeatedly review the same ingredients, degradation products and engineering questions, often with limited resources. Joint working groups could assess toxicological data, identify research priorities and agree on minimum evidence standards. Publication of reasoning would help industry and researchers understand where uncertainty remains. Such groups should include independent scientists and disclose conflicts of interest. They should not become closed committees that produce consensus without exposing disagreement. International cooperation gains legitimacy when it improves transparency rather than merely centralising decision-making.

Research coordination is equally important. Studies conducted in one market may not translate directly to another because products, consumer behaviour and smoking patterns differ. International projects can nevertheless use common protocols to compare nicotine delivery, youth uptake, switching, relapse and environmental effects across jurisdictions. Product identity must be precise so that researchers do not group materially different devices under one category. Shared core outcomes would make results more comparable, while local modules could reflect national conditions. This would produce stronger evidence than isolated surveys that cannot be integrated because definitions and measures differ.

Industry also has responsibilities within international cooperation. Manufacturers and importers should provide consistent technical data across markets rather than tailoring descriptions opportunistically to each regulator. Supplier changes, formulation updates and safety concerns should be communicated to all affected jurisdictions. A company that discovers a serious defect should not wait for each national authority to identify it independently.

Global recall plans, batch traceability and designated regulatory contacts should form part of responsible product stewardship. Commercial confidentiality deserves protection, but it cannot justify withholding information necessary to prevent harm.

Consumer and civil-society organisations should also participate. Users can identify product availability, illicit supply and unintended effects of regulation before official systems detect them. Public-health bodies can contribute population evidence, while environmental organisations may reveal failures in collection or recycling. Their participation should be structured so that anecdote does not substitute for evidence and political advocacy does not become confused with technical assessment. Transparent consultation and disclosure of interests are necessary on all sides. Cooperation should widen the evidence base without allowing any one stakeholder group to dominate it.

Capacity differences between countries present a major challenge. High-income regulators may have specialist laboratories, digital databases and trained enforcement teams, while lower-resource jurisdictions rely on general consumer-protection or customs staff. International systems should not impose reporting and testing models that only wealthy authorities can operate. Shared laboratories, regional centres, technical training and open-access methods can reduce inequality. Funding should support independent regulatory capacity rather than create dependence on industry or external donors. A global system is only as strong as its weakest enforcement points because illegal supply will move towards jurisdictions where oversight is limited.

Confidentiality, data protection and due process must remain central. Cross-border databases may contain formulations, commercial relationships, personal data and intelligence about suspected offences. Access should be limited, recorded and governed by clear legal agreements. Businesses and individuals should have routes to correct inaccurate information and challenge decisions based on shared alerts. A suspicion entered in one jurisdiction should not become an unquestionable global sanction. Cooperation must improve evidence, not remove accountability. Authorities should distinguish intelligence used to prioritise investigation from proof required for formal enforcement.

International cooperation should also include coordinated review of unintended consequences. A flavour restriction, nicotine limit or product ban in one country may displace demand into neighbouring markets or online supply. Seizure data, sales patterns and smoking trends should be examined across borders rather than nationally alone. This can reveal whether a policy reduced use, shifted product choice or created illicit trade. Joint evaluation does not require countries to reverse their policies together, but it allows each to understand consequences more accurately. Regulatory learning is stronger when governments compare outcomes rather than defend isolated decisions.

Future agreements should therefore be practical, modular and transparent. They may begin with common identifiers, analytical standards and alert protocols before moving towards broader recognition of audits, submissions or environmental data. International cooperation should not be measured by the number of committees created, but by whether products are identified faster, dangerous batches are removed sooner, duplicate testing is reduced and illegal networks are disrupted upstream. The objective is not a single global law of vaping. It is a connected regulatory system in which evidence can move as quickly as products, while national authorities remain responsible for the decisions they make.

The future nicotine market will be increasingly global even where laws remain national. Cooperation is therefore not an optional diplomatic exercise but part of competent domestic regulation. A country that cannot recognise foreign evidence, trace an overseas manufacturer or communicate a product failure beyond its borders will regulate only the final retail stage of a much larger system. Effective cooperation allows authorities to see the whole chain across regions, sectors and enforcement systems, compare evidence and respond before problems spread. Its success will depend on compatible data, trusted methods, clear governance and respect for legitimate national differences. Properly designed, it will make regulation more efficient without making it remote, and more consistent without pretending that every jurisdiction must reach the same conclusion.

Future Legislation

Future legislation will determine whether vaping regulation develops into a coherent system of risk control or continues as a collection of overlapping rules created in response to individual controversies. The first generation of law concentrated on product definition, nicotine concentration, container volume, notification, warning statements and advertising. Later measures added age restrictions, environmental controls, taxation, enforcement powers and prohibitions directed at particular formats. Each intervention addressed a concern, but cumulative legislation can produce fragmentation when departments define the same product differently, require separate registrations or pursue objectives that are not assessed together. Future law should therefore identify the regulatory architecture rather than add another isolated prohibition whenever political pressure rises. Those consequences should remain visible throughout review.

The central legislative challenge is to preserve clear legal obligations while avoiding definitions tied too closely to one generation of technology. Terms such as electronic cigarette, refill container, disposable device and nicotine product may appear precise when drafted, yet commercial innovation rapidly exposes their boundaries. Manufacturers can alter charging capability, component separation, liquid delivery or product presentation without changing the underlying consumer function. Technology-neutral drafting should focus on function, nicotine delivery, intended reuse and operational risk. Functional definitions are harder to evade than descriptions based solely on visible form, but they must remain precise enough for businesses, laboratories, enforcement officers and courts to apply consistently.

Primary legislation should establish enduring principles, powers and responsibilities, while secondary legislation and technical standards should manage details likely to change. Parliament or the relevant legislature should determine the scope of regulated products, the responsibilities of manufacturers and importers, the basis for enforcement, consumer protections and the conditions under which products may enter or remain on the market. More adaptable instruments can specify data formats, analytical methods, permitted substances, labelling presentation, digital identifiers and environmental performance. This division allows technical requirements to evolve without reopening the statutory framework. It also requires safeguards because significant market restrictions should not be introduced through obscure administrative changes without consultation, evidence and political accountability.

Future legislation should impose responsibility on the economic operator capable of controlling the product. Global supply chains often separate brand owner, manufacturer, importer, distributor, marketplace and retailer, allowing each to argue that another party held the decisive information. The law should identify a domestic responsible person or entity for every product placed on the market. That operator should maintain the technical file, verify notification status, control changes, cooperate with surveillance and organise corrective action. Where no responsible operator exists, the product should not be lawfully supplied. Online marketplaces and fulfilment providers should carry defined duties where they facilitate access to products from sellers outside the jurisdiction and cannot identify a compliant domestic operator.

Market-entry requirements should reflect product risk and regulatory purpose. A system that demands extensive scientific documentation for minor variants while failing to inspect products already in circulation misallocates resources. Future legislation could use tiered pathways based on formulation novelty, nicotine delivery, device complexity, environmental design and evidence of prior use. A flavour variation using assessed ingredients within an existing platform may not require the same review as a novel heating technology, synthetic nicotine form or high-delivery product. Tiering must not create loopholes through artificial classification, and businesses should provide enough information for regulators to determine the appropriate pathway. The objective is to concentrate scrutiny where uncertainty and potential consequence are greatest.

Notification systems should also become legally connected to lifecycle control. Submission should not end when a product number is issued. Legislation should require version management, significant-change assessment, periodic confirmation of market status and prompt reporting of safety concerns. A notified product should remain traceable to the formulation, hardware and packaging supplied. Material changes to ingredients, coil, battery, reservoir, manufacturing site or responsible operator should trigger defined obligations. Minor changes should be documented without unnecessary resubmission, while changes capable of affecting exposure, safety or identity should require regulatory review. Clear thresholds would reduce both silent product drift and excessive administrative burden.

Digital product passports are likely to require statutory support because voluntary systems cannot provide universal identity, interoperability or enforcement access. Legislation should define the minimum data attached to each product, the roles permitted to enter or amend information, the protection of confidential data and the legal meaning of verification status. A passport should not be allowed to imply absolute safety or approval where the system records only notification or registration. The law should also address counterfeit copying, data falsification and unauthorised access. Public authorities must retain control over legal status where private companies provide infrastructure, and businesses should be able to correct inaccurate records and challenge wrongful suspension.

Artificial intelligence will require legal discipline. Regulators may use automated tools to screen submissions, prioritise inspections, identify online sellers and detect unusual laboratory results. Businesses may use them to generate dossiers, assess ingredients and monitor manufacturing. Future legislation should require transparency proportionate to an automated decision's effect. A system that merely identifies missing fields needs fewer safeguards than one influencing market access or enforcement. High-impact decisions should remain attributable to a responsible human officer, supported by explainable reasons and subject to review. The law should prevent confidential submissions from being used for unrelated model training without authority and should establish standards for validation, audit, cybersecurity and correction of systematic error.

Environmental duties should be integrated into nicotine legislation rather than attached as an afterthought. Future law should define meaningful reusability, durability, repairability, battery accessibility, component availability and producer responsibility. A charging port alone should not establish that a product is reusable. Manufacturers should demonstrate service life and support replacement components for a defined period. Producers, importers and marketplaces should finance collection and treatment, while retailers should provide practical return routes. Environmental data should connect with product identity so that regulators can compare units placed on the market with quantities recovered. Requirements should encourage reduced material use without compromising nicotine containment, electrical safety or the availability of effective alternatives to smoking.

Nicotine controls will need a clearer legislative objective. If the purpose is to limit accidental poisoning, concentration and container limits may remain appropriate. If the objective is to control dependence or delivered dose, concentration alone is insufficient. Future law may need to combine formulation limits with performance requirements, standardised labelling and post-market evidence on delivery. Legislators should avoid embedding one numerical threshold where technology can alter exposure without changing stated concentration. Review powers should permit adjustment when evidence on compensation, youth use, adult switching or illegal supply changes. Any change should include transition periods, validated methods and assessment of whether the lawful market remains capable of replacing cigarettes for heavily dependent smokers.

Flavour legislation should distinguish ingredient safety from product presentation. A positive list of assessed flavouring substances, concentration conditions and supplier controls could provide greater scientific coherence than broad category bans. Separate restrictions may address names, imagery and promotion directed towards children. The law should require full composition disclosure to regulators while protecting legitimate trade secrets from public release. It should also define how sensory character is assessed where restrictions apply, because chemical analysis alone may not establish whether a product presents a prohibited flavour. Review should consider adult switching, youth initiation, illicit substitution and the development of less well-characterised replacement compounds.

Retail and online sales regulation will require stronger parity. Age verification, product-status checks, marketing restrictions and recall obligations should apply regardless of sales channel. Remote sellers should verify identity and age at purchase and, where appropriate, delivery. Marketplaces should verify sellers, preserve transaction records and remove repeat offenders rather than treating themselves as passive noticeboards. Social-media and messaging-based trade presents greater difficulty, but legislation can impose duties on commercial intermediaries, payment providers and fulfilment operations when they knowingly facilitate unlawful supply. The law should remain focused on commercial conduct rather than criminalising ordinary adult possession, unless possession itself creates a defined public-safety or tax concern.

Licensing may become a more prominent enforcement instrument. A retail or wholesale licence can create a clear privilege that is conditional on age controls, traceability, lawful sourcing and cooperation with inspection. Suspension or revocation may deter repeated non-compliance more effectively than small fines. Licensing must be designed carefully to avoid excluding responsible small businesses through excessive fees or bureaucracy. Criteria should be transparent, decisions appealable and enforcement consistent. A licence should not become evidence that every product within the premises is compliant; product-level verification remains necessary. Wholesale, import and online operations may require separate or enhanced conditions because their scale and upstream position create greater market consequences.

Future legislation should provide a graduated enforcement ladder. Advice, corrective notices and administrative penalties may be suitable for minor or first-time failures, while deliberate falsification, repeated youth sales, organised illegal importation and unsafe products require stronger sanctions. Penalties should reflect commercial gain, scale and persistence so that they do not become routine operating costs. Authorities need powers to inspect digital records, detain goods, require information, suspend listings, freeze distribution and coordinate with customs and tax bodies. These powers should be balanced by due process, evidential standards and routes of appeal. Regulatory effectiveness and legal fairness are not opposing objectives; both are necessary for durable enforcement.

Review clauses should be mandatory for major restrictions. Legislation should state the problem being addressed, the expected outcome, the indicators to be measured and the date of reassessment. Reviews should consider youth use, adult smoking, product substitution, illegal markets, business impact, environmental performance and enforcement cost. A policy should not be judged solely by the number of products removed or penalties issued. Sunset provisions may be appropriate for emergency measures, while permanent rules should require periodic renewal or formal evaluation. The willingness to amend or repeal ineffective provisions is a sign of competent government, not weakness.

Legislative development should also include structured consultation before the preferred solution is fixed. Manufacturers, laboratories, retailers, consumers, public-health bodies, enforcement authorities, waste operators and cessation services each hold different evidence. Consultation should require quantitative information where possible, disclose conflicts of interest and distinguish scientific evidence from policy preference. Governments should publish their reasoning, explain rejected alternatives and identify uncertainty. This makes legal change more defensible and helps businesses prepare. Consultation should not become a process in which thousands of submissions are collected but no practical evidence alters the final design.

International compatibility should be built into future law even where policy remains national. Common product identifiers, chemical terminology, laboratory methods and alert formats can reduce duplication and improve border control. Legislation should authorise secure exchange of product and enforcement data while protecting confidentiality and due process. Mutual recognition may be appropriate for accredited testing or manufacturing audits where standards are equivalent. It should not require automatic acceptance of another jurisdiction's policy decision. The aim is to make evidence portable while preserving national authority over nicotine limits, flavours, taxation and market access.

Transition arrangements will determine whether new legislation produces orderly compliance or sudden displacement. Businesses need time to redesign products, revise packaging, update systems, train staff and manage stock. Periods should be long enough for genuine implementation but not so generous that traders accelerate imports before a deadline. Different cut-off dates may be required for manufacture, importation, wholesale supply and retail sale. Unsold stock should enter controlled return or recycling pathways. Regulators should publish guidance early and maintain consistent interpretations, because uncertainty encourages overstocking, market withdrawal and opportunistic claims by suppliers that their products fall outside the new rule.

The strongest future legislation will not be the longest or most restrictive. It will be the framework that connects product identity, scientific evidence, market entry, post-market control, environmental responsibility and enforcement through clear lines of accountability. It will preserve adult access to credible alternatives to smoking while protecting children and non-users, demand evidence without making compliance an arbitrary barrier, and adapt technical requirements without sacrificing legal certainty. Most importantly, it will recognise that every prohibition, limit and duty changes behaviour throughout the market. Future law should therefore be written not only for the product visible today, but for the technological, commercial and behavioural responses that the law itself will create tomorrow.

Building Evidence-Based Regulation

Building evidence-based regulation requires more than placing scientific references beneath a predetermined policy. It requires a disciplined process in which the problem is defined clearly, relevant evidence is gathered systematically, uncertainty is made visible, competing interventions are compared and the consequences of action are measured after implementation. Vaping regulation has often been presented as a contest between science and politics, yet the relationship is more complex. Scientific evidence can describe chemistry, exposure, behaviour and population trends, but it cannot decide automatically how governments should balance adult harm reduction, youth protection, consumer autonomy, environmental responsibility and enforcement feasibility. Those balances contain ethical and political judgements. Evidence-based regulation does not remove judgement; it makes the basis of judgement explicit, proportionate and open to correction.

The first requirement is precise problem definition. A policy framed simply as reducing vaping may combine several distinct concerns: initiation among children, dependence among non-smokers, product defects, environmental waste, illegal supply or uncertainty about long-term inhalation. Each concern has different causes and demands different evidence. Youth access may be driven by retail practice, social supply, price, product presentation or online sales. Environmental harm may arise from battery design, short service life, low collection rates or poor producer responsibility. Product toxicity may involve ingredients, thermal degradation, metals, manufacturing variability or misuse. If these mechanisms are not separated, regulators may select a broad restriction that is visible politically but weakly connected to the actual source of harm.

Evidence should then be organised according to the question rather than treated as a single undifferentiated body of literature. Analytical chemistry can identify constituents and emissions. Toxicology can investigate hazard and biological effect. Clinical studies can assess symptoms, biomarkers and switching outcomes. Behavioural research can examine initiation, dependence, dual use and relapse. Market surveillance can reveal non-compliance, while economic evidence can estimate price responses and illicit incentives. No one discipline can answer every regulatory question. A laboratory study demonstrating a hazardous constituent does not establish population risk without realistic exposure information. A survey association does not prove causation. A randomised trial may establish efficacy under controlled conditions but fail to predict market behaviour. Evidence-based regulation depends on integrating these sources while respecting what each can and cannot establish.

Study quality matters more than rhetorical usefulness. Regulators should examine product relevance, sampling, controls, analytical validation, statistical power, conflicts of interest and whether conclusions are supported by results. Vaping technology changes rapidly, so findings from obsolete devices may have limited relevance to current products. Experimental conditions should reflect plausible use unless the purpose is explicitly to test failure or abuse. Extreme power settings, unrealistic puffing regimes or concentrations far above consumer exposure may identify theoretical hazards but should not be presented as direct evidence of ordinary risk. Conversely, industry-funded research should not be dismissed automatically because of its funding source. Its methods, data access and transparency should be assessed rigorously, just as publicly funded or advocacy-linked research should be.

Systematic review provides a stronger foundation than selective citation, but it too requires careful design. Search strategies, inclusion criteria, product definitions and outcome measures should be stated in advance. Reviews should distinguish between evidence on exclusive vaping, dual use, smoking cessation, youth experimentation and toxicological hazard. Combining unlike outcomes can create conclusions too broad to guide policy. Living reviews may be particularly useful because new studies and product types appear continuously. They allow evidence to be updated without restarting the entire assessment, although update procedures must remain transparent and protected from selective inclusion. Regulators should publish not only conclusions but the evidence map showing where confidence is high, moderate or weak.

Uncertainty should be described rather than hidden behind definitive language. Long-term epidemiological evidence will inevitably lag behind technology, while product diversity makes generalisation difficult. Absence of complete evidence does not justify inaction, but neither does it prove that the most restrictive response is proportionate. Regulators should identify the nature of uncertainty: whether it concerns hazard, exposure, causation, prevalence, behavioural substitution or enforcement outcomes. Different uncertainties imply different responses. A plausible acute safety risk may justify immediate precaution, while uncertainty about a modest long-term effect may justify monitoring, research and targeted controls. Policy should be capable of escalating or relaxing as evidence develops.

Comparators are essential. Vaping products are often evaluated against an ideal of no exposure, yet many users are current or former smokers whose realistic alternative may be continued combustible tobacco use. For those consumers, relative risk is central. For children and nicotine-naive adults, the relevant comparison is non-use. The same product can therefore have different implications across populations. Evidence-based regulation must preserve these distinctions rather than treating average risk as though it applies uniformly. A measure that reduces experimentation among non-users may also reduce switching among smokers. Whether that trade-off is acceptable cannot be answered by toxicology alone, but it must be informed by evidence on both effects.

Policy options should be compared before one is selected. If the concern is youth appeal, governments might consider age-verification enforcement, packaging controls, flavour naming restrictions, retail licensing, price measures or product bans. Each option carries different benefits, costs and risks of displacement. Impact assessment should examine likely behavioural responses, administrative burden, market concentration, illegal supply and effects on smoking. The comparison should include the option of improving enforcement under existing law rather than assuming that legislative expansion is always necessary. New rules may be attractive when existing powers are underused, but additional complexity can weaken compliance if enforcement resources remain unchanged.

Proportionality should link evidence strength to regulatory burden. Minor documentation defects should not be treated like serious safety failures, and uncertainty about presentation should not trigger the same response as confirmed contamination. Tiered controls allow authorities to escalate from guidance and monitoring to mandatory testing, restriction, withdrawal or prohibition. The least restrictive measure capable of achieving the objective should normally be preferred, although serious or irreversible risks may justify stronger precaution. Proportionality also requires consideration of cumulative burden. Individually reasonable requirements can combine into a system so costly or complex that only large firms remain, reducing competition without necessarily improving safety.

Real-world data are indispensable because premarket evidence cannot predict every consequence. Sales trends, complaints, laboratory surveillance, switching behaviour, youth use, environmental returns, seizures and retailer inspections should be linked to product identity and policy changes. Natural experiments created by different national rules can provide insight, but interpretation must account for background differences in smoking, enforcement, culture and market structure. A fall in legal sales may indicate reduced use, illegal substitution or movement to another nicotine category. Seizure totals may show enforcement activity rather than market contraction. Regulators should define outcome measures before implementation so that policy is not judged solely by whichever indicator later appears favourable.

Data quality and governance determine whether evidence can be trusted. Product databases should use standard identifiers, version histories and consistent units. Survey questions should distinguish occasional experimentation from regular use and separate exclusive vaping from dual use. Laboratory methods should report uncertainty and remain comparable across time. Commercial sales data may be valuable but incomplete where online, informal or cross-border markets are substantial. Personal data should be protected, while confidential industry information should be accessible to regulators where necessary. Public summaries should make clear which findings were independently verified and which were supplied by economic operators.

Stakeholder evidence should be welcomed but weighted appropriately. Manufacturers understand formulation, supply chains and technical feasibility. Retailers observe consumer demand and practical enforcement problems. Users can describe switching, satisfaction and unintended effects. Public-health organisations contribute population analysis, while schools, waste operators and enforcement officers observe harms not visible within product dossiers. Each participant also has interests and blind spots. Transparent declarations, publication of submissions and structured evaluation reduce the risk that consultation becomes either industry capture or symbolic participation. Regulators should explain how evidence influenced the final decision and why significant alternatives were rejected.

Conflicts of interest should be managed consistently. Commercial funding can influence research agendas and interpretation, but so can institutional ideology, campaign objectives and political pressure. Disclosure allows readers to judge potential influence, while preregistration, open methods and data access provide stronger protection than assumptions about motive. Regulators should avoid privileging evidence merely because it supports their existing policy or comes from a preferred source. Independent replication and methodological quality should carry greater weight than institutional identity. Evidence-based regulation loses credibility when similar weaknesses are condemned in one study and ignored in another because their conclusions differ politically.

Institutional competence is a prerequisite. Authorities need scientists, economists, behavioural researchers, lawyers, data specialists and enforcement professionals capable of interpreting complex evidence together. Outsourced reviews may support this work, but responsibility for the decision must remain within accountable institutions. Regulators should maintain access to laboratories, data systems and technical expertise rather than relying solely on manufacturer submissions or advocacy summaries. Training is required because evidence evolves, and decision-makers must understand analytical uncertainty, causal inference, market adaptation and the difference between hazard and risk. A large evidence base does not improve regulation if the institution cannot evaluate it critically.

Transparency should extend to reasoning, not merely publication of final rules. Authorities should state the problem, evidence considered, assumptions made, uncertainties identified, options rejected and outcomes expected. Technical annexes can provide detail while public summaries explain the logic accessibly. Where decisions rely partly on precaution, moral judgement or political priority, that should be acknowledged. Presenting value choices as unavoidable scientific conclusions weakens trust and makes later correction more difficult. Transparency also allows businesses, researchers and courts to challenge errors constructively before they become embedded.

Review mechanisms complete the evidence cycle. Major measures should include review dates, performance indicators and access to the data needed for evaluation. Reviews should examine intended and unintended effects, including smoking prevalence, youth uptake, illegal markets, environmental outcomes, compliance cost and product innovation. Authorities should be prepared to strengthen, amend or repeal rules. A policy that cannot be reconsidered when evidence changes is not evidence-based, regardless of how many studies supported its introduction. Sunset clauses may be useful for emergency measures, while periodic renewal can ensure that permanent controls remain justified.

Research priorities should be linked directly to regulatory uncertainty. Governments often call for more evidence without defining which evidence would change a decision. A better approach identifies the unanswered question, the decision threshold and the study design capable of resolving it. Priority areas may include nicotine delivery across product types, inhalation effects of flavour ingredients, determinants of youth progression, adult relapse after restrictions, environmental lifecycle performance and the scale of illicit substitution. Public funding should support independent work in areas where commercial incentives are weak, while industry should bear responsibility for product-specific evidence and post-market surveillance.

Evidence-based regulation also requires humility. Complex markets do not respond perfectly to law, and scientific models cannot predict every adaptation. Manufacturers redesign products, consumers substitute, retailers change channels and illegal suppliers exploit gaps. Regulators should expect these responses and monitor them rather than treating deviation from prediction as misconduct by the evidence. Policy failure may arise from an incorrect assumption, weak implementation or a changing market. Distinguishing among these causes is necessary before further intervention.

That standard also requires institutional memory, because repeated reforms are wasteful when earlier assumptions, failures and enforcement findings are forgotten. Decisions, datasets and review conclusions should remain accessible so that future policymakers can carefully distinguish genuinely new evidence from arguments already examined and previously rejected.

The objective is not to produce regulation free from politics, uncertainty or error. It is to create a system in which decisions are traceable to evidence, burdens are proportionate, outcomes are measured and correction remains possible. In vaping, this means protecting children and non-users without ignoring adults who smoke, controlling product hazards without confusing them with combustion, and improving enforcement without making the legal market less credible than the illegal one. Evidence should discipline policy rather than decorate it. Regulation becomes genuinely evidence-based when scientific findings, behavioural consequences, practical enforceability and ethical choices are examined together, stated honestly and revised when the real world demonstrates that the original judgement was incomplete.

CONCLUSION

The regulation of vaping has developed through an unusual combination of scientific uncertainty, technological change, political pressure, commercial adaptation and public-health ambition. It did not emerge from a settled understanding of what electronic nicotine products were or what place they should occupy within tobacco control. Governments were required to construct rules while products, evidence and patterns of use were changing around them. The resulting systems were therefore neither purely scientific nor purely political. They were negotiated structures intended to bring order, accountability and minimum standards to a market that had expanded beyond the capacity of existing medicines, tobacco, chemical and consumer-product law to control coherently. Across the chapters of this volume, that development has shown that effective regulation depends not simply on the existence of legislation, but on whether law remains connected to product chemistry, toxicology, manufacturing, evidence, consumer behaviour and the practical conditions of enforcement.

Government intervention was necessary because early vaping markets contained substantial variation in formulation, device construction, manufacturing control, labelling and technical documentation. Nicotine-containing liquids were being supplied through complex international chains, products were sold online across borders and responsibility for quality was not always clear. Existing electrical-safety rules could address batteries and chargers without resolving ingredient suitability or nicotine exposure. Chemical legislation could control hazardous substances without assessing the complete inhalation system. Medicines law could impose rigorous standards where therapeutic claims were made, but it did not fit easily around the rapid product cycles and consumer character of most of the market. General product-safety law provided broad obligations but lacked the nicotine-specific reporting, emissions and notification mechanisms that a growing category required. Regulation therefore began with a classification problem as much as a health problem: what was the product, which authority should control it and what evidence should be required before and after sale?

The European Tobacco Products Directive created one of the first durable answers. Article 20 established a specific pathway for nicotine-containing electronic cigarettes and refill containers that were not authorised as medicines.

The framework introduced notifications, ingredient and emissions information, nicotine and volume limits, packaging requirements, technical protections and ongoing responsibilities for producers. Its importance extended beyond the individual provisions. It gave consumer vaping products a defined legal identity, positioned them within tobacco-related legislation and created a common architecture across European markets. Manufacturers and importers could no longer rely solely on general assurances that products were safe or on documentation held loosely across suppliers. They were required to identify products, describe formulations, generate technical information and accept responsibility for what entered the market.

The Directive also demonstrated the compromises inherent in early regulation. Limits on nicotine concentration, refill-container volume and reservoir capacity offered clarity and enforceability, but they were imperfect proxies for exposure and risk. Nicotine delivery depends on formulation, device efficiency, aerosol generation and use behaviour, not concentration alone. A small reservoir does not determine daily consumption or environmental burden. A notified product is not automatically safe or independently approved. The legal precision of a numerical threshold can create an impression of scientific certainty greater than the evidence from which it arose. Nevertheless, regulators often require boundaries that laboratories can measure, businesses can understand and courts can enforce. The challenge is not to reject numerical controls entirely, but to recognise what they achieve and what they leave unresolved.

The role of the Medicines and Healthcare products Regulatory Agency illustrates this distinction between administration, scientific oversight and approval. Under the consumer-product pathway, the MHRA receives product information, manages the notification framework, publishes relevant product records and supports vigilance. This is not equivalent to granting a medicinal marketing authorisation. The producer remains responsible for the quality, safety and compliance of the product. Publication within a notification database should not be interpreted as proof that every formulation, emissions result or manufacturing process has been independently verified. The system creates regulatory visibility and accountability, but it depends on the accuracy of information supplied and on the ability of regulators and enforcement bodies to identify when the physical product differs from its notified record.

This distinction is central to understanding regulation as an operating system rather than a certificate. Compliance does not begin when a dossier is uploaded and does not end when a product appears on a register. It begins at concept stage, when the manufacturer or brand owner defines the product, intended market, nicotine strength, device architecture and formulation. Ingredient selection, supplier qualification, specifications, toxicological review, analytical strategy, packaging, stability, manufacturing tolerances and post-market control must be considered before commercial launch. A submission can only describe the system that already exists. Where the underlying development process is weak, regulatory documentation becomes an exercise in reconstructing evidence after decisions have been made.

Building a compliant product therefore requires control over identity. Every ingredient should be linked to a defined name, chemical identifier, supplier, specification and concentration. Every device component should be linked to controlled drawings, materials and performance requirements. The product described in the technical file must correspond with the product manufactured, imported and sold. This becomes difficult where flavour mixtures are proprietary, suppliers alter formulations without notice or contract manufacturers substitute components while retaining the same commercial part number. Regulatory responsibility cannot be delegated completely to a factory, flavour house or distributor. The economic operator placing the product on the market must retain sufficient knowledge and contractual authority to understand what has changed and whether the change affects safety, exposure or notification status.

Supplier qualification is consequently a scientific and regulatory function, not simply a purchasing exercise. A low price, certificate of analysis or general statement of conformity does not establish that a supplier can produce consistent material. Qualification requires assessment of manufacturing capability, quality systems, traceability, change control, analytical competence, impurity management and willingness to disclose information. Supplier documentation must be verified selectively rather than accepted automatically. Where a critical ingredient or component affects nicotine delivery, emissions, stability or electrical safety, reliance on an uncontrolled source creates a regulatory weakness that no later dossier can fully repair.

Specifications convert product intention into measurable requirements. They define what the product is expected to contain, how it should perform and which variations remain acceptable. A specification without an appropriate test method is incomplete, while a test method without justified acceptance criteria cannot establish conformity. Formulation quantities, nicotine strength, pH, density, fill volume, device resistance, battery performance, leak resistance and packaging features may all require defined limits. These limits should reflect product performance, manufacturing capability, analytical uncertainty and legal requirements. Tolerances should not be selected merely because the production process finds them convenient, nor should they be so narrow that normal method uncertainty creates artificial failure. Regulatory science requires the specification, process and method to be designed together.

Stability adds time to this identity. A product that meets specification on the date of manufacture may change through oxidation, evaporation, light exposure, temperature, interaction with packaging or degradation of flavour compounds. Nicotine strength, colour, pH, sensory profile, impurity levels and aerosol performance may shift during storage. Hardware can also change through seal degradation, corrosion, material migration or battery decline. Shelf-life claims must therefore be supported by evidence that the product remains within relevant chemical, physical and functional limits for the stated period. Stability is not a decorative date printed on a package. It is the demonstration that the product remains substantially the same product throughout its commercial life.

Toxicology provides the interpretive structure connecting formulation and exposure to regulatory judgement. Hazard identification is necessary, but the existence of a hazardous property does not establish the magnitude of risk under product conditions. Ingredient assessment must consider route, concentration, transfer into aerosol, frequency of exposure and possible degradation. Food use does not establish inhalation safety, and absence of inhalation data does not automatically prove unacceptable risk. The responsible approach uses available evidence, read-across, computational methods, exposure estimates, threshold concepts and weight-of-evidence reasoning while making uncertainty explicit.

Regulatory toxicology becomes particularly difficult where products contain complex flavour systems. A mixture may contain many compounds at low concentrations, some of which have limited inhalation information. Assessing every component as though it were an isolated high-dose chemical can exaggerate concern, while assuming that small amounts are automatically irrelevant can miss potent local effects or reactive substances. The assessment must consider chemical structure, respiratory hazards, concentration, aerosol transfer, thermal behaviour and cumulative exposure. Where evidence remains insufficient, uncertainty should lead to proportionate data requirements, formulation controls or monitoring rather than automatic reassurance or reflexive prohibition.

Read-across, threshold of toxicological concern, QSAR and non-animal methods can help prioritise evidence and reduce unnecessary animal testing, but they require scientific discipline. Structural similarity does not guarantee identical biological activity. A threshold framework is not appropriate for every chemical class or endpoint. Computational predictions depend on model domain, input quality and validation. In vitro results require consideration of exposure realism and biological relevance. These tools are most defensible when used as part of an integrated assessment rather than presented as isolated proof. Their future value will depend on transparent methods, clear uncertainty statements and regulatory acceptance grounded in performance rather than novelty.

Analytical science is equally essential because regulatory decisions cannot be stronger than the measurements supporting them. Emissions testing, nicotine verification, carbonyl analysis, metal assessment and stability testing require validated methods, controlled sampling, representative products and an understanding of uncertainty. Laboratories must specify puffing regimes, device conditioning, sample collection, calibration, recovery, detection limits and acceptance criteria. Differences in laboratory methods can produce apparently conflicting conclusions from the same product. A numerical value becomes meaningful only when the method, units, conditions and uncertainty are understood.

Laboratory accreditation supports competence but does not make every result automatically relevant. ISO/IEC 17025 provides an important framework for method validation, quality assurance, traceability and technical control, yet the method must still answer the regulatory question. Testing a device under conditions that consumers would not tolerate may reveal a failure mode without representing ordinary exposure. Testing only under gentle conditions may miss foreseeable intense use. Selecting one product unit from one batch may provide limited information about manufacturing consistency. Regulation therefore requires dialogue between laboratories, toxicologists, manufacturers and authorities so that test programmes reflect both scientific relevance and enforceability.

Carbonyls and metals demonstrate the need for this context. Formaldehyde, acetaldehyde and acrolein may be generated under particular thermal conditions, but their levels depend on device power, liquid composition, wick saturation, coil state and puffing regime. Metals may derive from coils, solder, materials, contamination or manufacturing residues and can vary across product life. Their detection should trigger quantitative assessment, comparison and investigation rather than automatic equivalence with cigarette smoke or automatic dismissal as trace chemistry. The objective is to identify avoidable exposure, understand the mechanism and improve design or control where necessary.

Nicotine verification appears simpler, yet it also reveals the importance of analytical discipline. A declared concentration must correspond reasonably with the measured product, accounting for method uncertainty and manufacturing variation. Incorrect nicotine strength can alter consumer exposure, satisfaction and regulatory status. A product labelled nicotine-free but containing nicotine presents a different problem from a product near a specification boundary. Enforcement should distinguish deliberate misrepresentation, poor quality control and results that cannot be interpreted confidently because sampling or methods are weak.

Quality systems provide the organisational structure through which scientific and regulatory controls remain effective over time. ISO 9001 principles, Good Manufacturing Practice, document control, CAPA, change management, supplier auditing, traceability, complaint handling and management review are often treated as administrative burdens. In reality, they determine whether a product can be reproduced consistently and whether failures lead to learning. A company can possess an impressive technical dossier while operating through weak manufacturing controls, undocumented changes and informal decision-making. Regulatory compliance is fragile where the quality system exists only to satisfy an audit.

Good Manufacturing Practice contributes discipline over facilities, personnel, hygiene, materials, equipment, production, release and records. The appropriate level of control should reflect the product and risk rather than imitate pharmaceutical manufacturing without purpose. Vaping products are not automatically medicines, but they are inhaled nicotine systems requiring stronger control than ordinary low-risk consumer goods. Mixing, filling, assembly, packaging and labelling operations should be managed to prevent contamination, mix-up, incorrect strength and release of non-conforming product. Production records should allow the business to reconstruct what was made, from which materials, under which conditions and where it was supplied.

CAPA distinguishes an organisation that records problems from one that corrects them. A complaint, test failure or audit finding should lead to investigation of root cause, not merely correction of the visible symptom. Replacing a label does not resolve the process that allowed the wrong label to be applied. Retesting a failed batch does not explain why it failed. Corrective action addresses the cause of an existing problem, while preventive action reduces the likelihood of recurrence or related failure. Effectiveness must be verified after implementation. Repeated occurrence of the same problem indicates that the original investigation or action was inadequate.

Change control is equally important because products do not remain static after notification. Suppliers change ingredients, factories alter processes, components become unavailable, packaging is redesigned and analytical methods improve. Some changes are minor and administrative; others affect exposure, safety, identity or regulatory status. A controlled system should describe the proposed change, assess technical and toxicological consequences, determine testing and submission requirements, approve implementation and maintain version history. Uncontrolled change creates product drift, in which the item sold gradually diverges from the formulation and device described in the original dossier.

Traceability converts documentation into practical control. Batch numbers, material lots, production records, shipment data and customer information allow a business to locate affected products when a problem emerges. Without traceability, complaints cannot be linked reliably, investigations cannot define scope and withdrawals become broad and inefficient. Traceability should extend through manufacturers, importers, distributors, fulfilment centres and retailers. Digital systems may improve speed, but they remain dependent on accurate data and disciplined use. A sophisticated database containing incorrect or incomplete records is not stronger than a simple system maintained properly.

Product notifications bring these elements together, but they also expose the limitations of regulatory databases. CAS-number management, ingredient records, toxicological summaries, emissions data and product descriptions must remain internally consistent. Complex submission platforms can encourage the belief that compliance is achieved by filling every field, even when the underlying evidence is weak. The purpose of a submission is not to satisfy software. It is to provide regulators with an accurate representation of the product, its composition, its emissions and the responsibilities attached to it.

Common submission failures frequently arise from poor source data rather than technical difficulty with the portal. Inconsistent ingredient names, incorrect identifiers, mismatched concentrations, generic toxicological statements, unclear emissions reports and untracked product variants make the regulatory record unreliable. Businesses should maintain a master product-data structure from which submissions, labels, specifications and safety assessments are generated. Re-entering information separately into multiple documents creates opportunities for contradiction. Data management is therefore part of product stewardship, particularly where products are supplied across jurisdictions with different formats and requirements.

Cross-border compliance demonstrates that notification in one market does not create universal legality. Countries differ in nicotine limits, flavours, labelling, language, taxation, registration and product classification. The same item may be permitted in one jurisdiction and prohibited or differently regulated in another. Manufacturers and importers must map requirements market by market and maintain controlled versions. Exporting packaging intended for one country into another without assessment can create legal and consumer confusion. International harmonisation can reduce duplication, but national policy differences will continue to shape market access.

The comparison of global regulatory models shows that no jurisdiction has resolved every tension. The European Union created a notification-based framework with harmonised limits and substantial national variation. The United Kingdom retained much of that architecture while increasingly developing its own policies on youth protection, environmental controls, taxation and presentation. The United States adopted the far more demanding Premarket Tobacco Product Application pathway, requiring applicants to demonstrate that marketing would be appropriate for the protection of public health. Australia placed vaping products within a restrictive therapeutic model. New Zealand adopted a more explicit harm-reduction orientation while introducing controls in response to youth use. Canada, Asian states, Middle Eastern jurisdictions and emerging markets have constructed different combinations of prohibition, licensing, tobacco regulation, medicinal control and consumer standards.

These differences reflect more than scientific disagreement. They reflect political culture, smoking prevalence, enforcement capability, healthcare systems, institutional history and tolerance of adult nicotine use. A jurisdiction that prioritises abstinence may treat any expansion of non-medical nicotine as a threat. One focused on reducing smoking-related disease may tolerate continuing nicotine use where combustion is displaced. A country with weak market surveillance may choose prohibition because it lacks the capacity to administer a sophisticated product framework, although prohibition itself may be difficult to enforce. Global models therefore reveal that regulation is never a direct output of toxicology alone.

Industry, politics and public health shape the interpretation of evidence before it becomes law. Public-health organisations, governments, manufacturers, trade associations, consumer groups, academics and media organisations all frame the issue through different objectives. Harm reduction advocates emphasise comparative risk and adult switching. Tobacco-control organisations may emphasise youth uptake, commercial influence and the danger of renormalising nicotine. Industry stresses innovation, consumer demand and the need for proportionate market access. Governments respond to public concern, electoral pressure, health objectives and the institutional need to demonstrate action.

Conflicts of interest are relevant across this system, but they should not be interpreted selectively. Commercial actors have financial interests, and their evidence and advocacy require scrutiny. Public-health organisations can also become committed to institutional positions, funding priorities or ideological interpretations. Researchers may be influenced by career incentives, publication bias or advocacy. Governments may favour measures that are publicly visible even where enforcement or evidence is weak. Disclosure is necessary, but evaluation should return to methods, data and reasoning rather than assume that institutional identity proves truth or falsehood.

Consultation should provide a mechanism for these perspectives to improve policy, not merely a formal stage after the decision has effectively been taken. Manufacturers and laboratories can explain technical feasibility. Retailers can describe market behaviour and enforcement weaknesses. Consumers can explain switching, relapse and product preference. Public-health bodies can provide population evidence. Schools and youth organisations can describe patterns of access. Waste operators can explain environmental consequences. Consultation becomes meaningful when government states the problem clearly, requests relevant evidence, considers alternatives and publishes how the evidence influenced the outcome.

The precautionary principle has often been invoked because long-term evidence remains incomplete. Properly applied, precaution allows proportionate intervention where credible risks exist and delay could cause harm. It should not treat uncertainty as proof of the most severe possibility, nor should it assess only the risk of permitting a product. Restriction also has consequences. It may reduce youth use, but it may also reduce adult switching, increase illegal supply, encourage home mixing or preserve cigarette consumption. Precaution should compare realistic options and their foreseeable effects rather than assume that intervention is risk-free.

Regulation in practice reveals whether these principles survive contact with the market. Retailers, importers and distributors are not merely commercial endpoints. They are control points through which product status, traceability, age restrictions and corrective action can be maintained or lost. Retailers should verify suppliers, examine products, control age-restricted sales, maintain records and respond to withdrawals. Importers should ensure that overseas manufacturers can provide accurate documentation and consistent products. Distributors should preserve batch identity and avoid mixing lawful and questionable stock. Online sellers require equivalent responsibility for product status, age verification, listings, fulfilment and consumer communication.

Enforcement must distinguish minor administrative errors from deliberate supply of unsafe, counterfeit or unauthorised products. Advice and corrective notices may be appropriate where responsible businesses cooperate and risk is limited. Repeated youth sales, false declarations, large-scale illegal importation and deliberate product falsification require stronger sanctions. Penalties must be large enough to alter commercial incentives. Where a fine is lower than the profit gained through non-compliance, it becomes another business expense rather than a deterrent.

Border control is crucial because products can enter in large consignments, small parcels or direct-to-consumer shipments. Customs declarations may conceal product identity, value or nicotine content. Effective border control requires product data, importer histories, intelligence sharing, physical examination and laboratory support. Customs compliance and product compliance are related but distinct: a correctly declared product may still be technically unlawful, while a compliant product may be imported without correct tax or documentation. Coordination between customs, health regulators, trading standards, tax authorities and environmental bodies is necessary if intervention is to occur before goods disperse through domestic supply chains.

Counterfeit and illegal markets demonstrate the limits of regulating compliant businesses while enforcement remains weak elsewhere. Counterfeit products sever the connection between brand, formulation, manufacturer and responsibility. Illegal markets include more than fake goods: they can involve unauthorised products, oversized devices, higher nicotine strengths, diverted stock, untaxed imports, false nicotine-free claims and sales through informal or online networks. Lawful and unlawful goods may coexist within the same shops and warehouses, making business identity an unreliable indicator of product status. Effective enforcement must follow invoices, payment flows, importer relationships and distribution networks rather than measure success only through visible retail seizures.

Illegal markets are sustained by demand as well as supply. Consumers may seek lower prices, higher capacities, particular flavours or products removed from lawful sale. Regulation does not create every illegal market, but cumulative restrictions, taxation and weak enforcement can increase the reward available to non-compliant suppliers. A credible lawful market must therefore remain capable of meeting adult demand within acceptable controls. Enforcement alone is unlikely to succeed where prohibited products remain widely preferred and easily obtained.

Product withdrawals and recalls show whether quality, traceability and regulatory responsibility remain connected after market entry. When a defect, analytical failure or safety concern emerges, businesses must identify affected batches, stop distribution, notify customers and regulators, recover stock where necessary and investigate root cause. A withdrawal should not be confused with routine commercial delisting. It is a structured corrective action requiring defined scope, communication, reconciliation and verification. Where products have reached consumers and present a material concern, public recall may be necessary. The speed and precision of the response depend on systems established long before the incident.

Regulatory case studies demonstrate that law becomes meaningful through evidence and follow-through. Laboratory testing of products labelled nicotine-free has revealed undeclared nicotine. Retail investigations have uncovered devices exceeding legal capacities alongside evidence of youth sales. Border examinations have identified engineering defects requiring redesign. Prohibitions on single-use products have forced regulators to distinguish genuine reuse from superficial technical compliance. United States enforcement has shown that demanding premarket authorisation does not prevent unauthorised products reaching retailers. Australian seizures have shown the scale of enforcement required under a restrictive market model. European safety alerts have shown how one national finding can support action elsewhere.

The lesson from these cases is that seizure totals and warning letters are not sufficient measures of regulatory success. Effective intervention should identify the responsible operator, disrupt the supply network, correct the product or behaviour and generate information that improves future control. A case that removes one batch but leaves the importer and distribution route untouched may create only temporary protection. Regulation becomes intelligent when each failure improves surveillance, product design, guidance or enforcement targeting.

The future of regulation will depend on whether these systems can adapt without becoming arbitrary. Technology changes more quickly than primary legislation. Fixed rules provide certainty but can become obsolete or invite circumvention. Broad principles offer flexibility but may create uncertainty and inconsistent enforcement. Adaptive regulation should preserve stable responsibilities while allowing technical standards, analytical methods, data requirements and market-surveillance priorities to evolve. Changes should remain transparent, evidence-based and reviewable. Flexibility without accountability becomes unpredictability; rigidity without review becomes stagnation.

Artificial intelligence may assist this adaptation by screening submissions, identifying inconsistent data, monitoring online markets, detecting manufacturing drift and synthesising scientific evidence. It can direct limited human attention towards higher-risk products and patterns. It cannot replace toxicological judgement, regulatory accountability or due process. Models may reproduce bias, misunderstand context or generate confident but unsupported conclusions. High-impact decisions must remain attributable to competent people, methods must be validated and businesses must be able to understand and challenge the evidence used against them.

Digital product passports may provide the infrastructure connecting physical products with notification, batch, import, duty, environmental and recall data. Their value lies in product identity, traceability and rapid verification. A code alone proves little if the underlying information is inaccurate or copied. Governance, cybersecurity, role-based access, version control and interoperability will determine whether passports improve regulation or merely add another symbol to the package. Properly implemented, they could make recalls faster, counterfeits easier to identify and regulatory status more transparent across supply chains.

Environmental regulation will increasingly shape product design. Vaping products combine electronics, plastics, metals, batteries, packaging and residual nicotine. The rise of low-cost single-use devices made this material footprint highly visible. Future control will need to assess durability, repairability, component availability, design for disassembly, take-back systems and producer responsibility. A charging port should not be sufficient evidence that a product is meaningfully reusable. Environmental regulation should reduce waste without weakening product safety or making lawful alternatives to smoking inaccessible. Lifecycle accountability must be integrated with nicotine and product regulation rather than imposed through separate systems that use incompatible definitions and data.

Nicotine and flavour controls will remain contested because they influence exposure, dependence, youth appeal and adult product acceptance. Concentration limits should be reviewed in relation to delivered dose, device performance and compensatory behaviour. Flavour regulation should distinguish chemical suitability, sensory character and youth-oriented presentation. Positive ingredient lists, supplier control and inhalation-relevant assessment may offer more scientific precision than broad category bans, while restrictions on branding and descriptors may address marketing without assuming that every flavour compound presents the same concern. Policy should measure substitution, illegal supply and smoking behaviour alongside intended effects.

International cooperation will become indispensable as products, data and illegal supply move across borders. Complete legal harmonisation is unlikely because countries differ in health priorities and political philosophy. Technical cooperation remains achievable through common identifiers, analytical methods, data formats, safety alerts and intelligence sharing. Evidence should be portable even where policy decisions differ. A laboratory result generated credibly in one country should not have to be rediscovered independently everywhere before regulators can act.

Future legislation should therefore be designed around accountability, product identity, lifecycle control and review. Primary law should define durable responsibilities and powers. Technical requirements capable of changing should sit within transparent secondary instruments or standards. Every product should have an identifiable responsible economic operator. Notifications should remain connected to the product after launch through change control, post-market surveillance and periodic confirmation. Major restrictions should contain explicit objectives, impact measures and review dates. Legislation should be strict where evidence justifies strictness and adaptable where product evolution makes fixed rules inadequate.

Evidence-based regulation does not mean that science will provide one politically neutral answer. Decisions about youth protection, adult autonomy, environmental cost and acceptable uncertainty involve values as well as data. The role of evidence is to constrain those decisions, expose likely consequences and prevent assumptions from being presented as fact. Governments should state when a measure reflects precaution or political priority rather than imply that science demanded one inevitable outcome. Transparency strengthens regulation because it allows later review to determine whether the original reasoning remained valid.

The central argument of this volume is therefore not that vaping should be lightly regulated. Modern nicotine products require serious controls over ingredients, manufacture, emissions, labelling, traceability, market conduct and youth access. Businesses should be expected to know what they sell, demonstrate control, report problems and remove defective products. Regulators should possess the scientific and legal competence to examine evidence and act against non-compliance. Enforcement should reach importers, wholesalers, online platforms and organised illegal supply rather than concentrating primarily on firms already attempting to comply.

Nor is the argument that every regulatory burden is justified because regulation serves public health. Poorly designed requirements can generate documentation without improving safety, consolidate markets around the largest firms, reduce lawful consumer choice and divert enforcement resources away from serious breaches. Restrictions can produce unintended substitution towards cigarettes, illegal products or other nicotine categories. A regulation should be judged by what it changes in the real world, not by the seriousness of its stated intention.

Competent regulation must hold several propositions together. Vaping is not harmless. Smoking remains substantially more harmful because it involves repeated inhalation of combustion-derived smoke. Young people and non-users should be protected from nicotine initiation. Adult smokers should not be denied truthful information or credible non-combustible alternatives. Industry should be required to demonstrate quality and responsibility. Regulators should remain open to evidence that challenges established policy. Illegal markets should not be allowed to benefit from restrictions imposed only on lawful businesses. These propositions are not mutually exclusive, although political debate frequently presents them as though they were.

The regulatory objective should be a market in which products are identifiable, documented, consistently manufactured and capable of correction when failures occur; in which adult consumers receive accurate information; in which youth access and irresponsible promotion are controlled; and in which enforcement is directed towards the conduct and products creating the greatest risk. Such a market will never be free from uncertainty or commercial pressure. It can nevertheless be more transparent, accountable and proportionate than one governed by either unrestricted sale or indiscriminate prohibition.

This volume began with the birth of modern regulation and ends at the point where regulation must become mature enough to learn from its own consequences. The first generation created categories, limits and notification systems. The next established quality, technical and enforcement expectations. The future will require a broader settlement concerning nicotine, public health, innovation, ethics and consumer choice. Regulation can define what products must contain, how they should be tested and who is responsible for them. It cannot alone decide how society should communicate comparative risk, how much autonomy adults should retain, how harm reduction should be valued or which compromises are ethically acceptable.

Those questions belong to the final stage of this series. Once the science has established the difference between combustion and non-combustion, and regulation has translated that distinction into product and market controls, the remaining task is to decide what future nicotine policy should seek to achieve. That task requires examination of behaviour, risk communication, economics, ethics, innovation, institutional power and informed choice. The question is no longer simply whether a product is compliant. It is whether the wider system reduces harm, preserves public trust and treats people as participants in health policy rather than merely objects of control.

Regulation is strongest when it remains connected to evidence and honest about its limits. It should protect without pretending that prohibition eliminates demand, demand evidence without confusing paperwork with safety, and adapt without sacrificing legal certainty. It should recognise that scientific uncertainty can justify monitoring and proportionate precaution, but not permanent ideological closure. It should distinguish the commercial interests of industry from the legitimate interests of adult consumers, and the protection of young people from the assumption that every adult choice must be removed in their name.

The regulation of vaping will continue to evolve because the products, evidence and politics surrounding it will continue to change. Its success will not be measured by the number of rules introduced, products prohibited or submissions received. It will be measured by whether unsafe and unlawful products are controlled, whether responsible products remain traceable and consistent, whether smoking-related harm declines, whether young people are protected, whether consumers understand relative risk and whether policy can correct itself when the evidence shows that its assumptions were incomplete.

That is the standard against which modern nicotine regulation should be judged. The purpose of law is not to create the appearance of control, nor to defend innovation for its own sake. It is to convert scientific knowledge into proportionate responsibility while remaining alert to the consequences of intervention. The scientific foundation has been established. The regulatory machinery has been examined. The final question is what kind of harm-reduction settlement should now be built upon them.

Evidence Interpretation Note

The scientific evaluation of vaping requires more than identifying chemicals, listing studies or comparing isolated findings. Evidence must be interpreted through mechanism, exposure, dose, route, biological relevance, product design and real-world behaviour. This volume therefore treats evidence as a structured body of information rather than a collection of disconnected claims.

The first distinction is between hazard and risk. A hazard is the intrinsic potential of a substance or condition to cause harm. Risk depends on whether exposure occurs, at what level, by which route, for how long, in which population and under what circumstances. A substance may be hazardous in principle while presenting low practical risk at sufficiently low exposure, and a product may reduce exposure to some toxicants while still requiring careful assessment of others.

The second distinction is between detection and significance. Modern analytical methods can detect very small quantities of many substances. Detection is scientifically useful, but it does not automatically establish toxicological concern. Interpretation requires concentration, uncertainty, toxicological endpoint, exposure frequency, comparator data and biological plausibility. A detected compound must be assessed in context rather than treated as self-explanatory evidence of harm.

The third distinction is between normal use, intense use and misuse. Emissions data generated under unrealistic heating conditions, dry-puff conditions or poorly controlled laboratory settings may identify possible degradation pathways, but such data should not be treated as representative of ordinary consumer exposure unless the use conditions are plausible. Conversely, normal-use testing should not ignore foreseeable patterns of intense use where those patterns are common enough to affect exposure.

Clinical evidence must also be read with care. Biomarker studies can provide useful evidence of exposure reduction, particularly when comparing smokers who switch to non-combustible products with those who continue smoking. However, biomarkers do not always translate directly into long-term disease outcomes. Cardiovascular, respiratory, cancer-related and population-level conclusions require longer timeframes, appropriate comparator groups and careful control of confounding factors.

In vitro studies, animal studies, human observational studies, clinical trials, emissions testing and mechanistic toxicology all contribute different kinds of evidence. None is sufficient alone. In vitro studies can identify biological activity under controlled conditions, but may not reflect realistic human exposure. Animal studies can provide toxicological insight, but species differences and exposure design matter. Human studies are directly relevant, but may be limited by duration, confounding, recruitment bias or self-reported behaviour.

Epidemiological interpretation is particularly vulnerable to error where smoking history, dual use, socioeconomic factors, previous disease, product type and duration of switching are not adequately considered. A person who vapes may also have smoked heavily for many years. Any health outcome observed in such a person cannot automatically be attributed to vaping without considering prior and concurrent tobacco exposure.

Behavioural science is therefore part of evidence interpretation, not an optional addition. The public health effect of a product depends on who uses it, why they use it, whether they switch completely, whether dual use continues, whether non-smokers initiate use, whether youth uptake changes, and whether former smokers relapse. A chemically lower-emission product may have limited harm reduction value if it fails to displace smoking, while a satisfying substitute may produce a larger population effect if it supports complete switching among adult smokers.

Uncertainty should be identified precisely. It is not scientifically adequate to use uncertainty as a blanket argument for either safety or prohibition. Missing long-term data, limited inhalation toxicology, evolving product design, incomplete flavour data and variable use patterns all matter. They justify continued research, surveillance, improved standards and cautious interpretation. They do not justify pretending that no evidence exists, nor that the evidence is complete.

This volume applies a weight-of-evidence approach. Greater weight is given to findings that are reproducible, biologically plausible, exposure-relevant, methodologically sound and consistent with established toxicological principles. Less weight is given to isolated results that depend on unrealistic conditions, poorly described products, weak comparators, inadequate controls or unsupported causal claims.

The central interpretive question throughout this book is comparative. Vaping should not be assessed as though the relevant comparator is clean air alone, nor as though absence of combustion automatically means absence of concern. For adult smokers, the most important scientific comparison is often between continued combustible tobacco smoking and complete switching to a non-combustible nicotine product. For non-smokers and young people, the comparison is different, and the tolerance for avoidable nicotine exposure is lower.

A credible scientific framework must therefore hold more than one conclusion at the same time. Combustion is a major driver of tobacco smoke toxicity. Aerosol products are chemically and toxicologically different from smoke. Vaping is not risk-free. Product design and formulation matter. Inhalation exposure requires specific assessment. Long-term evidence remains incomplete. Adult switching may reduce exposure to many smoke-related toxicants. Youth uptake and non-smoker initiation require serious prevention.

Evidence-based harm reduction depends on this discipline. It does not require certainty before any conclusion can be drawn, but it does require honesty about the limits of each conclusion. The purpose of this volume is to make that interpretation more transparent.

REFERENCES

This volume covers policy history, regulatory science, toxicology, analytical testing, quality systems, product notification, global regulation, public health politics, enforcement and future regulatory models.

Chapter 1: The Birth of Modern Regulation

The reference list below is arranged in the same chapter-end format used for Volume I, with legislation and institutional sources integrated alongside the scientific and policy literature supporting the chapter. It covers the full Chapter 1 manuscript.

European Parliament and Council of the European Union. Directive 2001/37/EC of 5 June 2001 on the approximation of the laws, regulations and administrative provisions of the Member States concerning the manufacture, presentation and sale of tobacco products. *Official Journal of the European Communities*. 2001;L194:26–35.

European Parliament and Council of the European Union. Directive 2014/40/EU of 3 April 2014 on the approximation of the laws, regulations and administrative provisions of the Member States concerning the manufacture, presentation and sale of tobacco and related products and repealing Directive 2001/37/EC. *Official Journal of the European Union*. 2014;L127:1–38.

European Commission. Proposal for a Directive of the European Parliament and of the Council concerning the manufacture, presentation and sale of tobacco and related products. COM(2012) 788 final. Brussels: European Commission; 2012.

European Commission. Commission Implementing Decision (EU) 2015/2183 of 24 November 2015 establishing a common format for the notification of electronic cigarettes and refill containers. *Official Journal of the European Union*. 2015;L309:15–27.

European Commission. Commission Implementing Decision (EU) 2016/586 of 14 April 2016 on technical standards for the refill mechanism of electronic cigarettes. *Official Journal of the European Union*. 2016;L101:15–16.

European Commission. *Implementing the Tobacco Products Directive: Directive 2014/40/EU*. Brussels: Directorate-General for Health and Food Safety.

European Commission. *EU Common Entry Gate: Step-by-Step Guide*. Brussels: Directorate-General for Health and Food Safety.

European Commission. Report from the Commission to the European Parliament, the Council, the European Economic and Social Committee and the Committee of the Regions on the application of Directive 2014/40/EU concerning the manufacture, presentation and sale of tobacco and related products. COM(2021) 249 final. Brussels: European Commission; 2021.

European Commission. *Evaluation of the Legislative Framework for Tobacco Control*. Brussels: Directorate-General for Health and Food Safety; 2026.

European Commission. *Europe's Beating Cancer Plan.* Brussels: European Commission; 2021.

European Commission. Communication from the Commission on the precautionary principle. COM(2000) 1 final. Brussels: European Commission; 2000.

Court of Justice of the European Union. *The Queen, on the application of Pillbox 38 (UK) Ltd, trading as Totally Wicked, v Secretary of State for Health.* Case C-477/14. Judgment of 4 May 2016.

Court of Justice of the European Union. *Poland v European Parliament and Council of the European Union.* Case C-358/14. Judgment of 4 May 2016.

Court of Justice of the European Union. *Philip Morris Brands SARL and Others v Secretary of State for Health.* Case C-547/14. Judgment of 4 May 2016.

UK Parliament. *Tobacco and Related Products Regulations 2016.* SI 2016/507. London: The Stationery Office; 2016.

UK Parliament. *Tobacco and Vapes Act 2026.* 2026 c.18. London: The Stationery Office; 2026.

UK Parliament. *Environmental Protection (Single-use Vapes) (England) Regulations 2024.* London: The Stationery Office; 2024.

Medicines and Healthcare products Regulatory Agency. *E-cigarettes: Regulations for Consumer Products.* London: MHRA.

Medicines and Healthcare products Regulatory Agency. *MHRA E-cigarette and Vape Products Guidance Hub.* London: MHRA; 2025.

Medicines and Healthcare products Regulatory Agency. *Licensing Procedure for Electronic Cigarettes as Medicines.* London: MHRA.

Medicines and Healthcare products Regulatory Agency. *Advice on Ingredients in Nicotine-containing Liquids in Electronic Cigarettes and Refill Containers.* London: MHRA.

Medicines and Healthcare products Regulatory Agency. *General Advice on Vigilance for Electronic Cigarette Devices and Refill Containers.* London: MHRA.

Medicines and Healthcare products Regulatory Agency. *Electronic Cigarette and Refill Container Notification Database.* London: MHRA.

Department of Health and Social Care. *Stopping the Start: Our New Plan to Create a Smokefree Generation.* London: HM Government; 2023.

Department of Health and Social Care. *Creating a Smokefree Generation and Tackling Youth Vaping: Government Response.* London: HM Government; 2024.

Department for Environment, Food and Rural Affairs. *Single-use Vapes Ban: Information for Businesses.* London: DEFRA; 2025.

HM Revenue and Customs. *Introduction of Vaping Products Duty from 1 October 2026.* London: HMRC; 2025.

HM Revenue and Customs. *Introduction of the Vaping Duty Stamps Scheme on 1 October 2026.* London: HMRC; 2025.

World Health Organization. *WHO Framework Convention on Tobacco Control.* Geneva: World Health Organization; 2003.

World Health Organization. *Electronic Nicotine Delivery Systems.* Report by WHO to the sixth session of the Conference of the Parties to the WHO Framework Convention on Tobacco Control. FCTC/COP/6/10 Rev.1. Geneva: WHO; 2014.

Conference of the Parties to the WHO Framework Convention on Tobacco Control. *Electronic Nicotine Delivery Systems and Electronic Non-nicotine Delivery Systems.* Decision FCTC/COP6(9). Geneva: WHO; 2014.

World Health Organization. *Electronic Nicotine Delivery Systems and Electronic Non-nicotine Delivery Systems.* Report to the seventh session of the Conference of the Parties. FCTC/COP/7/11. Geneva: WHO; 2016.

Conference of the Parties to the WHO Framework Convention on Tobacco Control. *Electronic Nicotine Delivery Systems and Electronic Non-nicotine Delivery Systems.* Decision FCTC/COP7(9). Geneva: WHO; 2016.

World Health Organization. *Guidelines for Implementation of Article 5.3 of the WHO Framework Convention on Tobacco Control: Protection of Public Health Policies with Respect to Tobacco Control from Commercial and Other Vested Interests of the Tobacco Industry.* Geneva: WHO; 2008.

World Health Organization. *WHO Position on Tobacco Control and Harm Reduction.* Geneva: World Health Organization; 2025.

World Health Organization. *Tobacco: E-cigarettes.* Geneva: World Health Organization.

European Commission. *Transparency Register: Annual Reports and Publications.* Brussels: European Commission and European Parliament.

European Commission. *Joint Action on Tobacco Control.* Brussels: Directorate-General for Health and Food Safety; 2017.

Vardavas CI, Kyriakos CN, Fernández E, et al. The European Tobacco Products Directive: assessing the impact of the implementation of tobacco control measures on smoking prevalence and tobacco consumption. *Tobacco Control.* 2022;31(2):198–204.

Farsalinos KE, Le Houezec J. Regulation in the face of uncertainty: the evidence on electronic nicotine delivery systems. *Risk Management and Healthcare Policy.* 2015;8:157–167.

McNeill A, Brose LS, Calder R, Simonavicius E, Robson D. *Vaping in England: An Evidence Update Including Vaping for Smoking Cessation.* London: Office for Health Improvement and Disparities; 2022.

McNeill A, Brose LS, Calder R, Bauld L, Robson D. *Evidence Review of E-cigarettes and Heated Tobacco Products 2018.* London: Public Health England; 2018.

Royal College of Physicians. *Nicotine Without Smoke: Tobacco Harm Reduction.* London: Royal College of Physicians; 2016.

Royal College of Physicians. *E-cigarettes and Harm Reduction: An Evidence Review.* London: Royal College of Physicians; 2024.

National Academies of Sciences, Engineering, and Medicine. *Public Health Consequences of E-cigarettes.* Washington, DC: National Academies Press; 2018.

Lindson N, Butler AR, McRobbie H, et al. Electronic cigarettes for smoking cessation. *Cochrane Database of Systematic Reviews.* 2025;Issue 1:CD010216.

Hajek P, Phillips-Waller A, Przulj D, et al. A randomised trial of e-cigarettes versus nicotine-replacement therapy. *New England Journal of Medicine.* 2019;380:629–637.

Hartmann-Boyce J, McRobbie H, Butler AR, et al. Electronic cigarettes for smoking cessation. *Cochrane Database of Systematic Reviews.* 2021;Issue 9:CD010216.

Gravely S, Fong GT, Cummings KM, et al. Awareness, trial and current use of electronic cigarettes in ten countries: findings from the International Tobacco Control Policy Evaluation Project. *International Journal of Environmental Research and Public Health.* 2014;11(11):11691–11704.

Glasser AM, Collins L, Pearson JL, et al. Overview of electronic nicotine delivery systems: a systematic review. *American Journal of Preventive Medicine.* 2017;52(2):e33–e66.

Abrams DB, Glasser AM, Pearson JL, Villanti AC, Collins LK, Niaura RS. Harm minimisation and tobacco control: reframing societal views of nicotine use to rapidly save lives. *Annual Review of Public Health.* 2018;39:193–213.

Levy DT, Borland R, Lindblom EN, et al. Potential deaths averted in the USA by replacing cigarettes with e-cigarettes. *Tobacco Control.* 2018;27(1):18–25.

Selya AS, Foxon F. Trends in electronic cigarette use and conventional smoking: quantifying a possible diversion effect among US adolescents. *Addiction.* 2021;116(7):1848–1858.

Stokes AC, Wilson AE, Lundberg DJ, et al. Association of cigarette and electronic cigarette use patterns with levels of inflammatory and oxidative stress biomarkers among US adults. *Circulation.* 2021;143(8):869–871.

National Institute for Health and Care Excellence. *Tobacco: Preventing Uptake, Promoting Quitting and Treating Dependence.* NICE Guideline NG209. London: NICE; 2021, updated 2025.

US Food and Drug Administration. *Premarket Tobacco Product Applications for Electronic Nicotine Delivery Systems: Guidance for Industry.* Silver Spring, MD: FDA; revised 2023.

US Food and Drug Administration. *Tobacco Products Marketing Orders.* Silver Spring, MD: FDA.

US Food and Drug Administration. *Enforcement Priorities for Electronic Nicotine Delivery Systems and Other Deemed Products on the Market Without Premarket Authorisation.* Silver Spring, MD: FDA; 2020.

Bialous SA, Glantz SA. Heated tobacco products: another tobacco-industry global strategy to slow progress in tobacco control. *Tobacco Control.* 2018;27(Suppl 1):s111–s117.

Smith KE, Savell E, Gilmore AB. What is known about tobacco-industry efforts to influence tobacco tax? A systematic review of empirical studies. *Tobacco Control.* 2013;22(2):144–153.

Savell E, Gilmore AB, Fooks G. How does the tobacco industry attempt to influence marketing regulations? A systematic review. *PLoS ONE.* 2014;9(2):e87389.

Fooks GJ, Smith J, Lee K, Holden C. Controlling corporate influence in health policy making? An assessment of the implementation of Article 5.3 of the WHO Framework Convention on Tobacco Control. *Globalization and Health.* 2017;13:12.

Smith MJ, Bansal-Travers M, Huang J, Barker D, Hyland AJ, Chaloupka F. Association between use of flavoured tobacco products and quit behaviours: findings from a cross-sectional survey of US adult tobacco users. *Tobacco Control.* 2016;25(Suppl 2):ii73–ii80.

Zare S, Nemati M, Zheng Y. A systematic review of consumer preference for e-cigarette attributes: flavour, nicotine strength and type. *PLoS ONE.* 2018;13(3):e0194145.

Russell C, McKeganey N, Dickson T, Nides M. Changing patterns of first e-cigarette flavour used and current flavours used by 20,836 adult frequent e-cigarette users in the United States. *Harm Reduction Journal.* 2018;15:33.

Etter JF. Gateway effects and electronic cigarettes. *Addiction.* 2018;113(10):1776–1783.

Kozlowski LT, Warner KE. Adolescents and e-cigarettes: objects of concern may appear larger than they are. *Drug and Alcohol Dependence.* 2017;174:209–214.

Warner KE. How to think—not feel—about tobacco harm reduction. *Nicotine & Tobacco Research.* 2019;21(10):1299–1309.

Fairchild AL, Bayer R, Colgrove J. The renormalisation of smoking? E-cigarettes and the tobacco endgame. *New England Journal of Medicine.* 2014;370:293–295.

Hall W, Gartner C, Forlini C. Ethical issues raised by a ban on the sale of electronic nicotine devices. *Addiction.* 2015;110(7):1061–1067.

Chapter 2: Building a Compliant Product

The following sources support the regulatory, quality-management, formulation-control, notification, risk-assessment and post-market principles applied throughout Chapter 2. The chapter itself covers the complete concept-to-compliance lifecycle, from regulatory strategy and supplier qualification through technical documentation, notification and continuing product stewardship.

European Parliament and Council of the European Union. Directive 2014/40/EU of 3 April 2014 on the approximation of the laws, regulations and administrative provisions of the Member States concerning the manufacture, presentation and sale of tobacco and related products. *Official Journal of the European Union.* 2014;L127:1–38.

European Commission. Commission Implementing Decision (EU) 2015/2183 of 24 November 2015 establishing a common format for the notification of electronic cigarettes and refill containers. *Official Journal of the European Union.* 2015;L309:15–27.

European Commission. Commission Implementing Decision (EU) 2016/586 of 14 April 2016 on technical standards for the refill mechanism of electronic cigarettes. *Official Journal of the European Union.* 2016;L101:15–16.

European Commission. *Providing Information on Tobacco Products, Electronic Cigarettes and Refill Containers: The EU Common Entry Gate.* Brussels: European Commission.

European Commission. *EU Common Entry Gate User Guide.* Brussels: Directorate-General for Health and Food Safety; 2020.

UK Government. *The Tobacco and Related Products Regulations 2016.* SI 2016/507. London: The Stationery Office; 2016.

UK Government. *The Electronic Cigarettes etc. (Fees) Regulations 2016.* SI 2016/521. London: The Stationery Office; 2016.

Medicines and Healthcare products Regulatory Agency. *E-cigarettes: Regulations for Consumer Products.* London: MHRA.

Medicines and Healthcare products Regulatory Agency. *MHRA E-cigarette and Vape Products Guidance Hub.* London: MHRA; 2025.

Medicines and Healthcare products Regulatory Agency. *Submitting a Notification for Electronic Cigarettes and Refill Containers.* London: MHRA.

Medicines and Healthcare products Regulatory Agency. *Guidance for Producers of Nicotine-containing Electronic Cigarettes and Refill Containers.* London: MHRA.

Medicines and Healthcare products Regulatory Agency. *E-cigarette and Vape Products Regulator Profile.* London: MHRA.

UK Government. *The General Product Safety Regulations 2005.* SI 2005/1803. London: The Stationery Office; 2005.

UK Government. *The Electrical Equipment (Safety) Regulations 2016.* SI 2016/1101. London: The Stationery Office; 2016.

UK Government. *The Electromagnetic Compatibility Regulations 2016.* SI 2016/1091. London: The Stationery Office; 2016.

UK Government. *The Waste Electrical and Electronic Equipment Regulations 2013.* SI 2013/3113. London: The Stationery Office; 2013.

UK Government. *The Environmental Protection (Single-use Vapes) (England) Regulations 2024.* SI 2024/1266. London: The Stationery Office; 2024.

Department for Environment, Food and Rural Affairs. *Single-use Vapes Ban: Information for Businesses.* London: DEFRA; 2025.

UK Parliament. *Tobacco and Vapes Act 2026.* London: The Stationery Office; 2026.

HM Revenue & Customs. *Prepare for Vaping Products Duty and the Vaping Duty Stamps Scheme.* London: HMRC; 2026.

International Organization for Standardization. *ISO 9001:2015: Quality Management Systems—Requirements.* Geneva: ISO; 2015.

International Organization for Standardization. *ISO 31000:2018: Risk Management—Guidelines.* Geneva: ISO; 2018.

International Organization for Standardization. *ISO 20768:2018: Vapour Products—Routine Analytical Vaping Machine—Definitions and Standard Conditions.* Geneva: ISO; 2018.

International Organization for Standardization. *ISO 20768:2018/Amd 1:2025: Vapour Products—Routine Analytical Vaping Machine—Definitions and Standard Conditions—Amendment 1.* Geneva: ISO; 2025.

International Organization for Standardization. *ISO 24197:2022: Vapour Products—Determination of E-liquid Vaporised Mass and Aerosol Collected Mass.* Geneva: ISO; 2022.

International Organization for Standardization. *ISO 24199:2022: Vapour Products—Determination of Nicotine in Vapour Product Emissions—Gas Chromatographic Method.* Geneva: ISO; 2022.

International Electrotechnical Commission. *IEC 62133-2:2017: Secondary Cells and Batteries Containing Alkaline or Other Non-acid Electrolytes—Safety Requirements for Portable Sealed Secondary Lithium Cells and Batteries.* Geneva: IEC; 2017.

International Council for Harmonisation. *ICH Q1A(R2): Stability Testing of New Drug Substances and Products*. Geneva: ICH; 2003.

International Council for Harmonisation. *ICH Q9(R1): Quality Risk Management*. Geneva: ICH; 2023.

International Council for Harmonisation. *ICH Q10: Pharmaceutical Quality System*. Geneva: ICH; 2008.

Allen JG, Flanigan SS, LeBlanc M, Vallarino J, MacNaughton P, Stewart JH, Christiani DC. Flavoring chemicals in electronic cigarettes: diacetyl, 2,3-pentanedione and acetoin in a sample of 51 products, including fruit-, candy- and cocktail-flavoured electronic cigarettes. *Environmental Health Perspectives*. 2016;124(6):733–739.

Behar RZ, Davis B, Wang Y, Bahl V, Lin S, Talbot P. Identification of toxicants in cinnamon-flavoured electronic cigarette refill fluids. *Toxicology in Vitro*. 2014;28(2):198–208.

Clapp PW, Pawlak EA, Lackey JT, et al. Flavoured e-cigarette liquids and cinnamaldehyde impair respiratory innate immune cell function. *American Journal of Physiology–Lung Cellular and Molecular Physiology*. 2017;313(2):L278–L292.

Farsalinos KE, Kistler KA, Gillman G, Voudris V. Evaluation of electronic cigarette liquids and aerosol for the presence of selected inhalation toxins. *Nicotine & Tobacco Research*. 2015;17(2):168–174.

Goniewicz ML, Knysak J, Gawron M, et al. Levels of selected carcinogens and toxicants in vapour from electronic cigarettes. *Tobacco Control*. 2014;23(2):133–139.

Kosmider L, Sobczak A, Fik M, et al. Carbonyl compounds in electronic cigarette vapours: effects of nicotine solvent and battery output voltage. *Nicotine & Tobacco Research*. 2014;16(10):1319–1326.

Lisko JG, Tran H, Stanfill SB, Blount BC, Watson CH. Chemical composition and evaluation of nicotine, tobacco alkaloids, pH and selected flavours in electronic cigarettes cartridges and refill solutions. *Nicotine & Tobacco Research*. 2015;17(10):1270–1278.

Olmedo P, Goessler W, Tanda S, et al. Metal concentrations in e-cigarette liquid and aerosol samples: the contribution of metallic coils. *Environmental Health Perspectives*. 2018;126(2):027010.

Sleiman M, Logue JM, Montesinos VN, et al. Emissions from electronic cigarettes: key parameters affecting the release of harmful chemicals. *Environmental Science & Technology*. 2016;50(17):9644–9651.

Stefaniak AB, LeBouf RF, Ranpara AC, Leonard SS. Toxicology of flavouring- and cannabis-containing e-liquids used in electronic delivery systems. *Pharmacology & Therapeutics*. 2021;224:107838.

Talih S, Salman R, Soule E, et al. Electrical features, nicotine yield and toxicant emissions from pod-like disposable electronic cigarettes. *Tobacco Control*. 2022;31(5):667–670.

Vas CA, Porter A, McAdam K. Acetoin is a precursor to diacetyl in electronic cigarette liquids. *Food and Chemical Toxicology*. 2019;133:110727.

Williams M, Villarreal A, Bozhilov K, Lin S, Talbot P. Metal and silicate particles including nanoparticles are present in electronic cigarette cartomizer fluid and aerosol. *PLoS ONE*. 2013;8(3):e57987.

Zhao D, Aravindakshan A, Hilpert M, et al. Metal and metalloid levels in electronic cigarette liquids, aerosols and human biosamples: a systematic review. *Environmental Health Perspectives.* 2020;128(3):036001.

Zhao J, Nelson J, Dada O, Pyrgiotakis G, Kavouras IG, Demokritou P. Assessing electronic cigarette emissions: linking physicochemical properties to product brand, e-liquid flavouring additives, operational voltage and user puffing patterns. *Inhalation Toxicology.* 2018;30(2):78–88.

El-Hellani A, El-Hage R, Baalbaki R, et al. Free-base and protonated nicotine in electronic cigarette liquids and aerosols. *Chemical Research in Toxicology.* 2015;28(8):1532–1537.

Etter JF, Zäther E, Svensson S. Analysis of refill liquids for electronic cigarettes. *Addiction.* 2013;108(9):1671–1679.

Flora JW, Meruva N, Huang CB, et al. Characterisation of potential impurities and degradation products in electronic cigarette formulations and aerosols. *Regulatory Toxicology and Pharmacology.* 2016;74:1–11.

National Academies of Sciences, Engineering, and Medicine. *Public Health Consequences of E-Cigarettes.* Washington, DC: National Academies Press; 2018.

World Health Organization. *Electronic Nicotine Delivery Systems and Electronic Non-Nicotine Delivery Systems: Report by WHO.* Geneva: World Health Organization; 2016.

The principal legal basis remains Article 20 of Directive 2014/40/EU and Part 6 of the Tobacco and Related Products Regulations 2016, while the MHRA guidance and EU-CEG materials define the practical notification architecture described in the chapter. ISO's vapour-product standards provide the principal standardised framework for routine aerosol generation and measurement, alongside broader quality and risk-management systems.

Chapter 3: Toxicology Within Regulation

The references below support the chapter's treatment of hazard identification, ingredient risk assessment, literature review, read-across, weight-of-evidence integration, exposure assessment, margin of exposure, missing inhalation data, non-animal methods and regulatory interpretation.

1- European Parliament and Council of the European Union. Directive 2014/40/EU of 3 April 2014 on the approximation of the laws, regulations and administrative provisions of the Member States concerning the manufacture, presentation and sale of tobacco and related products. Official Journal of the European Union. 2014;L127:1–38.

2- European Commission. Commission Implementing Decision (EU) 2015/2183 of 24 November 2015 establishing a common format for the notification of electronic cigarettes and refill containers. Official Journal of the European Union. 2015;L309:15–27.

3- UK Government. The Tobacco and Related Products Regulations 2016. SI 2016/507. London: The Stationery Office; 2016.

4- Medicines and Healthcare products Regulatory Agency. E-cigarettes: Regulations for Consumer Products. London: MHRA.

5- Medicines and Healthcare products Regulatory Agency. Advice on Ingredients in Nicotine-containing Liquids in Electronic Cigarettes and Refill Containers. London: MHRA.

6- Medicines and Healthcare products Regulatory Agency. Guidance for Producers of Nicotine-containing Electronic Cigarettes and Refill Containers. London: MHRA.

7- Medicines and Healthcare products Regulatory Agency. General Advice on Vigilance for Electronic Cigarette Devices and Refill Containers. London: MHRA.

8- European Chemicals Agency. Read-Across Assessment Framework. Helsinki: ECHA; 2017.

9- European Chemicals Agency. Read-Across Assessment Framework: Considerations on Multi-constituent Substances and Substances of Unknown or Variable Composition, Complex Reaction Products or Biological Materials. Helsinki: ECHA; 2017.

10- European Chemicals Agency. Practical Guide: How to Use Alternatives to Animal Testing to Fulfil Information Requirements for REACH Registration. Helsinki: ECHA; 2016.

11- European Chemicals Agency. Guidance on Information Requirements and Chemical Safety Assessment: Chapter R.4, Evaluation of Available Information. Helsinki: ECHA.

12- European Chemicals Agency. Guidance on Information Requirements and Chemical Safety Assessment: Chapter R.6, Quantitative Structure–Activity Relationships and Grouping of Chemicals. Helsinki: ECHA.

13- European Chemicals Agency. Guidance on Information Requirements and Chemical Safety Assessment: Chapter R.8, Characterisation of Dose–Concentration–Response for Human Health. Helsinki: ECHA.

14- Organisation for Economic Co-operation and Development. Guidance on Grouping of Chemicals. OECD Series on Testing and Assessment No. 194. Paris: OECD Publishing; 2014.

15- Organisation for Economic Co-operation and Development. Guidance Document for the Use of Adverse Outcome Pathways in Developing Integrated Approaches to Testing and Assessment. OECD Series on Testing and Assessment No. 260. Paris: OECD Publishing; 2016.

16- Organisation for Economic Co-operation and Development. Guidance Document on the Reporting of Defined Approaches and Individual Information Sources to Be Used within Integrated Approaches to Testing and Assessment. OECD Series on Testing and Assessment No. 255. Paris: OECD Publishing; 2017.

17- Organisation for Economic Co-operation and Development. Guidance Document for Describing Non-guideline In Vitro Test Methods. OECD Series on Testing and Assessment No. 211. Paris: OECD Publishing; 2014.

18- Organisation for Economic Co-operation and Development. Guidance Document on Good In Vitro Method Practices. OECD Series on Testing and Assessment No. 286. Paris: OECD Publishing; 2018.

19- Organisation for Economic Co-operation and Development. Test No. 497: Defined Approaches on Skin Sensitisation. OECD Guidelines for the Testing of Chemicals. Paris: OECD Publishing; 2023.

20- European Commission Joint Research Centre. Integrated Approaches to Testing and Assessment. Ispra: European Union Reference Laboratory for Alternatives to Animal Testing.

21- National Research Council. Toxicity Testing in the 21st Century: A Vision and a Strategy. Washington, DC: National Academies Press; 2007.

22- National Academies of Sciences, Engineering, and Medicine. Using 21st Century Science to Improve Risk-Related Evaluations. Washington, DC: National Academies Press; 2017.

23- National Academies of Sciences, Engineering, and Medicine. Public Health Consequences of E-Cigarettes. Washington, DC: National Academies Press; 2018.

24- International Programme on Chemical Safety. Environmental Health Criteria 170: Assessing Human Health Risks of Chemicals—Derivation of Guidance Values for Health-based Exposure Limits. Geneva: World Health Organization; 1994.

25- International Programme on Chemical Safety. Chemical-specific Adjustment Factors for Interspecies Differences and Human Variability: Guidance Document for Use of Data in Dose–Concentration–Response Assessment. Geneva: World Health Organization; 2005.

26- World Health Organization. Human Health Risk Assessment Toolkit: Chemical Hazards. IPCS Harmonization Project Document No. 8. Geneva: World Health Organization; 2010.

27- World Health Organization. Electronic Nicotine Delivery Systems and Electronic Non-Nicotine Delivery Systems: Report by WHO. Geneva: World Health Organization; 2016.

28- International Organization for Standardization. ISO 10993-17:2023: Biological Evaluation of Medical Devices—Part 17: Toxicological Risk Assessment of Medical Device Constituents. Geneva: ISO; 2023.

29- International Organization for Standardization. ISO 10993-18:2020: Biological Evaluation of Medical Devices—Part 18: Chemical Characterization of Medical Device Materials within a Risk Management Process. Geneva: ISO; 2020.

30- International Organization for Standardization. ISO 20768:2018: Vapour Products—Routine Analytical Vaping Machine—Definitions and Standard Conditions. Geneva: ISO; 2018.

31- International Organization for Standardization. ISO 24197:2022: Vapour Products—Determination of E-liquid Vaporised Mass and Aerosol Collected Mass. Geneva: ISO; 2022.

32- International Organization for Standardization. ISO 24199:2022: Vapour Products—Determination of Nicotine in Vapour Product Emissions—Gas Chromatographic Method. Geneva: ISO; 2022.

33- US Environmental Protection Agency. Guidelines for Carcinogen Risk Assessment. Washington, DC: US EPA; 2005.

34- US Environmental Protection Agency. A Review of the Reference Dose and Reference Concentration Processes. Washington, DC: US EPA; 2002.

35- US Food and Drug Administration. Premarket Tobacco Product Applications for Electronic Nicotine Delivery Systems: Guidance for Industry. Silver Spring, MD: FDA; 2023.

36- US Food and Drug Administration. Principles for Evaluating the Abuse Liability of Tobacco Products: Guidance for Industry. Silver Spring, MD: FDA; 2019.

37- European Food Safety Authority. Guidance on the Use of the Threshold of Toxicological Concern Approach in Food Safety Assessment. EFSA Journal. 2019;17(6):5708.

38- European Food Safety Authority Scientific Committee. Guidance on the Use of the Weight of Evidence Approach in Scientific Assessments. EFSA Journal. 2017;15(8):4971.

39- European Food Safety Authority Scientific Committee. Guidance on Uncertainty Analysis in Scientific Assessments. EFSA Journal. 2018;16(1):5123.

40- European Food Safety Authority Scientific Committee. Guidance on the Assessment of the Biological Relevance of Data in Scientific Assessments. EFSA Journal. 2017;15(8):4970.

41- Scientific Committee on Consumer Safety. The SCCS Notes of Guidance for the Testing of Cosmetic Ingredients and Their Safety Evaluation. 12th Revision. Luxembourg: European Commission; 2023.

42- Committee on Mutagenicity of Chemicals in Food, Consumer Products and the Environment. Guidance on a Strategy for Genotoxicity Testing of Chemical Substances. London: UK Health Security Agency; 2021.

43- Committee on Toxicity of Chemicals in Food, Consumer Products and the Environment. Guidance on the Use of the Threshold of Toxicological Concern Approach in Risk Assessment. London: Committee on Toxicity.

44- Benford D, Bolger PM, Carthew P, et al. Application of the margin of exposure approach to compounds in food which are both genotoxic and carcinogenic. Food and Chemical Toxicology. 2010;48(Suppl 1):S2–S24.

45- Barlow S, Renwick AG, Kleiner J, et al. Risk assessment of substances that are both genotoxic and carcinogenic: report of an international conference organised by EFSA and WHO. Food and Chemical Toxicology. 2006;44(10):1636–1650.

46- Boobis AR, Cohen SM, Dellarco V, et al. IPCS framework for analysing the relevance of a cancer mode of action for humans. Critical Reviews in Toxicology. 2006;36(10):781–792.

47- Meek ME, Boobis A, Cote I, et al. New developments in the evolution and application of the WHO/IPCS framework on mode of action and species concordance analysis. Journal of Applied Toxicology. 2014;34(1):1–18.

48- Rhomberg LR, Goodman JE, Bailey LA, et al. A survey of frameworks for best practices in weight-of-evidence analyses. Critical Reviews in Toxicology. 2013;43(9):753–784.

49- Linkov I, Loney D, Cormier S, Satterstrom FK, Bridges T. Weight-of-evidence evaluation in environmental assessment: review of qualitative and quantitative approaches. Science of the Total Environment. 2009;407(19):5199–5205.

50- Klimisch HJ, Andreae M, Tillmann U. A systematic approach for evaluating the quality of experimental toxicological and ecotoxicological data. Regulatory Toxicology and Pharmacology. 1997;25(1):1–5.

51- Hartung T. Toxicology for the twenty-first century. Nature. 2009;460:208–212.

52- Hartung T, McBride M. Food for thought on mapping the human toxome. ALTEX. 2011;28(2):83–93.

53- Leist M, Hasiwa N, Rovida C, et al. Consensus report on the future of animal-free systemic toxicity testing. ALTEX. 2014;31(3):341–356.

54- Rovida C, Hartung T. Re-evaluation of animal numbers and costs for in vivo tests to accomplish REACH legislation requirements for chemicals. ALTEX. 2009;26(3):187–208.

55- Clippinger AJ, Allen D, Behrsing H, et al. Pathway-based predictive approaches for non-animal assessment of acute inhalation toxicity. Toxicology in Vitro. 2018;52:131–145.

56- Clippinger AJ, Ahluwalia A, Allen D, et al. Expert consensus on an in vitro approach to assess pulmonary fibrogenic potential of aerosolised nanomaterials. Archives of Toxicology. 2016;90:1769–1783.

57- Aufderheide M. An efficient approach to study the toxicological effects of complex mixtures. Experimental and Toxicologic Pathology. 2008;60(2–3):163–180.

58- Paur HR, Cassee FR, Teeguarden J, et al. In-vitro cell exposure studies for the assessment of nanoparticle toxicity in the lung: a dialogue between aerosol science and biology. Journal of Aerosol Science. 2011;42(10):668–692.

59- Lenz AG, Karg E, Brendel E, et al. Inflammatory and oxidative stress responses of an alveolar epithelial cell line to airborne zinc oxide nanoparticles at the air–liquid interface: a comparison with conventional, submerged cell-culture conditions. BioMed Research International. 2013;2013:652632.

60- Thorne D, Adamson J. A review of in vitro cigarette smoke exposure systems. Experimental and Toxicologic Pathology. 2013;65(7–8):1183–1193.

61- Iskandar AR, Mathis C, Martin F, et al. 3-D nasal cultures: systems toxicological assessment of a candidate modified-risk tobacco product. Toxicology Letters. 2017;265:110–124.

62- Iskandar AR, Gonzalez-Suarez I, Majeed S, et al. A framework for in vitro systems toxicology assessment of e-liquids. Toxicology Mechanisms and Methods. 2016;26(6):389–413.

63- Neilson L, Mankus C, Thorne D, Jackson G, DeBay J, Meredith C. Development of an in vitro cytotoxicity model for aerosol exposure using 3D reconstructed human airway tissue. Toxicology in Vitro. 2015;29(7):1952–1962.

64- Bishop E, Haswell L, Adamson J, et al. An approach to testing undiluted e-cigarette aerosol in vitro using 3D reconstituted human airway epithelium. Toxicology in Vitro. 2019;54:391–401.

65- Azzopardi D, Haswell LE, Foss-Smith G, et al. Evaluation of an air–liquid interface cell culture model for studies on the inflammatory and cytotoxic effects of tobacco smoke aerosols. Toxicology in Vitro. 2015;29(7):1720–1728.

66- Misra M, Leverette RD, Cooper BT, Bennett MB, Brown SE. Comparative in vitro toxicity profile of electronic and tobacco cigarettes, smokeless tobacco and nicotine replacement therapy products. International Journal of Environmental Research and Public Health. 2014;11(11):11325–11347.

67- Cervellati F, Muresan XM, Sticozzi C, et al. Comparative effects between electronic and cigarette smoke in human keratinocytes and epithelial lung cells. Toxicology in Vitro. 2014;28(5):999–1005.

68- Scheffler S, Dieken H, Krischenowski O, Förster C, Branscheid D, Aufderheide M. Evaluation of e-cigarette liquid vapour and mainstream cigarette smoke after direct exposure of primary human bronchial epithelial cells. International Journal of Environmental Research and Public Health. 2015;12(4):3915–3925.

69- Leigh NJ, Lawton RI, Hershberger PA, Goniewicz ML. Flavourings significantly affect inhalation toxicity of aerosol generated from electronic nicotine delivery systems. Tobacco Control. 2016;25(Suppl 2):ii81–ii87.

70- Behar RZ, Davis B, Wang Y, Bahl V, Lin S, Talbot P. Identification of toxicants in cinnamon-flavoured electronic cigarette refill fluids. Toxicology in Vitro. 2014;28(2):198–208.

71- Behar RZ, Luo W, Lin SC, et al. Distribution, quantification and toxicity of cinnamaldehyde in electronic cigarette refill fluids and aerosols. Tobacco Control. 2016;25(Suppl 2):ii94–ii102.

72- Clapp PW, Pawlak EA, Lackey JT, et al. Flavoured e-cigarette liquids and cinnamaldehyde impair respiratory innate immune cell function. American Journal of Physiology–Lung Cellular and Molecular Physiology. 2017;313(2):L278–L292.

73- Clapp PW, Jaspers I. Electronic cigarettes: their constituents and potential links to asthma. Current Allergy and Asthma Reports. 2017;17:79.

74- Park HR, O'Sullivan M, Vallarino J, et al. Transcriptomic response of primary human airway epithelial cells to flavouring chemicals in electronic cigarettes. Scientific Reports. 2019;9:1400.

75- Allen JG, Flanigan SS, LeBlanc M, Vallarino J, MacNaughton P, Stewart JH, Christiani DC. Flavoring chemicals in electronic cigarettes: diacetyl, 2,3-pentanedione and acetoin in a sample of 51 products, including fruit-, candy- and cocktail-flavoured electronic cigarettes. Environmental Health Perspectives. 2016;124(6):733–739.

76- Farsalinos KE, Kistler KA, Gillman G, Voudris V. Evaluation of electronic cigarette liquids and aerosol for the presence of selected inhalation toxins. Nicotine & Tobacco Research. 2015;17(2):168–174.

77- Stefaniak AB, LeBouf RF, Ranpara AC, Leonard SS. Toxicology of flavouring- and cannabis-containing e-liquids used in electronic delivery systems. Pharmacology & Therapeutics. 2021;224:107838.

78- Effah F, Taiwo B, Baines D, Bailey A, Marczylo T. Pulmonary effects of e-liquid flavours: a systematic review. Journal of Toxicology and Environmental Health, Part B. 2022;25(7):343–371.

79- Callahan-Lyon P. Electronic cigarettes: human health effects. Tobacco Control. 2014;23(Suppl 2):ii36–ii40.

80- Cao DJ, Aldy K, Hsu S, McGetrick M, Verbeck G, De Silva I, Feng SY. Review of health consequences of electronic cigarettes and the outbreak of electronic cigarette, or vaping, product use-associated lung injury. Journal of Medical Toxicology. 2020;16(3):295–310.

81- Goniewicz ML, Knysak J, Gawron M, et al. Levels of selected carcinogens and toxicants in vapour from electronic cigarettes. Tobacco Control. 2014;23(2):133–139.

82- Kosmider L, Sobczak A, Fik M, et al. Carbonyl compounds in electronic cigarette vapours: effects of nicotine solvent and battery output voltage. Nicotine & Tobacco Research. 2014;16(10):1319–1326.

83- Sleiman M, Logue JM, Montesinos VN, et al. Emissions from electronic cigarettes: key parameters affecting the release of harmful chemicals. Environmental Science & Technology. 2016;50(17):9644–9651.

84- Jensen RP, Luo W, Pankow JF, Strongin RM, Peyton DH. Hidden formaldehyde in e-cigarette aerosols. New England Journal of Medicine. 2015;372:392–394.

85- Farsalinos KE, Voudris V, Poulas K. E-cigarettes generate high levels of aldehydes only in dry-puff conditions. Addiction. 2015;110(8):1352–1356.

86- Salamanca JC, Munhenzva I, Escobedo JO, Jensen RP, Shaw A, Campbell R, Luo W, Peyton DH, Strongin RM. Formaldehyde hemiacetal sampling, recovery and quantification from electronic cigarette aerosols. Scientific Reports. 2017;7:11044.

87- Flora JW, Meruva N, Huang CB, et al. Characterisation of potential impurities and degradation products in electronic cigarette formulations and aerosols. Regulatory Toxicology and Pharmacology. 2016;74:1–11.

88- Vas CA, Porter A, McAdam K. Acetoin is a precursor to diacetyl in electronic cigarette liquids. Food and Chemical Toxicology. 2019;133:110727.

89- El-Hellani A, El-Hage R, Baalbaki R, et al. Free-base and protonated nicotine in electronic cigarette liquids and aerosols. Chemical Research in Toxicology. 2015;28(8):1532–1537.

90- Lisko JG, Tran H, Stanfill SB, Blount BC, Watson CH. Chemical composition and evaluation of nicotine, tobacco alkaloids, pH and selected flavours in electronic cigarette cartridges and refill solutions. Nicotine & Tobacco Research. 2015;17(10):1270–1278.

91- Etter JF, Zäther E, Svensson S. Analysis of refill liquids for electronic cigarettes. Addiction. 2013;108(9):1671–1679.

92- Olmedo P, Goessler W, Tanda S, et al. Metal concentrations in e-cigarette liquid and aerosol samples: the contribution of metallic coils. Environmental Health Perspectives. 2018;126(2):027010.

93- Williams M, Villarreal A, Bozhilov K, Lin S, Talbot P. Metal and silicate particles including nanoparticles are present in electronic cigarette cartomizer fluid and aerosol. PLoS ONE. 2013;8(3):e57987.

94- Zhao D, Aravindakshan A, Hilpert M, et al. Metal and metalloid levels in electronic cigarette liquids, aerosols and human biosamples: a systematic review. Environmental Health Perspectives. 2020;128(3):036001.

95- Zhao J, Nelson J, Dada O, Pyrgiotakis G, Kavouras IG, Demokritou P. Assessing electronic cigarette emissions: linking physicochemical properties to product brand, e-liquid flavouring additives, operational voltage and user puffing patterns. Inhalation Toxicology. 2018;30(2):78–88.

96- Talih S, Balhas Z, Eissenberg T, et al. Effects of user puff topography, device voltage and liquid nicotine concentration on electronic cigarette nicotine yield. Chemical Research in Toxicology. 2015;28(7):1504–1512.

97- Talih S, Salman R, El-Hage R, et al. Characteristics and toxicant emissions of JUUL electronic cigarettes. Tobacco Control. 2019;28(6):678–680.

98- Gillman IG, Kistler KA, Stewart EW, Paolantonio AR. Effect of variable power levels on the yield of total aerosol mass and formation of aldehydes in e-cigarette aerosols. Regulatory Toxicology and Pharmacology. 2016;75:58–65.

99- Geiss O, Bianchi I, Barahona F, Barrero-Moreno J. Characterisation of mainstream and passive vapours emitted by selected electronic cigarettes. International Journal of Hygiene and Environmental Health. 2015;218(1):169–180.

100- Margham J, McAdam K, Forster M, et al. Chemical composition of aerosol from an e-cigarette: a quantitative comparison with cigarette smoke. Chemical Research in Toxicology. 2016;29(10):1662–1678.

101- Tayyarah R, Long GA. Comparison of select analytes in aerosol from e-cigarettes with smoke from conventional cigarettes and with ambient air. Regulatory Toxicology and Pharmacology. 2014;70(3):704–710.

102- Goniewicz ML, Gawron M, Smith DM, Peng M, Jacob P, Benowitz NL. Exposure to nicotine and selected toxicants in cigarette smokers who switched to electronic cigarettes: a longitudinal within-subjects observational study. Nicotine & Tobacco Research. 2017;19(2):160–167.

103- Shahab L, Goniewicz ML, Blount BC, et al. Nicotine, carcinogen and toxin exposure in long-term e-cigarette and nicotine-replacement-therapy users. Annals of Internal Medicine. 2017;166(6):390–400.

104- Hecht SS, Carmella SG, Kotandeniya D, et al. Evaluation of toxicant and carcinogen metabolites in the urine of e-cigarette users versus cigarette smokers. Nicotine & Tobacco Research. 2015;17(6):704–709.

105- McRobbie H, Phillips A, Goniewicz ML, et al. Effects of switching to electronic cigarettes with and without concurrent smoking on exposure to nicotine, carbon monoxide and acrolein. Cancer Prevention Research. 2015;8(9):873–878.

106- Farsalinos KE, Polosa R. Safety evaluation and risk assessment of electronic cigarettes as tobacco cigarette substitutes: a systematic review. Therapeutic Advances in Drug Safety. 2014;5(2):67–86.

107- Glasser AM, Collins L, Pearson JL, et al. Overview of electronic nicotine delivery systems: a systematic review. American Journal of Preventive Medicine. 2017;52(2):e33–e66.

108- National Academies of Sciences, Engineering, and Medicine. Public Health Consequences of E-Cigarettes. Washington, DC: National Academies Press; 2018.

109- Royal College of Physicians. Nicotine Without Smoke: Tobacco Harm Reduction. London: Royal College of Physicians; 2016.

110- McNeill A, Brose LS, Calder R, Simonavicius E, Robson D. Nicotine Vaping in England: 2022 Evidence Update. London: Office for Health Improvement and Disparities; 2022.

Chapter 4: Analytical Science and Laboratory Testing

These references cover the regulatory basis for emissions reporting, standardised aerosol generation, method validation, laboratory accreditation, repeatability and reproducibility, carbonyl and metal analysis, nicotine verification, batch consistency, measurement uncertainty and conformity decisions. The standards have been aligned with the current ISO vapour-product catalogue, including the 2025 amendment to ISO 20768, and with current Eurachem, ILAC and metrology guidance.

European Parliament and Council of the European Union. Directive 2014/40/EU of 3 April 2014 on the approximation of the laws, regulations and administrative provisions of the Member States concerning the manufacture, presentation and sale of tobacco and related products and repealing Directive 2001/37/EC. *Official Journal of the European Union.* 2014;L127:1–38.

European Commission. Commission Implementing Decision (EU) 2015/2183 of 24 November 2015 establishing a common format for the notification of electronic cigarettes and refill containers. *Official Journal of the European Union.* 2015;L309:15–27.

UK Government. *The Tobacco and Related Products Regulations 2016.* SI 2016/507.

Medicines and Healthcare products Regulatory Agency. *MHRA E-cigarette and Vape Products Guidance Hub.* London: MHRA; 2025.

Cooperation Centre for Scientific Research Relative to Tobacco. *CORESTA Recommended Method No. 81: Routine Analytical Machine for E-Cigarette Aerosol Generation and Collection — Definitions and Standard Conditions.* Paris: CORESTA; 2015.

Cooperation Centre for Scientific Research Relative to Tobacco. *Technical Guide No. 22: Technical Guide for the Selection of Appropriate Intense Vaping Regimes for E-Vapour Devices.* Paris: CORESTA; 2024.

International Organization for Standardization. *ISO 20768:2018. Vapour Products — Routine Analytical Vaping Machine — Definitions and Standard Conditions.* Geneva: ISO; 2018.

International Organization for Standardization. *ISO 20768:2018/Amd 1:2025. Vapour Products — Routine Analytical Vaping Machine — Definitions and Standard Conditions — Amendment 1: Correction of Puff Profile Requirements.* Geneva: ISO; 2025.

International Organization for Standardization. *ISO 20714:2019. E-Liquid — Determination of Nicotine, Propylene Glycol and Glycerol in Liquids Used in Electronic Nicotine Delivery Devices — Gas Chromatographic Method.* Geneva: ISO; 2019.

International Organization for Standardization. *ISO 24197:2022. Vapour Products — Determination of E-Liquid Vaporised Mass and Aerosol Collected Mass.* Geneva: ISO; 2022.

International Organization for Standardization. *ISO 24199:2022. Vapour Products — Determination of Nicotine in Vapour Product Emissions — Gas Chromatographic Method.* Geneva: ISO; 2022.

International Organization for Standardization. *ISO 24211:2022. Vapour Products — Determination of Selected Carbonyls in Vapour Product Emissions.* Geneva: ISO; 2022.

International Organization for Standardization and International Electrotechnical Commission. *ISO/IEC 17025:2017. General Requirements for the Competence of Testing and Calibration Laboratories.* Geneva: ISO; 2017.

International Organization for Standardization. *ISO 5725-1:2023. Accuracy (Trueness and Precision) of Measurement Methods and Results — Part 1: General Principles and Definitions.* Geneva: ISO; 2023.

International Organization for Standardization. *ISO 5725-2:2025. Accuracy (Trueness and Precision) of Measurement Methods and Results — Part 2: Basic Method for the Determination of Repeatability and Reproducibility of a Standard Measurement Method.* Geneva: ISO; 2025.

International Organization for Standardization. *ISO 5725-3:2023. Accuracy (Trueness and Precision) of Measurement Methods and Results — Part 3: Intermediate Precision and Alternative Designs for Collaborative Studies*. Geneva: ISO; 2023.

International Organization for Standardization. *ISO 21748:2017. Guidance for the Use of Repeatability, Reproducibility and Trueness Estimates in Measurement Uncertainty Evaluation*. Geneva: ISO; 2017.

International Council for Harmonisation of Technical Requirements for Pharmaceuticals for Human Use. *ICH Q2(R2): Validation of Analytical Procedures*. Geneva: ICH; 2023.

International Council for Harmonisation of Technical Requirements for Pharmaceuticals for Human Use. *ICH Q14: Analytical Procedure Development*. Geneva: ICH; 2023.

Cantwell H, ed. *The Fitness for Purpose of Analytical Methods: A Laboratory Guide to Method Validation and Related Topics*. 3rd ed. Eurachem; 2025.

Barwick V, Tsimillis KC, eds. *Eurachem/CITAC Guide to Quality in Analytical Chemistry: An Aid to Accreditation*. 4th ed. Eurachem; 2026.

Ellison SLR, Williams A, eds. *Eurachem/CITAC Guide: Quantifying Uncertainty in Analytical Measurement*. 3rd ed. Eurachem; 2012.

Williams A, Magnusson B, eds. *Eurachem/CITAC Guide: Use of Uncertainty Information in Compliance Assessment*. 2nd ed. Eurachem; 2021.

Bettencourt da Silva R, ed. *Eurachem/CITAC Guide: Evaluation of Measurement Uncertainty from In-House Precision and Recovery Data*. 1st ed. Eurachem; 2026.

Joint Committee for Guides in Metrology. *JCGM 100:2008. Evaluation of Measurement Data — Guide to the Expression of Uncertainty in Measurement*. Sèvres: Bureau International des Poids et Mesures; 2008.

Joint Committee for Guides in Metrology. *JCGM 106:2012. Evaluation of Measurement Data — The Role of Measurement Uncertainty in Conformity Assessment*. Sèvres: Bureau International des Poids et Mesures; 2012.

International Laboratory Accreditation Cooperation. *ILAC-G8:09/2019. Guidelines on Decision Rules and Statements of Conformity*. Silverwater, Australia: ILAC; 2019.

International Laboratory Accreditation Cooperation. *ILAC-G17:01/2021. ILAC Guidelines for Measurement Uncertainty in Testing*. Silverwater, Australia: ILAC; 2021.

Goniewicz ML, Knysak J, Gawron M, et al. Levels of selected carcinogens and toxicants in vapour from electronic cigarettes. *Tobacco Control*. 2014;23(2):133–139.

Goniewicz ML, Kuma T, Gawron M, Knysak J, Kosmider L. Nicotine levels in electronic cigarettes. *Nicotine & Tobacco Research*. 2013;15(1):158–166.

Cheng T. Chemical evaluation of electronic cigarettes. *Tobacco Control*. 2014;23(Suppl 2):ii11–ii17.

Famele M, Ferranti C, Abenavoli C, Palleschi L, Mancinelli R, Draisci R. The chemical components of electronic cigarette cartridges and refill fluids: review of analytical methods. *Nicotine & Tobacco Research*. 2015;17(3):271–279.

Tayyarah R, Long GA. Comparison of select analytes in aerosol from e-cigarettes with smoke from conventional cigarettes and with ambient air. *Regulatory Toxicology and Pharmacology*. 2014;70(3):704–710.

Margham J, McAdam K, Forster M, et al. Chemical composition of aerosol from an e-cigarette: a quantitative comparison with cigarette smoke. *Chemical Research in Toxicology*. 2016;29(10):1662–1678.

Uchiyama S, Ohta K, Inaba Y, Kunugita N. Determination of carbonyl compounds generated from the e-cigarette using coupled silica cartridges impregnated with hydroquinone and 2,4-dinitrophenylhydrazine, followed by high-performance liquid chromatography. *Analytical Sciences*. 2013;29(12):1219–1222.

Kosmider L, Sobczak A, Fik M, et al. Carbonyl compounds in electronic cigarette vapors: effects of nicotine solvent and battery output voltage. *Nicotine & Tobacco Research*. 2014;16(10):1319–1326.

Farsalinos KE, Voudris V, Poulas K. E-cigarettes generate high levels of aldehydes only in dry-puff conditions. *Addiction*. 2015;110(8):1352–1356.

Geiss O, Bianchi I, Barrero-Moreno J. Correlation of volatile carbonyl yields emitted by e-cigarettes with the temperature of the heating coil and the perceived sensorial quality of the generated vapours. *International Journal of Hygiene and Environmental Health*. 2016;219(3):268–277.

Sleiman M, Logue JM, Montesinos VN, et al. Emissions from electronic cigarettes: key parameters affecting the release of harmful chemicals. *Environmental Science & Technology*. 2016;50(17):9644–9651.

Wang P, Chen W, Liao J, et al. A device-independent evaluation of carbonyl emissions from heated electronic cigarette solvents. *PLoS ONE*. 2017;12(1):e0169811.

Flora JW, Wilkinson CT, Wilkinson JW, et al. Method for the determination of carbonyl compounds in e-cigarette aerosols. *Journal of Chromatographic Science*. 2017;55(2):142–148.

Williams M, Villarreal A, Bozhilov K, Lin S, Talbot P. Metal and silicate particles including nanoparticles are present in electronic cigarette cartomizer fluid and aerosol. *PLoS ONE*. 2013;8(3):e57987.

Olmedo P, Goessler W, Tanda S, et al. Metal concentrations in e-cigarette liquid and aerosol samples: the contribution of metallic coils. *Environmental Health Perspectives*. 2018;126(2):027010.

Zhao D, Aravindakshan A, Hilpert M, et al. Metal and metalloid levels in electronic cigarette liquids, aerosols and human biosamples: a systematic review. *Environmental Health Perspectives*. 2020;128(3):036001.

Etter JF, Zäther E, Svensson S. Analysis of refill liquids for electronic cigarettes. *Addiction*. 2013;108(9):1671–1679.

Lisko JG, Tran H, Stanfill SB, Blount BC, Watson CH. Chemical composition and evaluation of nicotine, tobacco alkaloids, pH and selected flavours in e-cigarette cartridges and refill solutions. *Nicotine & Tobacco Research*. 2015;17(10):1270–1278.

El-Hellani A, El-Hage R, Baalbaki R, Salman R, Talih S, Shihadeh A, Saliba NA. Free-base and protonated nicotine in electronic cigarette liquids and aerosols. *Chemical Research in Toxicology*. 2015;28(8):1532–1537.

Flora JW, Meruva N, Huang CB, et al. Characterisation of potential impurities and degradation products in electronic cigarette formulations and aerosols. *Regulatory Toxicology and Pharmacology*. 2016;74:1–11.

Peace MR, Mulder HA, Baird TR, et al. Evaluation of nicotine and the components of e-liquids generated from e-cigarette aerosols. *Journal of Analytical Toxicology*. 2018;42(8):537–543.

Cunningham A, Slayford S, Vas C, Gee J, Costigan S, Prasad K. Development, validation and application of a device to measure e-cigarette users' puffing topography. *Scientific Reports*. 2016;6:35071.

Felicione NJ, Robinson RJ, Hiler MM, Guo L, Naclerio R, Eissenberg T. Comparison of measurement methods for electronic cigarette puff topography. *Nicotine & Tobacco Research*. 2020;22(8):1343–1350.

National Academies of Sciences, Engineering, and Medicine. *Public Health Consequences of E-Cigarettes*. Washington, DC: National Academies Press; 2018.

Chapter 5: Quality Systems and Manufacturing

The standards list reflects the editions current in July 2026. ISO 9001:2015, incorporating Amendment 1:2024, remains the current published requirements standard pending the expected publication of its replacement in September 2026; ISO 9000:2026 and ISO 19011:2026 have already replaced their preceding editions.

International Organization for Standardization. *ISO 9000:2026. Quality Management — Fundamentals and Vocabulary*. Geneva: ISO; 2026.

International Organization for Standardization. *ISO 9001:2015. Quality Management Systems — Requirements*, incorporating *ISO 9001:2015/Amd 1:2024. Amendment 1: Climate Action Changes*. Geneva: ISO; 2015–2024.

International Organization for Standardization. *ISO 9004:2018. Quality Management — Quality of an Organization — Guidance to Achieve Sustained Success*. Geneva: ISO; 2018.

International Organization for Standardization. *ISO 10002:2018. Quality Management — Customer Satisfaction — Guidelines for Complaints Handling in Organizations*. Geneva: ISO; 2018.

International Organization for Standardization. *ISO 10005:2018. Quality Management — Guidelines for Quality Plans*. Geneva: ISO; 2018.

International Organization for Standardization. *ISO 10007:2017. Quality Management — Guidelines for Configuration Management*. Geneva: ISO; 2017.

International Organization for Standardization. *ISO 10013:2021. Quality Management Systems — Guidance for Documented Information*. Geneva: ISO; 2021.

International Organization for Standardization. *ISO 10014:2021. Quality Management Systems — Managing an Organization for Quality Results — Guidance for Realizing Financial and Economic Benefits*. Geneva: ISO; 2021.

International Organization for Standardization. *ISO 10015:2019. Quality Management — Guidelines for Competence Management and People Development*. Geneva: ISO; 2019.

International Organization for Standardization. *ISO 10017:2021. Quality Management — Guidance on Statistical Techniques for ISO 9001:2015*. Geneva: ISO; 2021.

International Organization for Standardization. *ISO 19011:2026. Guidelines for Auditing Management Systems*. Geneva: ISO; 2026.

International Organization for Standardization. *ISO 31000:2018. Risk Management — Guidelines*. Geneva: ISO; 2018.

International Organization for Standardization. *ISO 10377:2013. Consumer Product Safety — Guidelines for Suppliers*. Geneva: ISO; 2013.

International Organization for Standardization. *ISO 10393:2013. Consumer Product Recall — Guidelines for Suppliers*. Geneva: ISO; 2013.

International Organization for Standardization and International Electrotechnical Commission. *ISO/IEC 17025:2017. General Requirements for the Competence of Testing and Calibration Laboratories*. Geneva: ISO; 2017.

GS1. *GS1 Global Traceability Standard*. Release 2.0. Brussels: GS1 AISBL; 2017.

British Standards Institution. *PAS 7100:2022. Product Recall and Other Corrective Actions — Code of Practice*. London: BSI; 2022.

Office for Product Safety and Standards. *Product Safety and Noncompliance Notification Guidance for Business*. Version 3. London: Department for Business and Trade; 2026.

International Council for Harmonisation of Technical Requirements for Pharmaceuticals for Human Use. *ICH Q7: Good Manufacturing Practice Guide for Active Pharmaceutical Ingredients*. Geneva: ICH; 2000.

International Council for Harmonisation of Technical Requirements for Pharmaceuticals for Human Use. *ICH Q8(R2): Pharmaceutical Development*. Geneva: ICH; 2009.

International Council for Harmonisation of Technical Requirements for Pharmaceuticals for Human Use. *ICH Q9(R1): Quality Risk Management*. Geneva: ICH; 2023.

International Council for Harmonisation of Technical Requirements for Pharmaceuticals for Human Use. *ICH Q10: Pharmaceutical Quality System*. Geneva: ICH; 2008.

International Council for Harmonisation of Technical Requirements for Pharmaceuticals for Human Use. *ICH Q12: Technical and Regulatory Considerations for Pharmaceutical Product Lifecycle Management*. Geneva: ICH; 2019.

European Commission. *EudraLex Volume 4: EU Guidelines for Good Manufacturing Practice for Medicinal Products for Human and Veterinary Use. Part I, Chapter 1: Pharmaceutical Quality System*. Brussels: European Commission; 2013.

European Commission. *EudraLex Volume 4: EU Guidelines for Good Manufacturing Practice for Medicinal Products for Human and Veterinary Use. Part I, Chapter 2: Personnel*. Brussels: European Commission; 2014.

European Commission. *EudraLex Volume 4: EU Guidelines for Good Manufacturing Practice for Medicinal Products for Human and Veterinary Use. Part I, Chapter 3: Premises and Equipment*. Brussels: European Commission; 2015.

European Commission. *EudraLex Volume 4: EU Guidelines for Good Manufacturing Practice for Medicinal Products for Human and Veterinary Use. Part I, Chapter 4: Documentation.* Brussels: European Commission; 2011.

European Commission. *EudraLex Volume 4: EU Guidelines for Good Manufacturing Practice for Medicinal Products for Human and Veterinary Use. Part I, Chapter 5: Production.* Brussels: European Commission; 2015.

European Commission. *EudraLex Volume 4: EU Guidelines for Good Manufacturing Practice for Medicinal Products for Human and Veterinary Use. Part I, Chapter 6: Quality Control.* Brussels: European Commission; 2014.

European Commission. *EudraLex Volume 4: EU Guidelines for Good Manufacturing Practice for Medicinal Products for Human and Veterinary Use. Part I, Chapter 7: Outsourced Activities.* Brussels: European Commission; 2013.

European Commission. *EudraLex Volume 4: EU Guidelines for Good Manufacturing Practice for Medicinal Products for Human and Veterinary Use. Part I, Chapter 8: Complaints, Quality Defects and Product Recalls.* Brussels: European Commission; 2015.

European Commission. *EudraLex Volume 4: EU Guidelines for Good Manufacturing Practice for Medicinal Products for Human and Veterinary Use. Part I, Chapter 9: Self Inspection.* Brussels: European Commission; n.d.

European Commission. *EudraLex Volume 4: EU Guidelines for Good Manufacturing Practice for Medicinal Products for Human and Veterinary Use. Annex 11: Computerised Systems.* Revision 1. Brussels: European Commission; 2011.

European Commission. *EudraLex Volume 4: EU Guidelines for Good Manufacturing Practice for Medicinal Products for Human and Veterinary Use. Annex 15: Qualification and Validation.* Brussels: European Commission; 2015.

US Food and Drug Administration. *Quality Systems Approach to Pharmaceutical CGMP Regulations: Guidance for Industry.* Silver Spring, MD: FDA; 2006.

US Food and Drug Administration. *Process Validation: General Principles and Practices. Guidance for Industry.* Silver Spring, MD: FDA; 2011.

US Food and Drug Administration. *Investigating Out-of-Specification Test Results for Pharmaceutical Production: Guidance for Industry.* Silver Spring, MD: FDA; 2006.

US Food and Drug Administration. *Data Integrity and Compliance with Drug CGMP: Questions and Answers. Guidance for Industry.* Silver Spring, MD: FDA; 2018.

Medicines and Healthcare products Regulatory Agency. *MHRA GxP Data Integrity Guidance and Definitions.* Revision 1. London: MHRA; 2018.

Pharmaceutical Inspection Co-operation Scheme. *PE 009-17: Guide to Good Manufacturing Practice for Medicinal Products.* Geneva: PIC/S; 2023.

Pharmaceutical Inspection Co-operation Scheme. *PI 041-1: Good Practices for Data Management and Integrity in Regulated GMP/GDP Environments.* Geneva: PIC/S; 2021.

Pharmaceutical Inspection Co-operation Scheme. *PI 054-1: How to Evaluate and Demonstrate the Effectiveness of the Pharmaceutical Quality System with Regard to Risk-Based Change Management.* Geneva: PIC/S; 2021.

World Health Organization. *WHO Good Manufacturing Practices for Pharmaceutical Products: Main Principles*. WHO Technical Report Series No. 986, Annex 2. Geneva: WHO; 2014.

World Health Organization. *Guideline on Data Integrity*. WHO Technical Report Series No. 1033, Annex 4. Geneva: WHO; 2021.

Deming WE. *Out of the Crisis*. Cambridge, MA: Massachusetts Institute of Technology, Center for Advanced Engineering Study; 1986.

De Feo JA, ed. *Juran's Quality Handbook: The Complete Guide to Performance Excellence*. 7th ed. New York: McGraw-Hill Education; 2016.

Imai M. *Kaizen: The Key to Japan's Competitive Success*. New York: Random House; 1986.

Ishikawa K. *Guide to Quality Control*. 2nd revised ed. Tokyo: Asian Productivity Organization; 1986.

Montgomery DC. *Introduction to Statistical Quality Control*. 8th ed. Hoboken, NJ: John Wiley & Sons; 2020.

Oakland JS. *Total Quality Management and Operational Excellence: Text with Cases*. 4th ed. Abingdon: Routledge; 2014.

Chapter 6: Product Notifications and Compliance

Behar, R.Z., Luo, W., McWhirter, K.J., Pankow, J.F. and Talbot, P. (2018). Analytical and toxicological evaluation of flavour chemicals in electronic cigarette refill fluids. *Scientific Reports*, 8, 8288.

Carnicer-Pont, D., Tigova, O., Havermans, A., Remue, E., Ferech, M., Vejdovszky, K., Solimini, R. et al. (2022). Tobacco products in the European Union Common Entry Gate: a tool for monitoring the EU Tobacco Products Directive. *Tobacco Prevention & Cessation*, 8, 1–11.

Chemical Abstracts Service (CAS). *CAS REGISTRY: Chemical Substance Information and CAS Registry Numbers*. Columbus, Ohio: CAS, a division of the American Chemical Society.

Chemical Abstracts Service (CAS) (2007). *Naming and Indexing of Chemical Substances for Chemical Abstracts*. Columbus, Ohio: CAS.

Commission Implementing Decision (EU) 2015/2183 of 24 November 2015 establishing a common format for the notification of electronic cigarettes and refill containers. *Official Journal of the European Union*, L 309, 26 November 2015, 15–27.

Commission Implementing Decision (EU) 2016/586 of 14 April 2016 on technical standards for the refill mechanism of electronic cigarettes. *Official Journal of the European Union*, L 101, 16 April 2016, 15–16.

Directive 2014/40/EU of the European Parliament and of the Council of 3 April 2014 concerning the manufacture, presentation and sale of tobacco and related products and repealing Directive 2001/37/EC. *Official Journal of the European Union*, L 127, 29 April 2014, 1–38.

Electronic Cigarettes etc. (Fees) Regulations 2016, SI 2016/521. London: The Stationery Office.

EFSA Scientific Committee (2017). Guidance on the use of the weight of evidence approach in scientific assessments. *EFSA Journal*, 15(8), 4971.

Eshraghian, E.A. and Al-Delaimy, W.K. (2021). A review of constituents identified in electronic cigarette liquids and aerosols. *Tobacco Prevention & Cessation*, 7, 10.

Effah, F., Adragna, J., Luglio, D., Bailey, A., Marczylo, T. and Gordon, T. (2023). Toxicological assessment of electronic cigarette flavoured e-liquid aerosols using Calu-3 cells: a three-dimensional lung model approach. *Toxicology*, 500, 153683.

European Commission (2020). *EU Common Entry Gate User Guide.* Brussels: Directorate-General for Health and Food Safety.

European Commission. *EU Common Entry Gate: Step-by-Step Guide for Submitting Information on Tobacco Products, Electronic Cigarettes and Refill Containers.* Brussels: Directorate-General for Health and Food Safety.

European Commission (2021). *Report on the Application of Directive 2014/40/EU Concerning the Manufacture, Presentation and Sale of Tobacco and Related Products.* COM(2021) 249 final. Brussels: European Commission.

European Commission Scientific Committee on Health, Environmental and Emerging Risks (2021). *Opinion on Electronic Cigarettes.* Brussels: European Commission.

Food and Drug Administration (2023). *Premarket Tobacco Product Applications for Electronic Nicotine Delivery Systems: Guidance for Industry.* Silver Spring, Maryland: US Department of Health and Human Services.

Health Canada (2023). *Vaping Products Reporting Regulations*, SOR/2023-123. Ottawa: Government of Canada.

Health Canada (2024). *Industry Guide to Vaping Products Subject to the Canada Consumer Product Safety Act.* Ottawa: Government of Canada.

International Organization for Standardization (2015). *ISO 9001:2015: Quality Management Systems — Requirements.* Geneva: ISO.

International Organization for Standardization (2017). *ISO/IEC 17025:2017: General Requirements for the Competence of Testing and Calibration Laboratories.* Geneva: ISO.

International Organization for Standardization (2022). *ISO/IEC 27001:2022: Information Security, Cybersecurity and Privacy Protection — Information Security Management Systems — Requirements.* Geneva: ISO.

International Organization for Standardization (2018). *ISO 31000:2018: Risk Management — Guidelines.* Geneva: ISO.

International Organization for Standardization (2019). *ISO 20714:2019: E-Liquid — Determination of Nicotine, Propylene Glycol and Glycerol in Liquids Used in Electronic Nicotine Delivery Devices — Gas Chromatographic Method.* Geneva: ISO.

International Organization for Standardization (2018). *ISO 20768:2018: Vapour Products — Routine Analytical Vaping Machine — Definitions and Standard Conditions.* Geneva: ISO.

International Organization for Standardization (2022). *ISO 24197:2022: Vapour Products — Determination of E-Liquid Vaporised Mass and Aerosol Collected Mass.* Geneva: ISO.

International Organization for Standardization (2022). *ISO 24199:2022: Vapour Products — Determination of Nicotine in Vapour Product Emissions — Gas Chromatographic Method.* Geneva: ISO.

International Organization for Standardization (2022). *ISO 24211:2022: Vapour Products — Determination of Selected Carbonyls in Vapour Product Emissions*. Geneva: ISO.

Joint Action on Tobacco Control (2020). *WP5–D5.1: Report on What Data Is Public and Non-Confidential in the EU Common Entry Gate*. Brussels: European Union Joint Action on Tobacco Control.

Joint Action on Tobacco Control (2022). *WP7–D7.5: Second Report on Electronic Cigarette Product Analyses*. Brussels: European Union Joint Action on Tobacco Control.

Kassem, N.O.F., Strongin, R.M., Stroup, A.M., Brinkman, M.C., El-Hellani, A., Erythropel, H.C., Etemadi, A., Exil, V., Goniewicz, M.L. et al. (2024). A review of the toxicity of ingredients in electronic cigarettes, including ingredients having generally recognised as safe regulatory status for use in food. *Nicotine & Tobacco Research*, 26(11), 1445–1454.

Krüsemann, E.J.Z., Havermans, A., Pennings, J.L.A., de Graaf, K., Boesveldt, S. and Talhout, R. (2021). Comprehensive overview of common e-liquid ingredients and how they can be used to predict an e-liquid's flavour category. *Tobacco Control*, 30(2), 185–191.

Medicines and Healthcare products Regulatory Agency. *E-Cigarettes: Regulations for Consumer Products*. London: MHRA.

Medicines and Healthcare products Regulatory Agency (2024). *Submission and Content of Notifications for Great Britain*. London: MHRA.

Medicines and Healthcare products Regulatory Agency (2024). *Guidance on the Submission and Content of Notifications for Northern Ireland*. London: MHRA.

Medicines and Healthcare products Regulatory Agency (2024). *Chapter 1: Submission Type Guidance — Great Britain*. London: MHRA.

Medicines and Healthcare products Regulatory Agency (2025). *Chapter 2: Product Type Guidance — Great Britain*. London: MHRA.

Medicines and Healthcare products Regulatory Agency (2024). *Chapter 3: Emissions Guidance — Great Britain*. London: MHRA.

Medicines and Healthcare products Regulatory Agency (2024). *Chapter 6: Ingredient Guidance — Great Britain*. London: MHRA.

Medicines and Healthcare products Regulatory Agency (2024). *Chapter 7: Advice on Submitting Annual Reports for Electronic Cigarettes and Refill Containers — Great Britain*. London: MHRA.

Medicines and Healthcare products Regulatory Agency (2024). *Chapter 9: General Advice on Due Diligence — Great Britain*. London: MHRA.

Medicines and Healthcare products Regulatory Agency (2024). *Chapter 10: General Advice on Vigilance for Electronic Cigarette Devices and Refill Containers — Great Britain*. London: MHRA.

Medicines and Healthcare products Regulatory Agency (2022). *User Reference Guide: MHRA Electronic Cigarette Submissions*. London: MHRA.

Nyakutsikwa, B., Britton, J., Bogdanovica, I., Boobis, A. and Langley, T. (2021). Characterising vaping products in the United Kingdom: an analysis of Tobacco Products Directive notification data. *Addiction*, 116(9), 2521–2528.

New Zealand Ministry of Health. *Product Notifications for Manufacturers and Importers of Vaping and Other Notifiable Products*. Wellington: Ministry of Health.

Organisation for Economic Co-operation and Development (2018). *Test No. 412: Subacute Inhalation Toxicity — 28-Day Study*. OECD Guidelines for the Testing of Chemicals. Paris: OECD Publishing.

Organisation for Economic Co-operation and Development (2017). *Test No. 413: Subchronic Inhalation Toxicity — 90-Day Study*. OECD Guidelines for the Testing of Chemicals. Paris: OECD Publishing.

Sciuscio, D., Calvino-Martin, F., Kumar, A., Langston, T.B., Martin, E., Marescotti, D., Mathis, C., Hoeng, J., Peitsch, M.C., Smith, D.C. et al. (2022). Toxicological assessment of flavour ingredients in e-vapour products. *Frontiers in Toxicology*, 4, 878976.

Therapeutic Goods Administration (2021). *Therapeutic Goods (Standard for Therapeutic Vaping Goods) (TGO 110) Order 2021*, as amended. Canberra: Australian Government.

Tobacco and Related Products Regulations 2016, SI 2016/507, as amended. London: The Stationery Office.

Tobacco Products and Nicotine Inhaling Products (Amendment) (EU Exit) Regulations 2020, SI 2020/1316. London: The Stationery Office.

Chapter 7: Global Regulatory Models

European Parliament and Council (2014). Directive 2014/40/EU of 3 April 2014 concerning the manufacture, presentation and sale of tobacco and related products and repealing Directive 2001/37/EC. *Official Journal of the European Union*, L 127, 1–38.

European Commission (2015). Commission Implementing Decision (EU) 2015/2183 of 24 November 2015 establishing a common format for the notification of electronic cigarettes and refill containers. *Official Journal of the European Union*, L 309, 15–27.

European Commission (2016). Commission Implementing Decision (EU) 2016/586 of 14 April 2016 on technical standards for the refill mechanism of electronic cigarettes. *Official Journal of the European Union*, L 101, 15–16.

European Commission (2021). *Report on the Application of Directive 2014/40/EU Concerning the Manufacture, Presentation and Sale of Tobacco and Related Products*. COM(2021) 249 final. Brussels: European Commission.

Scientific Committee on Health, Environmental and Emerging Risks (2021). *Opinion on Electronic Cigarettes*. Brussels: European Commission.

European Commission (2026). *Commission Staff Working Document: Evaluation of the Legislative Framework for Tobacco Control*. Brussels: European Commission.

United Kingdom Parliament (2016). *The Tobacco and Related Products Regulations 2016*, SI 2016/507, as amended. London: The Stationery Office.

United Kingdom Parliament (2020). *The Tobacco Products and Nicotine Inhaling Products (Amendment) (EU Exit) Regulations 2020*, SI 2020/1316. London: The Stationery Office.

Medicines and Healthcare products Regulatory Agency (2025). *E-Cigarettes: Regulations for Consumer Products*. London: MHRA.

United Kingdom Parliament (2026). *Tobacco and Vapes Act 2026*. London: The Stationery Office.

HM Revenue and Customs (2026). *Prepare for Vaping Products Duty and the Vaping Duty Stamps Scheme*. London: HMRC.

United States Congress (2009). *Family Smoking Prevention and Tobacco Control Act*, Public Law 111-31, 123 Stat. 1776. Washington, DC: United States Government.

United States Food and Drug Administration (2016). Deeming tobacco products to be subject to the Federal Food, Drug, and Cosmetic Act, as amended by the Family Smoking Prevention and Tobacco Control Act. Final rule. *Federal Register*, 81, 28974–29106.

United States Food and Drug Administration (2021). Premarket tobacco product applications and recordkeeping requirements. Final rule. *Federal Register*, 86, 55300–55439.

United States Food and Drug Administration (2019). *Premarket Tobacco Product Applications for Electronic Nicotine Delivery Systems: Guidance for Industry*. Silver Spring, Maryland: FDA.

United States Food and Drug Administration (2026). *Flavored Electronic Nicotine Delivery Systems Premarket Applications: Considerations Related to Youth Risk*. Draft Guidance for Industry. Silver Spring, Maryland: FDA.

United States Food and Drug Administration (2026). *Enforcement Priorities for Certain New Tobacco Products Marketed Without Premarket Authorization: Guidance for Industry*. Silver Spring, Maryland: FDA.

Australian Parliament (2024). *Therapeutic Goods and Other Legislation Amendment (Vaping Reforms) Act 2024*. Canberra: Commonwealth of Australia.

Australian Government (2021). *Therapeutic Goods (Standard for Therapeutic Vaping Goods) (TGO 110) Order 2021*, as amended. Canberra: Commonwealth of Australia.

Therapeutic Goods Administration (2025). *Product Standards for Unapproved Therapeutic Vapes in Australia*. Canberra: Australian Government Department of Health and Aged Care.

Therapeutic Goods Administration (2026). *Notified Vape List: Goods for Smoking Cessation or Nicotine Dependence*. Canberra: Australian Government Department of Health and Aged Care.

New Zealand Parliament (1990). *Smokefree Environments and Regulated Products Act 1990*, as amended. Wellington: New Zealand Government.

New Zealand Government (2021). *Smokefree Environments and Regulated Products Regulations 2021*, as amended. Wellington: New Zealand Government.

New Zealand Ministry of Health (2025). *Product Notifications for Manufacturers and Importers of Vaping and Other Notifiable Products*. Wellington: Ministry of Health.

New Zealand Ministry of Health (2025). *Recent Changes to Smokefree Laws*. Wellington: Ministry of Health.

Parliament of Canada (2018). *Tobacco and Vaping Products Act*, SC 1997, c. 13, as amended. Ottawa: Government of Canada.

Government of Canada (2021). *Nicotine Concentration in Vaping Products Regulations*, SOR/2021-123. Ottawa: Government of Canada.

Government of Canada (2019). *Vaping Products Labelling and Packaging Regulations*, SOR/2019-353. Ottawa: Government of Canada.

Government of Canada (2023). *Vaping Products Reporting Regulations*, SOR/2023-123. Ottawa: Government of Canada.

Health Canada (2026). *Report of the Third Legislative Review of the Tobacco and Vaping Products Act.* Ottawa: Government of Canada.

Canada Revenue Agency (2024). *EDN95: Coordinated Vaping Duty System.* Ottawa: Government of Canada.

State Tobacco Monopoly Administration of the People's Republic of China (2022). *Measures for the Administration of Electronic Cigarettes.* Announcement No. 1 of 2022. Beijing: State Tobacco Monopoly Administration.

Standardization Administration of China (2022). *GB 41700-2022: Electronic Cigarettes.* Beijing: State Administration for Market Regulation and Standardization Administration of China.

Health Sciences Authority Singapore (2026). *Tobacco and Vaporisers Control Act: Tobacco Regulation and Vaping Enforcement.* Singapore: Health Sciences Authority.

Parliament of India (2019). *The Prohibition of Electronic Cigarettes (Production, Manufacture, Import, Export, Transport, Sale, Distribution, Storage and Advertisement) Act 2019*, Act No. 42 of 2019. New Delhi: Government of India.

Parliament of Malaysia (2024). *Control of Smoking Products for Public Health Act 2024*, Act 852. Putrajaya: Government of Malaysia.

Congress of the Philippines (2022). *Republic Act No. 11900: Vaporized Nicotine and Non-Nicotine Products Regulation Act.* Manila: Republic of the Philippines.

United Arab Emirates Ministry of Industry and Advanced Technology (2019). *UAE.S 5030: Electronic Nicotine Products—Mandatory UAE Regulation.* Abu Dhabi: Government of the United Arab Emirates.

Saudi Food and Drug Authority (2020). *SFDA.FD 5005:2020: E-Liquids and Heated Tobacco in Electronic Systems for Smoking.* Riyadh: Saudi Food and Drug Authority.

Israel Ministry of Health (2023). *Electronic Cigarettes: Regulation, Marketing Restrictions and Public-Health Requirements.* Jerusalem: Government of Israel.

World Health Organization (2003). *WHO Framework Convention on Tobacco Control.* Geneva: World Health Organization.

World Health Organization (2023). *Electronic Cigarettes: Call to Action.* Geneva: World Health Organization.

World Health Organization Regional Office for the Western Pacific (2026). *Electronic Cigarettes: Advocacy Brief.* Manila: World Health Organization.

International Organization for Standardization (2019). *ISO 20714:2019: E-Liquid—Determination of Nicotine, Propylene Glycol and Glycerol in Liquids Used in Electronic Nicotine Delivery Devices—Gas Chromatographic Method.* Geneva: ISO.

International Organization for Standardization (2018). *ISO 20768:2018: Vapour Products—Routine Analytical Vaping Machine—Definitions and Standard Conditions*, including Amendment 1:2025. Geneva: ISO.

International Organization for Standardization (2022). *ISO 24197:2022: Vapour Products—Determination of E-Liquid Vaporised Mass and Aerosol Collected Mass*. Geneva: ISO.

International Organization for Standardization (2022). *ISO 24199:2022: Vapour Products—Determination of Nicotine in Vapour Product Emissions—Gas Chromatographic Method*. Geneva: ISO.

International Organization for Standardization (2022). *ISO 24211:2022: Vapour Products—Determination of Selected Carbonyls in Vapour Product Emissions*. Geneva: ISO.

Kennedy, R.D., Awopegba, A., De León, E. and Cohen, J.E. (2017). Global approaches to regulating electronic cigarettes. *Tobacco Control*, 26(4), 440–445.

Campus, B., Fafard, P., St. Pierre, J. and Hoffman, S.J. (2021). Comparing the regulation and incentivization of e-cigarettes across 97 countries. *Social Science & Medicine*, 291, 114187.

Chapter 8: Industry, Politics and Public Health

World Health Organization (2003). *WHO Framework Convention on Tobacco Control*. Geneva: World Health Organization.

World Health Organization (2008). *Guidelines for Implementation of Article 5.3 of the WHO Framework Convention on Tobacco Control: Protection of Public Health Policies with Respect to Tobacco Control from Commercial and Other Vested Interests of the Tobacco Industry*. Geneva: World Health Organization.

World Health Organization (2008). *Tobacco Industry Interference with Tobacco Control*. Geneva: World Health Organization.

World Health Organization (2014). *Electronic Nicotine Delivery Systems: Report by WHO*. FCTC/COP/6/10 Rev.1. Geneva: World Health Organization.

World Health Organization (2016). *Electronic Nicotine Delivery Systems and Electronic Non-Nicotine Delivery Systems: Report by WHO*. FCTC/COP/7/11. Geneva: World Health Organization.

World Health Organization (2023). *Electronic Cigarettes: Call to Action*. Geneva: World Health Organization.

Royal College of Physicians (2016). *Nicotine Without Smoke: Tobacco Harm Reduction*. London: Royal College of Physicians.

National Academies of Sciences, Engineering, and Medicine (2018). *Public Health Consequences of E-Cigarettes*. Washington, DC: National Academies Press.

Britton, J. and Bogdanovica, I. (2014). *Electronic Cigarettes: A Report Commissioned by Public Health England*. London: Public Health England.

McNeill, A., Brose, L.S., Calder, R., Hitchman, S.C., Hajek, P. and McRobbie, H. (2015). *E-Cigarettes: An Evidence Update. A Report Commissioned by Public Health England*. London: Public Health England.

McNeill, A., Brose, L.S., Calder, R., Bauld, L. and Robson, D. (2018). *Evidence Review of E-Cigarettes and Heated Tobacco Products 2018*. London: Public Health England.

McNeill, A., Brose, L.S., Calder, R., Bauld, L. and Robson, D. (2019). *Vaping in England: An Evidence Update February 2019*. London: Public Health England.

McNeill, A., Brose, L.S., Calder, R., Simonavicius, E. and Robson, D. (2020). *Vaping in England: An Evidence Update Including Mental Health and Pregnancy, March 2020*. London: Public Health England.

McNeill, A., Brose, L.S., Calder, R., Simonavicius, E. and Robson, D. (2021). *Vaping in England: An Evidence Update February 2021*. London: Public Health England.

McNeill, A., Simonavicius, E., Brose, L.S., Taylor, E., East, K., Zuikova, E. and Calder, R. (2022). *Nicotine Vaping in England: 2022 Evidence Update*. London: Office for Health Improvement and Disparities.

Butler, A.R. et al. (2025). Electronic cigarettes for smoking cessation. *Cochrane Database of Systematic Reviews*, CD010216.

Hajek, P., Phillips-Waller, A., Przulj, D., Pesola, F., Myers Smith, K., Bisal, N., Li, J., Parrott, S., Sasieni, P., Dawkins, L., Ross, L., Goniewicz, M., Wu, Q. and McRobbie, H.J. (2019). A randomized trial of e-cigarettes versus nicotine-replacement therapy. *New England Journal of Medicine*, 380, 629–637.

Abrams, D.B., Glasser, A.M., Pearson, J.L., Villanti, A.C., Collins, L.K. and Niaura, R.S. (2018). Harm minimization and tobacco control: reframing societal views of nicotine use to rapidly save lives. *Annual Review of Public Health*, 39, 193–213.

Nutt, D.J., Phillips, L.D., Balfour, D., Curran, H.V., Dockrell, M., Foulds, J., Fagerström, K., Letlape, K., Milton, A., Polosa, R., Ramsey, J. and Sweanor, D. (2014). Estimating the harms of nicotine-containing products using the MCDA approach. *European Addiction Research*, 20(5), 218–225.

Warner, K.E. and Mendez, D. (2019). E-cigarettes: comparing the possible risks of increasing smoking initiation with the potential benefits of increasing smoking cessation. *Nicotine & Tobacco Research*, 21(1), 41–47.

Bell, K. and Keane, H. (2012). Nicotine control: e-cigarettes, smoking and addiction. *International Journal of Drug Policy*, 23(3), 242–247.

Farrimond, H. (2016). A typology of vaping: identifying differing beliefs, motivations for use, identity and political interest amongst e-cigarette users. *International Journal of Drug Policy*, 27, 102–108.

Farsalinos, K.E., Romagna, G., Tsiapras, D., Kyrzopoulos, S. and Voudris, V. (2014). Characteristics, perceived side effects and benefits of electronic cigarette use: a worldwide survey of more than 19,000 consumers. *International Journal of Environmental Research and Public Health*, 11(4), 4356–4373.

Etter, J.F. and Bullen, C. (2014). A longitudinal study of electronic cigarette users. *Addictive Behaviors*, 39(2), 491–494.

McKeganey, N. and Dickson, T. (2017). Why don't more smokers switch to using e-cigarettes: the views of confirmed smokers. *International Journal of Environmental Research and Public Health*, 14(6), 647.

Ward, E., Cox, S., Dawkins, L., Jakes, S., Holland, R. and Notley, C. (2018). A qualitative exploration of the role of vape shop environments in supporting smoking abstinence. *International Journal of Environmental Research and Public Health*, 15(2), 297.

Russell, C., McKeganey, N., Dickson, T. and Nides, M. (2018). Changing patterns of first e-cigarette flavor used and current flavors used by 20,836 adult frequent e-cigarette users in the USA. *Harm Reduction Journal*, 15, 33.

Rooke, C. and Amos, A. (2014). News media representations of electronic cigarettes: an analysis of newspaper coverage in the UK and Scotland. *Tobacco Control*, 23(6), 507–512.

Sun, S., Veltri, G.A. and Wang, F. (2018). Representations of electronic cigarettes in Chinese media. *BMC Public Health*, 18, 727.

Kasperson, R.E., Renn, O., Slovic, P., Brown, H.S., Emel, J., Goble, R., Kasperson, J.X. and Ratick, S. (1988). The social amplification of risk: a conceptual framework. *Risk Analysis*, 8(2), 177–187.

Entman, R.M. (1993). Framing: toward clarification of a fractured paradigm. *Journal of Communication*, 43(4), 51–58.

Scheufele, D.A. (1999). Framing as a theory of media effects. *Journal of Communication*, 49(1), 103–122.

Sumner, P., Vivian-Griffiths, S., Boivin, J., Williams, A., Venetis, C.A., Davies, A., Ogden, J., Whelan, L., Hughes, B., Dalton, B., Boy, F. and Chambers, C.D. (2014). The association between exaggeration in health-related science news and academic press releases: retrospective observational study. *BMJ*, 349, g7015.

Yavchitz, A., Boutron, I., Bafeta, A., Marroun, I., Charles, P., Mantz, J. and Ravaud, P. (2012). Misrepresentation of randomized controlled trials in press releases and news coverage: a cohort study. *PLoS Medicine*, 9(9), e1001308.

Brossard, D. (2013). New media landscapes and the science information consumer. *Proceedings of the National Academy of Sciences*, 110(Supplement 3), 14096–14101.

Blount, B.C., Karwowski, M.P., Shields, P.G., Morel-Espinosa, M., Valentin-Blasini, L., Gardner, M., Braselton, M., Brosius, C.R., Caron, K.T., Chambers, D., Corstvet, J., Cowan, E., De Jesús, V.R., Espinosa, P., Fernandez, C., Holder, C., Kuklenyik, Z., Kusovschi, J.D., Newman, C., Reis, G.B., Rees, J., Reese, C., Silva, L., Seyler, T., Song, M.A., Sosnoff, C., Spitzer, C.R., Tevis, D., Wang, L., Watson, C., Wewers, M.D., Xia, B., Heitkemper, D.T., Ghinai, I., Layden, J., Briss, P., King, B.A., Delaney, L.J., Jones, C.M., Baldwin, G.T., Patel, A., Meaney-Delman, D. and Rose, D. (2020). Vitamin E acetate in bronchoalveolar-lavage fluid associated with EVALI. *New England Journal of Medicine*, 382, 697–705.

Ulucanlar, S., Fooks, G.J. and Gilmore, A.B. (2016). The policy dystopia model: an interpretive analysis of tobacco industry political activity. *PLoS Medicine*, 13(9), e1002125.

Savell, E., Gilmore, A.B. and Fooks, G. (2014). How does the tobacco industry attempt to influence marketing regulations? A systematic review. *PLoS ONE*, 9(2), e87389.

Smith, K.E., Fooks, G., Collin, J., Weishaar, H., Mandal, S. and Gilmore, A.B. (2010). 'Working the system'—British American Tobacco's influence on the European Union Treaty and its implications for policy: an analysis of internal tobacco industry documents. *PLoS Medicine*, 7(1), e1000202.

Peeters, S. and Gilmore, A.B. (2013). Transnational tobacco company interests in smokeless tobacco in Europe: analysis of internal industry documents and contemporary industry materials. *PLoS Medicine*, 10(9), e1001506.

Hatchard, J.L., Fooks, G.J., Evans-Reeves, K.A., Ulucanlar, S. and Gilmore, A.B. (2014). A critical evaluation of the volume, relevance and quality of evidence submitted by the tobacco industry to oppose standardised packaging of tobacco products. *BMJ Open*, 4(2), e003757.

Fooks, G., Gilmore, A.B., Collin, J., Holden, C. and Lee, K. (2013). The limits of corporate social responsibility: techniques of neutralization, stakeholder management and political CSR. *Journal of Business Ethics*, 112(2), 283–299.

Bero, L.A. (2017). Addressing bias and conflict of interest among biomedical researchers. *JAMA*, 317(17), 1723–1724.

Lundh, A., Lexchin, J., Mintzes, B., Schroll, J.B. and Bero, L. (2017). Industry sponsorship and research outcome. *Cochrane Database of Systematic Reviews*, MR000033.

Lo, B. and Field, M.J. (eds.) (2009). *Conflict of Interest in Medical Research, Education, and Practice.* Washington, DC: National Academies Press.

Government Office for Science (2021). *Code of Practice for Scientific Advisory Committees and Councils.* London: HM Government.

Government Office for Science (2010). *Principles of Scientific Advice to Government.* London: HM Government.

Cabinet Office (2018). *Consultation Principles: Guidance.* London: HM Government.

Oliver, K., Innvar, S., Lorenc, T., Woodman, J. and Thomas, J. (2014). A systematic review of barriers to and facilitators of the use of evidence by policymakers. *BMC Health Services Research*, 14, 2.

Cairney, P. (2016). *The Politics of Evidence-Based Policy Making.* London: Palgrave Macmillan.

Chapter 9: Regulation in Practice

These sources correspond with Chapter 9's treatment of retail compliance, importation, distribution, online sales, enforcement, border control, counterfeit products, illegal markets, product withdrawals and regulatory case studies.

Department of Health. *The Tobacco and Related Products Regulations 2016*, SI 2016/507. London: The Stationery Office, 2016.

Department of Health. *The Nicotine Inhaling Products (Age of Sale and Proxy Purchasing) Regulations 2015*, SI 2015/895. London: The Stationery Office, 2015.

Department for Business, Innovation and Skills. *The Waste Electrical and Electronic Equipment Regulations 2013*, SI 2013/3113. London: The Stationery Office, 2013.

Department for Environment, Food and Rural Affairs. *The Environmental Protection (Single-use Vapes) (England) Regulations 2024*, SI 2024/1216. London: The Stationery Office, 2024.

European Parliament and Council of the European Union. *Directive 2014/40/EU on the Manufacture, Presentation and Sale of Tobacco and Related Products.* Official Journal of the European Union, L127, 2014.

European Commission. *Commission Implementing Decision (EU) 2015/2183 Establishing a Common Format for the Notification of Electronic Cigarettes and Refill Containers.* Official Journal of the European Union, L309, 2015.

European Commission. *Commission Implementing Decision (EU) 2016/586 on Technical Standards for the Refill Mechanism of Electronic Cigarettes.* Official Journal of the European Union, L101, 2016.

European Commission. *Providing Information on Tobacco Products, Electronic Cigarettes and Refill Containers through the EU Common Entry Gate.* Brussels: Directorate-General for Health and Food Safety.

European Commission. *EU Common Entry Gate User Guide.* Brussels: Directorate-General for Health and Food Safety, 2020.

European Commission. *Report on the Application of Directive 2014/40/EU Concerning the Manufacture, Presentation and Sale of Tobacco and Related Products.* COM(2021) 249 final. Brussels, 2021.

European Commission. *Evaluation of the Legislative Framework for Tobacco Control.* Brussels: Directorate-General for Health and Food Safety, 2026.

Medicines and Healthcare products Regulatory Agency. *E-cigarettes: Regulations for Consumer Products.* London: MHRA.

Medicines and Healthcare products Regulatory Agency. *MHRA E-cigarette and Vape Products Guidance Hub.* London: MHRA, 2025.

Medicines and Healthcare products Regulatory Agency. *E-cigarette and Vape Advice for Retailers and Producers.* London: MHRA, 2024.

Medicines and Healthcare products Regulatory Agency. *E-cigarette and Vape Products Regulator Profiles.* London: MHRA, 2025.

Medicines and Healthcare products Regulatory Agency. *Advice for Producers of E-cigarette and Vape Products.* London: MHRA, 2024.

Medicines and Healthcare products Regulatory Agency. *E-cigarettes and Refill Containers: Reporting Suspected Side Effects and Safety Concerns.* Drug Safety Update. London: MHRA, 2017.

Medicines and Healthcare products Regulatory Agency. *ECIG Dynamic Search: Published Electronic Cigarette and Refill-container Notifications.* London: MHRA.

Office for Product Safety and Standards. *Product Recalls and Alerts: Guidance for Consumers and Businesses.* London: Department for Business and Trade.

Office for Product Safety and Standards. *Product Safety and Noncompliance Notification Guidance for Business.* London: Department for Business and Trade, 2026.

British Standards Institution. *PAS 7100:2022—Product Recall and Other Corrective Actions: Code of Practice.* London: BSI, 2022.

Office for Product Safety and Standards. *OPSS Delivery Report 2024–2025.* London: Department for Business and Trade, 2025.

Office for Product Safety and Standards. *Product Safety Report: Hayati Twist 5000+ Puffs Electronic Vape, Juicy Peach.* Report 2407-0026. London: Department for Business and Trade, 2024.

Department for Environment, Food and Rural Affairs. *Single-use Vapes Ban: Information for Businesses.* London: Defra, 2025.

Department for Environment, Food and Rural Affairs. *Ban on the Sale and Supply of Disposable Vapes in England: Impact Assessment.* London: Defra, 2024.

Chartered Trading Standards Institute. *Annual Review 2024–2025.* Basildon: CTSI, 2025.

Devon, Plymouth, Somerset and Torbay Trading Standards Service. *Annual Performance Report 2024–2025.* Exeter: Heart of the South West Trading Standards Service, 2025.

Salford City Council. *'Nicotine-free' Vapes Falsely Advertised, Says Trading Standards Investigation.* Salford, 2025.

Surrey County Council. *Trading Standards Vapes Enforcement Update.* Guildford: Surrey County Council, 2024.

Enfield Council. *Illegal Vapes Seized by Enfield Trading Standards.* London Borough of Enfield, 2024.

HM Revenue & Customs. *Vaping Products Duty and Vaping Duty Stamps Scheme: Detailed Information.* London: HMRC, 2025–2026.

HM Revenue & Customs. *Importing and Exporting Vaping Products.* London: HMRC, 2026.

HM Revenue & Customs. *Handling Wholesale or Retail Vaping Products in the United Kingdom.* London: HMRC, 2026.

HM Revenue & Customs. *Vaping Products Duty and Vaping Duty Stamps: Record-keeping Requirements.* London: HMRC, 2026.

United States Food and Drug Administration. *Advisory and Enforcement Actions against Industry for Unauthorised Tobacco Products.* Silver Spring, Maryland: Center for Tobacco Products.

United States Food and Drug Administration. *FDA Issues Warning Letters to 80 Retailers for Selling Unauthorised Elf Bar and Lost Mary E-cigarettes.* Silver Spring, Maryland: FDA, 2024.

United States Food and Drug Administration. *FDA Issues Warning Letters to 14 Online Retailers for Selling Unauthorised E-cigarettes.* Silver Spring, Maryland: FDA, 2024.

United States Food and Drug Administration. *FDA Seeks Civil Money Penalties against 11 Retailers Selling Unauthorised E-cigarettes.* Silver Spring, Maryland: FDA, 2024.

United States Food and Drug Administration. *Import Alert 98-07: Detention without Physical Examination of Electronic Nicotine Delivery Systems Lacking Premarket Authorisation.* Silver Spring, Maryland: FDA, 2025.

United States Food and Drug Administration and United States Customs and Border Protection. *FDA and CBP Seize Nearly $34 Million Worth of Illegal E-cigarettes during Joint Operation.* Washington, DC, 2025.

Therapeutic Goods Administration. *Vapes: Compliance and Enforcement.* Canberra: Australian Government Department of Health, Disability and Ageing, 2026.

Therapeutic Goods Administration. *Business Surrender Scheme for Vaping Goods.* Canberra: Australian Government, 2024.

Therapeutic Goods Administration. *Vapes: Information for Retailers.* Canberra: Australian Government, 2024.

Therapeutic Goods Administration. *Vapes: Information for Wholesale, Transport, Logistics and Storage Facilities*. Canberra: Australian Government, 2024.

Therapeutic Goods Administration. *Vapes: Information for Sponsors, Importers and Manufacturers*. Canberra: Australian Government, 2025.

WHO Framework Convention on Tobacco Control Secretariat. *Global Progress Report on Implementation of the Protocol to Eliminate Illicit Trade in Tobacco Products*. Geneva: World Health Organization, 2025.

World Bank Group. *Confronting Illicit Tobacco Trade: A Global Review of Country Experiences*. Washington, DC: World Bank, 2019.

Romm, K. F., Berg, C. J., Henriksen, L., et al. "Rates of Age Verification for Cigarette and E-cigarette Purchases among United States Young Adults before and after Federal Tobacco 21 Implementation." *Nicotine & Tobacco Research*, 25(7), 2023, 1386–1390.

Aagesen, K., Moretti, A. and Demant, J. "Social Media Nicotine Markets: Criminogenic Affordances and Market Displacements." *International Journal of Drug Policy*, 145, 2025, 104943.

Guraka, A., Mierlea, S., Drake, S. J., et al. "A Comprehensive Toxicological Analysis of a Panel of Unregulated E-cigarettes to Human Health." *Toxicology*, 509, 2024, 153964.

Chapter 10: The Future of Regulation

United Kingdom Parliament. *Tobacco and Vapes Act 2026*. London: The Stationery Office, 2026.

Department of Health. *The Tobacco and Related Products Regulations 2016*, SI 2016/507. London: The Stationery Office, 2016.

Department for Environment, Food and Rural Affairs. *The Environmental Protection (Single-use Vapes) (England) Regulations 2024*, SI 2024/1216. London: The Stationery Office, 2024.

Department for Business, Innovation and Skills. *The Waste Electrical and Electronic Equipment Regulations 2013*, SI 2013/3113. London: The Stationery Office, 2013.

Department for Environment, Food and Rural Affairs. *The Waste Batteries and Accumulators Regulations 2009*, SI 2009/890. London: The Stationery Office, 2009.

European Parliament and Council of the European Union. *Directive 2014/40/EU on the Manufacture, Presentation and Sale of Tobacco and Related Products*. Official Journal of the European Union, L127, 2014.

European Parliament and Council of the European Union. *Regulation (EU) 2024/1781 Establishing a Framework for the Setting of Ecodesign Requirements for Sustainable Products*. Official Journal of the European Union, 2024.

European Parliament and Council of the European Union. *Regulation (EU) 2023/1542 Concerning Batteries and Waste Batteries*. Official Journal of the European Union, L191, 2023.

European Parliament and Council of the European Union. *Regulation (EU) 2024/1689 Laying Down Harmonised Rules on Artificial Intelligence*. Official Journal of the European Union, 2024.

European Commission. *Commission Launches Consultation on the Digital Product Passport*. Brussels: Directorate-General for Internal Market, Industry, Entrepreneurship and SMEs, 2025.

Organisation for Economic Co-operation and Development. *Recommendation of the Council for Agile Regulatory Governance to Harness Innovation.* Paris: OECD, 2021.

Organisation for Economic Co-operation and Development. *Risk and Regulatory Policy: Improving the Governance of Risk.* Paris: OECD Publishing, 2010.

Organisation for Economic Co-operation and Development. *OECD Regulatory Policy Outlook 2025.* Paris: OECD Publishing, 2025.

Organisation for Economic Co-operation and Development. *Governing with Artificial Intelligence: AI in Regulatory Design and Delivery.* Paris: OECD Publishing, 2025.

Organisation for Economic Co-operation and Development. *Recommendation of the Council on Artificial Intelligence: OECD AI Principles.* Paris: OECD, adopted 2019 and updated 2024.

Organisation for Economic Co-operation and Development. *OECD Due Diligence Guidance for Responsible AI.* Paris: OECD Publishing, 2026.

World Health Organization Framework Convention on Tobacco Control Secretariat. *Electronic Cigarettes.* Geneva: World Health Organization, 2024.

World Health Organization Study Group on Tobacco Product Regulation. *Report on the Scientific Basis of Tobacco Product Regulation: Eighth Report of a WHO Study Group.* WHO Technical Report Series. Geneva: World Health Organization, 2021.

World Health Organization Framework Convention on Tobacco Control. *Electronic Nicotine Delivery Systems and Electronic Non-Nicotine Delivery Systems: Report by WHO*, FCTC/COP/7/11. Geneva: World Health Organization, 2016.

World Health Organization Framework Convention on Tobacco Control. *Protocol to Eliminate Illicit Trade in Tobacco Products.* Geneva: World Health Organization, 2013.

World Health Organization Framework Convention on Tobacco Control Secretariat. *2025 Global Progress Report on Implementation of the WHO Framework Convention on Tobacco Control.* Geneva: World Health Organization, 2025.

World Health Organization Framework Convention on Tobacco Control. *Final Report of the Eleventh Session of the Conference of the Parties.* Geneva: World Health Organization, 2026.

Medicines and Healthcare products Regulatory Agency. *MHRA E-cigarette and Vape Products Guidance Hub.* London: MHRA, 2025.

Department of Health and Social Care. *Tobacco and Vapes: Evidence to Support Legislation.* London: Department of Health and Social Care, 2025.

Department of Health and Social Care. *Tobacco and Vapes: Packaging, Appearance and Display.* London: Department of Health and Social Care, 2026.

Department for Environment, Food and Rural Affairs. *Single-use Vapes Ban: Information for Businesses.* London: Defra, 2025.

Lindson, N., Butler, A. R., McRobbie, H., et al. "Electronic Cigarettes for Smoking Cessation." *Cochrane Database of Systematic Reviews*, 2025, CD010216. (

Voos, N., Goniewicz, M. L. and Eissenberg, T. "What Is the Nicotine Delivery Profile of Electronic Cigarettes?" *Expert Opinion on Drug Delivery*, 16, 2019, 1193–1203.

Dawkins, L., Cox, S., Goniewicz, M., et al. "'Real-world' Compensatory Behaviour with Low Nicotine Concentration E-liquid: Subjective Effects and Nicotine, Acrolein and Formaldehyde Exposure." *Addiction*, 113, 2018, 1874–1882.

Kosmider, L., Kimber, C. F., Kurek, J., Corcoran, O. and Dawkins, L. "Compensatory Puffing with Lower Nicotine Concentration E-liquids Increases Carbonyl Exposure in E-cigarette Aerosols." *Nicotine & Tobacco Research*, 20, 2018, 998–1003.

O'Connell, G., Pritchard, J. D., Prue, C., et al. "A Randomised, Open-label, Cross-over Clinical Study to Evaluate the Pharmacokinetic Profiles of Cigarettes and E-cigarettes with Nicotine-salt Formulations in Adult Smokers." *Internal and Emergency Medicine*, 2019.

Cho, Y. J., Mehta, T., Hinton, A., et al. "E-cigarette Nicotine Delivery among Young Adults by Nicotine Form, Concentration and Flavour: A Crossover Randomised Clinical Trial." *JAMA Network Open*, 7, 2024, e2426702.

Christen, S. E., Zhu, S. H., Galstyan, E., et al. "Pharmacokinetics and Pharmacodynamics of Inhaled Nicotine Salt and Free-base Formulations." *Nicotine & Tobacco Research*, 2024.

Harvanko, A. M., Havel, C. M., Jacob, P. and Benowitz, N. L. "Characterisation of Nicotine Salts in 23 Electronic Cigarette Refill Liquids." *Nicotine & Tobacco Research*, 22, 2020.

Jacobson, K., Martinez, J., Larroque, S., et al. "Nicotine Pharmacokinetics of Electronic Cigarettes: A Review of the Literature." *Regulatory Toxicology and Pharmacology*, 2021.

Notley, C., Gentry, S., Cox, S., et al. "Youth Use of E-liquid Flavours: A Systematic Review Exploring Patterns of Use and Associations with Continued Vaping, Tobacco Smoking Uptake or Cessation." *Addiction*, 117, 2022, 1258–1272.

Effah, F., Taiwo, B., Baines, D., Bailey, A. and Marczylo, T. "Pulmonary Effects of E-liquid Flavours: A Systematic Review." *Journal of Toxicology and Environmental Health, Part B*, 2022.

Soneji, S. S., Knutzen, K. E. and Villanti, A. C. "Use of Flavoured E-cigarettes among Adolescents, Young Adults and Older Adults: Findings from the Population Assessment for Tobacco and Health Study." *Public Health Reports*, 134, 2019.

Gravely, S., Cummings, K. M., Hammond, D., et al. "The Association of E-cigarette Flavours with Satisfaction, Enjoyment and Trying to Quit or Stay Abstinent from Smoking among Regular Adult Vapers." *Nicotine & Tobacco Research*, 22, 2020, 1831–1841.

Du, P., Bascom, R., Fan, T., et al. "Changes in Flavour Preference in a Cohort of Long-term Electronic Cigarette Users." *Annals of the American Thoracic Society*, 17, 2020.

Bold, K. W., Krishnan-Sarin, S., Stoney, C. M., et al. "Examining Associations of E-cigarette Flavour Restrictions with E-cigarette Use and Smoking Cessation among Adults." *Tobacco Control*, 2022.

Mosimann, A. F., Humair, J. P., Auer, R., et al. "E-liquid Flavours and Nicotine Concentration Choices over Six Months after a Smoking-cessation Attempt with Electronic Cigarettes." *Tobacco Prevention & Cessation*, 2025.

Ngambo, G., Hanna, E. G., Gannon, J., Marcus, H. and Lomazzi, M. "A Scoping Review on E-cigarette Environmental Impacts." *Tobacco Prevention & Cessation*, 9, 2023.

Reid, H. T., Fordham, A., Rasha, L., et al. "Up in Smoke: Considerations for Lithium-ion Batteries in Disposable E-cigarettes." *Joule*, 7, 2023, 2749–2759.

Gausden, A., Mayes, W. M., Fletcher, T. and Hagemann, N. "Single-use Vape Batteries: Investigating Their Potential as a Cause of Waste and Recycling Fires." *Batteries*, 10, 2024, 236.

Collins, L. G., Squires, H., Brennan, A., et al. "A Systematic Review of Modelling and Economic Evaluation Studies Assessing Regulatory Options for Electronic Cigarette Use." *International Journal of Drug Policy*, 2024.

Yan, D., Wang, Y., Huang, J., et al. "A Systematic Review of the Impacts of Global Approaches to Regulating Electronic Nicotine Products." *BMC Public Health*, 2023.

Moore, G., Hallingberg, B., Brown, R., et al. *Impacts of EU Tobacco Products Directive Regulations on Use of E-cigarettes in Adolescents in Great Britain: A Natural Experiment Evaluation.* Public Health Research, 11(5). Southampton: National Institute for Health and Care Research, 2023.

National Academies of Sciences, Engineering and Medicine. *Public Health Consequences of E-cigarettes.* Washington, DC: National Academies Press, 2018.

Balfour, D. J. K., Benowitz, N. L., Colby, S. M., et al. "Balancing Consideration of the Risks and Benefits of E-cigarettes." *American Journal of Public Health*, 111, 2021, 1661–1672.

ABOUT THE AUTHOR

Stephen Buss is a scientist, author and regulatory affairs specialist whose work has developed across formulation science, chemosensory research, consumer behaviour, toxicology, analytical interpretation, quality management and modern nicotine product regulation. His career has been shaped by a consistent interest in the point at which scientific evidence leaves the laboratory and begins to influence products, institutions, commercial decisions and public policy. Rather than remaining within a single technical discipline, he has worked across the connected stages through which scientific information is generated, interpreted, documented and converted into practical systems of control.

His formal scientific training began with a Higher National Diploma in Science at Guildford College of Technology, followed by a BSc (Hons) in Chemistry at Kingston University and later a BSc (Hons) in Psychology at the University of Portsmouth. That combination of chemistry and psychology gave him an unusually broad foundation for work involving both product composition and human response. Chemistry provided the basis for understanding formulation, analytical testing, material behaviour and experimental design, while psychology and sensory research developed his understanding of perception, consumer behaviour, product experience and the interpretation of qualitative and quantitative data. The two disciplines would later converge throughout his work in pharmaceutical development, tobacco science, consumer research and nicotine-product regulation.

He began his scientific career at SmithKline Beecham as a formulation scientist, working within a product-development environment in which experimental control, technical documentation and reproducibility were fundamental. His responsibilities included supporting senior scientists, conducting laboratory work, following defined test procedures, preparing technical reports and presenting findings objectively to project teams. This early experience established habits that continued throughout his later career: the need to understand what a method actually measures, to distinguish observation from interpretation and to ensure that scientific conclusions remain traceable to the data from which they were derived. Pharmaceutical formulation also provided an early appreciation of how apparently small changes in composition, process or storage can influence product performance, stability and user exposure.

From pharmaceutical science he moved into chemosensory research at British American Tobacco, where he worked on the sensory and consumer dimensions of product development. His role involved the design and management of strategic research, the development of sensory methods and the generation of data capable of describing how products were experienced by users. This required more than subjective opinion. Sensory science depends upon controlled methodology, careful panel design, appropriate statistical treatment and disciplined interpretation. It also requires an understanding of the relationship between chemistry, physical delivery and perception. During this period, he worked across quantitative and qualitative research, developed new evaluative methods and contributed to the training of research teams.

That work provided a detailed understanding of how formulation, aroma, taste, mouthfeel, nicotine delivery and product design interact with consumer behaviour. It also exposed the limits of relying on any single form of evidence. Analytical chemistry can identify constituents, but it does not explain why consumers accept or reject a product. Sensory research can describe perception, but it does not determine toxicological suitability. Consumer research can identify preference, but preference does not establish safety. Scientific interpretation becomes most useful when these evidence streams are examined together and their boundaries remain clear.

He later joined MMR Food and Drink Research Worldwide as a senior consumer research executive, managing and developing sensory and consumer projects for clients across the food, drink and tobacco sectors. The role broadened his experience of commercial research, supplier management, client communication and the translation of complex findings into decisions that could be understood by non-specialists. It also strengthened his appreciation of the difference between collecting data and producing evidence that is genuinely useful. Research can be technically sound yet operationally irrelevant if it does not address the decision that needs to be made. Conversely, commercially attractive conclusions can become unreliable if interpretation moves beyond the limits of the study.

Subsequent consultancy and management roles expanded this experience beyond the laboratory. He worked on business development, market evaluation, international operations, research strategy and the management of teams across different commercial and cultural environments. These roles required the same skills in another form: identifying the essential information within large volumes of material, defining priorities, communicating under pressure and converting broad objectives into structured programmes of work. They also reinforced the importance of systems. Scientific and regulatory performance does not depend only upon the competence of individual specialists. It depends upon whether organisations can document decisions, control suppliers, manage changes, investigate deviations and preserve traceability over time.

His return to specialist product science came through the rapidly developing electronic-cigarette sector. At a time when vaping products were expanding faster than the regulatory systems intended to govern them, he became involved in formulation development, flavour creation, laboratory management, product research, quality control and the interpretation of emerging European requirements. The sector presented a distinctive scientific problem because the product could not be understood through liquid composition alone. Formulation, device power, coil design, airflow, temperature, user behaviour and storage conditions all influenced the aerosol ultimately inhaled by the consumer. Product assessment therefore required chemistry, engineering, toxicology and behavioural interpretation to be considered as parts of one system.

As European regulation developed, his work increasingly moved towards product compliance and regulatory science. Through Vape Compliance Ltd, he worked with manufacturers, importers and distributors seeking to understand and meet the emerging requirements applied to electronic nicotine products. This included ingredient assessment, chemical identification, toxicological summaries, emissions data, product documentation, supplier records, analytical reports, packaging review and preparation for regulatory notification. The work required continual interpretation because legal requirements, technical guidance and regulator expectations did not always develop at the same speed.

The practical challenge was rarely the absence of information alone. More often, it was the absence of structure. A manufacturer might possess formulation records, laboratory reports, supplier certificates and packaging files, yet still lack a coherent dossier capable of demonstrating what the product contained, how it was made, how it had been assessed and whether the submitted data corresponded to the version placed on the market. His role involved organising these separate records into systems that could withstand technical and regulatory scrutiny.

This work also involved the interpretation of analytical evidence. Laboratory reports do not explain themselves. Results depend upon sampling, preparation, method selection, calibration, operating conditions, uncertainty and the relationship between the tested sample and the marketed product. A numerical value may appear definitive while remaining poorly suited to the regulatory question being asked. Stephen's approach developed around understanding the evidential chain: what was tested, under which conditions, using which method, against which specification and with what degree of confidence. This was especially important in vaping, where variations in power, puffing regime, coil condition and formulation can materially alter the results obtained from the same nominal product.

Toxicological interpretation formed another major part of this work. Ingredient names and CAS numbers provide identity, but identity alone does not determine suitability for inhalation. Assessment requires consideration of concentration, route of exposure, available toxicological data, likely thermal transformation and the contribution of the complete formulation. The absence of evidence of harm cannot be treated automatically as evidence of safety, while the detection of a hazardous substance does not by itself establish meaningful risk without consideration of dose and exposure. His work focused on maintaining that distinction between hazard identification and realistic risk assessment.

Quality systems provided the framework through which these scientific requirements could be maintained. Drawing upon ISO 9001 principles, he worked with documentation control, supplier qualification, change control, corrective and preventive action, traceability, complaint handling and continuous improvement. In a fast-moving market, these controls are not administrative additions to the science. They are the means by which the scientific identity of a product is preserved. A formulation cannot be assessed meaningfully if suppliers change without review, production records are incomplete or packaging no longer corresponds to the notified composition. Quality management connects the product described in a regulatory dossier with the product that reaches the consumer.

His experience therefore developed at the practical interface between science, regulation and industry. He worked during the period in which European vaping regulation moved from uncertainty and political negotiation into formal product limits, technical standards and notification requirements. This involved interpreting developing legislation while manufacturers were still designing products and regulators were still establishing procedures. Businesses needed to make decisions before every detail had been clarified, yet those decisions still required scientific justification, documentation and control. The period demonstrated how regulation is built in practice: not as a single moment of legal certainty, but through repeated interaction between legislation, guidance, laboratories, manufacturers, competent authorities and enforcement bodies.

As an author, Stephen writes longform scientific and non-fiction works concerned with evidence, regulation, public health, history, systems and contested knowledge. His writing is shaped by the same principles that informed his technical work. Complex subjects must be examined without losing the reader, but accessibility should not be achieved by removing the distinctions that give evidence meaning. Scientific language can clarify or conceal. Regulatory language can protect consumers or create the appearance of control without improving outcomes. Public-health arguments can be well intentioned while remaining incomplete if they ignore behaviour, market substitution or unintended consequences.

His work as an author therefore concentrates on the structures beneath public claims: how evidence is produced, how uncertainty is managed, how institutions define acceptable risk and how political or commercial pressures affect interpretation. He does not approach these subjects from the assumption that one sector possesses all relevant knowledge. Laboratories, regulators, manufacturers, clinicians, consumers and public-health organisations each see a different part of the same system. The quality of the final judgement depends upon whether those perspectives are integrated without allowing any one interest to dominate the evidence.

Evidence-Based Harm Reduction brings together this background in chemistry, formulation, psychology, sensory science, toxicology, analytical interpretation, quality systems and regulatory affairs. The series examines modern nicotine products through the distinction between combustion and non-combustion, while remaining attentive to product quality, youth protection, dependence, commercial conduct and scientific uncertainty. It treats harm reduction neither as unconditional support for an industry nor as a slogan capable of replacing evidence. It is approached as a disciplined method of comparison: an examination of what people use, what they are exposed to, what alternatives are realistically available and how regulation changes the choices made within the market.

The resulting work reflects a career spent moving between laboratory data, human behaviour, commercial systems and regulatory decision-making. It is written from the understanding that scientific evidence becomes valuable only when it is interpreted accurately, communicated honestly and applied in a form capable of improving real outcomes.

COMING SOON

The Evidence-Based Harm Reduction Library

A forthcoming collection of specialist titles examining the science, regulation, quality systems and consumer behaviour that shape modern nicotine products. Written for scientists, manufacturers, regulators, consultants, laboratories, legal teams and public-health professionals, each volume combines technical depth with practical interpretation, turning complex evidence and regulatory expectations into clear, usable guidance.

Science and Product Evaluation

The Toxicology of Vaping

Understanding hazard, exposure and regulatory evidence

A specialist examination of the toxicological principles used to evaluate modern vaping products. This volume explores ingredient assessment, inhalation exposure, dose–response relationships, toxicokinetics, read-across, threshold of toxicological concern, computational modelling, biomarkers and the interpretation of uncertainty.

Particular attention is given to the difference between hazard and real-world risk, the limitations of food-use assumptions, the importance of exposure context and the evidential standards expected within regulatory submissions. Designed for toxicologists, formulation scientists, regulators and technical teams, the book provides a structured framework for assessing ingredients and products without overstating either safety or uncertainty.

Vape Flavour Chemistry

From sensory design to inhalation toxicology

Flavour is one of the most technically complex and politically contested areas of vaping science. This volume examines the chemistry behind flavour creation and the scientific questions that arise when compounds traditionally used in foods are transferred into inhaled products.

The book considers ketones, aldehydes, esters, acids, sweeteners, cooling agents, flavour enhancers and complex mixtures, together with thermal degradation, ingredient interactions, analytical uncertainty and sensory performance. It also explores the limitations of GRAS status, the case for controlled flavour palettes and the future role of positive lists, pharmaceutical-grade flavour systems and inhalation-relevant assessment.

A detailed reference for flavour houses, product developers, toxicologists, laboratories and regulators.

Animal Testing Alternatives for Vape

The future of non-animal nicotine-product assessment

A scientific and regulatory review of the methods capable of reducing reliance on animal testing in vaping and nicotine-product evaluation.

The volume examines in vitro toxicology, computational modelling, read-across, QSAR, threshold-based assessment, exposure modelling, adverse outcome pathways, organotypic systems and emerging human-relevant methodologies. It considers where these approaches are already scientifically credible, where validation remains incomplete and how multiple lines of evidence can be integrated into a defensible regulatory strategy.

Written for toxicologists, regulators, laboratories and product developers, the book presents a practical route towards more ethical, efficient and scientifically relevant assessment.

Regulation and Quality

The Regulation Handbook

A practical operating guide for modern vape compliance

A comprehensive guide to the systems, documentation and decisions required to place and maintain vaping products on regulated markets.

The handbook covers product notifications, technical files, ingredient databases, toxicological summaries, laboratory evidence, supplier control, change management, post-market surveillance, corrective action and product withdrawal. It explains how compliance should operate across the full product lifecycle rather than as a one-time submission exercise.

Designed for regulatory-affairs teams, manufacturers, importers, distributors, laboratories and consultants, this volume translates legal and scientific requirements into practical compliance structures capable of standing up to regulatory scrutiny.

ISO 9001 for Vape Manufacturers

Building quality into products, processes and evidence

A dedicated quality-management guide for vaping manufacturers, importers and technical organisations.

This volume explains how ISO 9001 principles can be applied to formulation, filling, device assembly, supplier management, laboratory control and regulatory documentation. It covers process mapping, document control, CAPA, non-conformance, change control, supplier approval, traceability, complaints, internal auditing, management review and continuous improvement.

Rather than treating quality certification as a paperwork exercise, the book shows how an effective system can reduce product variation, prevent avoidable failures, strengthen regulatory evidence and protect the business throughout the product lifecycle.

European TPD Handbook

A practical guide to European vape regulation

A focused reference for businesses placing nicotine-containing vaping products on European markets.

The handbook explains product notification, EU-CEG submission, ingredient reporting, toxicological assessment, emissions data, nicotine limits, refill mechanisms, labelling, packaging, warnings, responsible-operator duties and continuing compliance. It also examines the practical challenges created by national interpretation, language requirements, market-specific fees and regulatory divergence across Europe.

Written for manufacturers, importers, distributors and regulatory professionals, the book provides a structured route through the Tobacco Products Directive and the systems required to maintain compliant products after notification.

FDA PMTA Guide

Understanding the United States premarket pathway

A structured introduction to the scientific, legal and strategic demands of the United States Premarket Tobacco Product Application process.

The book examines product chemistry, manufacturing information, toxicology, aerosol testing, clinical evidence, behavioural research, abuse liability, environmental assessment, population modelling and the demonstration that marketing a product would be appropriate for the protection of public health.

It also considers evidence planning, product comparators, deficiency responses, submission architecture and the commercial implications of the PMTA pathway. Designed for manufacturers, investors, scientists and regulatory teams, the volume provides a realistic account of one of the most demanding nicotine-product authorisation systems in the world.

Product Responsibility and Consumer Behaviour

Vape Product Stewardship

Responsible control across the complete product lifecycle

A lifecycle guide to the scientific, regulatory and commercial responsibilities attached to modern vaping products.

Beginning with concept development and formulation, the book follows the product through supplier qualification, manufacturing, testing, notification, distribution, retail, market surveillance, complaint handling, corrective action and withdrawal. It explains how technical ownership should continue long after a product first reaches the market.

The volume is designed for companies seeking to move beyond minimum compliance towards a defensible product-stewardship system capable of identifying risk, responding to evidence and maintaining control across complex international supply chains.

Vape Consumer Psychology

Understanding switching, satisfaction and long-term use

A behavioural-science examination of how consumers experience, adopt and continue using vaping products.

The book explores smoking behaviour, nicotine dependence, sensory satisfaction, flavour preference, habit formation, identity, product acceptance, dual use, relapse and complete switching. It considers why technically compliant products may still fail as alternatives to smoking and why product design, ritual, convenience and sensory performance matter alongside nicotine delivery.

Drawing together psychology, consumer research and harm-reduction evidence, the volume is written for product developers, researchers, public-health specialists and regulators seeking to understand the human behaviour behind market outcomes.

Vape Risk Communication

Communicating evidence without distortion

A practical guide to explaining vaping, nicotine and relative risk with accuracy, balance and credibility.

The book examines how scientific uncertainty, comparative risk and harm reduction can be communicated without exaggeration, dismissal, moral panic or false reassurance. It considers public-health messaging, media reporting, regulatory statements, consumer education, crisis communication and the language used to describe emerging evidence.

Particular attention is given to the difference between hazard and risk, the importance of realistic comparators and the consequences of messages that discourage smokers from switching. Written for scientists, regulators, manufacturers, journalists and public-health communicators, the volume provides a framework for responsible communication in a highly polarised field.

www.ingramcontent.com/pod-product-compliance
Lightning Source LLC
LaVergne TN
LVHW071049081126
851858LV00027B/134
* 9 7 8 1 9 1 9 4 5 6 7 7 5 *